Contents

Abbreviations

ACE	angiotensin-converting enzyme
ADR	adverse drug reaction
AIDS	acquired immunodeficiency syndrome
AV	atrioventricular
BP	British Pharmacopoeia
CNS	central nervous system
CSF	cerebrospinal fluid
DMARD	disease-modifying antirheumatic drug
ECG	electrocardiogram
EEG	electro-encephalogram
G6PD	glucose 6-phosphate dehydrogenase
GFR	glomerular filtration rate
HIV	human immunodeficiency virus
HRT	hormone replacement therapy
INR	international normalized ratio
MDI	metered dose inhaler
NSAID	nonsteroidal anti-inflammatory drug
spp.	species
SSRI	selective serotonin reuptake inhibitor
USP	Unites States Pharmacopeia
WHO	World Health Organization

WHO

MODEL

FORMULARY

2002

WORLD
HEALTH
ORGANIZATION

Editors

Mary R. Couper (1)
Dinesh K. Mehta (2)

(1) Department of Essential Drugs and Medicines Policy, World Health Organization, Geneva
(2) Royal Pharmaceutical Society of Great Britain, London

Acknowledgements

The WHO Model Formulary was developed over a period of several years and with the input of a large number of individuals and organizations.

The contributions and comments of the following persons are gratefully acknowledged: T.I.Bhutta (Pakistan), D.Birkett (Australia), H.Buschiazzo (Argentina), A.Chidarikire (Zimbabwe), I.Darmansjah (Indonesia), P.Folb (South Africa), H.Fraser (Barbados), T.Fukui (Japan), J.P.Giroud (France), A.Haeri (Iran), M.Hassar (Morocco), J.Idänpään-Heikkilä (WHO), K.Johnson (US Pharmacopeia), F.Juma (Kenya), O.Kasilo (Zimbabwe), G. P. Kilonzo (Tanzania), M. E. Kitler (WHO), M.Koulu (Finland), A.Kucers (Australia), V.Lepakhin (Russian Federation), Jia-Tai Li (China), P.Männistö (Finland), P.Mordujovich de Buschiazzo (Argentina), P.Neuvonen (Finland), G.O.Obiago (Nigeria), P.Paakari (Finland), J.H.Pater (Canada), L.Rago (Estonia), M.Reidenberg (USA), J.Reinstein (World Self-Medication Industry), H.Ruskoaho (Finland), B.Santoso (Indonesia), S.A.Shah (World Self-Medication Industry), M.Thomas (India), O.Tokola (Finland), H.Vapaatalo (Finland), K.Weerasuriya (Sri Lanka), H.Yasuhara (Japan), P.Ylitalo (Finland), Zhu Jun-ren (China).

The draft text of the formulary was reviewed by a team of the Royal Pharmaceutical Society of Great Britain, consisting of Mildred Davis, Ann M. Hargreaves, Sheenagh M. Townsend-Smith and Louise J. Whitley. Without their dedicated support this formulary could not have been published.

Priscilla Appiah, Eric I. Connor, Daphne Fresle, Charles Fry, Gerard P. Gallagher, Prakash Gotecha, Kath Hurst, Genevieve Meier, Balaji Ramachandran, Rachel S.M. Ryan, Li M. Wan, Ann Wilberforce and John Wilson all made valuable contributions to the production process.

The project was managed by Mary R. Couper and Hans V. Hogerzeil of the WHO Department of Essential Drugs and Medicines Policy with the secretarial assistance of Pam Jude.

The development of the WHO Model Formulary was partly funded through a grant received from the Finnish International Development Agency.

Introduction

In 1995 the WHO Expert Committee on the Use of Essential Drugs recommended development of a WHO Model Formulary which would complement the WHO Model List of Essential Drugs (the 'Model List') and that would be updated every two years. It was considered that such a Model Formulary would be a useful resource for countries wishing to develop their own national formulary.

After a first consultation in April 1996 work was started to draft sections of the text according to the therapeutic categories in the Model List. A second consultation was held in Helsinki in September 1997, at which several draft sections of the text were discussed. At a third consultation in October 1999 the full text was reviewed.

In November 1999 the Expert Committee on the Use of Essential Drugs reviewed progress in the project. It recommended that WHO accept an offer by the Royal Pharmaceutical Society of Great Britain (which, together with the British Medical Association, publishes the British National Formulary) to take responsibility for final data validation, editing and layout. Agreement to this effect was reached in early 2000.

During the validation process all statements in the draft text were compared with the original references and checked for consistency with other WHO documents and recommendations and reputable drug information sources. A full record of this validation and all ensuing technical and editorial changes to the draft text, with the underlying reasons and the relevant references, is available. As this was the first edition of a new reference text this work took almost two years and was completed by the end of 2001. During this process when necessary the text was updated to take into account new information that had become available since the time of writing. Monographs were included for the small number of essential drugs that had been added to the Model List in November 1999.

Although the initial plan was to maintain in the Model Formulary the section headings and numbering system of the Model List, this proved difficult in practice. The main reason was that the sections of the Model List are not always useful as therapeutic categories, and do not easily lend themselves to introductory evaluative statements. Small changes were therefore introduced. The Model Formulary has also been relatively generous in repeating the formulary text of essential drugs under other relevant therapeutic categories.

The lack of full concurrence with the numbering system of the Model List should not be a major problem for users. They will be able to access information readily either through the content list or through the main index which includes both drug names and disease terms. Dissemination of the Model List and the

Model Formulary will focus on electronic access through CD-ROMs and the WHO Medicines web site; the Model Formulary will be linked to the Model List.

The electronic version of the Model Formulary is also intended as a starting point for developing national or institutional formularies. Rather than having to start completely from the beginning, national or institutional formulary committees can adapt the text of the Model Formulary to their own needs by changing the text or aligning the formulary to their own list of essential drugs by adding or deleting entries.

Despite all efforts it is unavoidable that this first edition of the WHO Model Formulary may contain some omissions or errors. Every effort has been made to ensure that the information in the Model Formulary has international applicability, but inevitably there will be instances where the local management of conditions will be different to that advised here. All readers are encouraged to send their comments, corrections and suggestions to the Editor of the WHO Model Formulary, Department of Essential Drugs and Medicines Policy, World Health Organization, 1211 Geneva, Switzerland, fax 41-22-7914167.

General advice to prescribers

Rational approach to therapeutics

Drugs should only be prescribed when they are necessary, and in all cases the benefit of administering the medicine should be considered in relation to the risks involved. Bad prescribing habits lead to ineffective and unsafe treatment, exacerbation or prolongation of illness, distress and harm to the patient, and higher cost. The Guide to Good Prescribing. Geneva: WHO; 1994 provides undergraduates with important tools for training in the process of rational prescribing.

The following steps will help to remind prescribers of the rational approach to therapeutics.

1. **Define the patient's problem**

   Whenever possible, making the right diagnosis is based on integrating many pieces of information: the complaint as described by the patient; a detailed history; physical examination; laboratory tests; X-rays and other investigations. This will help in rational prescribing, always bearing in mind that diseases are evolutionary processes.

2. **Specify the therapeutic objective**

   Doctors must clearly state their therapeutic objectives based on the pathophysiology underlying the clinical situation. Very often physicians must select more than one therapeutic goal for each patient.

3. **Selecting therapeutic strategies**

   The selected strategy should be agreed with the patient; this agreement on outcome, and how it may be achieved, is termed concordance.

   The selected treatment can be non-pharmacological and/or pharmacological; it also needs to take into account the total cost of all therapeutic options.

   (a) *Non–pharmacological treatment*

   It is very important to bear in mind that the patient does not always need a drug for treatment of the condition. Very often, health problems can be resolved by a change in life style or diet, use of physiotherapy or exercise, provision of adequate psychological support, and other non–pharmacological treatments; these have the same importance as a prescription drug, and instructions must be written, explained and monitored in the same way.

   (b) *Pharmacological treatment*

   - *Selecting the correct group of drugs*

     Knowledge about the pathophysiology involved in the clinical situation of each patient and the pharmacodynamics of the chosen group of drugs, are two of the fundamental principles for rational therapeutics.

   - *Selecting the drug from the chosen group*

     The selection process must consider benefit/risk/cost information. This step is based on evidence about maximal clinical benfits of the drug for a given indication (efficacy) with the minimum production of adverse effects (safety).

     It must be remembered that each drug has adverse effects and it is estimated that up to 10% of hospital admissions in industrialized countries are due to adverse effects. Not all drug-induced injury can be prevented but much of it is caused by inappropriate selection of drugs. In cost comparisons between drugs, the cost of the total treatment and not only the unit cost of the drug must be considered.

   - *Verifying the suitability of the chosen pharmaceutical treatment for each patient*

     The prescriber must check whether the active substance chosen, its dosage form, standard dosage schedule and standard duration of treatment are suitable for each patient. Drug treatment should be individualized to the needs of each patient.

- *Prescription writing*

  The prescription is the link between the prescriber, the pharmacist (or dispenser) and the patient so it is important for the successful management of the presenting medical condition. This item is covered in more detail in the following section.

- *Giving information, instructions and warnings*

  This step is important to ensure patient adherence and is covered in detail in the following section.

- *Monitoring treatment*

  Evaluation of the follow up and the outcome of treatment allows the stopping of it (if the patient's problem is solved) or to reformulate it when necessary. This step gives rise to important information about the effects of drugs contributing to building up the body of knowledge of pharmacovigilance, needed to promote the rational use of drugs.

Variation in dose response

Success in drug treatment depends not only on the correct choice of drug but on the correct dose regimen. Unfortunately drug treatment frequently fails because the dose is too small or produces adverse effects because it is too large. This is because most texts, teachers and other drug information sources continue to recommend standard doses.

The concept of a standard or 'average' adult dose for every medicine is firmly rooted in the mind of most prescribers. After the initial 'dose ranging' studies on new drugs, manufacturers recommend a dosage that appears to produce the desired response in the majority of subjects. These studies are usually done on healthy, young male Caucasian volunteers, rather than on older men and women with illnesses and of different ethnic and environmental backgrounds. The use of standard doses in the marketing literature suggest that standard responses are the rule, but in reality there is considerable variation in drug response. As a result many prescribed doses are far too low or too high, leading to treatment failure or toxicity. There are many reasons for this variation which include adherence (see below), drug formulation, body weight and age, composition, variation in absorption, distribution, metabolism and excretion, variation in pharmacodynamics, disease variables, genetic and environmental variables.

Drug formulation

Poorly formulated drugs may fail to disintegrate or to dissolve. Enteric-coated drugs are particularly problematic, and have been known to pass through the gastrointestinal tract intact. Some drugs like digoxin or phenytoin have a track record of formulation problems, and dissolution profiles can vary not only from manufacturer to manufacturer but from batch to batch of the same company. The problem is worse if there is a narrow therapeutic to toxic ratio, as changes in absorption can produce sudden changes in drug concentration. For such drugs quality control surveillance should be carried out.

Body weight and age

Although the concept of varying the dose with the body weight or age of children has a long tradition, adult doses have been assumed to be the same irrespective of size or shape. Yet adult weights vary two to threefold, while a large fat mass can store large excesses of highly lipid soluble drugs compared to lean patients of the same weight.

Age changes can also be important. Adolescents may oxidize some drugs relatively more rapidly than adults, while the elderly may have reduced renal function and eliminate some drugs more slowly.

Physiological and pharmacokinetic variables

Drug absorption rates may vary widely between individuals and within the same individual at different times and in different physiological states. Drugs taken after a meal are delivered to the small intestine much more slowly than in the fasting state, leading to much lower drug concentrations. In the case of drugs like paracetamol with a high rate of metabolism on 'first pass' through the liver, this may render a standard dose completely ineffective. In pregnancy gastric emptying is also delayed, while some drugs may increase or decrease gastric emptying and affect absorption of other drugs.

Drug distribution

Drug distribution varies widely: fat soluble drugs are stored in adipose tissue, water soluble drugs are distributed chiefly in the extracellular space, acidic drugs bind strongly to plasma albumin and basic drugs to muscle cells. Hence variation in plasma albumin levels, fat content or muscle mass may all contribute to dose variation. With very highly albumin bound drugs like warfarin, a small change of albumin concentration can produce a big change in free drug and a dramatic change in drug effect.

Drug metabolism and excretion

Drug metabolic rates are determined both by genetic and environmental factors. Drug acetylation shows genetic polymorphism, whereby individuals fall clearly into either fast or slow acetylator types. Drug oxidation, however, is polygenic, and although a small proportion of the population can be classified as very slow oxidizers of some drugs, for most drugs and most subjects there is a normal distribution of drug metabolizing capacity, and much of the variation is under environmental control.

Many drugs are eliminated by the kidneys without being metabolized. Renal disease or toxicity of other drugs on the kidney can therefore slow excretion of some drugs.

Pharmacodynamic variables

There is significant variation in receptor response to some drugs, especially central nervous system responses, for example pain and sedation. Some of this is genetic, some due to tolerance, some due to interaction with other drugs and some due to addiction, for example, morphine and alcohol.

Disease variables

Both liver disease and kidney disease can have major effects on drug response, chiefly by the effect on metabolism and elimination respectively (increasing toxicity), but also by their effect on plasma albumin (increased free drug also increasing toxicity). Heart failure can also affect metabolism of drugs with rapid hepatic clearance (for example lidocaine, propranolol). Respiratory disease and hypothyroidism can both impair drug oxidation.

Enviromental variables

Many drugs and environmental toxins can induce the hepatic microsomal enzyme oxidizing system (MEOS) or cytochrome P450 oxygenases, leading to more rapid metabolism and elimination and ineffective treatment. Environmental pollutants, anaesthetic drugs and other compounds such as pesticides can also induce metabolism. Diet and nutritional status also impact on pharmacokinetics. For example in infantile malnutrition and in malnourished elderly populations drug oxidation rates are decreased, while high protein diets, charcoal cooked foods and certain other foods act as metabolizing enzyme inducers. Chronic alcohol use induces oxidation of other drugs, but in the presence of high circulating alcohol concentrations drug metabolism may be inhibited.

Adherence (compliance) with drug treatment

It is often assumed that once the appropriate drug is chosen, the prescription correctly written and the medication correctly dispensed, that it will be taken correctly and treatment will be successful. Unfortunately this is very often not the case, and physicians overlook one of the most important reasons for treatment failure—poor adherence (compliance) with the treatment plan.

There are sometimes valid reasons for poor adherence—the drug may be poorly tolerated, may cause obvious adverse effects or may be prescribed in a toxic dose. Failure to adhere with such a prescription has been described as 'intelligent non-compliance'. Bad prescribing or a dispensing error may also create a problem, which patients may have neither the insight nor the courage to question. Even with rational prescribing, failure to adhere to treatment is common. Factors may be related to the patient, the disease, the doctor, the prescription, the pharmacist or the health system and can often be avoided.

Patient reasons

In general, women tend to be more adherent than men, younger patients and the very elderly are less adherent, and people living alone are less adherent than those with partners or spouses. Specific education interventions have been shown to improve adherence. Patient failings such as illiteracy, poor eyesight or cultural attitudes (for example preference for traditional or alternative medicines and suspicion of modern medicine) may be very important in some individuals or societies. Such attitudes need to be discussed and brought in to the open.

Disease reasons

Conditions with a known worse prognosis (for example cancer) or painful conditions (for example rheumatoid arthritis) elicit better adherence rates than asymptomatic 'perceived as benign' conditions such as hypertension. Doctors need to realize that in most settings less than half of patients started for the first time on antihypertensive drug treatment are still taking it a year later. Similarly, in epilepsy, where events may occur at long intervals, adherence is notoriously unsatisfactory.

Doctor reasons

Doctors may cause poor adherence in many ways—by failing to inspire confidence in the treatment offered, by giving too little or no explanation, by thoughtlessly prescribing too many medications, by making errors in prescribing, or by their overall attitude to the patient.

The doctor-patient interaction

There is considerable evidence that this is crucial to concordance. 'Satisfaction with the interview' has been consistently shown to be one of the highest predictors of good adherence. Patients are often well informed and expect a greater say in their health care. If they are in doubt or dissatisfied there are more options, including 'alternative medicines'. There is no doubt that the drug 'doctor' has a powerful effect to encourage confidence and perhaps contribute directly to the healing process.

Prescription reasons

Many aspects of the prescription may lead to non-adherence. It may be illegible or inaccurate; it may get lost; it may not be refilled as intended or instructed for a chronic disease. And it may be too complex; it has been shown that the greater the number of medications the poorer the adherence, while multiple doses also decrease adherence if more than two doses per day are given. Not surprisingly adverse effects like drowsiness, impotence or nausea negatively influence adherence and patients may not admit to the problem.

Pharmacist reasons

The pharmacist's personality and professional manner, like the doctor's, may have a positive impact, supporting adherence, or a negative one, raising suspicions or concerns. This has been reported especially in relation to generic drugs when substituted for brand name drugs. Pharmacist information and advice can be a valuable reinforcement, as long as it tallies with the doctor's advice.

The health care system

The health care system may be the biggest hindrance to adherence. Long waiting times, uncaring staff, uncomfortable environment, exhausted drug supplies and so on, are all common problems in developing countries, and have a major impact on adherence. An important problem is the distance and accessibility of the clinic from the patient. Some studies have confirmed the obvious, that patients furthest from the clinic are least likely to adhere to treatment in the long term.

Recommendations

- Review the prescription to be sure it is correct.
- Spend time explaining the problem and the reason for the drug.
- Establish a good relationship with the patient, rather than a hurried or brusque manner with little eye contact.
- Explore problems, for example reading the label, getting the prescription filled.
- Insist that patients bring their medication to the clinic 'for checking', so that tablet counts can be made unobtrusively.
- Insist that patients learn the names of their tablets, and review their regimen with them. Write notes for them.
- Keep treatment regimens simple.
- Communicate with the pharmacist, to develop teamwork and collaboration in helping and advising the patient.
- Involve the partner or another family member,
- Listen to the patient.

Adverse effects and interactions

Adverse drug reactions

An adverse drug reaction (ADR) may be defined as 'any response to a drug which is noxious, unintended and occurs at doses normally used for prophylaxis, diagnosis, or therapy...'. ADRs are therefore unwanted or unintended effects of a medicine, including idiosyncratic effects, which occur during its proper use. They differ from accidental or deliberate excessive dosage or drug maladministration, (see section 4 for the treatment of poisoning).

ADRs may be directly linked to the properties of the drug in use, the so-called 'A' type reactions. An example is hypoglycaemia induced by an antidiabetic drug. ADRs may also be unrelated to the known pharmacology of the drug, the 'B' type reactions including allergic effects, for example anaphylaxis with **penicillins**.

Thalidomide marked the first recognized public health disaster related to the introduction of a new drug. It is now recognized that clinical trials, however thorough, cannot be guaranteed to detect all adverse effects likely to be caused by a drug. Health workers are thus encouraged to record and report to their national pharmacovigilance centre any unexpected adverse effects with any drug to achieve faster recognition of serious related problems. For example, from reports received in one country recently, a relationship was established between **thioacetazone** and Stevens-Johnson syndrome when the drug was used in HIV infection, leading to the withdrawal of the drug in that country.

Major factors predisposing to adverse effects

It is well known that different patients often respond differently to a given treatment regimen. For example, in a sample of 2422 patients who had been taking combinations of drugs known to interact, only 7 (0.3%) showed any clinical evidence of interactions. In addition to the pharmaceutical properties of the drug therefore, there are characteristics of the patient which predispose to ADRs.

EXTREMES OF AGE. The very old and the very young are more susceptible to ADRs. Drugs which commonly cause problems in the elderly include hypnotics, diuretics, non-steroidal anti-inflammatory drugs, antihypertensives, psychotropics and digoxin.

All children, and particularly neonates, differ from adults in the way they respond to drugs. Some drugs are likely to cause problems in neonates (for example **morphine**), but are generally tolerated in children. Other drugs (for example **valproic acid**) are associated with increased risk of ADRs in children of all ages. Other drugs associated with problems in children include **chloramphenicol** (grey baby syndrome), **antiarrhythmics** (worsening of arrhythmias), **aspirin** (Reye syndrome).

INTERCURRENT ILLNESS. If besides the condition being treated the patient also suffers from another disease, such as kidney, liver or heart disease, special precautions are necessary to prevent ADRs. Remember also that, as well as the above factors, the genetic make-up of the individual patient may predispose to ADRs.

DRUG INTERACTIONS. Interactions (see also Appendix 1) may occur between drugs which compete for the same receptor or act on the same physiological system. They may also occur indirectly when a drug-induced disease or a change in fluid or electrolyte balance alters the response to another drug.

Interactions may occur when one drug alters the absorption, distribution or elimination of another drug, such that the amount which reaches the site of action is increased or decreased.

Drug-drug interactions are some of the commonest causes of adverse effects. When two drugs are administered to a patient, they may either act independently of each other, or interact with each other. Interaction may increase or decrease the effects of the drugs concerned and may cause unexpected toxicity. As newer and more potent drugs become available, the number of serious drug interactions is likely to increase. Remember that interactions which modify the effects of a drug may involve non-prescription drugs, non-medicinal chemical agents, and social drugs such as **alcohol, marijuana, and traditional remedies,** as well as certain types of food. The physiological changes in individual patients, caused by such factors as age and gender, also influence the predisposition to ADRs resulting from drug interactions.

The following table is designed as a teaching and reference tool for physicians and health care providers who wish to avoid drug interactions in their patients.

The table lists drugs in columns under the designation of specific cytochrome P450 isoforms. A drug appears in a column if there is published evidence that it is metabolized, at least in part, via that isoform. Alterations in the rate of the metabolic reaction catalyzed by that isoform are likely to have effects on the pharmacokinetics of the drug.

CYTOCHROME P450 DRUG INTERACTION TABLE.

SUBSTRATES

CYP1A2	CYP2C9	CYP2C19	CYP2D6	CYP2E1	CYP3A4
Amitriptyline	Amitripty-line	Cyclophosphamide	Codeine	Alcohol	Carbamazepine
Clomipramine	Ibuprofen	Diazepam	Haloperidol	Halothane	Chlorphenamine
Haloperidol	Phenytoin	Omeprazole	Propranolol		Ciclosporin
Propranolol	Tamoxifen	Proguanil	Timolol		Cyclophosphamide
Theophylline	s-Warfarin				Diazepam
Verapamil					Erythromycin
					Ethosuximide
					Etoposide
					Haloperidol
					Nifedipine
					Testosterone
					Verapamil
					Vinblastine
					Vincristine

INHIBITORS

1A2	2C9	2C19	2D6	2E1	3A4
Cimetidine	Isoniazid	Cimetidine	Chlorphenamine		Cimetidine
Ciprofloxacin			Clomipramine		Ciprofloxacin
			Cimetidine		Erythromycin
			Quinidine		Grapefruit juice

INDUCERS

1A2	2C9	2C19	2D6	2E1	3A4
Tobacco	Rifampicin	Rifampicin		Alcohol	Carbamazepine
				Isoniazid	Glucocorticoids
					Phenobarbital
					Phenytoin
					Rifampicin

Incompatibilities between drugs and IV fluids

Drugs should not be added to blood, amino acid solutions or fat emulsions. Certain drugs, when added to IV fluids, may be inactivated by pH changes, by precipitation or by chemical reaction. **Benzylpenicillin** and **ampicillin** lose potency after 6–8 hours if added to dextrose solutions, due to the acidity of these solutions. Some drugs bind to plastic containers and tubing, for example **diazepam** and **insulin**. **Aminoglycosides** are incompatible with **penicillins** and **heparin**. **Hydrocortisone** is incompatible with **heparin**, **tetracycline**, and **chloramphenicol**.

Adverse effects caused by traditional medicines

Patients who have been or are taking traditional herbal remedies may develop ADRs. It is not always easy to identify the responsible plant or plant constituent. Refer to the drug and toxicology information service if available and/or to suitable literature.

The effect of food on drug absorption

Food delays gastric emptying and reduces the rate of absorption of many drugs; the total amount of drug absorbed may or may not be reduced. However, some drugs are preferably taken with food, either to increase absorption or to decrease the irritant effect on the stomach.

Prescription writing

A prescription is an instruction from a prescriber to a dispenser. The prescriber is not always a doctor but can also be a paramedical worker, such as a medical assistant, a midwife or a nurse. The dispenser is not always a pharmacist, but can be a pharmacy technician, an assistant or a nurse. Every country has its own standards for the minimum information required for a prescription, and its own laws and regulations to define which drugs require a prescription and who is entitled to write it. Many countries have separate regulations for prescriptions for controlled drugs such as opioid analgesics.

The following guidelines will help to ensure that prescriptions are correctly interpreted and leave no doubt about the intention of the prescriber. The guidelines are relevant for primary care prescribing; they may, however, be adapted for use in hospitals or other specialist units.

Prescription form

The most important requirement is that the prescription be clear. It should be legible and indicate precisely what should be given. The local language is preferred.

The following details should be shown on the form:

- The prescriber's name, address and telephone number. This will allow either the patient or the dispenser to contact the prescriber for any clarification or potential problem with the prescription.
- Date of the prescription. In many countries the validity of a prescription has no time limit, but in some countries pharmacists do not dispense drugs on prescriptions older than 3 to 6 months.
- Name, form and strength of the drug. The International Nonproprietary Name of the drug should always be used. If there is a specific reason to prescribe a special brand, the trade name can be added. Generic substitution is allowed in some countries. The pharmaceutical form (for example 'tablet', 'oral solution', 'eye ointment') should also be stated.
- The strength of the drug should be stated in standard units using abbreviations that are consistent with the Système Internationale (SI). 'Microgram' and 'nanogram' should not, however, be abbreviated. Also, 'units' should not be abbreviated. Avoid decimals whenever possible. If unavoidable, a zero should be written in front of the decimal point.
- Specific areas for filling in details about the patient including name, address and age.

Directions

Directions specifying the route, dose and frequency should be clear and explicit; use of phrases such as 'take as directed' or 'take as before' should be **avoided**.

For preparations which are to be taken on an 'as required' basis, the minimum dose interval should be stated together with, where relevant, the maximum daily dose. It is good practice to qualify such prescriptions with the purpose of the medication (for example 'every 6 hours as required for pain', 'at night as required to sleep').

It is good practice to explain the directions to the patient; these directions will then be reinforced by the label on the medicinal

product and possibly by appropriate counselling by the
dispenser. It may be worthwhile giving a written note for
complicated regimens although it must be borne in mind that the
patient may lose the separate note.

Quantity to be dispensed

The quantity of the medicinal product to be supplied should be
stated such that it is not confused with either the strength of the
product or the dosage directions.

Alternatively, the length of the treatment course may be stated
(for example 'for 5 days').

Wherever possible, the quantity should be adjusted to match
the pack sizes available.

For liquid preparations, the quantity should be stated in
millilitres (abbreviated as 'ml') or litres (preferably not
abbreviated since the letter 'l' could be confused with the
figure '1').

Narcotics and controlled substances

The prescribing of a medicinal product that is liable to abuse
requires special attention and may be subject to specific
statutory requirements. Practitioners may need to be authorized
to prescribe controlled substances; in such cases it might be
necessary to indicate details of the authority on the prescription.

In particular, the strength, directions and the quantity of the
controlled substance to be dispensed should be stated clearly,
with all quantities written in words as well as in figures to
prevent alteration. Other details such as patient particulars and
date should also be filled in carefully to avoid alteration.

Sample prescription

PRESCRIPTION

Dr B Who
Geneva
Switzerland
Tel: 791 2111

Date: _____

Name of patient _____   Date of birth _____

Address _____   Sex _____

_____

_____

R_x

For use by dispensary

Section 1: Drugs used in Anaesthesia

This section describes drugs used in anaesthesia. The reader is referred to WHO. Model Prescribing Information. Drugs used in Anaesthesia. Geneva: WHO; 1989 for more detailed information.

To produce a state of prolonged full surgical anaesthesia reliably and safely, a variety of drugs is needed. Special precautions and close monitoring of the patient are required. These drugs may be fatal if used inappropriately and should be used by non–specialized personnel only as a last resort. Irrespective of whether a general or conduction (regional or local) anaesthetic technique is used, it is essential that facilities for intubation and mechanically assisted ventilation are available. A full preoperative assessment is required including, if necessary, appropriate fluid replacement.

Anaesthesia may be induced with an intravenous barbiturate, parenteral ketamine, or a volatile agent. Maintenance is with inhalational agents often supplemented by other drugs given intravenously. Specific drugs may be used to produce muscle relaxation. Various drugs may be needed to modify normal physiological functions or otherwise to maintain the patient in a satisfactory condition during surgery.

1.1   General anaesthetics and oxygen

1.1.1   Intravenous agents

Intravenous anaesthetics may be used alone to produce anaesthesia for short surgical procedures but are more commonly used for induction only. They can produce apnoea and hypotension and thus facilities for adequate resuscitation must be available. They are contraindicated if the anaesthetist is not confident of being able to maintain an airway. Before intubation is attempted, a muscle relaxant must be given. Individual requirements vary considerably; lesser dosage is indicated in the elderly, debilitated or hypovolaemic patients.

Intravenous induction using **thiopental** is rapid and excitement does not usually occur. Anaesthesia persists for about 4–7 minutes; large or repeated doses severely depress respiration and delay recovery.

Anaesthesia with **ketamine** persists for up to 15 minutes after a single intravenous injection and is characterized by profound analgesia. It may be used as the sole agent for diagnostic and minor surgical interventions. Subanaesthetic concentrations of ketamine may be used to provide analgesia for painful procedures of short duration such as the dressing of burns, radiotherapeutic procedures, marrow sampling and minor orthopaedic procedures. It is of particular value in children.

Thiopental sodium

Thiopental is a representative intravenous anaesthetic. Various drugs can serve as alternatives

Injection, powder for solution, thiopental sodium, 0.5 g, 1 g, and 2 g ampoules

Uses: induction of anaesthesia prior to administration of inhalational anaesthetic; anaesthesia of short duration

Contraindications: inability to maintain airway; hypersensitivity to barbiturates; cardiovascular disease; dyspnoea or obstructive respiratory disease; porphyria

Precautions: local extravasation can result in extensive tissue necrosis and sloughing; intra-arterial injection causes intense pain and may result in arteriospasm; hepatic impairment (Appendix 5); pregnancy (Appendix 2); **interactions:** Appendix 1

SKILLED TASKS. Warn patient not to perform skilled tasks, for example operating machinery, driving, for 24 hours and also to avoid alcohol for 24 hours

Dosage:

Induction, *by intravenous injection* over 10–15 seconds, ADULT 100–150 mg, followed by a further quantity if necessary according to response after 30–60 seconds; CHILD 2–7 mg/kg

RECONSTITUTION. Solutions containing 25 mg/ml should be freshly prepared by mixing 20 ml of water for injections with the contents of the 0.5-g ampoule, 40 ml with the 1-g ampoule or 100 ml with the 2.5-g ampoule. Any solution made up over 24 hours previously or in which cloudiness, precipitation or crystallization is evident should be discarded

Adverse effects: rapid injection may result in severe hypotension and hiccup; cough, laryngeal spasm, allergic reactions

Ketamine

Injection, ketamine (as hydrochloride) 50 mg/ml, 10-ml ampoule

Uses: induction and maintenance of anaesthesia; analgesia for painful procedures of short duration

Contraindications: thyrotoxicosis; hypertension (including pre-eclampsia); history of cerebrovascular accident, cerebral trauma, intracerebral mass or haemorrhage or other cause of raised intracranial pressure; eye injury and increased intraocular pressure; psychiatric disorders, particularly hallucinations

Precautions: supplementary analgesia often required in surgical procedures involving visceral pain pathways (morphine may be used but addition of nitrous oxide will often suffice); during recovery, patient must remain undisturbed but under observation; pregnancy (Appendix 2); **interactions:** Appendix 1

SKILLED TASKS. Warn patient not to perform skilled tasks, for example operating machinery or driving, for 24 hours and also to avoid alcohol for 24 hours

Dosage:

Induction, *by intramuscular injection,* ADULT and CHILD 6–8 mg/kg (duration of anaesthesia up to 25 minutes)

By intravenous injection over at least 1 minute, ADULT and CHILD 1–4.5 mg/kg (duration of anaesthesia 5–10 minutes after 2 mg/kg dose)

By intravenous infusion of a solution containing 1 mg/ml, ADULT and CHILD total induction dose 0.5–2 mg/kg; maintenance (using microdrip infusion), 10–45 micrograms/kg/minute, rate adjusted according to response

Analgesia, *by intramuscular injection,* ADULT and CHILD initially 4 mg/kg

DILUTION AND ADMINISTRATION. According to manufacturer's directions

Adverse effects: emergence reactions during recovery possibly accompanied by irrational behaviour (effects rarely persist for more than few hours but recurrences can occur at any time within 24 hours); transient elevation of pulse rate and blood pressure common, arrhythmias have occurred; hypotension and bradycardia occasionally reported

1.1.2   Volatile inhalational agents

One of the volatile anaesthetics, ether, halothane (with or without nitrous oxide), must be used for induction when intravenous agents are contraindicated and particularly when intubation is likely to be difficult.

Full muscle relaxation is achieved in deep anaesthesia with **ether**. Excess bronchial and salivary secretion can be avoided by premedication with atropine. Laryngeal spasm may occur during induction and intubation. Localized capillary bleeding can be troublesome and postoperative nausea and vomiting are frequent; recovery time is slow particularly after prolonged administration.

If intubation is likely to be difficult, **halothane** is preferred. It does not augment salivary or bronchial secretions and the incidence of postoperative nausea and vomiting is low. Severe hepatitis, which may be fatal, sometimes occurs; it is more likely in patients who are repeatedly anaesthetized with halothane within a short period of time.

Ether, anaesthetic

> Drug subject to international control under the United Nations Convention against Illicit Traffic in Narcotic Drugs and Psychotropic Substances (1988)

Volatile liquid

Uses: induction and maintenance of anaesthesia (administered from many types of vaporizers)

Contraindications: severe liver disease

Precautions: risk of potentially fatal convulsions in febrile patients; pregnancy (Appendix 2); **interactions:** Appendix 1

FIRE HAZARD. Diathermy must not be used when ether/oxygen mixtures in use and operating theatre and its equipment should be designed to minimize risk of static discharge, particularly in hot, dry climates

Dosage:

Induction, ADULT and CHILD, up to 15% in inspired gases

Maintenance of light anaesthesia, 3–5% in air (with or without muscle relaxants); up to 10% for deep anaesthesia

Adverse effects: transient postoperative effects include impairment of liver function and leukocytosis; nausea and vomiting; capillary bleeding

---

Halothane
Volatile liquid

Uses: induction and maintenance of anaesthesia

Contraindications: history of unexplained jaundice or pyrexia following previous exposure to halothane; family history of malignant hyperthermia; raised cerebrospinal fluid pressure; porphyria

Precautions: anaesthetic history should be carefully taken to determine previous exposure and previous reactions to halothane (at least 3 months should be allowed to elapse between each re-exposure); pregnancy and breastfeeding (Appendices 2 and 3); **interactions:** Appendix 1

Dosage:

Induction, using gas flow containing at least oxygen 30%, gradually increase inspired gas concentration to 2–3% (ADULT) or 1.5–2% (CHILD)

Maintenance, ADULT and CHILD 0.5–1.5%

Adverse effects: arrhythmias; bradycardia; respiratory depression; hepatic damage

1.1.3   Inhalational gases

Nitrous oxide is used for the maintenance of anaesthesia. It is too weak to be used alone, but it allows the dosage of other anaesthetic agents to be reduced. It has a strong analgesic action.

Oxygen should be added routinely during anaesthesia with inhalational agents, even when air is used as the carrier gas, to protect against hypoxia.

Identification of cylinders for inhalation gases. An ISO standard (International Standard 32, Gas cylinders for medical use, 1977) requires that cylinders containing nitrous oxide should bear the name of the contents in legible and permanent characters and, preferably, also the chemical symbol N_2O. The neck, from the valve to the shoulder, should be coloured blue. Cylinders containing oxygen intended for medical use should bear the name of the contents in legible and permanent characters and, preferably, also the chemical symbol O_2. The neck, from the valve to the shoulder, should be coloured white. Cylinders containing nitrous oxide and oxygen mixtures should be similarly labelled, and the neck coloured white and blue.

Nitrous oxide
Inhalation gas

Uses: maintenance of anaesthesia in combination with other anaesthetic agents (halothane, ether, or ketamine) and muscle relaxants; analgesia for obstetric practice, for emergency management of injuries, during postoperative physiotherapy and for refractory pain in terminal illness

---

Contraindications: demonstrable collection of air in pleural, pericardial or peritoneal space; intestinal obstruction; occlusion of middle ear; arterial air embolism; decompression sickness; chronic obstructive airway disease, emphysema

Precautions: minimize exposure of staff; pregnancy (Appendix 2); **interactions:** Appendix 1

Dosage:

Anaesthesia, ADULT and CHILD 70% nitrous oxide mixed with at least 30% oxygen

Analgesia, 50% nitrous oxide mixed with 50% oxygen

Adverse effects: nausea and vomiting; after prolonged administration megaloblastic anaemia, depressed white cell formation; peripheral neuropathy

---

Oxygen

Inhalation gas

Uses: to maintain an adequate oxygen tension in inhalational anaesthesia

FIRE HAZARD. Avoid use of cautery when oxygen is used with ether; reducing valves on oxygen cylinders **must not** be greased (risk of explosion)

Precautions: interactions: Appendix 1

Dosage:

Concentration of oxygen in inspired anaesthetic gases should never be less than 21%

Adverse effects: concentrations greater than 80% have a toxic effect on the lungs leading to pulmonary congestion, exudation and atelectasis

---

1.2   Local anaesthetics

Drugs used for conduction anaesthesia (also termed local or regional anaesthesia) act by causing a reversible block to conduction along nerve fibres. Local anaesthetics are used very widely in dental practice, for brief and superficial interventions, for obstetric procedures, and for specialized techniques of regional anaesthesia calling for highly developed skills. Where patient cooperation is required the patient must be psychologically prepared to accept the proposed procedure. Facilities and equipment for resuscitation should be readily available at all times. Care must always be taken to avoid inadvertent intravascular injection.

LOCAL INFILTRATION. Many simple surgical procedures that neither involve the body cavities nor require muscle relaxation can be performed under local infiltration anaesthesia. Lower-segment caesarean section can also be performed under local infiltration anaesthesia. The local anaesthetic drug of choice is **lidocaine** 0.5% with or without epinephrine. No more than 4 mg/kg of plain lidocaine or 7 mg/kg of lidocaine with epinephrine should be administered on any one occasion. The addition of **epinephrine** (adrenaline) diminishes local blood flow, slows the rate of absorption of the local anaesthetic, and prolongs its effect. Care is necessary when using epinephrine for this purpose since, in excess, it may produce ischaemic necrosis. It should **not** be added to injections used in digits or appendages.

SURFACE ANAESTHESIA. Topical preparations of **lidocaine** are available and topical eye drop solutions of **tetracaine** (section 21.3) are used for local anaesthesia of the cornea and conjunctiva.

REGIONAL BLOCK. A regional nerve block can provide safe and effective anaesthesia but its execution requires considerable training and practice. Nevertheless, where the necessary skills are available, techniques such as axillary or ankle blocks can be invaluable. Either **lidocaine** 1% or **bupivacaine** 0.5% is suitable. Bupivacaine has the advantage of a longer duration of action.

SPINAL ANAESTHESIA. This is one of the most useful of all anaesthetic techniques and can be used widely for surgery of the abdomen and the lower limbs. It is a major procedure requiring considerable training and practice. Either **lidocaine** 5% in glucose or **bupivacaine** 0.5% in glucose can be used but the latter is often chosen because of its longer duration of action.

Bupivacaine hydrochloride

Bupivacaine is a representative local anaesthetic. Various drugs can serve as alternatives

Injection, bupivacaine hydrochloride 2.5 mg/ml (0.25%), 10-ml ampoule; 5 mg/ml (0.5%), 10-ml ampoule; 5 mg/ml (0.5%) with glucose 75 mg/ml (7.5%), 4-ml ampoule

Uses: infiltration anaesthesia; peripheral and sympathetic nerve block; spinal anaesthesia; postoperative pain relief

Contraindications: adjacent skin infection; concomitant anticoagulant therapy; severe anaemia or heart disease; spinal or epidural anaesthesia in dehydrated or hypovolaemic patient

Precautions: respiratory impairment; hepatic impairment (Appendix 5); epilepsy; porphyria; myasthenia gravis; pregnancy and breastfeeding (Appendices 2 and 3); **interactions:** Appendix 1

Dosage:

Maximum cumulative safe dose for adults and children of a 0.25% solution of bupivacaine is 1.5 mg/kg

Local infiltration, using 0.25% solution, ADULT up to 150 mg (up to 60 ml)

Peripheral nerve block, using 0.5% solution, ADULT up to 150 mg (up to 30 ml)

Dental anaesthesia, using 0.5% solution, ADULT 9–18 mg (1.8–3.6 ml)

Spinal anaesthesia, using 0.75% solution (with glucose 7.5%), ADULT 7.5–11.25 mg (1–1.5 ml)

NOTE. Use lower doses for debilitated, elderly, epileptic, or acutely ill patients

0.75% **contraindicated** for epidural use in obstetrics

Do not use solutions containing preservatives for spinal, epidural, caudal or intravenous regional anaesthesia

---

Adverse effects: with excessive dosage or following intravascular injection, light-headedness, dizziness, blurred vision, restlessness, tremors and, occasionally, convulsions rapidly followed by drowsiness, unconsciousness and respiratory failure; cardiovascular toxicity includes hypotension, heart block and cardiac arrest; hypersensitivity and allergic reactions also occur; epidural anaesthesia occasionally complicated by urinary retention, faecal incontinence, headache, backache or loss of perineal sensation; transient paraesthesia and paraplegia very rare

---

Lidocaine hydrochloride

Lidocaine is a representative local anaesthetic. Various drugs can serve as alternatives

Injection, lidocaine hydrochloride 5 mg/ml (0.5%), 20-ml ampoule; 10 mg/ml (1%), 20-ml ampoule; 50 mg/ml (5%), 2-ml ampoule to be mixed with glucose 75 mg/ml (7.5%)

Injection with epinephrine, lidocaine hydrochloride 10 mg/ml (1%) with epinephrine 5 micrograms/ml (1 in 200 000), 20-ml ampoule

Injection with epinephrine (dental use), lidocaine hydrochloride 20 mg/ml (2%) with epinephrine 12.5 micrograms/ml (1 in 80 000), 2.2-ml dental cartridge

Topical gel or *solution*, lidocaine hydrochloride 20–40 mg/ml (2–4%)

Uses: surface anaesthesia of mucous membranes; infiltration anaesthesia; peripheral and sympathetic nerve block; dental anaesthesia; spinal anaesthesia; intravenous regional anaesthesia; arrhythmias (section 12.2)

Contraindications: adjacent skin infection; concomitant anticoagulant therapy; severe anaemia or heart disease; spinal or epidural anaesthesia in dehydrated or hypovolaemic patient

Precautions: respiratory impairment; hepatic impairment (Appendix 5); epilepsy; porphyria; myasthenia gravis; pregnancy (Appendix 2); breastfeeding (Appendix 3); **interactions:** Appendix 1

Dosage:

Maximum safe doses of lidocaine for adults and children are: 0.5%, 1% lidocaine 4 mg/kg; 0.5%, 1% lidocaine + epinephrine 5 micrograms/ml (1 in 200 000) 7 mg/kg

Plain Solutions

Local infiltration and peripheral nerve block, using 0.5% solution, ADULT up to 250 mg (up to 50 ml)

Local infiltration and peripheral nerve block, using 1% solution, ADULT up to 250 mg (up to 25 ml)

Surface anaesthesia of pharynx, larynx, trachea, using 4% solution, ADULT 40–200 mg (1–5 ml)

Surface anaesthesia of urethra, using 4% solution, ADULT 400 mg (10 ml)

Spinal anaesthesia, using 5% solution (with glucose 7.5%), ADULT 50–75 mg (1–1.5 ml)

Solutions containing epinephrine

Local infiltration and peripheral nerve block, using 0.5% solution with epinephrine, ADULT up to 400 mg (up to 80 ml)

Local infiltration and peripheral nerve block, using 1% solution with epinephrine, ADULT up to 400 mg (up to 40 ml)

Dental anaesthesia, using 2% solution with epinephrine, ADULT 20–100 mg (1–5 ml)

NOTE. Use lower doses for debilitated, elderly, epileptic, or acutely ill patients

Do not use solutions containing preservatives for spinal, epidural, caudal or intravenous regional anaesthesia

Adverse effects: with excessive dosage or following intravascular injection, light-headedness, dizziness, blurred vision, restlessness, tremors and, occasionally, convulsions rapidly followed by drowsiness, unconsciousness and respiratory failure; cardiovascular toxicity includes hypotension, heart block and cardiac arrest; hypersensitivity and allergic reactions also occur; epidural anaesthesia occasionally complicated by urinary retention, faecal incontinence, headache, backache or loss of perineal sensation; transient paraesthesia and paraplegia very rare

Vasoconstrictors

Ephedrine hydrochloride

Injection, ephedrine hydrochloride 30 mg/ml, 1-ml ampoule

Uses: prevent hypotension during delivery under spinal anaesthesia

Precautions: hyperthyroidism; diabetes mellitus; ischaemic heart disease, hypertension; angle-closure glaucoma; renal impairment (Appendix 4); pregnancy and breastfeeding (Appendices 2 and 3); **interactions:** Appendix 1

Dosage:

By slow intravenous injection of solution containing 3 mg/ml, ADULT 3–6 mg (maximum single dose 9 mg), repeated if necessary every 3–4 minutes; maximum cumulative dose 30 mg

Adverse effects: anorexia, hypersalivation, nausea, vomiting; tachycardia (also in fetus), arrhythmias, anginal pain, vasoconstriction with hypertension, vasodilation with hypotension; dyspnoea; headache, dizziness, anxiety, restlessness, confusion, tremor; difficulty in micturition; sweating, flushing; changes in blood-glucose concentration

Epinephrine (adrenaline)

Uses: vasoconstrictor to retard systemic absorption of infiltrated local anaesthetics

Contraindications: ring block of digits, penis or other situations where there is risk of local ischaemia

Precautions: hypertension, atherosclerotic heart disease, cerebral vascular insufficiency, heart block; thyrotoxicosis or diabetes mellitus; **interactions:** Appendix 1

Dosage:

Final concentration 5 micrograms/ml (1 in 200 000); in dental surgery, in which small volumes are injected, concentrations of up to 12.5 micrograms/ml (1 in 80 000) commonly used

1.3   Preoperative medication and sedation

Pre-anaesthetic medication is often advisable prior to both conduction and general anaesthetic procedures.

Sedatives improve the course of subsequent anaesthesia in apprehensive patients. Diazepam, promethazine and chloral are effective. **Diazepam** can be administered by mouth or by rectum. **Promethazine**, which has antihistaminic and antiemetic properties as well as a sedative effect, is of particular value in children, as is **chloral hydrate**.

Potent analgesics such as **morphine** or **pethidine** should be administered preoperatively to patients in severe pain or to provide analgesia during and after surgery. Sedatives should then be withheld since they may cause restlessness or confusion.

Anticholinergic (more correctly antimuscarinic) drugs such as **atropine** are additionally used prior to general anaesthetic procedures. They inhibit excessive bronchial and salivary secretions induced, in particular, by ether and ketamine. Intramuscular administration is most effective, but oral administration is more convenient in children. Lower doses should be used in cardiovascular disease or hyperthyroidism.

Atropine sulfate

Tablets, atropine sulfate 1 mg
Injection, atropine sulfate 600 micrograms/ml, 1-ml ampoule

Uses: to inhibit salivary secretions; to inhibit arrhythmias resulting from excessive vagal stimulation; to block the parasympathomimetic effects of anticholinesterases such as neostigmine; organophosphate poisoning (section 4.2.3); antispasmodic (section 17.5); mydriasis and cycloplegia (section 21.5)

Contraindications: angle-closure glaucoma; myasthenia gravis; paralytic ileus, pyloric stenosis; prostatic enlargement

Precautions: Down syndrome, children, elderly; ulcerative colitis, diarrhoea; hyperthyroidism; heart failure, hypertension; pregnancy and breastfeeding (Appendices 2 and 3); **interactions:** Appendix 1

Dosage:

Premedication, *by mouth* 2 hours before induction, CHILD 20 micrograms/kg; *by intramuscular injection* 30–60 minutes before induction, ADULT and CHILD 20 micrograms/kg; *by intravenous injection* immediately before induction, ADULT up to max. 500 micrograms

Inhibition of bradycardia, *by intravenous injection,* ADULT 0.4–1 mg, CHILD 10–30 micrograms/kg

Reversal of neuromuscular block, *by intravenous injection* 2–3 minutes before anticholinesterase, ADULT 0.6–1.2 mg, CHILD 20 micrograms/kg

Adverse effects: dry mouth; blurred vision, photophobia; flushing and dryness of skin, rash; difficulty in micturition; less commonly arrhythmias, tachycardia, palpitations; confusion (particularly in elderly); heat prostration and convulsions, especially in febrile children

---

Chloral hydrate

Oral solution (Elixir), chloral hydrate 200 mg/5 ml

Uses: preoperative sedation

Contraindications: hepatic or renal impairment; cardiac disease

Precautions: respiratory disease; pregnancy and breastfeeding (Appendices 2 and 3); **interactions:** Appendix 1
SKILLED TASKS. Warn patient not to perform skilled tasks, for example operating machinery, driving, for 24 hours

Dosage:
By mouth 30 minutes before surgery, ADULT 30 mg/kg (maximum 2 g); CHILD 30 mg/kg (maximum 1 g)

Adverse effects: gastric irritation; rash

Diazepam

Drug subject to international control under the Convention on Psychotropic Substances (1971)

Diazepam is a representative benzodiazepine. Various drugs can serve as alternatives
Tablets, diazepam 2 mg, 5 mg
Injection, diazepam 5 mg/ml, 2-ml ampoule

Uses: premedication before major or minor surgery; sedation with amnesia for endoscopic procedures and surgery under local anaesthesia; in combination with pethidine, when anaesthetic not available, for emergency reduction of fractures; epilepsy (section 5.1); anxiety disorders (section 24.3)

Contraindications: central nervous system depression or coma; shock; respiratory depression; acute alcohol intoxication

Precautions: elderly or debilitated patients (adverse effects more common in these groups); hepatic impairment (Appendix 5) or renal failure (Appendix 4); chronic pulmonary insufficiency or sleep apnoea; pregnancy and breastfeeding (Appendices 2 and 3); **interactions:** Appendix 1
SKILLED TASKS. Warn patient not to perform skilled tasks, for example operating machinery, driving, for 24 hours

Dosage:
Premedication, *by mouth* 2 hours before surgery, ADULT and CHILD over 12 years, 5–10 mg

Sedation, *by slow intravenous injection* immediately before procedure, ADULT and CHILD over 12 years, 200 micrograms/kg
ADMINISTRATION. Absorption following intramuscular injection slow and erratic; route should only be used if oral or intravenous administration not possible

Slow intravenous injection into large vein reduces risk of thrombophlebitis

Resuscitation equipment must be available

Adverse effects: central nervous system effects common and include drowsiness, sedation, confusion, vertigo, and ataxia; hypotension, bradycardia, or cardiac arrest, particularly in elderly or severely ill patients; also paradoxical reactions, including irritability, excitability, hallucinations, sleep disturbances

---

Promethazine hydrochloride

Promethazine is a representative sedative antihistamine. Various drugs can serve as alternatives

Tablets, promethazine hydrochloride 10 mg, 25 mg
Oral solution (Elixir), promethazine hydrochloride 5 mg/5 ml
Injection, promethazine hydrochloride 25 mg/ml, 2-ml ampoule

Uses: premedication prior to surgery; antiemetic (section 17.2)

Contraindications: child under 1 year; impaired consciousness due to cerebral depressants or of other origin; poryphyria

Precautions: prostatic hypertrophy, urinary retention; glaucoma; hepatic impairment (Appendix 5); pregnancy and breastfeeding (Appendices 2 and 3); **interactions:** Appendix 1
SKILLED TASKS. Warn patient not to perform skilled tasks, for example operating machinery, driving, for 24 hours

Dosage:

By mouth 1 hour before surgery, CHILD over 1 year 0.5–1 mg/kg

By deep intramuscular injection 1 hour before surgery, ADULT 25 mg

Adverse effects: drowsiness (rarely paradoxical stimulation in children); headache; anticholinergic effects such as dry mouth, blurred vision, urinary retention

---

1.4   Muscle relaxants and cholinesterase inhibitors

Muscle relaxants used in surgery are classified according to their mode of action as depolarizing or non–depolarizing neuromuscular blocking drugs. Their use allows abdominal surgery to be carried out under light anaesthesia. They should never be given until it is certain that general anaesthesia has been established and ventilation must be mechanically assisted until they have been completely inactivated.

Suxamethonium is the only widely used depolarizing muscle relaxant. It produces rapid, complete paralysis, which is very short-lasting in most patients and is of particular value for laryngoscopy and intubation. Should paralysis be prolonged, ventilation must be assisted until muscle function is fully restored. Suxamethonium normally produces a phase 1 (depolarizing) neuromuscular block. After high doses or prolonged use, the nature of the block changes to a phase II (non-depolarizing) block; this phase II block (also known as dual block) is associated with prolonged neuromuscular blockade and apnoea.

Alcuronium is a non-depolarizing muscle relaxant with a duration of action of about 30 minutes. Its effects may be rapidly reversed after surgery by the anticholinesterase neostigmine, provided atropine is given to prevent excessive autonomic activity. **Vecuronium**, another relatively new and expensive non-depolarizing muscle relaxant, has a shorter duration of action (20–30 minutes); it causes minimal adverse cardiovascular effects

REVERSAL OF BLOCK. Cholinesterase inhibitors, such as **neostigmine**, are used at the end of an operation to reverse the muscle paralysis produced by non-depolarizing blocking drugs, such as alcuronium and vercuronium. Neostigmine must not be used with depolarizing blocking drugs, such as suxamethonium, since neostigmine will prolong the muscle paralysis. Neostigmine is also used to treat postoperative non-obstructive urinary retention.

For use of cholinesterase inhibitors in myasthenia gravis, see section 20.1.

Alcuronium chloride

Alcuronium is a representative non-depolarizing muscle relaxant. Various drugs can serve as alternatives

Injection, alcuronium chloride 5 mg/ml, 2-ml ampoule

Uses: muscle relaxation during surgery

Contraindications: respiratory insufficiency or pulmonary disease; dehydrated or severely ill patients; myasthenia gravis or other neuromuscular disorders

Precautions: renal or hepatic impairment (see Appendices 4 and 5); possibly increase dose in patient with burns; electrolyte disturbances; possibly decrease dose in respiratory acidosis or hypokalemia; history of asthma; pregnancy and breastfeeding (Appendices 2 and 3); **interactions:** Appendix 1

Dosage:

By intravenous injection, ADULT initially 200–250 micrograms/kg, then 50 mg/kg as required for maintenance; CHILD initially 125–200 mg/kg, then 50 mg/kg for maintenance

Adverse effects: histamine release, causing allergic reactions, such as wheal and flare effects at site of injection, flushing, bronchospasm (anaphylactoid reactions reported); transient hypotension, slight increase in heart rate or decreased pulse rate

---

Vecuronium bromide

Vecuronium is a complementary non-depolarizing muscle relaxant

Injection (Powder for solution for injection), vecuronium chloride, 10-mg vial

Uses: muscle relaxation during surgery

Contraindications: respiratory insufficiency or pulmonary disease; dehydrated or severely ill patients; myasthenia gravis or other neuromuscular disorders

Precautions: renal impairment (Appendix 4); hepatic impairment; possibly increase dose in patient with burns; electrolyte disturbances; possibly decrease dose in respiratory acidosis or hypokalemia; history of asthma; severe obesity (maintenance of adequate airway and ventilation support); pregnancy and breastfeeding (Appendices 2 and 3); **interactions:** Appendix 1

Dosage:

Intubation, *by intravenous injection,* ADULT and CHILD over 5 months, 80–100 micrograms/kg, reduced for maintenance to 20–30 micrograms/kg; CHILD under 4 months, initially 10–20 micrograms/kg, followed by increments according to response

By intravenous infusion, ADULT, initial bolus 40–100 micrograms/kg then 0.8–1.4 micrograms/kg/minute

Adverse effects: minimal release of histamine (rarely hypersensitivity reactions including bronchospasm, hypotension, tachycardia, oedema, erythema, pruritus)

Suxamethonium chloride

Injection, suxamethonium chloride 50 mg/ml, 2-ml ampoule

Injection (Powder for solution for injection), suxamethonium chloride

NOTE. Powder formulation recommended; liquid requires refrigerated storage

Uses: brief muscular paralysis during endotracheal intubation, endoscopy and electroconvulsive therapy

Contraindications: inability to maintain clear airway; personal or family history of malignant hyperthermia; myasthenia gravis; glaucoma, ocular surgery; liver disease; burns; genetically determined disorder of plasma pseudocholinesterase; hyperkalaemia

Precautions: digitalis toxicity or recent digitalization; degenerative neuromuscular disease, paraplegia, spinal cord inury, or severe trauma; prolonged apnoea on repeated injection (infusion preferred for long surgical procedures); hepatic impairment (Appendix 5); renal impairment; pregnancy (Appendix 2); children; **interactions:** Appendix 1

Dosage:

By intramuscular injection, INFANT up to 4–5 mg/kg; CHILD up to 4 mg/kg; maximum 150 mg

By intravenous injection, ADULT and CHILD 0.3–1 mg/kg, followed if necessary by supplements of 300 micrograms/kg; INFANT 2 mg/kg

By intravenous infusion, ADULT and CHILD 2–5 mg/minute of solution containing 1–2 mg/ml

Adverse effects: postoperative muscle pain, particularly in patients ambulant after operation, and more common in females; prolonged apnoea; increases intra-ocular pressure; hyperkalaemia; bradycardia, hypotension, arrhythmias, particularly with halothane (however, with repeated doses tachycardia, hypertension); increases salivary, bronchial and gastric secretions; transient rise in intragastric pressure; hypersensitivity reactions including flushing, rash, urticaria, bronchospasm, and shock (more common in women, in history of allergy, or in asthmatics); rarely, malignant hyperthermia (often fatal)

Neostigmine metilsulfate

Neostigmine is a representative anticholinesterase. Various drugs can serve as alternatives

Injection, neostigmine metilsulfate 500 micrograms/ml, 1-ml ampoule; 2.5 mg/ml, 1-ml ampoule

Uses: counteract effect of non-depolarizing muscle relaxants administered during surgery; postoperative non-obstructive urinary retention; myasthenia gravis (section 20.1)

Contraindications: recent intestinal or bladder surgery; mechanical intestinal or urinary tract obstruction; after suxamethonium; pneumonia; peritonitis

Precautions: asthma; urinary tract infections; cardiovascular disease, including arrhythmias (especially bradycardia or atrioventricular block); hypotension; peptic ulcer; epilepsy; parkinsonism; avoid before halothane administration has been stopped; maintain adequate ventilation (respiratory acidosis predisposes to arrhythmias); renal impairment (Appendix 4); pregnancy and breastfeeding (Appendices 2 and 3); **interactions:** Appendix 1

Dosage:

Reversal of non-depolarizing block, *by intravenous injection* over 1 minute, ADULT 2.5 mg, followed if necessary by supplements of 500 micrograms to maximum total dose of 5 mg; CHILD 40 micrograms/kg (titrated using peripheral nerve stimulator)

NOTE. To reduce muscarinic effects atropine sulfate *by intravenous injection* (ADULT 0.6–1.2 mg, CHILD 20 micrograms/kg) with or before neostigmine

Postoperative urinary retention, *by subcutaneous or intramuscular injection,* ADULT 500 micrograms (catheterization required if urine not passed within 1 hour)

Adverse effects: increased salivation and bronchial secretions, nausea and vomiting, abdominal cramps, diarrhoea; allergic reactions, hypotension

---

1.5   Analgesics and opioid antagonists

Opioid analgesics, **morphine** and **pethidine,** may be used to supplement general anaesthesia, usually in combination with nitrous oxide–oxygen and a muscle relaxant. Repeated doses of intra-operative analgesics should be given with care, since respiratory depression may persist into the postoperative period.

The specific opioid antagonist **naloxone** will immediately reverse this respiratory depression but the dose may need to be repeated. Other resuscitative measures must also be available. It is important to remember that naloxone will also antagonize the *analgesic* effect of opioids.

For further information on opioid analgesics, see section 2.2.

Morphine

> Drug subject to international control under the Single Convention on Narcotic Drugs (1961)

Morphine is a representative opioid analgesic. Various drugs can serve as alternatives

Injection, morphine (as hydrochloride or sulfate) 10 mg/ml, 1-ml ampoule

Uses: adjunct during major surgery; postoperative analgesia; pain, myocardial infarction, acute pulmonary oedema (section 2.2)

Contraindications: acute respiratory depression; increased intracranial pressure, head injury or brain tumour; severe hepatic impairment (Appendix 5); adrenocortical insufficiency; hypothyroidism; convulsive disorders; acute alcoholism, delirium tremens; diverticulitis and other spastic conditions of colon; recent surgery on biliary tract; diarrhoea due to toxins

Precautions: asthma, emphysema, or heart failure secondary to chronic lung disease; ability to maintain airway; if used in biliary colic, antispasmodic needed; renal impairment (Appendix 4); pregnancy (Appendix 2); breastfeeding (Appendix 3); **overdosage:** see section 4.2.2; **interactions:** Appendix 1

Dosage:

Premedication, *by subcutaneous or intramuscular injection* 1 hour before surgery, ADULT 150–200 micrograms/kg; *by intramuscular injection* 1 hour before surgery, CHILD 50–100 micrograms/kg

Intra-operative analgesia, *by intravenous injection,* ADULT and CHILD 100 micrograms/kg, repeated every 40–60 minutes as required

Postoperative analgesia, *by intramuscular injection,* ADULT 150–300 micrograms/kg every 4 hours, CHILD 100–200 micrograms/kg; or *by intravenous infusion* ADULT 8–10 mg over 30 minutes, then 2–2.5 mg/hour

---

Adverse effects: respiratory depression; anorexia, nausea, vomiting, constipation; euphoria, dizziness, drowsiness, confusion, headache; dry mouth; spasm of urinary and biliary tract; circulatory depression, hypotension, bradycardia, palpitations; miosis; allergic reactions; physical dependence

---

Pethidine hydrochloride

> Drug subject to international control under the Single Convention on Narcotic Drugs (1961)

Pethidine is a representative opioid analgesic. Various drugs can serve as alternatives

Injection, pethidine hydrochloride 50 mg/ml, 1-ml ampoule

Uses: preoperative management of musculoskeletal and visceral pain; adjunct during major surgery; postoperative and obstetric analgesia; in combination with diazepam, and in the absence of other agents, for reduction of fractures and other minor interventions; pain (section 2.2)

Contraindications: increased intracranial pressure, head injury or brain tumour; severe hepatic impairment; adrenocortical insufficiency, hypothyroidism; acute respiratory depression; convulsive disorders; acute alcoholism, delirium tremens; diarrhoea due to toxins

Precautions: asthma, emphysema, or heart failure secondary to chronic lung disease; ability to maintain airway; renal impairment (Appendix 4); hepatic impairment (Appendix 5); pregnancy (Appendix 2); breastfeeding (Appendix 3); **overdosage:** see section 4.2.2; **interactions:** Appendix 1

Dosage:

Premedication, *by subcutaneous or intramuscular injection* 1 hour before surgery, ADULT 50–100 mg; *by intramuscular injection* 1 hour before surgery, CHILD over 1 year 1 mg/kg

Intra-operative analgesia, *by slow intravenous injection,* ADULT and CHILD over 1 year 250 micrograms/kg, repeated every 40–60 minutes as required

Postoperative analgesia, *by subcutaneous injection,* CHILD 1–2 mg/kg; *or by intramuscular injection,* ADULT 50–150 mg every 4 hours, CHILD over 1 year 1–2 mg/kg; *or by intravenous infusion,* ADULT 15–35 mg/hour

Obstetric analgesia, *by subcutaneous or intramuscular injection,* ADULT 1 mg/kg, repeated as required (last dose preferably 1–3 hours before delivery to reduce neonatal depression)

NOTE. Give intravenous injections slowly over several minutes with patient recumbent to reduce hypotension and respiratory depression

ADMINISTRATION. According to manufacturer's directions

Adverse effects: respiratory depression; nausea, vomiting; dizziness, drowsiness and confusion; circulatory depression, hypotension, bradycardia and palpitations; convulsions; allergic reactions; physical dependence

---

Naloxone hydrochloride
Injection, naxolone hydrochloride 400 micrograms/ml, 1-ml ampoule

Uses: to counteract respiratory depression induced by opioids during anaesthesia; opioid overdosage (see also section 4.2.2)

Precautions: dependence on opioids; cardiovascular disease

Dosage:

Opioid-induced respiratory depression, *by intravenous injection,* ADULT 100–200 micrograms, repeated every 2–3 minutes to obtain required response; CHILD initially 10 micrograms/kg, if no response followed by 100 micrograms/kg

Opioid-induced respiratory depression at birth, *by subcutaneous, intramuscular, or intravenous injection,* NEONATE 10 micrograms/kg immediately after delivery

Opioid overdosage, *by intravenous injection,* ADULT 0.4–2 mg, repeated every 2–3 minutes according to response to maximum total dose of 10 mg

Adverse effects: nausea and vomiting; hypertension and hypotension reported; left ventricular failure; pulmonary oedema; seizures; arrhythmias such as ventricular tachycardia or fibrillation, particularly in pre-existing cardiac disease

1.6   Blood substitutes and solutions for correcting fluid imbalance

Fluid requirements must be assessed before, during and after major surgery. Replacement fluids should correspond as nearly as possible in volume and composition to those lost. Blood transfusion is essential to restore oxygen-carrying capacity when more than 15% of the circulating blood volume is lost but should be avoided whenever screening for human immunodeficiency viruses and hepatitis B virus is impracticable. Isotonic sodium chloride solution may be used for short-term volume replacement. Plasma expanders such as dextran 70 or polygeline may be useful. Provided renal function is maintained, fluid is most simply replaced by intravenous administration of **sodium chloride solution** (sodium chloride 9 mg/ml, 0.9%) or the more physiologically appropriate **compound solution of sodium lactate**. In emergency cases, there is usually an existing fluid deficit, which must be assessed and corrected before surgery. Isotonic **glucose/sodium chloride** mixtures (most commonly glucose 4%/ sodium chloride 0.18%) are preferred in children to avoid the danger of sodium overload and hypoglycaemia. When fluids are administered intravenously for more than 24 hours, potassium chloride is required to prevent potassium depletion. In order to avoid serious arrhythmias, especially in patients with impaired renal function, the required dose of potassium should be determined, whenever possible, by monitoring plasma concentrations of potassium.

See also sections 11.1 (plasma substitutes) and 26.2 (solutions correcting water, electrolyte, and acid-base disturbances).

Section 2: Analgesics, antipyretics, nonsteroidal anti-inflammatory drugs, drugs used to treat gout, and disease-modifying antirheumatic drugs

Pain can be classified as acute or chronic. Acute pain is usually of short duration and the cause often identifiable (disease, trauma). Chronic pain persists after healing is expected to be complete, or is caused by a chronic disease. Pain may be modified by psychological factors and attention to these is essential in pain management. Drug treatment aims to modify the peripheral and central mechanisms involved in the development of pain. Neurogenic pain generally responds poorly to conventional analgesics; treatment can be difficult and includes the use of carbamazepine (section 5.1) for trigeminal neuralgia and amitriptyline (section 24.2.1) for diabetic neuropathy and postherpetic neuralgia.

Non-opioid analgesics (section 2.1) are particularly suitable for pain in musculoskeletal conditions whereas the opioid analgesics (section 2.2) are more suitable for moderate to severe visceral pain. Those non-opioid analgesics which also have anti-inflammatory actions include salicylates and NSAIDs (nonsteroidal anti-inflammatory drugs); they can reduce both pain and inflammation of chronic inflammatory disorders such as rheumatoid arthritis, but they do not alter or modify the disease process itself. For the management of rheumatoid arthritis DMARDs (disease-modifying antirheumatic drugs) may favourably influence the outcome of the disease (section 2.4). The pain and inflammation of an acute attack of gout is treated with an NSAID or colchicine (section 2.3.1); a xanthine-oxidase inhibitor (section 2.3.2) is used for long-term control of gout.

2.1   Non-opioid analgesics

Non-opioid analgesics with anti-inflammatory activity include salicylates such as acetylsalicylic acid and other nonsteroidal anti-inflammatory drugs such as ibuprofen. Non-opioid analgesics with little or no anti-inflammatory activity include paracetamol.

2.1.1   Acetylsalicylic acid

The principal effects of **acetylsalicylic acid** are anti-inflammatory, analgesic, antipyretic and antiplatelet. Oral doses are absorbed rapidly from the gastrointestinal tract; rectal absorption is less reliable but suppositories are useful in patients unable to take oral dosage forms. Acetylsalicylic acid is used for the management of mild to moderate pain such as headache, acute migraine attacks (section 7.1), transient musculoskeletal pain and dysmenorrhoea, and for reducing fever. Although it may be used in higher doses in the management of pain and inflammation of rheumatoid arthritis, other NSAIDs are preferred because they are likely to be better tolerated. Acetylsalicylic acid is also used for its antiplatelet properties (section 12.5). Adverse effects with analgesic doses are generally mild but include a high incidence of gastrointestinal irritation with slight blood loss, bronchospasm and skin reactions in hypersensitive patients, and increased bleeding time. Anti-inflammatory doses are associated with a much higher incidence of adverse reactions, and they also cause mild chronic salicylism which is characterized by tinnitus and deafness. Acetylsalicylic acid is contraindicated for children under 12 years, unless specifically indicated for juvenile arthritis, because of an association with Reye syndrome (encephalopathy and liver damage).

Acetylsalicylic acid

Tablets, acetylsalicylic acid 300 mg
Dispersible tablets, acetylsalicylic acid 300 mg
Suppositories, acetylsalicylic acid 150 mg, 300 mg

Uses: mild to moderate pain including dysmenorrhoea, headache; pain and inflammation in rheumatic disease and other musculoskeletal disorders (including juvenile arthritis); pyrexia; also acute migraine attack (section 7.1); antiplatelet (section 12.5)

Contraindications: hypersensitivity (including asthma, angioedema, urticaria or rhinitis) to acetylsalicylic acid or any other NSAID; children under 12 years (Reye syndrome) unless for juvenile arthritis (Still disease); gastrointestinal ulceration; haemophilia and other bleeding disorders; gout

Precautions: asthma, allergic disease; impaired renal or hepatic function (Appendices 4 and 5); pregnancy (Appendix 2); breastfeeding (Appendix 3); elderly; to avoid risk of haemorrhage do not administer within 7 days of surgery; G6PD-deficiency; dehydration; **interactions:** see Appendix 1

Dosage:

Mild to moderate pain, pyrexia, *by mouth* with or after food, ADULT 300–900 mg every 4–6 hours if necessary; maximum 4 g daily; CHILD contraindicated under 12 years

Mild to moderate pain, pyrexia, *by rectum*, ADULT 600–900 mg inserted every 4 hours if necessary; maximum 3.6 g daily; CHILD contraindicated under 12 years

Inflammatory arthritis, *by mouth* with or after food, ADULT 4–8 g daily in divided doses in acute conditions; up to 5.4 g daily may be sufficient in chronic conditions

Juvenile arthritis, *by mouth* with or after food, CHILD up to 130 mg/kg body weight daily in 5–6 divided doses in acute conditions; 80–100 mg/kg body weight daily in divided doses for maintenance

Adverse effects: generally mild and infrequent for lower doses, but common with anti-inflammatory doses; gastrointestinal discomfort or nausea, ulceration with occult bleeding (occasionally major haemorrhage); also other haemorrhage (including subconjunctival); hearing disturbances such as tinnitus (rarely deafness), vertigo, confusion, hypersensitivity reactions (angioedema, bronchospasm and rash); increased bleeding time; rarely oedema, myocarditis, blood disorders (particularly thrombocytopenia)

2.1.2 Paracetamol

Paracetamol is similar in analgesic and antipyretic efficacy to
acetylsalicylic acid. It is used for mild to moderate pain
including headache and acute migraine attacks (section 7.1) and
for reducing fever, including post-immunization pyrexia. Paracetamol is particularly useful in patients in whom salicylates or
other NSAIDs are contraindicated, such as asthmatics and those
with a history of peptic ulcer, or for children under the age of 12
years in whom salicylates are contraindicated because of the
risk of Reye syndrome. It is generally preferred to acetylsalicylic acid, particularly in the elderly, because it is less irritant
to the stomach. Unlike acetylsalicylic acid and other NSAIDs,
paracetamol has little anti-inflammatory activity which limits its
usefulness for long-term treatment of pain associated with
inflammation; however it is useful in the management of
osteoarthritis, a condition with only a small inflammatory
component. In normal doses adverse effects are rare, but
overdosage with a single dose of 10–15 g is particularly
dangerous because it may cause hepatocellular necrosis and,
less frequently, renal tubular necrosis.

Paracetamol

Tablets, paracetamol 500 mg
Dispersible tablets, paracetamol 120 mg, 500 mg
Oral solution, paracetamol 120 mg/5 ml, 250 mg/5 ml
Suppositories, paracetamol 60 mg, 100 mg, 125 mg, 250 mg, 500 mg

Uses: mild to moderate pain including dysmenorrhoea, headache; pain relief in osteoarthritis and soft tissue lesions;
pyrexia including post-immunization pyrexia; also acute
migraine attack (section 7.1)

Precautions: hepatic impairment (Appendix 5); renal impairment; alcohol dependence; pregnancy and breastfeeding
(Appendices 2 and 3); **overdosage:** see section 4.2.1;
interactions: see Appendix 1

Dosage:

Post-immunization pyrexia, *by mouth*, INFANT 2–3 months,
60 mg followed by a second dose, if necessary, 4–6 hours
later; warn parents to seek medical advice if pyrexia persists
after second dose

Mild to moderate pain, pyrexia, *by mouth,* ADULT 0.5–1 g every
4–6 hours, maximum 4 g daily; CHILD 3 months–1 year 60–
120 mg, 1–5 years 120–250 mg, 6–12 years 250–500 mg,
these doses may be repeated every 4–6 hours if necessary
(maximum 4 doses in 24 hours)

Mild to moderate pain, pyrexia, *by rectum,* ADULT 0.5–1g; CHILD
1–5 years 125–250 mg, 6–12 years 250–500 mg; doses
inserted every 4–6 hours if necessary, maximum 4 doses in
24 hours

NOTE. Infants under the age of 3 months should not be given paracetamol
unless advised by a doctor; a dose of 10 mg/kg (5 mg/kg if jaundiced) is
suitable

Adverse effects: rare, but rashes, blood disorders; acute pancreatitis reported after prolonged use; **important:** liver damage (and less frequently renal damage) following overdosage

2.1.3 NSAIDs (nonsteroidal anti-inflammatory drugs)

NSAIDs, including **ibuprofen**, have analgesic, anti-inflammatory and antipyretic properties. In single doses NSAIDs have analgesic activity comparable to that of paracetamol. In regular full dosage, they have a lasting analgesic and anti-inflammatory effect, which makes them useful for continuous or regular pain due to inflammation. Differences in anti-inflammatory activity between different NSAIDs are small but there is considerable variation in individual patient response and in the incidence and type of adverse effects. Ibuprofen has fewer adverse effects than other NSAIDs but its anti-inflammatory properties are weaker. Ibuprofen is used in the treatment of mild to moderate pain and in the management of pain and inflammation in rheumatoid arthritis and juvenile arthritis. It may also be of value in the less well-defined conditions of back pain and soft-tissue disorders. Ibuprofen is also used to reduce pain and fever in children. With all NSAIDs caution should be exercised in the treatment of the elderly, in allergic disorders, during pregnancy and breastfeeding. In patients with renal, cardiac or hepatic impairment, the dose should be kept as low as possible and renal function should be monitored. NSAIDs should not be given to patients with active peptic ulceration and used with caution in those with a history of the disease. The commonest adverse effects are generally gastrointestinal including nausea, vomiting, diarrhoea, dyspepsia; hypersensitivity reactions including anaphylaxis, bronchospasm, rash; also fluid retention.

Ibuprofen

Ibuprofen is a representative nonsteroidal anti-inflammatory drug (NSAID). Various drugs can serve as alternatives

Tablets, ibuprofen 200 mg, 400 mg, 600 mg, 800 mg

Oral suspension, ibuprofen 100 mg/5 ml

Uses: pain and inflammation in rheumatic disease and other musculoskeletal disorders including juvenile arthritis; mild to moderate pain including dysmenorrhoea, headache; fever and pain in children; also acute migraine attack (section 7.1)

Contraindications: hypersensitivity (including asthma, angioedema, urticaria or rhinitis) to acetylsalicylic acid or any other NSAID; active peptic ulceration

Precautions: renal and hepatic impairment (Appendices 4 and 5); history of peptic ulceration; cardiac disease; elderly; pregnancy and breastfeeding (Appendices 2 and 3); coagulation defects; allergic disorders; **interactions:** see Appendix 1

Dosage:

Mild to moderate pain, pyrexia, inflammatory musculoskeletal disorders, *by mouth* with or after food, ADULT 1.2–1.8 g daily in 3–4 divided doses, increased if necessary to maximum 2.4 g daily; maintenance dose of 0.6–1.2 g daily may be sufficient

Juvenile arthritis, *by mouth* with or after food, CHILD over 7 kg, 30–40 mg/kg body weight daily in 3–4 divided doses

Fever and pain in children (not recommended for child under 7 kg body weight), *by mouth* with or after food, 20–30 mg/kg body weight daily in divided doses *or* 1–2 years 50 mg 3–4 times daily, 3–7 years 100 mg 3–4 times daily, 8–12 years 200 mg 3–4 times daily

Adverse effects: gastrointestinal disturbances including nausea, diarrhoea, dyspepsia, gastrointestinal haemorrhage; hypersensitivity reactions including rash, angioedema, bronchospasm; headache, dizziness, vertigo, tinnitus, photosensitivity, haematuria; fluid retention, renal failure; rarely hepatic damage, alveolitis, pulmonary eosinophilia, pancreatitis, visual disturbances, erythema multiforme (Stevens-Johnson syndrome), toxic dermal necrolysis (Lyell syndrome), colitis, aseptic meningitis

2.2 Opioid analgesics

Morphine and **pethidine** are opioid analgesics which are effective in relieving moderate to severe pain, particularly of visceral origin; there is a large variation in patient response. Weaker opioids such as **codeine** are suitable for mild to moderate pain.

Morphine remains the most valuable analgesic for severe pain. In addition to pain relief it confers a state of euphoria and mental detachment; repeated administration may cause dependence and tolerance, but this should not be a deterrent in the control of pain in terminal illness (see also section 8.4). In normal doses common adverse effects include nausea, vomiting, constipation and drowsiness; larger doses produce respiratory depression and hypotension.

Pethidine produces prompt but short-acting analgesia; it is less constipating than morphine, but even in high doses it is less effective. A neurotoxic metabolite, norpethidine, accumulates during repeated administration and can cause central nervous system excitation, including myoclonus and seizures. These adverse effects together with the short duration of analgesic action make pethidine unsuitable for severe, continuing pain. It is used for analgesia in labour; however other opioid analgesics such as morphine are often preferred.

Codeine is an opioid analgesic much less potent than morphine and much less liable, in normal doses, to produce adverse effects including dependency. It is effective for mild to moderate pain but is too constipating for long-term use.

Morphine salts

Drug subject to international control under the Single Convention on Narcotic Drugs (1961)

Morphine is a representative opioid analgesic. Various drugs can serve as alternatives

Tablets, morphine sulfate 10 mg

Oral solution, morphine hydrochloride or sulfate 10 mg/5 ml

Injection, morphine sulfate 10 mg/ml, 1-ml ampoule

Uses: severe pain (acute and chronic); myocardial infarction, acute pulmonary oedema; also adjunct during major surgery and postoperative analgesia (section 1.5)

Contraindications: acute respiratory depression, acute alcoholism, where risk of paralytic ileus; acute abdomen; raised intracranial pressure or head injury (interferes with respiration, also affects pupillary responses vital for neurological assessment); avoid injection in phaeochromocytoma

Precautions: renal and hepatic impairment (Appendices 4 and 5); reduce dose or avoid in elderly and debilitated; dependence (severe withdrawal symptoms if withdrawn abruptly); hypothyroidism; convulsive disorders; decreased respiratory reserve and acute asthma; hypotension; prostatic hypertrophy; pregnancy and breastfeeding (Appendices 2 and 3); **overdosage:** see section 4.2.2; **interactions:** see Appendix 1

Dosage:

Acute pain, *by subcutaneous injection* (not suitable for oedematous patients) *or by intramuscular injection* ADULT 10 mg every 4 hours if necessary (15 mg for heavier well-muscled patients); INFANT up to 1 month 150 micrograms/kg body weight, 1–12 months 200 micrograms/kg body weight; CHILD 1–5 years 2.5–5 mg, 6–12 years 5–10 mg

Chronic pain, *by mouth or by subcutaneous injection* (not suitable for oedematous patients) *or by intramuscular injection* 5–20 mg regularly every 4 hours; dose may be increased according to need; oral dose should be approximately double corresponding intramuscular dose

Myocardial infarction, *by slow intravenous injection* (2 mg/minute), 10 mg followed by a further 5–10 mg if necessary; elderly or debilitated patients, reduce dose by half

Acute pulmonary oedema, *by slow intravenous injection* (2 mg/minute), 5–10 mg

NOTE. The doses stated above refer equally to morphine sulfate and hydrochloride

Adverse effects: nausea, vomiting (particularly in initial stages) constipation; drowsiness; also dry mouth, anorexia, spasm of urinary and biliary tract; bradycardia, tachycardia, palpitations, euphoria, decreased libido, rash, urticaria, pruritus, sweating, headache, facial flushing, vertigo, postural hypotension, hypothermia, hallucinations, confusion, dependence, miosis; larger doses produce respiratory depression and hypotension

---

Pethidine hydrochloride

> Drug subject to international control under the Single Convention on Narcotic Drugs (1961)

Pethidine is a representative opioid analgesic. Various drugs can serve as alternatives
Tablets, pethidine hydrochloride 50 mg, 100 mg
Injection, pethidine hydrochloride 50 mg/ml, 1-ml ampoule

Uses: moderate to severe pain; also adjunct during major surgery and postoperative analgesia, obstetric analgesia (section 1.5)

Contraindications: severe renal impairment; acute respiratory depression, acute alcoholism, where risk of paralytic ileus; acute abdomen; raised intracranial pressure or head injury (interferes with respiration, also affects pupillary responses vital for neurological assessment); avoid injection in phaeochromocytoma (risk of pressor response to histamine release)

Precautions: not suitable for severe continuing pain; hepatic impairment (Appendix 5), moderate renal impairment (Appendix 4); reduce dose or avoid in elderly and debilitated; dependence (severe withdrawal symptoms if withdrawn abruptly); hypothyroidism; convulsive disorders; asthma and decreased respiratory reserve; hypotension; prostatic hypertrophy; pregnancy (Appendix 2); breastfeeding (Appendix 3); **overdosage:** see section 4.2.2; **interactions:** see Appendix 1

Dosage:

Acute pain, *by mouth*, ADULT 50–150 mg every 4 hours; CHILD 0.5–2 mg/kg body weight

By subcutaneous or intramuscular injection ADULT 25–100 mg, repeated after 4 hours; CHILD *by intramuscular injection,* 0.5–2 mg/kg body weight

By slow intravenous injection, 25–50 mg, repeated after 4 hours

Adverse effects: nausea, vomiting (particularly in initial stages), constipation; drowsiness; also dry mouth, anorexia, spasm of urinary and biliary tract; bradycardia, tachycardia, palpitations, euphoria, decreased libido, rash, urticaria, pruritus, sweating, headache, facial flushing, vertigo, postural hypotension, hypothermia, hallucinations, confusion, dependence, miosis; larger doses produce respiratory depression and hypotension; **important:** convulsions reported in overdosage

Codeine phosphate

> Drug subject to international control under the Single Convention
> on Narcotic Drugs (1961)

Tablets, codeine phosphate, 30 mg

Uses: mild to moderate pain; also diarrhoea (section 17.7.2)

Contraindications: respiratory depression, obstructive airways
disease, acute asthma attack; where risk of paralytic ileus

Precautions: renal and hepatic impairment (Appendices 4 and
5); dependence; pregnancy (Appendix 2); breastfeeding
(Appendix 3); **overdosage:** see section 4.2.2; **interactions:**
see Appendix 1

Dosage:

Mild to moderate pain, *by mouth*, ADULT 30–60 mg every 4 hours
when necessary to a maximum of 240 mg daily; CHILD 1–12
years, 3 mg/kg daily in divided doses

Adverse effects: constipation particularly troublesome in long-
term use; dizziness, nausea, vomiting; difficulty with
micturition; ureteric or biliary spasm; dry mouth, headaches,
sweating, facial flushing; in therapeutic doses, codeine is
much less liable than morphine to produce tolerance,
dependence, euphoria, sedation or other adverse effects

2.3 Drugs used in gout

2.3.1 Acute gout

Acute attacks of gout are usually treated with high doses of an
NSAID such as indometacin (150–200 mg daily in divided
doses); ibuprofen has weaker anti-inflammatory properties than
other NSAIDs and is therefore unsuitable for treatment of gout.
Salicylates, including acetylsalicylic acid are also not suitable
because they may increase plasma-urate concentrations. **Colchicine** is an alternative for those patients in whom NSAIDs are
contraindicated. Its use is limited by toxicity with high doses. It
does not induce fluid retention and can therefore be given to
patients with heart failure; it can also be given to patients
receiving anticoagulants.

Colchicine

Tablets, colchicine 500 micrograms

Uses: acute gout; short-term prophylaxis during initial therapy
with allopurinol

Contraindications: pregnancy; breastfeeding (Appendix 3)

Precautions: elderly; gastrointestinal disease; cardiac impairment; hepatic impairment; renal impairment (Appendix 4);
interactions: see Appendix 1

Adverse reactions include blood disorders (bone marrow suppression), hepatotoxicity, skin reactions and gastrointestinal disturbances.

Methotrexate, an immunosuppressant, is considered to be a first-line DMARD; at the low doses used for rheumatoid arthritis it is well tolerated but there remains the risk of blood disorders (bone marrow suppression) and of hepatic and pulmonary toxicity. Other immunosuppressant drugs, including **cyclophospamide** and **azathioprine**, are generally reserved for use in patients with severe disease who have failed to respond to other DMARDs, especially in those with extra-cellular manifestations such as vasculitis. Immunosuppressants are used in psoriatic arthritis. Adverse reactions include blood disorders, alopecia, nausea and vomiting.

Penicillamine is not a first-line drug and its use is limited by a significant incidence of adverse effects including blood disorders (bone marrow suppression), proteinuria and rash.

Corticosteroids (section 18.1) are potent anti-inflammatory drugs but their place in the treatment of rheumatoid arthritis remains controversial. Their usefulness is limited by adverse effects and their use should be controlled by specialists. Corticosteroids are usually reserved for use in patients with severe disease which has failed to respond to other antirheumatics, or where there are severe extra-articular effects such as vasculitis. Corticosteroids are also used to control disease activity during initial therapy with DMARDs. Although corticosteroids are associated with bone loss this appears to be dose-related; recent studies have suggested that a low dose of a corticosteroid started during the first two years of moderate to severe rheumatoid arthritis may reduce the rate of bone destruction. The smallest effective dose should be used, such as oral prednisolone 7.5 mg daily for 2–4 years only, and at the end of treatment the dose should be tapered off slowly to avoid possible long term adverse effects. Relatively high doses of a corticosteroid, with cyclophosphamide, may be needed to control vasculitis.

Azathioprine
Tablets, azathioprine 50 mg

Uses: rheumatoid arthritis in cases that have failed to respond to chloroquine or penicillamine; psoriatic arthritis; also transplant rejection (section 8.1); inflammatory bowel disease (section 17.4)

Contraindications: hypersensitivity to azathioprine or mercaptopurine

Precautions: monitor throughout treatment including blood counts; hepatic impairment (Appendix 5); renal impairment (Appendix 4); elderly (reduce dose); pregnancy (Appendix 2); breastfeeding (Appendix 3); warn patient to report immediately any unexplained symptoms including bleeding, bruising, purpura, infection, sore throat or fever; **interactions:** see Appendix 1

Dosage:

Administered on expert advice

Rheumatoid arthritis, *by mouth*, initially, 1.5–2.5 mg/kg body weight daily in divided doses, adjusted according to response; maintenance 1–3 mg/kg body weight daily; consider withdrawal if no improvement within 3 months

Adverse effects: hypersensitivity reactions requiring immediate and permanent withdrawal include malaise, dizziness, vomiting, diarrhoea, fever, rigors, myalgia, arthralgia, disturbed liver function, cholestatic jaundice, arrhythmias, rash, hypotension and interstitial nephritis; dose-related bone marrow suppression; hair loss and increased suceptibility to infections and colitis in patients also receiving corticosteroids; nausea; rarely pancreatitis and pneumonitis

---

Chloroquine salts

Tablets, chloroquine sulfate 200 mg; chloroquine phosphate 250 mg

NOTE. Chloroquine base 150 mg is approximately equivalent to chloroquine sulfate 200 mg or chloroquine phosphate 250 mg

Uses: rheumatoid arthritis (including juvenile arthritis); also malaria (section 6.4.3)

Contraindications: psoriatic arthritis

Precautions: monitor visual acuity throughout treatment; warn patient to report immediately any unexplained visual disturbances; hepatic impairment; renal impairment (Appendix 4); pregnancy and breastfeeding (Appendices 2 and 3); neurological disorders including epilepsy; severe gastrointestinal disorders; G6PD deficiency; elderly; may exacerbate psoriasis and aggravate myasthenia gravis; porphyria; **interactions:** see Appendix 1

Dosage:

Administered on expert advice

Rheumatoid arthritis, *by mouth*, ADULT chloroquine base 150 mg daily; maximum 2.5 mg/kg body weight daily; CHILD chloroquine base up to 3 mg/kg body weight daily

NOTE. To avoid excessive dosage in obese patients the dose of chloroquine should be calculated on the basis of lean body weight

Adverse effects: gastrointestinal disturbances, headache, skin reactions (rash, pruritus); less frequently ECG changes, convulsions, visual changes, retinal damage, keratopathy, ototoxicity, hair depigmentation, alopecia, discoloration of skin and mucous membranes; rarely blood disorders (including thrombocytopenia, agranulocytosis, aplastic anaemia); mental changes (including emotional disturbances, psychosis), myopathy (including cardiomyopathy), acute generalised exanthematous pustulosis, exfoliative dermatitis, erythema multiforme (Stevens-Johnson syndrome) and hepatic damage; **important**: arrhythmias and convulsions in overdosage

---

Cyclophosphamide

Tablets, cyclophosphamide 25 mg

Uses: rheumatoid arthritis (with severe systemic manifestations) which has failed to respond to penicillamine or chloroquine; also malignant disease (section 8.2)

Contraindications: bone marrow aplasia; urothelial toxicity; acute systemic or urinary infection; pregnancy and breastfeeding (Appendices 2 and 3)

Precautions: monitor throughout treatment including blood counts; reduce dose or withdraw if acute infection develops; renal and hepatic impairment (Appendices 4 and 5); for woman or man, contraception during and for at least 3 months after treatment; ensure adequate fluid intake; elderly or debilitated; diabetes mellitus; adrenalectomy; porphyria; warn patient to report immediately any unexplained symptoms including bleeding, bruising, purpura, infection, sore throat or fever; **interactions:** see Appendix 1

Dosage:

Administered on expert advice

Rheumatoid arthritis, *by mouth*, ADULT 1–1.5 mg/kg body weight daily

Adverse effects: bone marrow suppression (withdraw treatment), nausea and vomiting, alopecia, haemorrhagic cystitis, hepatotoxicity

Methotrexate

Tablets, methotrexate 2.5 mg

Uses: severe rheumatoid arthritis which has failed to respond to penicillamine or chloroquine; also malignant disease (section 8.2)

Contraindications: pregnancy and breastfeeding (Appendices 2 and 3); immunodeficiency syndromes; significant pleural effusion or ascites

Precautions: monitor throughout treatment including blood counts and hepatic and renal function tests; renal and hepatic impairment (avoid if severe, see also Appendices 4 and 5); reduce dose or withdraw if acute infection develops; for woman or man, contraception during and for at least 6 months after treatment; peptic ulceration, ulcerative colitis, diarrhoea, ulcerative stomatitis; advise patient to avoid self-medication with salicylates or other NSAIDs; warn patient to report immediately any unexplained symptoms including bleeding, bruising, purpura, infection, sore throat or fever; warn patient with rheumatoid arthritis to report cough or dyspnoea; **interactions:** see Appendix 1

Dosage:

Administered on expert advice

Rheumatoid arthritis, *by mouth*, ADULT 7.5 mg once *weekly* (as a single dose *or* divided into 3 doses of 2.5 mg given at intervals of 12 hours), adjusted according to response; maximum total *weekly* dose 20 mg

Adverse effects: blood disorders (bone marrow suppression), liver damage, pulmonary toxicity; gastrointestinal disturbances—if stomatitis and diarrhoea occur, stop treatment; renal failure, skin reactions, alopecia, osteoporosis, arthralgia, myalgia, ocular irritation, precipitation of diabetes

---

Penicillamine

Tablets, penicillamine 125 mg, 250 mg

Uses: severe rheumatoid arthritis; also copper and lead poisoning (section 4.2.5)

Contraindications: hypersensitivity; lupus erythematosus

Precautions: monitor throughout treatment including blood counts and urine tests; renal impairment (Appendix 4); pregnancy (Appendix 2); avoid concurrent gold, chloroquine or immunosuppressive treatment; avoid oral iron within 2 hours of a dose; warn patient to report immediately any unexplained symptoms including bleeding, bruising, purpura, infection, sore throat or fever; **interactions:** see Appendix 1

Dosage:

Administered on expert advice

Rheumatoid arthritis, *by mouth,* ADULT initially 125–250 mg daily before food for 1 month, increased by similar amounts at intervals of not less than 4 weeks to usual maintenance of 500–750 mg daily in divided doses; maximum 1.5 g daily; ELDERLY initially up to 125 mg daily before food for 1 month increased at intervals of not less than 4 weeks; maximum 1 g daily; CHILD 8–12 years initially 2.5–5 mg/kg body weight daily, gradually increased to usual maintenance of 15–20 mg/kg body weight daily at intervals of 4 weeks over a period of 3–6 months

Adverse effects: initially nausea (less of a problem if taken before food or on retiring, and if initial dose is only gradually increased), anorexia, fever; taste loss (mineral supplements not recommended); blood disorders including thrombocytopenia, neutropenia, agranulocytosis and aplastic anaemia; proteinuria, rarely haematuria (withdraw immediately); haemolytic anaemia, nephrotic syndrome, lupus erythematosus-like syndrome, myasthenia-like syndrome, polymyositis (rarely with cardiac involvement), dermatomyositis, mouth ulcers, stomatitis, alopecia, bronchiolitis and pneumonitis, pemphigus, glomerulonephritis (Goodpasture syndrome) and erythema multiforme (Stevens-Johnson syndrome) also reported; male and female breast enlargement reported; rash (early rash disappears on withdrawing treatment—reintroduce at lower dose and increase gradually; late rash is more resistant—either reduce dose or withdraw treatment)

Sulfasalazine

Tablets (gastro-resistant), sulfasalazine 500 mg

Uses: severe rheumatoid arthritis; also ulcerative colitis and Crohn disease (section 17.4)

Contraindications: hypersensitivity to salicylates and sulphon-amides; severe renal impairment; children

Precautions: monitor during first 3 months of treatment including blood counts and hepatic and renal function tests; renal impairment (Appendix 4); pregnancy and breastfeeding (Appendices 2 and 3); history of allergy; G6PD deficiency; slow acetylator status; porphyria; warn patient to report immediately any unexplained symptoms including bleeding, bruising, purpura, infection, sore throat or fever; **interactions:** see Appendix 1

Dosage:

Administered on expert advice

Rheumatoid arthritis, *by mouth* as gastro-resistant tablets, ADULT initially 500 mg daily, increased by 500 mg at intervals of 1 week to a maximum of 2–3 g daily in divided doses

Adverse effects: nausea, diarrhoea, headache, loss of appetite; fever; blood disorders (including Heinz body anaemia, megaloblastic anaemia, leukopenia, neutropenia, thrombocytopenia); hypersensitivity reactions (including rash, urticaria, erythema multiforme (Stevens-Johnson syndrome), exfoliative dermatitis, epidermal necrolysis, pruritus, photosensitization, anaphylaxis, serum sickness, interstitial nephritis, lupus erythematosus-like syndrome); lung complications (including eosinophilia, fibrosing alveolitis); ocular complications (including periorbital oedema); stomatitis, parotitis; ataxia, aseptic meningitis, vertigo, tinnitus, alopecia, peripheral neuropathy, insomnia, depression, hallucinations; kidney reactions (including proteinuria, crystalluria, haematuria); oligospermia; rarely acute pancreatitis, hepatitis; urine may be coloured orange; some soft contact lenses may be stained

Section 3: Antiallergics and drugs used in anaphylaxis

3.1   Antiallergics and drugs used in anaphylaxis

The H_1-receptor antagonists are generally referred to as antihistamines. They inhibit the wheal, pruritus, sneezing and nasal secretion responses that characterize allergy. Antihistamines thus relieve the symptoms of allergic reactions, such as urticaria, allergic rhinitis, and allergic conjunctivitis; they also control pruritus in skin disorders, such as eczema. Antihistamines are used to treat drug allergies, food allergies, insect stings and some of the symptoms of anaphylaxis and angioedema. Drug treatment and other supportive care should not be delayed in critically ill patients (see Allergic Emergencies below). Specific precipitants should be sought and if identified, further exposure avoided and desensitization considered.

Drowsiness and sedation are particular disadvantages of the early antihistamines and the patient should be warned against driving or operating machinery. Other central nervous depressants, including alcohol, barbiturates, hypnotics, opioid analgesics, anxiolytics and neuroleptics, may enhance the sedative effects of antihistamines. Since antihistamines interfere with skin tests for allergy, they should be stopped at least one week before conducting a skin test.

Chlorphenamine is a typical sedative antihistamine. Newer antihistamines do not cause significant sedation. In practice, all antihistamines are equally effective in relieving the symptoms of allergic reactions and differ mainly in the intensity of sedative and anticholinergic (more correctly antimuscarinic) effects. Selection of an antihistamine should thus be based on the intended therapeutic use, the adverse reaction profile, and the cost.

Corticosteroids, such as **dexamethasone**, **hydrocortisone**, or **prednisolone**, suppress or prevent almost all symptoms of inflammation associated with allergy. The route of administration depends on the particular type of allergic condition. For example, for a mild allergic skin reaction, the best therapy may be the use of a corticosteroid ointment or cream. If the skin reaction does not respond to topical corticosteroid therapy, it may be necessary to give a corticosteroid orally.

Allergic reactions of limited duration and with mild symptoms, such as urticaria or allergic rhinitis, usually require no treatment. If on the other hand, symptoms become persistent, antihistamines constitute the mainstay of treatment. However, oral corticosteroids may be required for a few days in an acute attack of urticaria or for severe skin reactions. Oral corticosteroids are also used to relieve severe exacerbations in chronic urticaria, but long-term use should be avoided.

Corticosteroids may be used topically to reduce inflammation in allergic rhinitis but should only be used systemically for this condition when symptoms are disabling.

Adverse effects associated with long-term use of corticosteroids include inhibition of growth in children, disturbances of electrolyte balance leading to oedema, hypertension and hypokalaemia, with osteoporosis, spontaneous fractures, skin thinning, increased susceptibility to infection, mental disturbances and diabetes mellitus. For further information on the disadvantages of corticosteroids, see section 18.1.

Allergic emergencies

Anaphylactic shock and conditions such as angioedema are medical emergencies that can result in cardiovascular collapse and/or death. They require prompt treatment of possible laryngeal oedema, bronchospasm or hypotension. Atopic individuals are particularly susceptible. Insect bites and certain foods including eggs, fish, peanuts and nuts are also a risk for sensitized persons. Therapeutic substances particularly associated with anaphylaxis include blood products, vaccines, hyposensitizing (allergen) preparations, antibiotics (especially penicillins), iron injections, heparin, and neuromuscular blocking drugs. Acetylsalicylic acid and other nonsteroidal anti-inflammatory drugs (NSAIDs) may cause bronchoconstriction in leukotriene-sensitive patients. In the case of drug allergy, anaphylaxis is more likely to occur after parenteral administration. Resuscitation facilities should always be available when injecting a drug associated with a risk of anaphylactic reactions.

First-line treatment of a severe allergic reaction includes administering epinephrine (adrenaline), keeping the airway open (with assisted respiration if necessary), and restoring blood pressure. Epinephrine (adrenaline) should immediately be given by intramuscular injection to produce vasoconstriction and bronchodilation and injections should be repeated every 10 minutes until blood pressure and pulse have stabilized. If there is cardiovascular shock with inadequate circulation, epinephrine (adrenaline) must be given cautiously by slow intravenous injection of a dilute solution.

An antihistamine such as chlorphenamine is a useful adjunctive treatment given after epinephrine (adrenaline) injection and continued for 24 to 48 hours to reduce the severity and duration of symptoms and to prevent relapse. An intravenous corticosteroid such as hydrocortisone has an onset of action that is delayed by several hours but should be given to help prevent later deterioration in severely affected patients.

Further treatment of anaphylaxis may include intravenous fluids, oxygen, an intravenous vasopressor such as dopamine, intravenous aminophylline or injected or nebulized bronchodilator, such as salbutamol.

Steps in anaphylaxis:

1. **Sympathomimetic**
   Epinephrine (adrenaline) *by intramuscular injection* using epinephrine injection 1 in 1000, ADULT and ADOLESCENT, 500 micrograms (0.5 ml); INFANT under 6 months 50 micrograms (0.05 ml); CHILD 6 months–6 years 120 micrograms (0.12 ml), 6–12 years 250 micrograms (0.25 ml)

   NOTE. The above doses may be repeated several times if necessary at 5-minute intervals, according to blood pressure, pulse, and respiratory function

   If circulation inadequate, *by slow intravenous injection* using epinephrine injection 1 in 10 000 (given at a rate of 1 ml/minute), ADULT 500 micrograms (5 ml); CHILD 10 micrograms/kg (0.1 ml/kg), given over several minutes

2. **Vital functions**
   Maintain an open airway; give oxygen by mask, restore blood pressure (lay patient flat, raise feet)

3. **Antihistamine** such as chlorphenamine *by slow intravenous injection* over 1 minute, ADULT 10–20 mg, repeated if required (maximum total dose 40 mg in 24 hours)

4. **Corticosteroids** such as hydrocortisone *by slow intravenous injection*, ADULT 100–300 mg; CHILD up to 1 year, 25 mg; 1–5 years, 50 mg; 6–12 years, 100 mg

5. **Intravenous fluids:** start infusion with sodium chloride (0.5–1 litre during the first hour)

6. If the patient has asthma-like symptoms, give salbutamol 2.5–5 mg by nebulization or aminophylline 5 mg/kg by intravenous injection over at least 20 minutes.

Antihistamine

Chlorphenamine maleate

Chlorphenamine is a representative sedative antihistamine. Various drugs can serve as alternatives

Tablets, chlorphenamine maleate 4 mg
Oral solution (Elixir), chlorphenamine maleate 2 mg/5 ml
Injection, chlorphenamine maleate 10 mg/ml, 1-ml ampoule

Uses: symptomatic relief of allergy, allergic rhinitis (hay fever) and conjunctivitis, urticaria, insect stings and pruritus of allergic origin; adjunct in the emergency treatment of anaphylactic shock and severe angioedema

Contraindications: prostatic enlargement, urinary retention; ileus or pyloric stenosis; glaucoma; child under 1 year

Precautions: pregnancy and breastfeeding (Appendices 2 and 3); renal and hepatic impairment (Appendices 4 and 5); **interactions:** Appendix 1

SKILLED TASKS. May impair ability to perform skilled tasks, for example operating machinery, driving

Dosage:

By mouth, ADULT 4 mg every 4–6 hours (maximum 24 mg daily); CHILD not recommended under 1 year, 1–2 years 1 mg twice daily, 2–5 years 1 mg every 4–6 hours (maximum 6 mg daily), 6–12 years 2 mg every 4–6 hours (maximum 12 mg daily)

By subcutaneous, intramuscular, or slow intravenous injection over 1 minute, ADULT 10–20 mg, repeated if required (maximum 40 mg in 24 hours); *by subcutaneous injection* CHILD 87.5 micrograms/kg, repeated if necessary up to 4 times daily

Adverse effects: drowsiness (rarely paradoxical stimulation with high doses, or in children or elderly), hypotension, headache, palpitations, psychomotor impairment, urinary retention, dry mouth, blurred vision, gastrointestinal disturbances; liver dysfunction; blood disorders; also rash and photosensitivity reactions, sweating and tremor, hypersensitivity reactions (including bronchospasm, angiodema, anaphylaxis); injections may be irritant

Sympathomimetic

Epinephrine (adrenaline)
Injection, epinephrine (as hydrochloride or hydrogen tartrate) 1 mg/1 ml; 1-ml ampoule

Uses: severe anaphylactic reaction; severe angioedema; cardiac arrest (section 12.2)

Precautions: hyperthyroidism, hypertension, diabetes mellitus, ischaemic heart disease, arrhythmias, cerebrovascular disease, elderly; **interactions:** Appendix 1

Dosage:

Caution: Different dilutions of epinephrine injection are used for different routes of administration

Intramuscular or subcutaneous injection use 1:1000 epinephrine injection, see Steps in Anaphylaxis for doses

Slow intravenous injection use 1:10 000 epinephrine injection. This route should be reserved for severely ill patients when there is doubt about the adequacy of circulation and absorption from the intramuscular site, see Steps in Anaphylaxis for doses

Adverse effects: tachycardia and arrhythmias, hypertension, tremor, anxiety, sweating, nausea, vomiting, weakness, dizziness, pulmonary oedema have all been reported; headache common

Corticosteroids

Dexamethasone
Dexamethasone is a representative corticosteroid. Various drugs can serve as alternatives

Tablets, dexamethasone 500 micrograms, 4 mg

Injection, dexamethasone phosphate (as sodium salt), 4 mg/ml, 1-ml ampoule

Uses: adjunct in the emergency treatment of anaphylaxis; short-term suppression of inflammation in allergic disorders; for other indications see section 18.1

Contraindications: untreated systemic infection (unless condition life-threatening); administration of live virus vaccines

Precautions: increased susceptibility to and severity of infection; activation or exacerbation of tuberculosis, amoebiasis, strongyloidiasis; risk of severe chickenpox in nonimmune patient (varicella-zoster immunoglobulin required if exposed to chickenpox); avoid exposure to measles (normal immunoglobulin possibly required if exposed); diabetes mellitus; peptic ulcer; hypertension; for further precautions relating to long-term use of corticosteroids see section 18.1

Dosage:

By mouth, ADULT and CHILD, usual range 0.5–10 mg daily as a single dose in the morning

By slow intravenous injection or infusion, ADULT 0.5–20 mg; CHILD 200–500 micrograms/kg

Adverse effects: nausea, dyspepsia, malaise, hiccups; hypersensitivity reactions including anaphylaxis; perineal irritation after intravenous administration; for adverse effects associated with long-term corticosteroid treatment see section 18.1

Hydrocortisone

Powder for injection, hydrocortisone (as sodium succinate), 100-mg vial

Uses: adjunct in the emergency treatment of anaphylaxis; inflammatory skin conditions (section 13.3); inflammatory bowel disease (section 17.4); adrenocortical insufficiency (section 18.1)

Contraindications: not relevant to emergency use but for contra-indications relating to long-term use see section 18.1

Precautions: not relevant to emergency use but for precautions relating to long-term use see section 18.1

Dosage:

Anaphylactic emergency, *by slow intravenous injection* as a single dose, see Steps in Anaphylaxis

---

Prednisolone

Prednisolone is representative corticosteroid. Various drugs can serve as alternatives

Tablets, prednisolone 5 mg

Uses: short-term suppression of inflammation in allergic disorders; longer-term suppression (section 18.1); malignant disease (section 8.3); eye (section 21.2)

Contraindications: untreated systemic infection; administration of live virus vaccines

Precautions: increased susceptibility to and severity of infection; activation or exacerbation of tuberculosis, amoebiasis, strongyloidiasis; risk of severe chickenpox in non-immune patient (varicella-zoster immunoglobulin required if exposed to chickenpox); avoid exposure to measles (normal immunoglobulin possibly required if exposed); diabetes mellitus; peptic ulcer; hypertension; for further precautions relating to long-term use of corticosteroids see section 18.1

Dosage:

By mouth, ADULT and CHILD, initially up to 10–20 mg daily as a single dose in the morning (in severe allergy up to 60 mg daily as a short course of 5–10 days)

Adverse effects: nausea, dyspepsia, malaise, hiccups; hypersensitivity reactions including anaphylaxis; for adverse effects associated with long-term corticosteroid treatment see section 18.1

Section 4: Antidotes and other substances used in poisonings

These notes are only guidelines and it is strongly recommended that poisons information centres be consulted in cases where there is doubt about the degree of risk or about appropriate management.

4.1   General care and non-specific treatment

All patients who show features of poisoning should generally be admitted to hospital. Patients who have taken poisons with delayed actions should also be admitted, even if they appear well; delayed-action poisons include acetylsalicylic acid, iron, lithium, paracetamol, paraquat, tricyclic antidepressants and warfarin. This also applies to modified-release preparations. However, it is often impossible to establish with certainty the identity of the poison and the size of the dose but information on the nature of the poison may be useful for carrying out symptomatic management. Few patients require active removal of the poison.

Most patients must be treated symptomatically and monitored. Particular care must be given to maintenance of respiration and blood pressure. Assisted ventilation may be required. Cardiac conduction defects and arrhythmias often respond to correction of underlying hypoxia or acidosis. Hypothermia which may develop in patients who have been unconscious for some hours is best treated by wrapping the patient in blankets to conserve body heat. Convulsions which are prolonged or recurrent may be controlled by intravenous diazepam. In some situations removal of the poison from the stomach by gastric lavage may be appropriate (see below). Activated charcoal can bind many poisons in the stomach and therefore prevent absorption. Active elimination techniques such as repeated administration of activated charcoal can enhance the elimination of some drugs after they have been absorbed (see below). Other techniques to enhance elimination of poisons after their absorption are only practical in hospital and are only suitable for a small number of patients and only to a limited number of poisons. Methods include haemodialysis and haemoperfusion. Alkalinization of urine can be used to increase the elimination of salicylates. Forced alkaline diuresis is no longer recommended.

Gastric lavage

The dangers of attempting to empty the stomach have to be balanced against the toxicity of the ingested poison, as assessed by the quantity ingested, the inherent toxicity of the poison, and the time since ingestion. Gastric emptying is clearly unnecessary if the risk of toxicity is small or if the patient presents too late. Emptying the stomach may be of value if undertaken within 1–2 hours after ingestion. The main risk is with inhalation of stomach contents and gastric lavage should not be undertaken in drowsy or comatose patients without assistance of an anaesthetist so that the airway can be protected by a cuffed endotracheal tube. Gastric lavage must not be attempted after corrosive poisoning or for petroleum products.

Emesis

Emesis induced by **ipecacuanha** has been widely used in adults and children but its use is controversial. It should only be considered if the patient is fully conscious, if the poison ingested is neither corrosive nor a petroleum distillate, if the poison is not adsorbed by activated charcoal or, if gastric lavage is inadvisable or refused.

Prevention of absorption

Given by mouth **activated charcoal** can bind many poisons in the stomach, thereby reducing their absorption. The sooner it is given, the more effective it is, but it may be effective for as long as 2 hours after ingestion. It may be effective several hours after poisoning with modified-release preparations or drugs with anticholinergic (antimuscarinic) properties. It is safe and particularly useful for prevention of absorption of poisons which are toxic in small amounts, for example, antidepressants. Furthermore, repeated doses of activated charcoal enhance the faecal elimination of some drugs (that undergo enterohepatic or enteroenteric recycling) several hours after ingestion and after they have been absorbed, for example phenobarbital, theophylline.

Activated charcoal

Activated charcoal is used to treat poisoning. Various agents can serve as alternatives

Powder for oral suspension, activated charcoal

Uses: treatment of acute poisoning

Contraindications: poisoning by corrosive substances (strong alkali or acid); concurrent administration with specific oral antidotes or oral emetics

Precautions: unconscious patients—risk of aspiration (intubate before administration via a nasogastric or gastric tube); gastric lavage or oral emesis—if required, before administration; concurrent medication should be given parenterally; ensure adequate fluid intake after administration if poison has diuretic properties

Dosage:

Poisoning (prevention of absorption), *by mouth*, ADULT 50–100 g as a single dose, as soon as possible after ingestion of poison; INFANT 1 g/kg as a single dose; CHILD 1–12 years, 25 g as a single dose (50 g in severe poisoning)

Poisoning (active elimination), *by mouth*, ADULT and CHILD over 1 year, 25–50 g initially, then 25–50 g every 4–6 hours; INFANTS 1 g/kg every 4–6 hours

Adverse effects: vomiting, constipation or diarrhoea; pneumonitis—due to aspiration

---

Ipecacuanha
Syrup, ipecacuanha (14 mg total alkaloids calculated as emetine)/10 ml

Uses: treatment of acute poisoning, particularly of slowly absorbed poisons

Contraindications: drowsiness, unconsciousness, convulsions, shock or other conditions which increase risk of aspiration; poisoning with corrosive or petroleum products; children under 6 months

Precautions: cardiac disorders—risk if ipecacuanha absorbed

Dosage:

Acute poisoning, *by mouth*, ADULT 30 ml; CHILD 6–18 months, 10 ml, 18 months–12 years, 15 ml

ADMINISTRATION. Dose should be followed by 100–200 ml of water; if vomiting does not occur within 20–30 minutes a second dose may be given. If appropriate, activated charcoal may be given after emesis has occurred, or if emesis has not occurred 30 minutes after second dose

Adverse effects: excessive vomiting—may cause fluid and electrolyte loss; mucosal damage; cardiac effects if absorbed

4.2   Specific antidotes

4.2.1   Paracetamol overdosage
As little as 10–15 g of paracetamol may cause severe liver damage. Patients who have taken an overdosage of paracetamol should be transferred to hospital urgently.

Administration of activated charcoal should be considered if paracetamol in excess of 150 mg/kg or 12 g, whichever is smaller, is thought to have been ingested within the previous hour.

Acetylcysteine or **methionine** protect the liver if given within 10–12 hours of ingesting paracetamol. Acetylcysteine, given intravenously is most effective within 8 hours of overdosage, but is effective for up to and possibly beyond 24 hours. Alternatively, methionine may be given by mouth provided the overdose was ingested within 10–12 hours and the patient is not vomiting. However, acetylcysteine is the preferred treatment. Concurrent use of activated charcoal and specific oral antidotes should be avoided.

In remote areas methionine should be given, since administration of acetylcysteine outside hospital is not generally practicable. Once the patient is in hospital the need to continue antidote treatment can be assessed from plasma-paracetamol concentrations.

Acetylcysteine
Injection (Concentrate for dilution for infusion), acetylcysteine 200 mg/ml, 10-ml ampoule

Uses: paracetamol overdosage

Precautions: asthma

Dosage:

Paracetamol overdosage, *by intravenous infusion*, ADULT and CHILD initially, 150 mg/kg in 200 ml glucose 5% over 15 minutes, followed by 50 mg/kg in 500 ml glucose 5% over 4 hours, then 100 mg/kg in 1000 ml glucose 5% over 16 hours

NOTE. Children are given the same doses of acetylcysteine as adults, but the volume of infusion may need to be reduced to avoid fluid overload

Adverse effects: rashes, anaphylaxis

DL-Methionine

DL-Methionine is an amino acid used as an antidote to paracetamol overdosage. Various drugs can serve as alternatives

Tablets, DL-methionine 250 mg

Uses: paracetamol overdosage

Precautions: severe liver disease—may precipitate hepatic encephalopathy; avoid concurrent use with activated charcoal

Dosage:

Paracetamol overdosage, *by mouth*, ADULT 2.5 g initially, followed by 3 further doses of 2.5 g every 4 hours

Adverse effects: nausea, vomiting, drowsiness, irritability

4.2.2   Opioid analgesic overdosage

Opioids cause varying degrees of coma, respiratory depression and pinpoint pupils. **Naloxone** is a specific antidote indicated if there is coma or bradypnoea. Naloxone has a shorter duration of action than many opioids so close monitoring and repeated injections are required depending on respiratory rate and depth of coma. The effects of some opioids such as buprenorphine are only partially reversed by naloxone.

Acute withdrawal syndromes may be precipitated by the use of naloxone in patients with a physical dependence on opioids or in overdosage with large doses; a withdrawal syndrome may occur in neonates of opioid-dependent mothers.

Naloxone hydrochloride

Injection (Solution for injection), naloxone hydrochloride 400 micrograms/ml, 1-ml ampoule

Uses: opioid overdosage; postoperative respiratory depression (section 1.5)

Precautions: physical dependence on opioids or other situations where acute withdrawal syndrome may be precipitated (see above); pregnancy (Appendix 2); breastfeeding (Appendix 3); cardiovascular disease

Dosage:

Overdosage of opioids, *by intravenous injection*, ADULT 0.8–2 mg repeated at intervals of 2–3 minutes to a maximum of 10 mg, if respiratory function does not improve, question diagnosis; CHILD 10 micrograms/kg; a subsequent dose of 100 micrograms/kg if no response

NOTE. Naloxone hydrochloride may be administered in the same doses by intramuscular or subcutaneous injection, but only if the intravenous route is not feasible (slower onset of action)

Adverse effects: nausea, vomiting, sweating; hypertension, tremor, convulsions, hyperventilation; cardiac arrest

4.2.3 Organophosphate and carbamate poisoning

Initial treatment of organophosphate or carbamate poisoning includes prevention of further absorption by emptying the stomach by gastric lavage, moving patient to fresh air supply, removing contaminated clothing and washing contaminated skin. A clear airway must be maintained.

Organophosphates inhibit cholinesterases and thus prolong the effects of acetylcholine. **Atropine** will reverse the muscarinic effects of acetylcholine and is used (in conjunction with oximes such as pralidoxime) with additional symptomatic treatment.

Additional treatment for carbamate poisoning is generally symptomatic and supportive. **Atropine** may be given but may not be required because of the rapidly reversible type of cholinesterase inhibition produced (oximes should not be given).

Atropine sulfate

Injection (Solution for injection), atropine sulfate 1 mg/ml, 1-ml ampoule

Uses: organophosphate and carbamate poisoning; premedication (section 1.3); antispasmodic (section 17.5); mydriasis and cycloplegia (section 21.5)

Precautions: children, elderly, Down syndrome; angle-closure glaucoma; myasthenia gravis; gastrointestinal disorders; prostatic enlargement; cardiac disorders; pyrexia; pregnancy (Appendix 2); breastfeeding (Appendix 3); **interactions:** Appendix 1

Dosage:

Organophosphate poisoning, *by intramuscular or intravenous injection* (depending on severity of poisoning), ADULT 2 mg every 20–30 minutes until the skin becomes flushed and dry and tachycardia develops

4.2.4 Iron poisoning and iron and aluminium overload

Mortality due to iron poisoning is reduced by specific therapy with **deferoxamine** which chelates iron. The stomach should be emptied by gastric lavage before administration of deferoxamine. Deferoxamine is also used to diagnose and treat iron or aluminium overload in patients on maintenance haemodialysis.

Deferoxamine mesilate

Injection (Powder for solution for injection or infusion), deferoxamine mesilate 500-mg vial

Uses: acute iron poisoning; iron or aluminium overload

Precautions: renal impairment (Appendix 4); eye and ear examinations before and at 3-month intervals during treatment; aluminium encephalopathy (may exacerbate neurological dysfunction); pregnancy (Appendix 2); breastfeeding (Appendix 3); children under 3 years (may retard growth)

Dosage:

Acute iron poisoning, *by slow intravenous infusion*, ADULT and CHILD initially, 15 mg/kg/hour, reduced after 4–6 hours so that total dose does not exceed 80 mg/kg in 24 hours

Chronic iron overload, *by subcutaneous or intravenous infusion*, ADULT and CHILD lowest effective dose, usually within range of 20–60 mg/kg/day on 4–7 days a week

Aluminium overload in end-stage renal failure, *by intravenous infusion*, ADULT and CHILD 5 mg/kg, once a week during last hour of dialysis

Diagnosis of iron overload, *by intramuscular injection*, ADULT and CHILD 500 mg

Diagnosis of aluminium overload, *by intravenous infusion*, ADULT and CHILD 5 mg/kg during last hour of dialysis

RECONSTITUTION AND ADMINISTRATION. According to manufacturer's directions. For full details and warnings relating to administration for therapeutic or diagnostic purposes, see manufacturer's literature

Adverse effects: anaphylaxis; flushing, urticaria, arrhythmias, hypotension, shock (especially if given by too rapid intravenous infusion); gastrointestinal disturbances; hepatic and renal impairment; dizziness, convulsions; Yersinia infection more frequent; visual disturbances (including lens opacity and retinopathy) and hearing loss; rash; rarely, growth retardation (in young children); rarely, adult respiratory distress syndrome (following excessively high intravenous doses); pain on intramuscular injection; local irritation on subcutaneous infusion; reddish-brown discoloration of urine

4.2.5 Heavy metal poisoning

Heavy metal poisoning may be treated with a range of antidotes including **dimercaprol, penicillamine, potassium ferric hexacyanoferrate** and **sodium calcium edetate**. Penicillamine is also used to promote excretion of copper in Wilson disease.

Dimercaprol

Oily injection (Solution for injection), dimercaprol 50 mg/ml in arachis (peanut) oil, 2-ml ampoule

Uses: acute poisoning by antimony, arsenic, bismuth, gold, mercury, possibly thallium; adjunct (with sodium calcium edetate) in lead poisoning

Contraindications: not indicated for iron, selenium or cadmium poisoning; severe hepatic impairment (unless due to arsenic poisoning)

Precautions: hypertension; renal impairment (discontinue or use with extreme caution if renal failure occurs during treatment); any abnormal reaction such as hyperpyrexia should be assessed; elderly; pregnancy; breastfeeding

Dosage:

Poisoning by heavy metals, *by intramuscular injection*, ADULT 400–800 mg in divided doses on first day, then 200–400 mg daily in divided doses on the second and third days, then 100–200 mg daily in divided doses on subsequent days (single doses generally should not exceed 3 mg/kg, but in severe

poisoning initial single doses up to 5 mg/kg may be required);
CHILD calculate on basis of body-weight using same unit dose/
kg as for adult in similar clinical circumstances

Adverse effects: hypertension, tachycardia; malaise, nausea,
vomiting, abdominal pain, salivation, lacrimation, sweating,
burning sensation in the mouth, throat and eyes; feeling of
constriction in throat and chest; headache, muscle spasms,
tingling of the extremities; fever in children; local pain and
abscess at injection site

Penicillamine

Tablets, penicillamine 125 mg, 250 mg

Uses: poisoning by heavy metals, particularly lead and copper;
Wilson disease; severe rheumatoid arthritis (section 2.4)

Contraindications: hypersensitivity; lupus erythematosus

Precautions: monitor throughout treatment including blood
counts and urine tests; renal impairment (Appendix 4);
pregnancy (Appendix 2); avoid concurrent gold, chloroquine
or immunosuppressive treatment; avoid oral iron within 2
hours of a dose; **interactions:** Appendix 1

PATIENT ADVICE. Warn patient to tell doctor immediately if sore throat, fever,
infection, non-specific illness, unexplained bleeding and bruising, purpura,
mouth ulcers or rash develop

Dosage:

Heavy metal poisoning, *by mouth,* ADULT 1–2 g daily in 4
divided doses before food (continue until urinary lead
stabilised at less than 500 micrograms/day); CHILD 20–
25 mg/kg daily in divided doses

Wilson disease, *by mouth,* ADULT 1.5–2 g daily in divided doses
before food; maximum 2 g daily for 1 year then maintenance
0.75–1 g daily; ELDERLY 20 mg/kg daily in divided doses
adjusted according to response; CHILD up to 20 mg/kg daily in
divided doses; minimum 500 mg daily

Adverse effects: initially nausea (less of a problem if taken with
food and on retiring), anorexia, fever; taste loss (mineral
supplements not recommended); blood disorders including
thrombocytopenia, neutropenia, agranulocytosis and aplastic
anaemia; proteinuria, rarely haematuria (withdraw immediately); haemolytic anaemia, nephrotic syndrome, lupus
erythematosus-like syndrome, myasthenia-like syndrome,
polymyositis (rarely with cardiac involvement), dermatomyositis, mouth ulcers, stomatitis, alopecia, bronchiolitis and
pneumonitis, pemphigus, Goodpasture syndrome and Stevens-Johnson syndrome also reported; male and female breast
enlargement reported; rash early in treatment (usually allergic—may need temporary withdrawal), late rashes (reduce
dose or withdraw treatment)

Potassium ferric hexacyanoferrate

Prussian blue

Powder for oral solution, potassium ferric hexacyanoferrate

Uses: thallium poisoning

Contraindications: constipation; paralytic ileus; renal failure

Dosage:

Treatment of thallium poisoning, *by duodenal tube*, ADULT 125 mg/kg in 100 ml of mannitol 15% twice daily (until urinary thallium stabilized at 500 micrograms or less/day)

Sodium calcium edetate

Infusion (Concentrate for solution for infusion), sodium calcium edetate 200 mg/ml, 5-ml ampoule

Uses: lead poisoning

Precautions: renal impairment

Dosage:

Treatment of lead poisoning, *by intravenous infusion*, ADULT and CHILD up to 40 mg/kg twice daily for up to 5 days; repeated if necessary after interval of 48 hours

DILUTION AND ADMINISTRATION. According to manufacturer's directions

Adverse effects: renal tubular necrosis; nausea, diarrhoea, abdominal cramps, thrombophlebitis (if given too rapidly or as too concentrated a solution); fever, malaise, headache, myalgia, thirst, chills, histamine-like responses (sneezing, nasal congestion, lacrimation) and transient hypotension

---

4.2.6 **Methaemoglobinaemia**

Methylthioninium chloride can lower the levels of methaemoglobin in red blood cells and is used in the treatment of methaemoglobinaemia. In large doses, it may cause methaemoglobinaemia and therefore methaemoglobin levels should be monitored during treatment.

Methylthioninium chloride

Methylene blue

Injection (Solution for injection), methylthioninium chloride, 10 mg/ml, 10-ml ampoule

Uses: acute methaemoglobinaemia

Contraindications: severe renal impairment; methaemoglobinaemia due to chlorate or induced by sodium nitrite in treatment of cyanide poisoning

Precautions: G6PD deficiency—may cause haemolytic anaemia; monitor blood methaemoglobin throughout treatment; pregnancy; breastfeeding

Dosage:

Acute methaemoglobinaemia, *by slow intravenous injection* over several minutes ADULT and CHILD 1–2 mg/kg as a single dose; may be repeated after 1 hour if required

ADMINISTRATION. According to manufacturer's directions

Adverse effects: nausea, vomiting, abdominal pain, chest pain, headache, dizziness, confusion, profuse sweating; hypertension or hypotension reported; haemolytic anaemia—in G6PD deficiency; methaemoglobinaemia—with high dosage; bluish skin discoloration; blue saliva, urine and faeces

4.2.7 Cyanide poisoning

Cyanide poisoning may be treated with **sodium nitrite** followed by **sodium thiosulfate**.

Sodium nitrite

Injection (Solution for injection), sodium nitrite 30 mg/ml, 10-ml ampoule

Uses: cyanide poisoning (together with sodium thiosulfate)

Precautions: monitor plasma methaemoglobin levels; severe cardiovascular or cerebrovascular disease

Dosage:

Cyanide poisoning, *by intravenous injection* over 3–5 minutes, ADULT 300 mg (followed by sodium thiosulfate); further dose of 150 mg after 30 minutes if symptoms recur

Adverse effects: hypotension, vasodilatation resulting in syncope, methaemoglobinaemia, cyanosis, flushing, dyspnoea, tachypnoea, tachycardia, headache, nausea, vomiting and abdominal pain

---

Sodium thiosulfate

Injection (Solution for injection), sodium thiosulfate 250 mg/ml, 50-ml ampoule

Uses: (together with sodium nitrite); pityriasis versicolor (section 13.1)

Dosage:

Cyanide poisoning, after sodium nitrite, *by slow intravenous injection* over about 10 minutes, ADULT 12.5 g; further dose of 6.25 g after 30 minutes if symptoms recur

Section 5: Anticonvulsants/ antiepileptics

5.1   Control of epilepsy

Treatment should always be started with a single drug, but the choice of an anticonvulsant can only be made on an individual basis and will depend on the efficacy of the drug and the patient's tolerance of treatment. If one drug fails to control the seizures after it has been used in full therapeutic dosage for an adequate period, or if it is not well tolerated, it should be gradually substituted with another. If monotherapy is ineffective, two drugs should be given in combination and several regimens may need to be tried before the most appropriate is found.

Initial dose of the drug of choice should be determined on the basis of the degree of urgency, the size and age of the patient. It should be increased gradually until an effective response is obtained. All antiepileptics commonly produce neurological adverse effects at too high a dose, and should be monitored for the earliest signs to help in accurate dose titration. Where the necessary laboratory facilities exist, it can be useful to measure plasma concentrations as an aid to dose adjustment or to determine whether the patient is complying with treatment. Non-compliance because of inappropriate dosing and over-dosing is a major impediment to effective antiepileptic treatment. Patients should ideally remain under supervision throughout treatment.

WITHDRAWAL. Treatment is normally continued for a minimum of two years after the last seizure. Withdrawal should be extended over a period of several months since abrupt withdrawal can lead to complications such as status epilepticus. Abrupt discontinuation is therefore never warranted. Many adult patients relapse once treatment is withdrawn and it may be justified to continue treatment indefinitely, particularly when the patient's livelihood or lifestyle can be endangered by recurrence of a seizure.

PREGNANCY AND BREASTFEEDING. Untreated epilepsy during pregnancy may cause harm to the fetus; there is therefore no justification for abrupt withdrawal of treatment although withdrawal of therapy may be an option if the patient has been seizure-free for at least 2 years; resumption of treatment may be considered after the first trimester. If antiepileptics are continued in pregnancy, monotherapy with the lowest effective dose is preferred, with adjustment made to take account of changes in plasma levels associated with pregnancy. There is an increased risk of birth defects with the use of anticonvulsants, particularly **carbamazepine**, **valproate** and **phenytoin**. However, if there is good seizure control, there is probably no advantage in changing pregnant patients' antiepileptic drugs. In view of the risks of neural tube and other defects, patients who may become pregnant should be informed of the risks and referred for advice, and pregnant patients should be offered counselling and antenatal screening. To counteract the risk of neural tube defects, adequate **folate** supplements are advised for women before and during pregnancy. In view of the risk of neonatal bleeding associated with **carbamazepine, phenobarbital** and **phenytoin**, prophylactic **phytomenadione (vitamin K$_1$)** is recommended for the neonate and the mother before delivery. Antiepileptic drugs can be continued during breast-feeding (see also Appendix 3).

DRIVING. Regulations are in place in many countries which may, for example, restrict driving by patients with epilepsy to those whose seizures are controlled. Further, antiepileptic drugs may cause CNS depression, particularly in the early stages of treatment and patients affected by adverse effects such as drowsiness or dizziness should not operate machinery or drive.

Choice of antiepileptic in management of convulsive disorders

GENERALIZED TONIC-CLONIC, SIMPLE PARTIAL AND COMPLEX PARTIAL SEIZURES. **Carbamazepine, phenobarbital, phenytoin**, and **valproate** are widely used in the treatment of these conditions. However, each of these drugs is associated with dose-related and idiosyncratic adverse effects and monitoring of haematological and hepatic function is often advised, particularly for carbamazepine and valproate.

ABSENCE SEIZURES. Both **ethosuximide** and **valproate** are widely used in the treatment of absence seizures (petit mal) and are usually well tolerated. However, ethosuximide can, rarely, cause lupus erythematosus and psychoses which call for immediate, but cautious, discontinuation. Absence seizures are commonly associated with tonic-clonic seizures and valproate is preferred since it is effective in both disorders.

TONIC SEIZURES, ATONIC SEIZURES AND ATYPICAL ABSENCE SEIZURES. **Phenobarbital** or **phenytoin** is widely used for tonic seizures, **valproate** or **clonazepam** for atonic seizures, and **clonazepam** for atypical absence seizures.

MYOCLONIC SEIZURES. **Valproate** is widely used and most effective for juvenile myoclonic seizures. However, both valproate and this type of seizure are associated with a high relapse rate and it is often necessary to continue therapy indefinitely. Other myoclonic seizures are often resistant to treatment and some do not have an epileptic basis. **Valproate** or **clonazepam** can be of value in this case and other antiepileptic drugs may be useful in intractable cases. Both drugs are generally well accepted, although tolerance to clonazepam has been reported.

INFANTILE SPASM (INFANTILE MYOCLONIC EPILEPSY). Infantile spasms, which are often associated with severe brain damage, can be resistant to antiepileptic drugs. **Clonazepam** is sometimes of value in resistant cases.

FEBRILE CONVULSIONS. Febrile convulsions usually respond to sponging with tepid water and antipyretics such as paracetamol. Rectal **diazepam** is needed for severe attacks. Prolonged treatment is advisable when first seizures occur during the first 18 months of life, when the child has evident neurological abnormalities or has had previous prolonged or focal convulsions. **Phenobarbital** is used for this purpose but careful clinical monitoring and dosage adjustment are necessary to minimize the risk of adverse effects. **Valproate**, although also effective, is not recommended because of the greater risk of hepatotoxicity in this age group. Alternatively, intermittent prophylaxis with rectal diazepam during febrile episodes can also be effective.

Status epilepticus

Status epilepticus is a medical emergency which carries a high mortality rate. Maintenance of the airway and assisted ventilation are crucial even when the seizures are controlled, since the drugs used in its management may also depress respiration. Unresponsive patients require intensive care. Intravenous **diazepam** or **clonazepam** is often effective. Diazepam, which is rapid-acting, should be administered first and should be followed immediately by a loading dose of **phenytoin** which has a longer-acting effect. When cannulation is impossible, diazepam may be administered rectally as a solution (absorption from suppositories is too slow for treatment of status epilepticus). Intravenous **phenobarbital** is also effective but is more likely to cause respiratory depression; it is used in refractory cases but should be avoided in patients who have recently received oral phenobarbital. Rectal paraldehyde may also be used; it causes little respiratory depression and is therefore useful where facilities for resuscitation are poor. If seizures continue despite treatment, general anaesthesia may be required. The underlying cause must be identified and remedied in all cases.

Carbamazepine
Tablets, carbamazepine 100 mg, 200 mg

Uses: generalized tonic-clonic and partial seizures; trigeminal neuralgia; bipolar disorder (section 24.2.2)

Contraindications: atrioventricular conduction abnormalities; history of bone-marrow depression; porphyria

Precautions: hepatic impairment (Appendix 5); renal impairment (Appendix 4); cardiac disease (see also Contraindications); skin reactions (see Adverse effects); history of blood disorders (blood counts before and during treatment); glaucoma; pregnancy (**important** see notes above; Appendix 2); breastfeeding (see notes above; Appendix 3); avoid sudden withdrawal; **interactions:** Appendix 1

BLOOD, HEPATIC OR SKIN DISORDERS. Patients or their carers should be told how to recognize signs of blood, liver or skin disorders, and advised to seek immediate medical attention if symptoms such as fever, sore throat, rash, mouth ulcers, bruising or bleeding develop. Leukopenia which is severe, progressive and associated with clinical symptoms requires withdrawal (if necessary under cover of suitable alternative)

SKILLED TASKS. May impair ability to perform skilled tasks, for example operating machinery, driving; see also notes above

Dosage:

Generalized tonic-clonic seizures, partial seizures, *by mouth*, ADULT initially 100 mg twice daily, increased gradually according to response to usual maintenance dose of 0.8–1.2 g daily in divided doses; ELDERLY reduce initial dose; CHILD 10–20 mg/kg daily in divided doses

Trigeminal neuralgia, *by mouth*, ADULT initially 100 mg 1–2 times daily increased gradually according to response; usual dose 200 mg 3–4 times daily with up to 1.6 g daily in some patients

NOTE. Plasma concentration for optimum response 4–12 mg/litre (17–50 micromol/litre)

Adverse effects: dizziness, drowsiness, headache, ataxia, blurred vision, diplopia (may be associated with high plasma levels); gastrointestinal intolerance including nausea and vomiting, anorexia, abdominal pain, dry mouth, diarrhoea or constipation; commonly, mild transient generalized erythematous rash (withdraw if worsens or is accompanied by other symptoms); leukopenia and other blood disorders (including thrombocytopenia, agranulocytosis and aplastic anaemia); cholestatic jaundice, hepatitis, acute renal failure, Stevens-Johnson syndrome (erythema multiforme), toxic epidermal necrolysis, alopecia, thromboembolism, arthralgia, fever, proteinuria, lymph node enlargement, arrhythmias, heart block and heart failure, dyskinesias, paraesthesia, depression, impotence, male infertility, gynaecomastia, galactorrhoea, aggression, activation of psychosis, photosensitivity, pulmonary hypersensitivity, hyponatraemia, oedema, disturbances of bone metabolism with osteomalacia also reported; confusion and agitation in elderly

Clonazepam

Drug subject to international control under the Convention on Psychotropic Substances (1971)

Clonazepam is a representative benzodiazepine anticonvulsant. Various drugs can serve as alternatives

Clonazepam is a complementary drug

Tablets, clonazepam 500 micrograms

Uses: atonic seizures; myoclonic seizures; atypical absence seizures; absence seizures resistant to ethosuximide or valproate; infantile spasms

Contraindications: respiratory depression; acute pulmonary insufficiency; myasthenia gravis

Precautions: respiratory disease; hepatic impairment (Appendix 5); renal impairment (Appendix 4); elderly and debilitated; pregnancy (see notes above; Appendix 2); breastfeeding (see notes above; Appendix 3); avoid sudden withdrawal; porphyria; **interactions:** Appendix 1

SKILLED TASKS. May impair ability to perform skilled tasks, for example operating machinery, driving; effects of alcohol enhanced; see also notes above

Dosage:

Epilepsy (see Uses above), *by mouth*, ADULT initially 1 mg at night for 4 nights, increased gradually over 2–4 weeks to a usual maintenance dose of 4–8 mg daily in divided doses; ELDERLY (or debilitated patients) initial dose 500 micrograms increased as above; CHILD up to 1 year 250 micrograms increased as above to 0.5–1 mg daily in divided doses; 1–5 years initially 250 micrograms increased to 1–3 mg daily in divided doses; 5–12 years initially 500 micrograms increased to 3–6 mg daily in divided doses

Adverse effects: drowsiness, lethargy, ataxia, paradoxical aggression, irritability and mental changes; rarely blood disorders, abnormal hepatic function tests, excessive salivation

---

Diazepam

Drug subject to international control under the Convention on Psychotropic Substances (1971)

Diazepam is a representative benzodiazepine anticonvulsant. Various drugs can serve as alternatives

Injection (Solution for injection), diazepam 5 mg/ml, 2-ml ampoule

Rectal solution, diazepam 2 mg/ml, 1.25- and 2.5-ml tube; 4 mg/ml, 2.5-ml tube

Uses: status epilepticus; emergency management of recurrent seizures; febrile convulsions; seizures associated with poisoning and drug withdrawal; adjunct in acute alcohol withdrawal; premedication (section 1.3); anxiety disorders (section 24.3)

Contraindications: respiratory depression; acute pulmonary insufficiency; sleep apnoea; severe hepatic impairment; myasthenia gravis

Precautions: respiratory disease, muscle weakness, history of alcohol or drug abuse, marked personality disorder; pregnancy (see notes above; Appendix 2); breastfeeding (see notes above; Appendix 3); reduce dose in elderly or debilitated and in hepatic impairment (avoid if severe,

Appendix 5), renal impairment (Appendix 4); avoid prolonged use and abrupt withdrawal; when given intravenously facilities for reversing respiratory depression with mechanical ventilation must be at hand (see below); porphyria; **interactions:** Appendix 1

PRECAUTIONS FOR INTRAVENOUS INFUSION. Intravenous infusion of diazepam is potentially hazardous (especially if prolonged) calling for close and constant observation and best carried out in a specialist centre with intensive care facilities. Prolonged intravenous infusion requires special caution according to manufacturer's directions

SKILLED TASKS. May impair ability to perform skilled tasks, for example operating machinery, driving; see also notes above

Dosage:

Status epilepticus or emergency management of recurrent epileptic seizures, *by slow intravenous injection* (at rate of 5 mg/minute), ADULT 10–20 mg, repeated if necessary after 30–60 minutes; may be followed *by intravenous infusion* to maximum 3 mg/kg over 24 hours; *by slow intravenous injection*, CHILD 200 to 300 micrograms/kg (*or* 1 mg per year of age); *by rectum* as solution, ADULT and CHILD over 10 kg, 500 micrograms/kg; ELDERLY 250 micrograms/kg; repeated if necessary every 12 hours; if convulsions not controlled, other measures should be instituted

Febrile convulsions (preferred treatment), *by rectum* as solution, CHILD over 10 kg, 500 micrograms/kg (maximum 10 mg), with dose repeated if necessary

Febrile convulsions (alternative treatment), *by slow intravenous injection*, CHILD 200–300 micrograms/kg (*or* 1 mg per year of age)

Drug or alcohol withdrawal, *by slow intravenous injection* (at rate of 5 mg/minute), ADULT 10 mg; higher doses may be required depending on severity of symptoms

Seizures associated with poisoning, *by slow intravenous injection* (at rate of 5 mg/minute), ADULT 10–20 mg

Adverse effects: drowsiness and lightheadedness the next day; confusion and ataxia (especially in the elderly); amnesia; dependence; paradoxical increase in aggression; muscle weakness; occasionally headache, vertigo, salivation changes, gastrointestinal disturbances, rashes, visual disturbances, dysarthria, tremor, changes in libido, incontinence, urinary retention; blood disorders and jaundice; raised liver enzymes; hypotension and apnoea, pain and thrombophlebitis (with injection)

Ethosuximide
Capsules, ethosuximide 250 mg
Syrup, ethosuximide 250 mg/5 ml

Uses: absence seizures

Precautions: hepatic or renal function impairment; blood counts and hepatic and renal function tests recommended; pregnancy (see notes above; Appendix 2); breastfeeding (see notes above; Appendix 3); avoid sudden withdrawal; porphyria; **interactions:** Appendix 1

BLOOD DISORDERS. Patients or their carers should be told how to recognize signs of blood disorders, and advised to seek immediate medical attention if symptoms such as fever, sore throat, mouth ulcers, bruising or bleeding develop

SKILLED TASKS. May impair ability to perform skilled tasks, for example operating machinery, driving; see also notes above

Dosage:

Absence seizures, *by mouth,* ADULT and CHILD over 6 years initially 500 mg daily, increased by 250 mg at intervals of 4–7 days to a usual dose of 1–1.5 g daily (occasionally, up to maximum of 2 g daily); CHILD under 6 years initially 250 mg daily, increased gradually to usual dose of 20 mg/kg daily

PATIENT ADVICE. Daily doses of 1 g and above should be taken as 2 or more divided doses

NOTE. Plasma concentration for optimum response 40–100 mg/litre (300–700 micromol/litre)

Adverse effects: gastrointestinal disturbances including anorexia, hiccups, nausea and vomiting, epigastric pain (particularly during initial treatment); weight loss, drowsiness, dizziness, ataxia, headache, depression, mild euphoria; rarely, rash including Stevens-Johnson syndrome (erythema multiforme), systemic lupus erythematosus, disturbances of liver and renal function (see Precautions), haematological disorders including leukopenia, agranulocytosis, aplastic anaemia, thrombocytopenia, pancytopenia; gum hyperplasia, swelling of tongue, irritability, hyperactivity, sleep disturbances, night terrors, aggressiveness, psychosis, increased libido, myopia, vaginal bleeding, also reported

---

Phenobarbital

> Drug subject to international control under the Convention on Psychotropic Substances (1971)

Tablets, phenobarbital 15 mg, 30 mg, 60 mg, 100 mg
Oral solution (Elixir), phenobarbital 15 mg/5 ml
Injection (Concentrate for solution for injection), phenobarbital sodium 200 mg/ml

Uses: generalized tonic-clonic seizures; partial seizures; neonatal seizures; febrile convulsions; status epilepticus (see notes above)

Contraindications: porphyria; absence seizures

Precautions: elderly, debilitated, children (may cause behavioural changes); impaired renal function (Appendix 4) or hepatic function (Appendix 5), respiratory depression

---

(avoid if severe); pregnancy (see notes above; Appendix 2); breastfeeding (see notes above; Appendix 3); avoid sudden withdrawal; **interactions:** Appendix 1

SKILLED TASKS. May impair ability to perform skilled tasks, for example operating machinery, driving; see also notes above

Dosage:

Generalized tonic-clonic seizures, partial seizures, *by mouth*, ADULT 60–180 mg at night; CHILD up to 8 mg/kg daily

Febrile convulsions, *by mouth*, CHILD up to 8 mg/kg daily

Neonatal seizures, *by intravenous injection* (dilute injection 1 in 10 with water for injections), NEONATE 5–10 mg/kg every 20–30 minutes up to plasma concentration of 40 mg/litre

Status epilepticus, *by intravenous injection* (dilute injection 1 in 10 with water for injections), ADULT 10 mg/kg at a rate of not more than 100 mg/minute (up to maximum total dose of 1 g); CHILD 5–10 mg/kg at a rate of not more than 30 mg/minute

NOTE. For therapeutic purposes phenobarbital and phenobarbital sodium may be considered equivalent in effect.

Plasma concentration for optimum response 15–40 mg/litre (65–170 micromol/litre)

Adverse effects: sedation, mental depression, ataxia, nystagmus; allergic skin reactions including rarely, exfoliative dermatitis, toxic epidermal necrolysis, Stevens-Johnson syndrome (erythema multiforme); paradoxical excitement, restlessness and confusion in the elderly; irritability and hyperactivity in children; megaloblastic anaemia (may be treated with folic acid); osteomalacia; status epilepticus (on treatment withdrawal); hypotension, shock, laryngospasm and apnoea (with intravenous injection)

Phenytoin sodium

Tablets, phenytoin sodium 25 mg, 50 mg, 100 mg

Capsules, phenytoin sodium 25 mg, 50 mg, 100 mg

Injection (Solution for injection), phenytoin sodium 50 mg/ml, 5-ml ampoule

Uses: generalized tonic-clonic seizures; partial seizures; status epilepticus

Contraindications: porphyria; avoid parenteral use in sinus bradycardia, sino-atrial block, second- and third-degree heart block, Stokes-Adams syndrome

Precautions: hepatic impairment (reduce dose; Appendix 5); pregnancy (**important**, see notes above; Appendix 2); breastfeeding (see notes above; Appendix 3); diabetes mellitus; monitor blood counts; hypotension and heart failure (caution with parenteral use); intravenous administration—resuscitation facilities must be available; injection solution alkaline (irritant to tissues); **interactions:** Appendix 1

BLOOD OR SKIN DISORDERS. Patients or their carers should be told how to recognize signs of blood or skin disorders and advised to seek immediate medical attention if symptoms such as sore throat, rash, mouth ulcers, bruising or bleeding develop. Leukopenia which is severe, progressive or associated with clinical symptoms requires withdrawal (if necessary under cover of suitable alternative)

SKILLED TASKS. May impair ability to perform skilled tasks, for example operating machinery, driving; see notes above

Dosage:

Generalized tonic-clonic seizures, partial seizures, *by mouth*, ADULT initially 3–4 mg/kg daily (as a single dose *or* in 2 divided doses), increased gradually by 25 mg at intervals of 2 weeks as necessary (with plasma-phenytoin concentration monitoring); usual dose 200–500 mg daily; CHILD initially 5 mg/kg daily in 2 divided doses; usual dose range 4–8 mg/kg daily (maximum 300 mg)

NOTE. Plasma concentration for optimum response 10–20 mg/litre (40–80 micromol/litre)

PATIENT ADVICE. Preferably taken with or after food

Status epilepticus, *by slow intravenous injection or by intravenous infusion* (with blood pressure and ECG monitoring), ADULT 15 mg/kg at a rate of not more than 50 mg/minute, as a loading dose; maintenance doses of about 100 mg *by mouth* or *by slow intravenous injection* should be given thereafter at intervals of 6–8 hours, monitored by measurement of plasma concentrations; rates and dose reduced according to weight; CHILD 15 mg/kg as a loading dose at rate of 0.5–1.5 mg/kg/minute; NEONATE 15–20 mg/kg as a loading dose at rate of 1–3 mg/kg/minute

DILUTION AND ADMINISTRATION. According to manufacturer's directions

Adverse effects: gastric intolerance, headache, sleeplessness, agitation (during initial phase); sedation, confusion, blurred vision, ataxia, nystagmus, diplopia, slurred speech, cerebellar-vestibular symptoms, behavioural disorders, hallucinations, hyperglycaemia (may be signs of overdosage); gingival hyperplasia, acne, coarse facies, hirsutism, fever, hepatitis, neurological changes (peripheral neuropathy, choreiform movements, impaired cognition, increased seizure frequency); osteomalacia, rickets (associated with reduced plasma calcium levels); lymph-node enlargement; rashes (discontinue; if mild re-introduce cautiously, but discontinue if recurrence); very rarely, Stevens-Johnson syndrome (erythema multiforme), systemic lupus erythematosus, toxic epidermal necrolysis; rarely blood disorders including megaloblastic anaemia (may be treated with folic acid), leukopenia, thrombocytopenia, agranulocytosis with or without bone marrow depression; intravenous administration—cardiovascular and CNS depression (particularly if administered too rapidly) with arrhythmias, hypotension and cardiovascular collapse, alterations in respiratory function (including respiratory collapse)

Sodium valproate

Gastro-resistant tablets (Enteric-coated tablets), sodium valproate 200 mg, 500 mg

Uses: generalized tonic-clonic seizures; partial seizures; atonic seizures; absence seizures; myoclonic seizures; acute mania (section 24.2.2)

Contraindications: active liver disease, family history of severe hepatic dysfunction; pancreatitis; porphyria

Precautions: monitor liver function before and during first 6 months of therapy (Appendix 5), especially in patients at most risk (children under 3 years of age, those with metabolic disorders, degenerative disorders, organic brain disease or severe seizure disorders associated with mental retardation, or multiple antiepileptic therapy); ensure no undue potential for bleeding before starting and before major surgery or anticoagulant therapy; renal impairment (Appendix 4); pregnancy (**important** see notes above; Appendix 2 (neural tube screening)); breastfeeding (see notes above; Appendix 3); systemic lupus erythematosus; false-positive urine tests for ketones; avoid sudden withdrawal; **interactions:** Appendix 1

BLOOD OR HEPATIC DISORDERS. Patients or their carers should be told how to recognize signs of blood or liver disorders, and advised to seek immediate medical attention if symptoms including loss of seizure control, malaise, weakness, anorexia, lethargy, oedema, vomiting, abdominal pain, drowsiness, jaundice, or spontaneous bruising or bleeding develop

SKILLED TASKS. Restrictions on driving in patients with epilepsy, see notes above

Dosage:

Generalized tonic-clonic seizures, partial seizures, absence seizures, atonic seizures; myoclonic seizures, *by mouth*, ADULT initially 600 mg daily in 2 divided doses, preferably after food, increased by 200 mg daily at 3-day intervals to maximum of 2.5 g daily in divided doses; usual maintenance dose 1–2 g daily (20–30 mg/kg daily); CHILD up to 20 kg, initially 20 mg/kg daily in divided doses, may be increased provided plasma concentrations monitored (above 40 mg/kg daily also monitor clinical chemistry and haematological parameters); CHILD over 20 kg, initially 400 mg daily in divided doses, increased until control (usually in range of 20–30 mg/kg daily); maximum 35 mg/kg daily

NOTE. Plasma concentrations in therapeutic range of 40–100 mg/litre (280 to 700 micromol/litre); not generally considered useful in assessing control, but higher levels associated with increased incidence of adverse effects; indicator of compliance, dose change or co-medication

Adverse effects: gastrointestinal irritation, nausea, increased appetite and weight gain, hyperammonaemia; ataxia, tremor; transient hair loss (regrowth may be curly); oedema, thrombocytopenia, inhibition of platelet aggregation; impaired hepatic function and rarely fatal hepatic failure (see Precautions—withdraw treatment immediately if malaise, weakness, lethargy, oedema, abdominal pain, vomiting, anorexia, jaundice, drowsiness or loss of seizure control); sedation reported and also increased alertness; behavioural disturbances; rarely pancreatitis (measure plasma amylase if acute abdominal pain), leukopenia, pancytopenia, red cell hypoplasia, fibrinogen reduction; irregular periods, amenorrhoea, gynaecomastia, hearing loss, Fanconi syndrome, dementia, toxic epidermal necrolysis, Stevens-Johnson syndrome (erythema multiforme) and vasculitis reported

Section 6: Anti-infective drugs

6.1   Anthelminthics

6.1.1   Intestinal anthelminthics

6.1.1.1   Cestode infections

Cestode infections (tapeworms) include intestinal taeniasis and cysticercosis, hymenolepiasis (dwarf tapeworm), diphyllobothriasis and echinococcosis (hydatid disease). Cysticercosis is a systemic infection caused by the larval form (cysticercus) of *Taenia solium*.

Neurocysticercosis occurs when the infection involves the brain. In man, echinococcosis is due to the larval stage of *Echinococcus granulosus* or *E. multilocularis*. The larvae (oncospheres) develop by expansion (cystic echinococcosis) or tumour-like infiltration (alveolar echinococcosis), respectively, in the liver, lungs, or other organs.

TAENIASIS. In taeniasis, **praziquantel** is well tolerated and extensively absorbed and kills adult intestinal taenia worms in a single dose. Praziquantel also kills *T. solium* cysticerci when taken for 14 days in high doses. It thus offers the prospect of a cure for neurocysticercosis, which has been treatable only by surgery, anti-inflammatory corticosteroids and anticonvulsants. However, because dying and disintegrating cysts may induce localized cerebral oedema, treatment with praziquantel must always be undertaken in a hospital setting. In addition, a corticosteroid is usually given to reduce the inflammatory response. **Albendazole** also kills neurocysticerci when given daily for one month; a corticosteroid or an antihistamine is also given to reduce any inflammatory reaction. The longer-established **niclosamide** acts only against the adult intestinal worms. Cestode infections, due to *T. solium*, occurring during pregnancy should always be treated immediately (with praziquantel or niclosamide, but not with albendazole) because of the risk of cysticercosis.

HYMENOLEPIASIS. In hymenolepiasis, **praziquantel** is more effective than **niclosamide**, although resistance to praziquantel has been reported. Repeated treatment may be necessary to cure intense infections or to eliminate the parasite within a family group or institution.

DIPHYLLOBOTHRIASIS. In diphyllobothriasis, **niclosamide** or **praziquantel** in a single dose is highly effective. Hydroxocobalamin injections and folic acid supplements may also be required.

ECHINOCOCCOSIS. In echinococcosis, although surgery is still the treatment of choice for operable cystic disease due to *Echinococcus granulosus* chemotherapy with benzimidazoles, such as **mebendazole** and **albendazole**, may be of value as adjunctive therapy. Alveolar echinococcosis due to *E. multilocularis* requires both surgery and long-term treatment with either mebendazole or albendazole to inhibit metastatic spread. In *animal* studies, albendazole and mebendazole have been found to be teratogenic. They are contraindicated for the treatment of cestode infections in pregnancy; pregnancy should be excluded before treatment with albendazole (non-hormonal contraception during and for 1 month after treatment). For single dose or short-term use in pregnancy, see 6.1₁1.2.

Albendazole
Chewable tablets, albendazole 400 mg

Uses: *Echinococcus multilocularis* and *E. granulosus* infections prior to or not amenable to surgery; neurocysticercosis; nematode infections (sections 6.1.1.2 and 6.1.1.3); filariasis (6.1.2.2)

Contraindications: pregnancy (Appendix 2; see notes above and Precautions)

Precautions: liver function tests and blood counts before treatment and twice during each cycle; exclude pregnancy before starting treatment (non-hormonal contraception during and for 1 month after treatment); breastfeeding

Dosage:
Cystic echinococcosis, *by mouth*, ADULT over 60 kg, 800 mg daily in 2 divided doses for 28 days followed by 14 tablet-free days; ADULT less than 60 kg, 15 mg/kg daily in two divided doses (to a maximum daily dose of 800 mg) for 28 days followed by 14 tablet-free days; up to 3 courses may be given

Alveolar echinococcosis, *by mouth*, ADULT as for cystic echinococcosis, but treatment cycles may need to be continued for months or years

Neurocysticercosis, *by mouth*, ADULT over 60 kg, 800 mg daily in 2 divided doses for 8–30 days; ADULT less than 60 kg, 15 mg/kg daily in two divided doses (to a maximum daily dose of 800 mg) for 8 to 30 days

Adverse effects: gastrointestinal disturbances, headache, dizziness; increases in liver enzymes; reversible alopecia; rash; fever; leukopenia and rarely, pancytopenia; allergic shock if cyst leakage; convulsions and meningism in cerebral disease

Mebendazole
Mebendazole is a representative benzimidazole carbamate derivative anthelminthic. Various drugs can serve as alternatives
Chewable tablets, mebendazole 100 mg, 500 mg

Uses: *Echinococcus granulosus* and *E. multilocularis* infections prior to or not amenable to surgery; nematode infections (sections 6.1.1.2 and 6.1.1.3)

Contraindications: pregnancy (Appendix 2; see also notes above)

Precautions: blood counts and liver function tests (with high-dose regimens); breastfeeding (Appendix 3); **interactions:** Appendix 1

Dosage:

Cystic echinococcosis, alveolar echinococcosis, *by mouth*, ADULT 4.5 g daily in 3 divided doses for 6 months; in alveolar echinococcosis, treatment may be required for up to 2 years after radical surgery, or indefinitely in inoperable cases

PATIENT ADVICE. Doses should be taken between meals

Adverse effects: gastrointestinal disturbances, headache, dizziness; with high doses, allergic reactions, raised liver enzymes, alopecia, bone marrow depression

---

Niclosamide

Chewable tablets, niclosamide 500 mg

Uses: *Taenia saginata, T. solium, Hymenolepis nana*, and *Diphyllobothrium latum* infections

Precautions: chronic constipation (restore regular bowel movement before treatment); antiemetic before treatment; not effective against larval worms; pregnancy (Appendix 2)

Dosage:

Taenia solium infection, *by mouth*, ADULT and CHILD over 6 years 2 g as a single dose after a light breakfast, followed by a purgative after 2 hours; CHILD under 2 years 500 mg, 2–6 years 1 g

T. saginata and *Diphyllobothrium latum* infections, *by mouth*, as for *T. solium* but half the dose may be taken after breakfast and the remainder 1 hour later followed by a purgative 2 hours after last dose

Hymenolepis nana infection, *by mouth*, ADULT and CHILD over 6 years 2 g as a single dose on first day then 1 g daily for 6 days; CHILD under 2 years 500 mg on the first day then 250 mg daily for 6 days, 2–6 years, 1 g on first day then 500 mg daily for 6 days

PATIENT ADVICE. Tablets should be chewed thoroughly (or crushed) before washing down with water

Adverse effects: nausea, retching, abdominal pain; light-headedness; pruritus

---

Praziquantel

Tablets, praziquantel 150 mg, 600 mg

Uses: *Taenia saginata, T. solium, Hymenolepis nana* and *Diphyllobothrium latum* infections; trematode infections (sections 6.1.3.1 and 6.1.3.2)

Contraindications: ocular cysticercosis

Precautions: neurocysticercosis (corticosteroid cover with monitoring, in hospital); pregnancy (Appendix 2); breastfeeding (avoid during and for 72 hours after treatment); **interactions:** Appendix 1

SKILLED TASKS. May impair ability to perform skilled tasks, for example operating machinery, driving

---

Dosage:

Taenia saginata and *T. solium* infections, *by mouth*, ADULT and CHILD over 4 years 5–10 mg/kg as a single dose

Hymenolepis nana infection, *by mouth*, ADULT and CHILD over 4 years, 15–25 mg/kg as a single dose

Diphyllobothrium latum infection, *by mouth,* ADULT and CHILD over 4 years, 10–25 mg/kg as a single dose

Cysticercosis, *by mouth*, ADULT and CHILD over 4 years, 50 mg/kg daily in 3 divided doses for 14 days with prednisolone (or similar corticosteroid) given 2–3 days before and throughout treatment period

Dermal cysticercosis, *by mouth,* ADULT and CHILD over 4 years, 60 mg/kg daily in 3 divided doses for 6 days

Adverse effects: abdominal discomfort, nausea, vomiting, malaise; headache, dizziness, drowsiness; rarely hypersensitivity reactions including fever, urticaria, pruritus, eosinophilia (may be due to dead and dying parasites); in neurocysticercosis, headache, hyperthermia, seizures, intracranial hypertension (inflammatory response to dead and dying parasites in CNS)

6.1.1.2   Intestinal nematode infections

Intestinal nematode infections include ascariasis, hookworm infection, strongyloidiasis, enterobiasis, trichuriasis, trichostrongyliasis and capillariasis.

HOOKWORM INFECTIONS. Hookworm infections are caused by *Ancylostoma duodenale* (ancylostomiasis) and *Necator americanus* (necatoriasis); they are a major cause of iron-deficiency anaemia in the tropics and sub-tropics. Ideally all cases of hookworm infection should be treated. However, when this is impracticable, priority should be given to women in second- and third-trimester pregnancy, children and debilitated patients. In hookworm, broad-spectrum anthelminthics are preferred wherever other nematode infections are endemic. Both **mebendazole** and **albendazole** are effective.

In *animal* studies, **albendazole** and **mebendazole** have been found to be teratogenic. There is some evidence to suggest that the use of mebendazole in pregnancy is not associated with an increased incidence of adverse effects on the fetus. However, neither mebendazole nor albendazole should be used during the first trimester of pregnancy to treat nematode infections. Both drugs are contraindicated for the treatment of cestode infections in pregnancy (see section 6.1.1.1).

Levamisole is effective in the treatment of mixed *Ascaris* and hookworm infections and **pyrantel** has been highly effective in some community-based control programmes, although several doses are often needed to eliminate *Necator americanus* infection. Patients with iron-deficiency anaemia caused by hookworm infection require supplementary iron salts and should receive ferrous sulfate (200 mg for adults daily) for at least 3 months after the haemoglobin concentration of 12 g/100 ml is obtained.

ASCARIASIS. Ascariasis is an infection, usually of the small intestine, caused by *Ascaris lumbricoides* (roundworm). Single doses of **levamisole** or **pyrantel** are effective; the broad-spectrum anthelminthics, **albendazole** or **mebendazole** are also effective.

STRONGYLOIDIASIS. Strongyloidiasis is an infection of the small intestine caused by *Strongyloides stercoralis*. All infected patients should be treated. **Ivermectin** in a single dose of 200 micrograms/kg or 200 micrograms/kg/day on two consecutive days is now the treatment of choice for chronic strongyloidiasis but it may not be available in all countries. **Albendazole** 400 mg, administered for 3 consecutive days is well tolerated by both adults and children aged over 2 years and it may eradicate up to 80% of infections. **Mebendazole** has also been used but, to be effective, it must be administered for longer periods as it has a limited effect on larvae and hence the prevention of autoinfection.

ENTEROBIASIS. Enterobiasis is an infection of the large intestine caused by *Enterobius vermicularis* (pinworm, threadworm). All household members should be treated concurrently with a single dose of **mebendazole**, **albendazole** or **pyrantel**. Since reinfection readily occurs, at least one further dose should be given 2–4 weeks later. Piperazine is also effective but must be taken regularly for at least 7 consecutive days.

TRICHURIASIS. Trichuriasis is an infection of the large intestine caused by *Trichuris trichiura*. Chemotherapy is required whenever symptoms develop or when faecal samples are found to be heavily contaminated (up to 10 000 eggs per gram). A single dose of **albendazole** (400 mg) or **mebendazole** (500 mg) can be effective in mild to moderate infections; heavier infections require a 3-day course.

TRICHOSTRONGYLIASIS. Trichostrongyliasis is an infection of the small intestine caused by *Trichostrongylus* spp. In symptomatic trichostrongyliasis, a single dose of **pyrantel** (10 mg/kg) or **albendazole** (400 mg) is effective.

CAPILLARIASIS. Capillariasis is caused by infection of the intestine with *Capillaria philippinensis*. Prolonged treatment with **mebendazole** or **albendazole** offers the only prospect of cure.

Albendazole

Chewable tablets, albendazole 200 mg, 400 mg

Uses: ascariasis, hookworm infections, strongyloidiasis, entero-biasis, trichuriasis, trichostrongyliasis, and capillariasis; cestode infections (section 6.1.1.1); tissue nematode infections (section 6.1.1.3); filariasis (6.1.2.2)

Precautions: pregnancy (see notes above and Appendix 2; also section 6.1.1.1)

Dosage:

Ascariasis, hookworm infections, enterobiasis, and trichostron-gyliasis, *by mouth,* ADULT and CHILD over 2 years, 400 mg as a single dose

Trichuriasis, *by mouth,* ADULT and CHILD over 2 years, 400 mg as a single dose (for moderate infections) or 400 mg daily for 3 days (severe infections)

Strongyloidiasis, *by mouth,* ADULT and CHILD over 2 years, 400 mg daily for 3 days

Capillariasis, *by mouth,* ADULT and CHILD over 2 years, 400 mg daily for 10 days

Adverse effects: gastrointestinal discomfort, headache; adverse effects associated with use in cestode infections (section 6.1.1.1)

Levamisole

Tablets, levamisole (as hydrochloride) 40 mg, 50 mg, 150 mg

Uses: ascariasis, hookworm, and mixed ascariasis with hook-worm infections; malignant disease (section 8.2)

Contraindications: breastfeeding (Appendix 3)

Precautions: pregnancy (Appendix 2); **interactions:** consult manufacturer's literature

Dosage:

Ascariasis, hookworm, and mixed ascariasis with hookworm infections, *by mouth,* ADULT and CHILD 2.5 mg/kg as a single dose; in severe hookworm infection, a second dose may be given after 7 days

Adverse effects: abdominal pain, nausea, vomiting, dizziness, and headache

Mebendazole

Mebendazole is a representative benzimidazole carbamate derivative anthelminthic. Various drugs can serve as alternatives

Chewable tablets, mebendazole 100 mg, 500 mg

Uses: ascariasis, hookworm infections, enterobiasis, trichur-iasis, and capillariasis; cestode infections (section 6.1.1.1); tissue nematode infections (section 6.1.1.3)

Precautions: pregnancy (Appendix 2; see also notes above and section 6.1.1.1); breastfeeding (Appendix 3); **interactions:** Appendix 1

Dosage:

Ascariasis, *by mouth,* ADULT and CHILD over 2 years, 500 mg as a single dose *or* 100 mg twice daily for 3 days

Hookworm infections, trichuriasis, *by mouth*, ADULT and CHILD over 2 years, 100 mg twice daily for 3 days; if eggs persist in the faeces, second course after 3–4 weeks; alternatively (especially for mass treatment control programmes), *by mouth*, ADULT and CHILD over 2 years, 500 mg as a single dose

Enterobiasis, *by mouth*, ADULT and CHILD over 2 years, 100 mg as a single dose, repeated after interval of 2–3 weeks; all household members over 2 years should be treated at the same time

Capillariasis, *by mouth*, ADULT and CHILD over 2 years, 200 mg daily for 20–30 days; for mass treatment control programmes, *by mouth*, ADULT and CHILD over 2 years, 500 mg as a single dose 4 times a year

PATIENT ADVICE. Doses should be taken between meals

Adverse effects: gastrointestinal disturbances, headache, and dizziness; adverse effects associated with use in cestode infections (section 6.1.1.1)

Pyrantel

Chewable tablet, pyrantel (as embonate) 250 mg
Oral suspension, pyrantel (as embonate) 50 mg/ml

Uses: ascariasis, hookworm infections, enterobiasis, and trichostrongyliasis; tissue nematode infections (6.1.1.3)

Precautions: pregnancy; breastfeeding; liver disease (reduce dose)

Dosage:

Ascariasis, trichostrongyliasis, *by mouth*, ADULT and CHILD 10 mg/kg as a single dose

Hookworm infections, *by mouth*, ADULT and CHILD 10 mg/kg as a single dose; in severe infections, 10 mg/kg daily for 4 days

Enterobiasis, *by mouth*, ADULT and CHILD 10 mg/kg as a single dose with a second dose after 2–4 weeks

Adverse effects: mild gastrointestinal disturbances, headache, dizziness, drowsiness, insomnia, rash

6.1.1.3 Tissue nematode infections

Tissue nematode infections include dracunculiasis, trichinellosis, cutaneous larva migrans, visceral larva migrans, anisakiasis and angiostrongyliasis.

DRACUNCULIASIS. Dracunculiasis (dracontiasis, guinea-worm infection) is caused by infection with *Dracunculus medinensis*, acquired through drinking water containing larvae that develop in small freshwater crustaceans. **Metronidazole** (25 mg/kg daily for 10 days, with a daily maximum of 750 mg for children) provides rapid symptomatic relief. It also weakens the anchorage of the worms in the subcutaneous tissues, and they can then be removed by traction. However, since it has no effect on the larvae of pre-emergent worms, it does not immediately prevent transmission.

TRICHINELLOSIS. Trichinellosis (trichinosis) is caused by infection with the larvae of *Trichinella spiralis*. Each case of confirmed or even suspected trichinellosis infection should be treated in order to prevent the continued production of larvae. In both adults and children, **mebendazole** (200 mg for 5 days), **albendazole** (400 mg for 3 days), and **pyrantel** (10 mg/kg daily for 5 days) are all effective. Prednisolone (40–60 mg daily) may be needed to alleviate the allergic and inflammatory symptoms.

CUTANEOUS LARVA MIGRANS. Cutaneous larva migrans (creeping eruption) is caused by infection with larvae of animal hookworms, usually *Ancylostoma braziliense* and *A. caninum* which infect cats and dogs. **Albendazole** in a single dose of 400 mg is effective.

VISCERAL LARVA MIGRANS. Visceral larva migrans (toxocariasis) is caused by infection with the larval forms of *Toxocara canis* and less commonly, *T. cati* (which infect dogs and cats). Treatment should be reserved for symptomatic infections. A 3-week oral course of **diethylcarbamazine** kills the larvae and arrests the disease, but established lesions are irreversible. To reduce the intensity of allergic reactions induced by dying larvae, dosage is commonly commenced at 1 mg/kg twice daily and raised progressively to 3 mg/kg twice daily (adults and children). Ocular larva migrans occurs when larvae invade the eye, causing a granuloma which may result in blindness. In order to suppress allergic inflammatory responses in patients with ophthalmic lesions, prednisolone should be administered concurrently, either topically or systemically.

ANISAKIASIS. Anisakiasis is caused by infection with seafood containing larvae of *Anisakis*, *Contracaecum*, or *Pseudoterranova* spp. In anisakiasis, anthelminthic treatment is rarely necessary. Prevention is dependent upon informing communities of the hazards of eating raw or inadequately prepared salt-water fish; and early evisceration of fish after capture and freezing of seafood at −20°C for at least 60 hours before sale.

ANGIOSTRONGYLIASIS. Angiostrongyliasis is caused by infection with the larvae of the rat lungworm, *Parastrongylus cantonensis* (*Angiostrongylus cantonensis*). Symptomatic treatment pending spontaneous recovery is often all that is required.

6.1.2   Antifilarials

6.1.2.1   Loiasis

Loiasis is an infection with the filarial nematode *Loa loa* and is transmitted by the biting tabanid fly *Chrysops*. **Diethylcarbamazine** is effective against both adult worms and larvae; a single weekly dose is normally effective as prophylaxis. During individual treatment, particularly of persons with heavy microfilaraemia (>50 000 microfilariae/ml blood), a condition simulating meningoencephalitis occasionally occurs. This probably results from sludging of moribund microfilariae within cerebral capillaries. The frequency of meningoencephalitis associated with diethylcarbamazine therapy of loiasis is reported as 1.25%, with a mortality rate of about 50% in affected patients. Permanent cerebral damage is common among patients who survive and this possibility should be considered when deciding on treatment. Treatment of heavily infected patients should thus begin at low dosage and corticosteroid and antihistamine cover should be provided for the first 2 to 3 days.

Diethylcarbamazine citrate

Tablets, diethylcarbamazine citrate 50 mg

Uses: treatment of loiasis; prophylaxis of loiasis in temporary residents in endemic areas; tissue nematode infections (6.1.1.3); lymphatic filariasis (6.1.2.2)

Contraindications: pregnancy (delay treatment until after delivery); infants, elderly, debilitated (usually excluded from mass treatment programmes; see also Precautions)

Precautions: renal impairment (reduce dose; Appendix 4); cardiac disorders; other severe acute diseases—delay diethylcarbamazine treatment until after recovery; risk of meningoencephalitis in severe infection (see notes above)

Dosage:

Loiasis, treatment, *by mouth,* ADULT 1 mg/kg as a single dose on the first day, doubled on two successive days, then adjusted to 2–3 mg/kg 3 times daily for a further 18 days

Loiasis, prophylaxis, *by mouth,* ADULT 300 mg weekly for as long as exposure occurs

PATIENT ADVICE. Complete the prescribed course as directed to mimimize allergic reactions to dying parasites

Adverse effects: headache, dizziness, drowsiness, nausea and vomiting; immunological reactions, within a few hours of the first dose, subsiding by fifth day of treatment, and including fever, headache, joint pain, dizziness, anorexia, malaise, nausea and vomiting, urticaria, and asthma in asthmatics (similar to Mazzotti reaction—see section 6.1.2.3), induced by disintegrating microfilariae; microencephalitis (with heavy microfilaraemia, see notes above); reversible proteinuria

6.1.2.2 Lymphatic filariasis

Lymphatic filariasis is caused by infection with *Wuchereria bancrofti* (bancroftian filariasis), *Brugia malayi* or *B. timori* (brugian filariasis). Occult filariasis (tropical pulmonary eosinophilia) is a clinical variant of *W. bancrofti* infection. Individual treatment with **diethylcarbamazine** which has both microfilaricidal and macrofilaricidal activity is effective. Total cumulative dosages of 72 mg/kg are generally recommended for *Wuchereria bancrofti* infections with half this dose used for *Brugia malayi* and *B. timori* infections. In all cases treatment should be initiated with smaller doses for 2–3 days to avoid the danger of immunological reactions. Rigorous hygiene to the affected limbs with adjunctive measures to minimize infection and promote lymph flow are important for reducing acute episodes of inflammation.

In communities where filariasis is endemic, annual administration of single doses of **ivermectin**, 400 micrograms/kg may be effective in reducing transmission. This treatment must be continued for at least 4–6 years. **Albendazole** 600 mg with either diethylcarbamazine or ivermectin may also be used. Trials in India and China have shown that the consistent use for 6–12 months of table salt containing diethylcarbamazine 0.1% can eliminate *W. bancrofti;* a concentration of 0.3% for 3–4 months may be required where *B. malayi* is endemic.

Diethylcarbamazine citrate

Tablets, diethylcarbamazine citrate 50 mg

Uses: systemic lymphatic filariasis and occult filariasis; loiasis (6.1.2.1); tissue nematode infections (6.1.1.3)

Contraindications: pregnancy (delay treatment until after delivery)

Precautions: renal impairment (reduce dose; Appendix 4); cardiac disorders; other severe acute disease—delay diethylcarbamazine treatment until after recovery

Dosage:

Lymphatic filariasis (bancroftian), *by mouth*, ADULT and CHILD over 10 years, 6 mg/kg daily, preferably in divided doses after meals, for 12 days; CHILD under 10 years, half the adult dose; mass treatment control programmes, ADULT and CHILD over 10 years, 6 mg/kg in divided doses over 24 hours, once a year; CHILD under 10 years, half the adult dose

Lymphatic filariasis (brugian), *by mouth*, ADULT and CHILD over 10 years, 3–6 mg/kg, preferably in divided doses after meals, for 6–12 days; CHILD under 10 years, half the adult dose; mass treatment control programmes, ADULT and CHILD over 10 years, 3–6 mg/kg in divided doses over 24 hours, 6 times at weekly or monthly intervals; CHILD under 10 years, half the adult dose

Occult filariasis, *by mouth*, ADULT 8 mg/kg daily for 14 days, repeated as necessary if symptoms return

NOTE. The above dose regimens are intended only as a guide, since many countries have developed specific treatment regimens

Adverse effects: headache, dizziness, drowsiness, nausea and vomiting; immunological reactions, within a few hours of the first dose, subsiding by fifth day of treatment, including fever, headache, joint pain, dizziness, anorexia, malaise, transient haematuria, urticaria, vomiting, asthma in asthmatics (similar to Mazzotti reaction—see section 6.1.2.3) induced by disintegrating microfilariae; nodules (palpable subcutaneously and along spermatic cord—formed by recently killed worms); transient lymphangitis and exacerbation of lymphoedema

6.1.2.3   Onchocerciasis

Onchocerciasis (river blindness) is caused by infection with the filarial nematode *Onchocerca volvulus*. The vector is the blackfly which breeds near fast-flowing rivers. **Ivermectin** has transformed suppressive treatment of onchocerciasis and is now used extensively in control programmes in many countries. Its microfilaricidal action is more persistent and less liable to provoke adverse reactions than that of diethylcarbamazine. A single oral dose reduces the microfilarial count to low levels for up to a year. It appears both to kill microfilariae and to inhibit their expulsion from the uterus of female worms. A single annual dose may suppress the microfilaraemia to a degree that prevents development of clinical disease. Although the drug is generally well tolerated, it is advisable to have medical support available during treatment programmes. Patients with a heavy microfilarial load occasionally react adversely and, rarely, transient severe postural hypotension has occurred within 12–24 hours of treatment.

Treatment of pregnant women with ivermectin should be limited to those situations where the risk of complications from untreated onchocerciasis exceeds the potential risk to the fetus from treatment. Mass treatment programmes should not include children under 15 kg, pregnant patients or those with severe illness.

Diethylcarbamazine is now largely superseded as a microfilaricide in onchocerciasis because of the frequency with which it induces severe host (Mazzotti) reactions characterized by itching, rash, oedema, pain and swelling of the lymph nodes, fever and severe eye lesions.

Suramin is the only macrofilaricide that is currently available for use against *Onchocerca volvulus*. Administered intravenously over a period of several weeks suramin also kills microfilariae. It is, however, one of the most toxic substances used in clinical medicine and should always be given under medical supervision in a hospital. A careful assessment must always be made of the patient's capacity to withstand the effects of suramin treatment both before and during administration.

Ivermectin
Tablets, ivermectin 3 mg, 6 mg

Uses: suppressive treatment of onchocerciasis; filariasis (6.1.2.2)

Contraindications: pregnancy (delay treatment until after delivery)

Precautions: breastfeeding (avoid treating mother until infant is 1 week old)

Dosage:

Suppression of microfilariae, *by mouth*, ADULT and CHILD over 5 years (and weighing over 15 kg), 150 micrograms/kg as a single dose once a year

PATIENT ADVICE. Avoid food or alcohol for at least 2 hours before and after a dose

Adverse effects: mild ocular irritation; somnolence; raised liver enzymes; rarely postural hypotension; mild Mazzotti reaction within 3 days of treatment, resulting from death of microfilariae—fever, headache, pruritus, rash, conjunctivitis, arthralgia, myalgia, lymphadenopathy, lymphadenitis, oedema, weakness, tachycardia, nausea and vomiting, diarrhoea

---

Suramin sodium

Suramin sodium is a complementary drug
Injection (Powder for solution for injection), suramin sodium 1-g vial

Uses: curative treatment of onchocerciasis; trypanosomiasis (section 6.4.4.1)

Contraindications: previous anaphylaxis or suramin sensitivity; pregnancy (delay treatment until after delivery); severe liver or renal function impairment; elderly or debilitated; total blindness (unless required for relief from intensely itchy lesions)

Precautions: administer only under close medical supervision in hospital and with general condition of patient improved as far as possible before treatment (see notes above); first dose—possible loss of consciousness (see under Dosage, below); maintain satisfactory food and fluid intake during treatment; urine tests before and weekly during treatment—reduce dose if moderate albuminuria, discontinue immediately if severe albuminuria or casts in urine

Dosage:

Curative treatment of onchocerciasis, *by slow intravenous injection*, ADULT 3.3 mg/kg as a single dose (see First (Test) Dose administration, below), followed at weekly intervals by incremental doses of 6.7 mg/kg, 10.0 mg/kg, 13.3 mg/kg, 16.7 mg/kg, and 16.7 mg/kg on weeks 2 to 6 respectively (total dose 66.7 mg/kg over 6 weeks)

RECONSTITUTION OF INJECTION. Reconstitute in water for injections to produce a final concentration of 10%

FIRST (TEST) DOSE. Administer first dose with particular caution; wait at least 1 minute after injecting the first few microlitres; inject the next 0.5 ml over 30 seconds and wait 1 minute; inject the remainder over several minutes

Adverse effects: rarely, immediate and potentially fatal reaction with nausea, vomiting, shock and loss of consciousness during first dose—see First (Test) Dose, above; albuminuria; abdominal pain; severe diarrhoea; stomal ulceration; exfoliative dermatitis; fever; tiredness; anorexia; malaise; polyuria; thirst; raised liver enzyme values; paraesthesia and hyperaesthesia of palms and soles; swelling, tenderness and abscess formation around adult worms; urticopapular rash, painful hip, hand and foot joints, inflammatory and degenerative changes in optic nerve and retina—due to dying microfilariae

6.1.3 Trematode infections

6.1.3.1 Schistosomiasis

Schistosomiasis, a waterborne parasitic infection, is caused by several species of trematode worms (blood flukes). Its socio-economic impact as a parasitic disease is outstripped only by that of malaria. Intestinal schistosomiasis is caused principally by *Schistosoma mansoni* as well as *S. japonicum, S. mekongi,* and *S. intercalatum.* Urinary schistosomiasis is caused by *S. haematobium.* The latter is an important predisposing cause of squamous cell cancer of the bladder.

Praziquantel has transformed the treatment of schistosomiasis and is often effective in a single dose, against all species of the parasite. It can be of particular value in patients with mixed infections and those who do not respond adequately to other drugs. It is also extremely well tolerated and well suited for mass treatment control programmes. Extensive use over several years has provided no evidence of serious adverse effects or long-term toxicity, nor has mutagenic or carcinogenic activity been shown in experimental animals.

Drugs still widely used in the treatment of schistosomiasis include **oxamniquine**, which is effective against *S. mansoni.* Strains resistant to oxamniquine, which have been reported in South America, have been effectively treated with praziquantel. It is preferable to delay treatment with oxamniquine in pregnant women until after delivery unless immediate intervention is essential. Due to lack of information on whether oxamniquine is excreted in breast milk, it is preferable not to administer it to nursing mothers.

Praziquantel
Tablets, praziquantel 600 mg

Uses: intestinal schistosomiasis; urinary schistosomiasis; cestode infections (section 6.1.1.1); fluke infections (section 6.1.3.2)

Contraindications: ocular cysticercosis (see section 6.1.1.1)

Precautions: pregnancy (unless immediate treatment required, delay treatment until after delivery; Appendix 2); breastfeeding (avoid during and for 72 hours after treatment); areas endemic for cysticercosis—possible oedematous reaction; **interactions:** Appendix 1

SKILLED TASKS. May impair ability to perform skilled tasks, for example operating machinery, driving

Dosage:

Schistosomiasis, *by mouth,* ADULT and CHILD over 4 years 40–60 mg/kg as a single dose; alternatively 3 doses of 20 mg/kg on one day at intervals of 4–6 hours

---

Adverse effects: abdominal discomfort, nausea, vomiting, malaise, headache, dizziness, drowsiness, rectal bleeding; rarely hypersensitivity reactions, including fever, pruritus, eosinophilia (may be due to dead and dying parasites)

Oxamniquine

Oxamniquine is a complementary drug

Capsules, oxamniquine 250 mg

Oral suspension, oxamniquine 250 mg/5 ml

Uses: intestinal schistosomiasis due to *Schistosoma mansoni* (acute stage and chronic hepatosplenic disease)

Precautions: epilepsy—close observation, may precipitate seizures; pregnancy (see notes above); breastfeeding (see notes above)

SKILLED TASKS. May impair ability to perform skilled tasks, for example operating machinery, driving

Dosage:

Intestinal schistosomiasis due to *S. mansoni* (West Africa, South America, Caribbean islands), *by mouth*, ADULT 15 mg/kg as a single dose; CHILD under 30 kg body-weight, 20 mg/kg in 2 divided doses

Intestinal schistosomiasis due to *S. mansoni* (East and central Africa, Arabian peninsula), *by mouth*, ADULT and CHILD 30 mg/kg in 2 divided doses

Intestinal schistosomiasis due to *S. mansoni* (Egypt and southern Africa), ADULT and CHILD 60 mg/kg in divided doses over 2–3 days (maximum single dose 20 mg/kg)

Adverse effects: commonly, dizziness and drowsiness; headache, vomiting, diarrhoea; intense reddish discoloration of urine; rarely, urticaria, hallucinations, epileptiform convulsions; raised liver enzyme values; transient fever, eosinophilia, scattered pulmonary infiltrates (Loeffler syndrome)—after 3-day course in patients in Egypt and eastern Mediterranean

6.1.3.2   Fluke infections

The intestinal flukes include *Fasciolopsis buski, Metagonimus yokogawai, Heterophyes heterophyes, Echinostoma* spp. and *Gastrodiscoides hominis*. The liver flukes include *Clonorchis sinensis, Opisthorchis viverrini, O. felineus* and *Fasciola hepatica*. In some areas *C. sinensis* and *Opisthorchis* spp. infections are strongly associated with cholangiocarcinoma (cancer of the bile ducts). The lung flukes are of the genus *Paragonimus*.

Praziquantel has transformed the therapy of most fluke infections. Parasitological cure has been obtained in virtually all cases (with the exception of *Fasciola* infections) without significant adverse effect but it needs to be taken for several days in the treatment of *Paragonimus* infections.

Triclabendazole, a benzimidazole compound is highly effective and well tolerated, as a single dose or two divided doses, for both *Fasciola* and *Paragonimus* infections.

Praziquantel

Tablets, praziquantel 600 mg

Uses: intestinal flukes, liver flukes, and lung flukes; cestode infections (section 6.1.1.1); schistosomiasis (section 6.1.3.1)

Contraindications: ocular cysticercosis (see section 6.1.1.1)

Precautions: *Paragonimus* infections—treatment in hospital as may be central nervous system involvement; pregnancy (unless immediate treatment required, delay treatment until after delivery; Appendix 2); breastfeeding (avoid during and for 72 hours after treatment); areas endemic for cysticercosis—possible oedematous reaction; **interactions:** Appendix 1

SKILLED TASKS. May impair ability to perform skilled tasks, for example operating machinery, driving

Dosage:

Intestinal fluke infections, *by mouth*, ADULT and CHILD over 4 years, 25 mg/kg as a single dose

Liver and lung fluke infections, *by mouth*, ADULT and CHILD over 4 years, 25 mg/kg 3 times daily for 2 consecutive days; alternatively 40 mg/kg as a single dose; treatment may need to be extended for several days in paragonimiasis

Adverse effects: abdominal discomfort, nausea, vomiting, malaise, headache, dizziness, drowsiness, rectal bleeding; rarely hypersensitivity reactions, including fever, pruritus

---

Triclabendazole

Tablets, triclabendazole 250 mg

Uses: fascioliasis; paragonimiasis

Precautions: *Paragonimus* infections—treatment in hospital as may be central nervous system involvement; severe fascioliasis—biliary colic, due to obstruction by dying worms

Dosage:

Fascioliasis, *by mouth*, ADULT and CHILD over 4 years, 10 mg/kg as a single dose

Paragonimiasis, *by mouth*, ADULT and CHILD over 4 years, 20 mg/kg given in 2 divided doses

Adverse effects: gastrointestinal discomfort; headache

6.2   Antibacterials

6.2.1   Beta-lactam drugs

Beta-lactam antibiotics including penicillins, cefalosporins and carbapenems share a common structure; they are bactericidal, their mechanism of action resulting from inhibition of peptidoglycan, a mucopeptide in bacterial cell walls. **Benzylpenicillin** and **phenoxymethylpenicillin** are active against susceptible strains of Gram-positive bacteria and Gram-negative bacteria, spirochaetes, and actinomycetes, but are inactivated by penicillinase and other beta-lactamases. **Benzathine benzylpenicillin** and **procaine benzylpenicillin** are long-acting preparations which slowly release benzylpenicillin on injection. A range of penicillins with improved stability to gastric acid and penicillinases have been produced by substitution of the 6-amino position of 6-aminopenicillanic acid. **Cloxacillin** is an isoxazoyl penicillin which is resistant to staphylococcal penicillinase. Broad-spectrum penicillins such as **ampicillin** are acid-stable and active against Gram-positive and Gram-negative bacteria, but are inactivated by penicillinase. Beta-lactamase inhibitors such as **clavulanic acid** are often necessary to provide activity against beta-lactamases produced by a wide range of both Gram-negative and Gram-positive bacteria.

Cefalosporins are classified by generation, with the first generation agents having Gram-positive and some Gram-negative activity; the second generation drugs have improved Gram-negative activity and the third generation cefalosporins have a wider spectrum of activity, although may be less active against Gram-positive bacteria than first generation drugs, but they are active against Gram-negative Enterobacteriaceae and *Pseudomonas aeruginosa*.

Carbapenems are semisynthetic derivatives of *Streptomyces cattleya*. They have a broad spectrum of activity and are stable to most penicillinases. They should be reserved for severe infections resistant to other antibiotics.

Penicillins may cause encephalopathy due to cerebral irritation. This rare, but serious adverse effect may result from very high doses or in severe renal failure. Penicillins should not be given by intrathecal injection because they can cause encephalopathy which may be fatal.

HYPERSENSITIVITY. The most important adverse effect of penicillins is hypersensitivity which causes rashes and, occasionally anaphylaxis, which can be fatal. A careful history should be taken with regard to previous allergic reactions. If rashes develop, another antimicrobial should be substituted. Patients who are allergic to one penicillin will be allergic to them all and about 10% of penicillin-sensitive patients will be allergic to cefalosporins and other beta-lactams. However, very few penicillin-allergic patients are at risk of anaphylaxis; a penicillin should not be withheld unnecessarily for severe infections; however, facilities should be available for treating anaphylaxis.

6.2.1.1 Benzylpenicillins and phenoxymethylpenicillin

Benzylpenicillin remains an important and useful antibiotic but it is inactivated by bacterial beta-lactamases. It is effective for many streptococcal, (including pneumococcal), gonococcal and meningococcal infections and also for anthrax, diphtheria, gas gangrene, leptospirosis, tetanus and treatment of Lyme disease in children. Pneumococci, meningococci and gonococci often have decreased sensitivity to penicillin and benzylpenicillin is no longer the first choice for pneumococcal meningitis. Benzylpenicillin is given by injection as it is inactivated by gastric acid and absorption from the intestinal tract is low.

Depot preparations are used when therapeutic concentrations need to be sustained for several hours. **Benzathine benzylpenicillin** or **procaine benzylpenicillin** provides a tissue depot from which the drug is slowly absorbed over a period of 12 hours to several days. They are the preferred choice for the treatment of syphilis or yaws.

Phenoxymethylpenicillin is suitable for oral administration; it has a similar spectrum of activity but is less effective than benzylpenicillin. It should not be used for serious infections because absorption can be unpredictable and plasma concentrations variable.

Benzylpenicillin

Injection (Powder for solution for injection), benzylpenicillin sodium 600-mg vial (1 million units), 3-g vial (5 million units)

Uses: pneumonia; throat infections; otitis media; Lyme disease in children; streptococcal endocarditis; meningococcal meningitis; necrotizing enterocolitis; necrotizing fasciitis; leptospirosis; neurosyphilis; anthrax; actinomycosis; brain abscess; gas gangrene; cellulitis; osteomyelitis

Contraindications: penicillin hypersensitivity (see notes above); avoid intrathecal route (see notes above)

Precautions: history of allergy (see notes above); renal failure (Appendix 4); heart failure; pregnancy and breastfeeding (Appendices 2 and 3); **interactions:** Appendix 1

Dosage:

Mild to moderate infections due to sensitive organisms, *by intramuscular injection or by slow intravenous injection or by intravenous infusion*, ADULT 0.6–2.4 g daily in 2–4 divided doses, with higher doses in severe infections and duration of treatment depending on disease (see also below); NEONATE 50 mg/kg daily in 2 divided doses; INFANT 1 to 4 weeks, 75 mg/kg daily in 3 divided doses; CHILD 1 month to 12 years, 100 mg/kg daily in 4 divided doses, with higher doses in severe infections (see also below)

Bacterial endocarditis, *by slow intravenous injection or by intravenous infusion*, ADULT up to 7.2 g daily in 6 divided doses

Meningococcal meningitis, *by slow intravenous injection or by intravenous infusion*, ADULT up to 14.4 g daily in divided doses; PREMATURE INFANT and NEONATE 100 mg/kg daily in 2 divided doses; INFANT 150 mg/kg daily in 3 divided doses; CHILD 1 month to 12 years, 180–300 mg/kg daily in 4–6 divided doses

Suspected meningococcal disease (before transfer to hospital), *by intramuscular injection or by slow intravenous injection*, ADULT and CHILD over 10 years, 1.2 g; CHILD 1 to 9 years, 600 mg; CHILD under 1 year, 300 mg

Neurosyphilis, *by slow intravenous injection*, ADULT 1.8–2.4 g every 4 hours for 2 weeks

Congenital syphilis, *by intramuscular injection or by slow intravenous injection*, CHILD up to 2 years, 30 mg/kg daily in 2 divided doses for 10 days; CHILD over 2 years, 120–180 mg/kg (to a maximum of 1.44 g) daily in divided doses for 14 days

RECONSTITUTION AND ADMINISTRATION. According to manufacturer's directions

Adverse effects: hypersensitivity reactions including urticaria, fever, joint pains, rashes, angioedema, anaphylaxis, serum sickness-like reactions, haemolytic anaemia, interstitial nephritis (see also notes above); diarrhoea, antibiotic-associated colitis; neutropenia, thrombocytopenia, coagulation disorders, central nervous system toxicity, including convulsions, coma, and encephalopathy (associated with high dosage, or severe renal failure); electrolyte disturbances; Jarisch-Herxheimer reaction (during treatment for syphilis and other spirochaete infections, probably due to release of endotoxins); inflammation, phlebitis or thrombophlebitis at injection sites

---

Benzathine benzylpenicillin

Injection (Powder for solution for injection), benzathine benzylpenicillin, 1.8-g vial (equivalent to benzylpenicillin 1.44 g, 2.4 million units)

Uses: streptococcal pharyngitis; diphtheria carrier state; syphilis and other treponemal infections (yaws, pinta, bejel); rheumatic fever prophylaxis

Contraindications: penicillin hypersensitivity (see notes above); intravascular injection; neurosyphilis

Precautions: history of allergy (see notes above); renal failure (Appendix 4); pregnancy and breastfeeding (Appendices 2 and 3); **interactions:** Appendix 1

Dosage:

Streptococcal pharyngitis; primary prophylaxis of rheumatic fever, *by deep intramuscular injection*, ADULT and CHILD over 30 kg body-weight, 900 mg as a single dose; CHILD under 30 kg body-weight, 450–675 mg as a single dose

Secondary prophylaxis of rheumatic fever, *by deep intramuscular injection*, ADULT and CHILD over 30 kg body-weight, 900 mg once every 3–4 weeks; CHILD under 30 kg body-weight, 450 mg once every 3–4 weeks

Early syphilis, *by deep intramuscular injection*, ADULT 1.8 g as a single dose, divided between 2 sites

Late syphilis, *by deep intramuscular injection*, ADULT 1.8 g, divided between two sites, once weekly for 3 consecutive weeks

Congenital syphilis (where no evidence of CSF involvement), *by deep intramuscular injection*, CHILD up to 2 years, 37.5 mg/kg as a single dose

Yaws, pinta, and bejel, *by deep intramuscular injection*, ADULT 900 mg as a single dose; CHILD 450 mg as a single dose

RECONSTITUTION AND ADMINISTRATION. According to manufacturer's directions

---

Adverse effects: hypersensitivity reactions including urticaria, fever, joint pains, rashes, angioedema, anaphylaxis, serum sickness-like reaction, haemolytic anaemia, interstitial nephritis (see also notes above); neutropenia, thrombocytopenia, coagulation disorders and central nervous system toxicity (associated with high dosage or severe renal failure); Jarisch-Herxheimer reaction (during treatment for syphilis and other spirochaete infections, probably due to release of endotoxins); rarely, non-allergic (embolic-toxic) reactions; pain and inflammation at injection site

---

Procaine benzylpenicillin

Injection (Powder for solution for injection), procaine benzylpenicillin 1-g vial (1 million units), 3-g vial (3 million units)

Uses: syphilis; anthrax; childhood pneumonia; diphtheria carrier state; cellulitis; mouth infections; bites

Contraindications: hypersensitivity to penicillins (see notes above); intravascular injection

Precautions: history of allergy (see notes above); renal failure (Appendix 4); **interactions:** Appendix 1

Dosage:

Infections due to sensitive organisms, *by deep intramuscular injection*, ADULT 0.6 to 1.2 g daily

Pneumonia, *by deep intramuscular injection*, CHILD 50 mg/kg daily for 10 days

Syphilis, *by deep intramuscular injection*, ADULT 1.2 g daily for 10 to 15 days, or up to 3 weeks in late syphilis

Congenital syphilis, *by deep intramuscular injection*, CHILD up to 2 years, 50 mg/kg daily for 10 days

RECONSTITUTION AND ADMINISTRATION. According to manufacturer's directions

Adverse effects: hypersensitivity reactions including urticaria, fever, joint pains, rashes, angioedema, anaphylaxis, serum sickness-like reaction, haemolytic anaemia, interstitial nephritis (see also notes above); neutropenia, thrombocytopenia, coagulation disorders and central nervous system toxicity (associated with high doses and severe renal failure); Jarisch-Herxheimer reaction (during treatment for syphilis and other spirochaete infections, probably due to release of endotoxins); rarely, non-allergic (embolic-toxic) reactions; pain and inflammation at injection site

---

Phenoxymethylpenicillin

Tablets, phenoxymethylpenicillin (as potassium salt) 250 mg
Oral suspension (Powder for oral suspension), phenoxymethylpenicillin (as potassium salt) 250 mg/5 ml

Uses: streptococcal pharyngitis; otitis media; erysipelas; mouth infections; secondary prophylaxis of rheumatic fever; post-splenectomy prophylaxis

Contraindications: hypersensitivity to penicillins (see notes above); serious infections (see notes above)

Precautions: history of allergy (see notes above); pregnancy and breastfeeding (Appendices 2 and 3); **interactions:** Appendix 1

Dosage:

Infections due to sensitive organisms, *by mouth*, ADULT 500–750 mg every 6 hours; CHILD up to 1 year, 62.5 mg every 6 hours; CHILD 1–5 years, 125 mg every 6 hours; CHILD 6–12 years, 250 mg every 6 hours

Secondary prophylaxis of rheumatic fever, *by mouth*, ADULT 500 mg twice daily; CHILD 1–5 years, 125 mg twice daily; CHILD 6–12 years, 250 mg twice daily

PATIENT ADVICE. Phenoxymethylpenicillin should be taken at least 30 minutes before or 2 hours after food

Adverse effects: hypersensitivity reactions including urticaria, joint pain, rash, angioedema, anaphylaxis (see notes above); nausea and diarrhoea

6.2.1.2   Cloxacillin, ampicillin, amoxicillin, and amoxicillin with clavulanic acid

Cloxacillin is used to treat infections due to penicillinase-producing staphylococci which are resistant to benzylpenicillin. It is acid-stable and may therefore be given by mouth as well as by injection.

Ampicillin is active against certain Gram-positive and Gram-negative organisms. It is used to treat a wide range of infections including otitis media, respiratory-tract and urinary-tract infections, and gonorrhoea due to susceptible bacteria. However, ampicillin is inactivated by penicillinases including those produced by *Staphylococcus aureus* and by common Gram-negative bacilli such as *Escherichia coli*; many strains of *Haemophilus influenzae*, *Moraxella catarrhalis*, *Neisseria gonorrhoea*, and *Salmonella* and *Shigella* spp. are resistant. There are geographical variations in the incidence of resistance and an awareness of local patterns is important. In some areas, oral use should be restricted to treatment of *Shigella* infections; it is given in an oral dose of 1 g every 6 hours for 7–10 days.

Amoxicillin has a similar spectrum of activity to ampicillin, but is also inactivated by penicillinases. However, it is better absorbed after oral administration than ampicillin and higher plasma and tissue levels are achieved. Amoxicillin is preferred to ampicillin for the treatment of some infections including otitis media and respiratory-tract and urinary-tract infections.

Clavulanic acid is a beta-lactamase inhibitor. It has no significant antibacterial activity but in combination with **amoxicillin** widens amoxicillin's spectrum of activity and allows its use against amoxicillin-resistant strains of bacteria. It is used in respiratory-tract, genito-urinary and abdominal infections, cellulitis, animal bites, and dental infections.

These antibiotics may also be administered with an aminoglycoside to increase their spectrums of activity. The penicillin and aminoglycoside should not be mixed before or during administration, because loss of aminoglycoside activity can occur on mixing.

Amoxicillin

Amoxicillin is a representative broad-spectrum penicillin. Various drugs can serve as alternatives
Capsules, amoxicillin 250 mg, 500 mg
Oral suspension (Powder for oral suspension), amoxicillin 125 mg/5 ml

Uses: urinary-tract infections, upper respiratory-tract infections, bronchitis; pneumonia; otitis media; dental abscess; osteomyelitis; Lyme disease in children; endocarditis prophylaxis; post-splenectomy prophylaxis; gynaecological infections; gonorrhoea; *Helicobacter pylori* eradication (section 17.1)

Contraindications: hypersensitivity to penicillins (see notes above)

Precautions: history of allergy (see notes above); renal impairment (Appendix 4); erythematous rashes common in glandular fever, chronic lymphatic leukaemia, and possibly HIV infection; pregnancy and breastfeeding (Appendices 2 and 3); **interactions:** Appendix 1

Dosage:

Infections due to sensitive organisms, *by mouth*, ADULT and CHILD over 10 years, 250 mg every 8 hours, doubled in severe infections; CHILD up to 10 years, 125 mg every 8 hours, doubled in severe infections

Severe or recurrent purulent respiratory-tract infections, *by mouth*, ADULT 3 g every 12 hours

Dental abscess (short course), *by mouth*, ADULT 3 g repeated once after 8 hours

Urinary-tract infections (short course), *by mouth*, ADULT 3 g repeated once after 10–12 hours

Gonorrhoea (short course), *by mouth*, ADULT 3 g as a single dose

Otitis media (short course), *by mouth*, CHILD aged 3–10 years, 750 mg twice daily for 2 days

Adverse effects: nausea and vomiting, diarrhoea; rashes (hypersensitivity or toxic response; may be serious reaction—discontinue treatment); hypersensitivity reactions including urticaria, angioedema, anaphylaxis, serum sickness-like reactions, haemolytic anaemia, interstitial nephritis (see also notes above); rarely, antibiotic-associated colitis; neutropenia, thrombocytopenia, coagulation disorders; rarely, central nervous system disorders including convulsions—associated with high doses or impaired renal function

Ampicillin

Injection (Powder for solution for injection), ampicillin (as sodium salt) 500-mg vial

Uses: mastoiditis; gynaecological infections; septicaemia; peritonitis; endocarditis; meningitis; cholecystitis; osteomyelitis

Contraindications: hypersensitivity to penicillins (see notes above)

Precautions: history of allergy (see notes above); renal impairment (Appendix 4); erythematous rashes common in glandular fever, chronic lymphatic leukaemia, and possibly HIV infection; pregnancy and breastfeeding (Appendices 2 and 3); **interactions:** Appendix 1

Dosage:

Severe infections due to sensitive organisms, *by intramuscular, by slow intravenous injection or by intravenous infusion,* ADULT 500 mg every 4–6 hours; CHILD under 10 years, half the adult dose

Meningitis, *by slow intravenous injection,* ADULT 1–2 g every 3–6 hours (maximum 14 g daily); CHILD 150–200 mg/kg daily in divided doses

RECONSTITUTION AND ADMINISTRATION. According to manufacturer's directions

Adverse effects: nausea and vomiting, diarrhoea; rashes (hypersensitivity or toxic response—may be serious reaction, discontinue treatment); hypersensitivity reactions including urticaria, angioedema, anaphylaxis, serum sickness-like reaction, haemolytic anaemia, interstitial nephritis (see also notes above); rarely, antibiotic-associated colitis; neutropenia, thrombocytopenia, coagulation disorders

Amoxicillin with clavulanic acid

Amoxicillin is a representative broad-spectrum penicillin and clavulanic acid is a beta-lactamase inhibitor. Various drug combinations can serve as alternatives.

Amoxicillin with clavulanic acid is available for restricted use

Tablets, amoxicillin (as trihydrate) 500 mg with clavulanic acid (as potassium salt) 125 mg

Oral suspension (Powder for oral suspension), amoxicillin (as trihydrate) 125 mg with clavulanic acid (as potassium salt) 31 mg

Oral suspension (Powder for oral suspension), amoxicillin (as trihydrate) 250 mg with clavulanic acid (as potassium salt) 62 mg

Injection (Powder for solution for injection), amoxicillin (as sodium salt) 0.5 g or 1 g with clavulanic acid (as potassium salt) 100 mg or 200 mg respectively

Uses: infections due to beta-lactamase producing bacteria (where amoxicillin alone not appropriate) including respiratory-tract infections, genito-urinary and abdominal infections, cellulitis, animal bites, severe dental infections, and surgical prophylaxis

Contraindications: hypersensitivity to penicillins (see notes above); history of penicillin- or amoxicillin with clavulanic acid-associated jaundice or hepatic dysfunction

Precautions: history of allergy (see notes above); renal impairment (Appendix 4); erythematous rashes common in glandular fever, chronic lymphatic leukaemia, and possibly HIV infection; hepatic impairment (Appendix 5); pregnancy (Appendix 2); breastfeeding (Appendix 3); **interactions:** Appendix 1

Dosage:

NOTE. All doses expressed as amoxicillin

Infections due to susceptible beta-lactamase producing organisms, *by mouth*, ADULT and CHILD over 12 years, 250 mg every 8 hours, doubled in severe infections; CHILD 1–6 years, 125 mg every 8 hours; 6–12 years, 250 mg every 8 hours

Severe dental infections, *by mouth*, ADULT 250 mg every 8 hours for 5 days

Infections due to susceptible beta-lactamase producing organisms, *by slow intravenous injection*, ADULT and CHILD over 12 years, 1 g every 8 hours, increased to 1 g every 6 hours in severe infections; NEONATE and PREMATURE INFANT 25 mg/kg every 12 hours; INFANT up to 3 months, 25 mg/kg every 8 hours; CHILD 3 months to 12 years, 25 mg/kg every 6 hours

Surgical prophylaxis, *by intravenous injection*, ADULT 1 g at induction, with a further doses every 8 hours for 24 hours (or longer, if increased risk of infection)

RECONSTITUTION AND ADMINISTRATION. According to manufacturer's directions

Adverse effects: nausea and vomiting, diarrhoea; rashes (hypersensitivity or toxic response—may be serious, discontinue treatment); hypersensitivity reactions including urticaria, angioedema, anaphylaxis, serum sickness-type reaction, haemolytic anaemia, interstitial nephritis (see also notes above); rarely, antibiotic-associated colitis; neutropenia, thrombocytopenia, coagulation disorders; dizziness, headache, convulsions (particularly with high doses or in renal impairment); hepatitis, cholestatic jaundice; erythema multiforme (including Stevens-Johnson syndrome), toxic epidermal necrolysis, exfoliative dermatitis, vasculitis reported; superficial staining of teeth with suspension; phlebitis at injection site

---

Cloxacillin

Cloxacillin is a representative penicillinase-resistant penicillin. Various drugs can serve as alternatives

Capsules, cloxacillin (as sodium salt) 500 mg

Oral solution (Powder for oral solution), cloxacillin (as sodium salt) 125 mg/5 ml

Injection (Powder for solution for injection), cloxacillin (as sodium salt) 500-mg vial

Uses: infections due to beta-lactamase-producing staphylococci including impetigo, cellulitis and other soft-tissue infections; staphylococcal endocarditis, septicaemia, pneumonia and osteomyelitis

Contraindications: hypersensitivity to penicillins (see notes above)

Precautions: history of allergy (see notes above); renal and hepatic impairment (Appendices 4 and 5); heart failure; pregnancy and breastfeeding (Appendices 2 and 3); **interactions:** Appendix 1

Dosage:
Infections due to susceptible beta-lactamase-producing staphylococci, *by mouth*, ADULT 500 mg 4 times daily, doubled in severe infection; *by intramuscular injection*, 250 mg every 4–6 hours, doubled in severe infection; *by slow intravenous injection or intravenous infusion*, 1–2 g every 6 hours; CHILD up to 2 years, quarter adult dose; CHILD 2–10 years, half adult dose

RECONSTITUTION AND ADMINISTRATION. According to manufacturer's directions

Adverse effects: nausea and vomiting, diarrhoea; hypersensitivity reactions including urticaria, fever, joint pain, rashes, angioedema, anaphylaxis, serum sickness-like reactions, haemolytic anaemia, interstitial nephritis (see also notes above); neutropenia, thrombocytopenia, coagulation disorders; antibiotic-associated colitis; hepatitis and cholestatic jaundice—may be delayed in onset; electrolyte disturbances; pain, inflammation, phlebitis or thrombophlebitis at injection sites

6.2.1.3 Cefalosporins and imipenem with cilastatin

Ceftazidime and **ceftriaxone** are third generation cefalosporins. Ceftriaxone is used for serious infections such as septicaemia, pneumonia and meningitis; it is used as a reserve antimicrobial to treat meningitis due to *Streptococcus pneumoniae* in some areas where penicillin resistance is found. Ceftazidime is active against *Pseudomonas aeruginosa* and other Gram-negative bacteria; it is used in the treatment of pseudomonas infections and in some areas is restricted to use only where gentamicin resistance is high.

Imipenem is a broad-spectrum antibiotic. As it is partially inactivated by enzymatic activity in the kidney, it is administered with **cilastatin** which inhibits the renal metabolism of imipenem. It is active against many aerobic and anaerobic Gram-positive and Gram-negative bacteria; in some areas it is reserve agent for the treatment of infections due to *Acinetobacter* spp. and *Ps aeruginosa*, which are resistant to other more usual treatments.

Ceftazidime
Ceftazidime is available for restricted use
Injection (Powder for solution for injection), ceftazidime (as pentahydrate) 250-mg vial

Uses: infections due to sensitive bacteria, especially those due to *Pseudomonas* spp. and including those resistant to aminoglycosides

Contraindications: cefalosporin hypersensitivity (see section 6.2.1); porphyria

Precautions: penicillin sensitivity (see section 6.2.1); renal impairment (Appendix 4); pregnancy and breastfeeding (but appropriate to use, see Appendices 2 and 3); false positive urinary glucose (if tested for reducing substances) and false positive Coombs' test; **interactions:** Appendix 1

Dosage:

Infections due to susceptible organisms, *by deep intramuscular injection or by intravenous injection or intravenous infusion*, ADULT 1 g every 8 hours *or* 2 g every 12 hours, or in severe infections (including immunocompromised), 2 g every 8–12 hours (ELDERLY usual maximum 3 g daily); *by intravenous injection or intravenous infusion*, NEONATE and INFANT up to 2 months, 25–60 mg/kg daily in 2 divided doses; CHILD over 2 months, 30–100 mg/kg daily in 2–3 divided doses

Pseudomonal lung infection in cystic fibrosis, *by deep intramuscular injection or by intravenous injection or intravenous infusion*, ADULT with normal renal function, 100–150 mg/kg daily in 3 divided doses

Infections in immunocompromised, cystic fibrosis, or meningitis, *by intravenous injection or intravenous infusion*, CHILD up to 150 mg/kg daily in 3 divided doses (maximum 6 g daily)

RECONSTITUTION AND ADMINISTRATION. According to manufacturer's directions. Intramuscular doses over 1 g divided between more than one site

Adverse effects: diarrhoea, nausea, vomiting, abdominal discomfort, headache; rarely, antibiotic-associated colitis (particularly with higher doses); allergic reactions (see notes above) including rashes, pruritus, urticaria, serum sickness-like reaction, fever and arthralgia, and anaphylaxis; erythema multiforme, toxic epidermal necrolysis reported; disturbances in liver enzymes, transient hepatitis, cholestatic jaundice; eosinophilia and blood disorders (including thrombocytopenia, leukopenia, agranulocytosis, aplastic anaemia, and haemolytic anaemia); reversible interstitial nephritis; nervousness, sleep disturbances, confusion, hypertonia, and dizziness

---

Ceftriaxone

Ceftriaxone is available for restricted use

Ceftriaxone is a representative third generation cefalosporin antibiotic. Various drugs can serve as alternatives

Injection (Powder for solution for injection), ceftriaxone (as sodium salt) 250-mg vial

Uses: serious infections due to sensitive bacteria, including septicaemia, pneumonia, and meningitis; surgical prophylaxis; prophylaxis of meningococcal meningitis; gonorrhoea

Contraindications: cefalosporin hypersensitivity (see section 6.2.1); porphyria; neonates with jaundice, hypoalbuminaemia, acidosis or impaired bilirubin binding

Precautions: penicillin sensitivity (see section 6.2.1); severe renal impairment (Appendix 4); hepatic impairment if accompanied by renal impairment (Appendix 5); premature neonates; may displace bilirubin from serum albumin; pregnancy and breastfeeding (but appropriate to use, see

Appendices 2 and 3); false positive urinary glucose (if tested for reducing substances) and false positive Coombs' test; **interactions:** Appendix 1

Dosage:

Infections due to susceptible organisms, *by deep intramuscular injection, by slow intravenous injection* (over 3–4 minutes) *or by intravenous infusion,* ADULT 1 g daily; severe infections 2–4 g daily; INFANT and CHILD 20–50 mg/kg daily; up to 80 mg/kg daily in severe infections; *by intravenous infusion* (over 60 minutes), NEONATES 20–50 mg/kg daily

Uncomplicated gonorrhoea, *by deep intramuscular injection,* ADULT 250 mg as a single dose

Surgical prophylaxis, *by deep intramuscular injection or by intravenous injection* (over at least 2–4 minutes), ADULT 1 g as a single dose

Colorectal surgery (with antibacterial active against anaerobes), *by deep intramuscular injection or by intravenous injection* (over at least 2–4 minutes), *or by intravenous infusion,* 2 g as a single dose

RECONSTITUTION AND ADMINISTRATION. According to manufacturer's directions. Intramuscular doses over 1 g divided between more than one site. Administer by intravenous infusion over 60 minutes in neonates (see also Contraindications)

Adverse effects: diarrhoea, nausea and vomiting, abdominal discomfort, headache; antibiotic-associated colitis (particularly with higher doses); allergic reactions including rashes, pruritus, urticaria, serum sickness-like reactions, fever and arthralgia, and anaphylaxis (see notes above); erythema multiforme, toxic epidermal necrolysis reported; disturbances in liver enzymes, transient hepatitis and cholestatic jaundice; eosinophilia and blood disorders (including thrombocytopenia, leukopenia, agranulocytosis, aplastic anaemia, and haemolytic anaemia); reversible interstitial nephritis, hyperactivity, nervousness, sleep disturbances, confusion, hypertonia and dizziness; calcium ceftriaxone precipitates in urine (particularly in very young, dehydrated, or those who are immobilized) or in gall bladder—consider discontinuation if symptomatic; rarely prolongation of prothrombin time, pancreatitis

---

Imipenem with cilastatin

Imipenem with cilastatin is available for restricted use

Injection (Powder for solution for intramuscular injection), imipenem (as monohydrate) 500 mg with cilastatin (as sodium salt) 500 mg

Infusion (Powder for solution for intravenous infusion), imipenem (as monohydrate) 250 mg or 500 mg with cilastatin (as sodium salt) 250 mg or 500 mg, respectively

Uses: severe aerobic and anaerobic Gram-positive and Gram-negative infections in hospital (not indicated for CNS infections), including infections caused by resistant *Pseudomonas* and *Acinetobacter* spp.

Contraindications: hypersensitivity to imipenem or cilastatin

Precautions: hypersensitivity to other beta-lactam antibiotics (see section 6.2.1); renal impairment (Appendix 4); CNS disorders, such as epilepsy; pregnancy (Appendix 2); breast-feeding (Appendix 3)

Dosage:

NOTE. All doses are in terms of imipenem

Infections due to susceptible organisms, *by intravenous infusion*, ADULT 1–2 g daily (in 3–4 divided doses); less susceptible organisms, ADULT up to 50 mg/kg daily (maximum 4 g daily); CHILD 3 months and older, 60 mg/kg daily (maximum 2 g daily) in 4 divided doses

RECONSTITUTION AND ADMINISTRATION. According to manufacturer's directions.

The intramuscular   preparation must **not** be administered intravenously.

The infusion preparation must **not** be administered intramuscularly

Adverse effects: nausea, vomiting, diarrhoea; antibiotic-associated colitis; taste disturbances; blood disorders, positive Coombs' test; allergic reactions (see section 6.2.1) including rash, pruritus, urticaria, fever, anaphylactic reactions, rarely toxic epidermal necrolysis; myoclonic activity, convulsions, confusion, and mental disturbances; slight increases in liver enzymes and bilirubin; increases in serum creatinine and blood urea; red coloration of urine in children; erythema, pain and induration, and thrombophlebitis at injection sites

6.2.2   Other antibacterials

6.2.2.1   Chloramphenicol

Chloramphenicol is a potent broad-spectrum antibiotic. It is associated with serious haematological adverse effects and should be reserved for the treatment of severe infections, particularly those caused by *Haemophilus influenzae* and typhoid fever. The oily suspension shold be reserved for use in situations of catastrophic epidemics of meningococcal meningitis occurring mainly in sub-Saharan Africa, during which the medical services are overwhelmed by the epidemic and in which the overwhelming scale of the epidemic precludes any other form of antimicrobial therapy.

Chloramphenicol

Chloramphenicol is a representative broad-spectrum antibiotic. Various drugs can serve as alternatives

Chloramphenicol (oily injection) is a complementary drug

Capsules, chloramphenicol 250 mg

Oral suspension, chloramphenicol (as palmitate) 150 mg/5 ml

Injection (Powder for solution for injection), chloramphenicol (as sodium succinate) 1-g vial

Oily injection (Suspension for injection), chloramphenicol (as sodium succinate) 500 mg/ml, 2-ml ampoule

Uses: severe life-threatening infections, particularly those caused by *Haemophilus influenzae*, and typhoid fever; also, cerebral abscess; mastoiditis; relapsing fever; gangrene;

granuloma inguinale; listeriosis; severe melioidosis; plague; psitticosis; tularaemia; Whipple disease; septicaemia; empirical treatment of meningitis

Contraindications: pregnancy (Appendix 2); porphyria

Precautions: avoid repeated courses and prolonged use; reduce dose in hepatic impairment (Appendix 5) and renal failure (Appendix 4); blood counts required before and during treatment; monitor plasma concentrations in neonates (see below); breastfeeding (Appendix 3); **interactions:** Appendix 1

Dosage:

Infections due to susceptible organisms (not susceptible to other antimicrobials), *by mouth or by intravenous injection or intravenous infusion,* ADULT and CHILD 50 mg/kg daily in 4 divided doses; up to 100 mg/kg daily in divided doses, in severe infections such as meningitis, septicaemia, and haemophilus epiglottitis (reduce high doses as soon as clinically indicated); INFANTS under 2 weeks, 25 mg/kg daily in 4 divided doses, 2 weeks to 1 year, 50 mg/kg daily in 4 divided doses

Epidemics of meningococcal meningitis, *by intramuscular injection* (of oily injection), ADULT 0.5–1 g daily; CHILD 25 mg/kg daily

RECONSTITUTION AND ADMINISTRATION. According to manufacturer's directions. The oily injection is for intramuscular use only (see notes above)

NOTE. Plasma concentration monitoring required in neonates and preferred in those under 4 years of age; recommended peak plasma concentration (measured approximately 1 hour after intravenous injection or infusion) 15–25 mg/litre; pre-dose 'trough' concentration should not exceed 15 mg/litre

Adverse effects: bone marrow depression—reversible and irreversible aplastic anaemia (with reports of leukaemia), anaemia, leukopenia and thrombocytopenia; nocturnal haemoglobinuria; peripheral neuritis and optic neuritis; nausea, vomiting, diarrhoea, stomatitis, glossitis; hypersensitivity reactions including, rashes, fever, angioedema and rarely anaphylaxis; grey syndrome (vomiting, greenish diarrhoea, abdominal distension, hypothermia, pallid cyanosis, irregular respiration, circulatory collapse) may follow excessive doses in neonates with immature hepatic metabolism; also reported in infants born to mothers treated in late pregnancy

6.2.2.2 Quinolones

Ciprofloxacin is active against both Gram-positive and Gram-negative bacteria. It is particularly active against salmonella, shigella, campylobacter, neisseria and pseudomonas. It is also active against chlamydia and some mycobacteria. Most anaerobic organisms are not susceptible. Ciprofloxacin is used with doxycycline and metronidazole to treat pelvic inflammatory disease. **Nalidixic acid** is an older quinolone effective in uncomplicated urinary-tract infections and, in the treatment of shigella in areas where it remains susceptible.

Precautions. Quinolones should be used with caution in patients with a history of epilepsy or conditions predisposing to seizures; convulsions may be induced in patients with or without a history of convulsions; also, use with caution in G6PD deficiency, pregnancy (Appendix 2) or breastfeeding (Appendix 3); use in children or adolescents is generally not recommended (quinolones cause arthropathy in weight-bearing joints in young *animals*), although in some specific circumstances, short-term use may be justified. Exposure to sunlight should be avoided (discontinue if photosensitivity occurs).

Adverse effects. Adverse effects of quinolones include nausea, vomiting, dyspepsia, abdominal pain, diarrhoea, and rarely, antibiotic-associated colitis; headache, dizziness, sleep disorders, rash (rarely Stevens-Johnson syndrome and toxic epidermal necrolysis), and pruritus; less commonly, anorexia, transient disturbances in liver enzymes and bilirubin and increases in blood urea and creatinine; drowsiness, restlessness, depression, confusion, hallucinations, convulsions, paraesthesia; photosensitivity; hypersensitivity reactions including fever, urticaria, angioedema, arthralgia, myalgia, and anaphylaxis; blood disorders; disturbances in vision, taste, hearing, and smell; isolated reports of tendon inflammation and damage; if psychiatric, neurological, or hypersensitivity reactions occur—discontinue drug.

Ciprofloxacin

Ciprofloxacin is a representative quinolone antibacterial. Various drugs can serve as alternatives

Tablets, ciprofloxacin (as hydrochloride) 250 mg

Uses: gastroenteritis—including cholera, shigellosis, travellers' diarrhoea, campylobacter and salmonella enteritis; typhoid; gonorrhoea; chancroid; legionnaires' disease; meningitis (including meningococcal meningitis prophylaxis); respiratory-tract infections—including pseudomonal infections in cystic fibrosis, but not pneumococcal pneumonia; urinary-tract infections; bone and joint infections; septicaemia; skin infections; prophylaxis in surgery

Precautions: see notes (above); hepatic impairment (Appendix 5); renal failure (Appendix 4); avoid excessive alkalinity of urine and ensure adequate fluid intake as risk of crystalluria; **interactions:** Appendix 1

SKILLED TASKS. May impair ability to perform skilled tasks, for example operating machinery, driving

Dosage:

Infections due to susceptible organisms, *by mouth*, ADULT 250–750 mg twice daily

Acute uncomplicated cystitis, *by mouth*, ADULT 100 mg twice daily for 3 days

Gonorrhoea, chancroid, shigellosis, or cholera, *by mouth*, 500 mg as a single dose

Pseudomonal lower respiratory-tract infection in cystic fibrosis, *by mouth*, ADULT 750 mg twice daily; CHILD 5–17 years (see Precautions) up to 20 mg/kg twice daily (maximum 1.5 g daily)

Surgical prophylaxis, *by mouth*, ADULT 750 mg 60–90 minutes before procedure

Prophylaxis of meningococcal meningitis, *by mouth*, ADULT 500 mg as a single dose

Adverse effects: see notes above; flatulence, dysphagia, tremor, altered prothrombin concentration, jaundice and hepatitis, renal failure, nephritis, vasculitis, erythema nodosum, petechiae, haemorrhagic bullae, tinnitus, tenosynovitis, and tachycardia, also reported

---

Nalidixic acid
Tablets, nalidixic acid 250 mg, 500 mg

Uses: urinary-tract infections; shigellosis

Precautions: see notes above; porphyria; hepatic impairment (Appendix 5); renal failure (Appendix 4); false positive urinary glucose (if tested for reducing substances); monitor blood counts, renal and liver function if treatment exceeds 2 weeks; **interactions:** Appendix 1

Dosage:

Urinary-tract infections, *by mouth*, ADULT 1 g every 6 hours for 7 days, reduced in chronic infections to 500 mg every 6 hours; CHILD over 3 months, maximum 50 mg/kg daily in divided doses, reduced in prolonged treatment to 30 mg/kg daily

Shigellosis, *by mouth*, ADULT 1 g every 6 hours for 5 days; CHILD over 3 months, 15 mg/kg every 6 hours for 5 days
PATIENT ADVICE. Take on an empty stomach, preferably one hour before a meal

Adverse effects: see notes above; toxic psychosis, weakness, increased intracranial pressure, cranial nerve palsy, cholestasis, and metabolic acidosis also reported

6.2.2.3   Tetracyclines

Doxycycline is a tetracycline and is a broad-spectrum antibiotic effective for conditions caused by chlamydia, rickettsia, brucella and the spirochaete, *Borrelia burgdorferi* (Lyme disease). It is the preferred tetracycline since it has a more favourable pharmacokinetic profile than tetracycline. It is deposited in growing bone and teeth causing staining and occasionally dental hypoplasia. It should not be given to children under 8 years or pregnant women; in some countries, use in children under 12 years is contraindicated.

Doxycycline

Doxycycline is a representative broad-spectrum antibiotic. Various drugs can serve as alternatives

Capsules, doxycycline (as hydrochloride) 100 mg

Uses: respiratory-tract infections, including pneumonia and chronic bronchitis; urinary-tract infections; syphilis; chlamydia, mycoplasma, and rickettsia; prostatitis; lymphogranuloma venereum; pelvic inflammatory disease (with metronidazole); Lyme disease; brucellosis (with rifampicin); leptospirosis, scrub typhus and travellers' diarrhoea; psittacosis; cholera; melioidosis; plague; anthrax; Q fever; malaria (section 6.4.3)

Contraindications: pregnancy (Appendix 2); children (see notes above); porphyria; systemic lupus erythematosus

Precautions: avoid exposure to sunlight or sunlamps—photosensitivity reported; hepatic impairment (Appendix 5); breast-feeding (Appendix 3); **interactions:** Appendix 1

Dosage:

Infections due to susceptible organisms, *by mouth*, ADULT and CHILD over 8 years, 200 mg on first day then 100 mg daily; in severe infections, 200 mg daily

Syphilis, *by mouth*, 200–300 mg daily in 1–2 divided doses

Uncomplicated genital chlamydia, non-gonococcal urethritis, *by mouth*, 100 mg twice daily

Louse and tick-borne relapsing fevers, *by mouth*, 100 mg or 200 mg as a single dose

Cholera, *by mouth,* ADULT 300 mg as a single dose; CHILD over 8 years, 100 mg as a single dose

PATIENT ADVICE. Capsules should be swallowed whole with plenty of fluid while sitting or standing to prevent oesophageal irritation. May be given with milk or food to counter gastric irritation

Adverse effects: gastrointestinal disturbances; erythema (discontinue treatment); photosensitivity; headache and visual disturbances; hepatotoxicity, pancreatitis, and antibiotic-associated colitis reported; staining of growing teeth and occasional dental hypoplasia

6.2.2.4 Macrolides

Erythromycin is a macrolide; it has an antibacterial spectrum that is similar but not identical to penicillin and is used as an alternative in penicillin-allergic patients. It is effective in respiratory infections, whooping cough, legionnaires' disease and campylobacter enteritis.

Erythromycin

Erythromycin is a representative macrolide antibiotic. Various drugs can serve as alternatives

Tablets, erythromycin (as stearate) 250 mg; erythromycin (as ethyl succinate) 500 mg

Gastro-resistant tablets, erythromycin 250 mg

Gastro-resistant capsules, erythromycin 250 mg

Oral suspension, erythromycin (as stearate) 125 mg/5 ml; erythromycin (as ethyl succinate) 125 mg/5 ml

Infusion (Powder for solution for infusion), erythromycin (as lactobionate) 1-g vial

Uses: alternative to penicillin in hypersensitive patients; pneumonia; legionnaires' disease; syphilis; chancroid; non-gonococcal urethritis; prostatitis; lymphogranuloma venereum; campylobacter enteritis; relapsing fever; diphtheria and whooping cough prophylaxis

Contraindications: hypersensitivity to erythromycin or other macrolides; porphyria

Precautions: hepatic impairment (Appendix 5) and renal failure (Appendix 4); prolongation of the QT interval (tachycardia reported); pregnancy (not known to be harmful); breastfeeding (Appendix 3); **interactions:** Appendix 1

Dosage:

Infections due to sensitive organisms, *by mouth*, ADULT and CHILD over 8 years, 250–500 mg every 6 hours; up to 4 g daily in severe infections; CHILD up to 2 years, 125 mg every 6 hours, doubled in severe infections; CHILD 2–8 years, 250 mg every 6 hours, doubled in severe infections

Early syphilis, *by mouth*, ADULT 500 mg 4 times daily for 14 days

Non-gonococcal urethritis, *by mouth*, ADULT 500 mg 4 times daily for 7 days

Severe infections, *by intravenous infusion*, ADULT and CHILD 50 mg/kg daily by continuous infusion *or* in divided doses every 6 hours

PATIENT ADVICE. Gastro-resistant tablets and capsules should be swallowed whole

Adverse effects: nausea, vomiting, abdominal discomfort, diarrhoea (and antibiotic-associated colitis); urticaria, rashes, and other allergic reactions (rarely, anaphylaxis); reversible hearing loss after large doses; cholestatic jaundice and cardiac effects (including chest pain and arrhythmias)

6.2.2.5 Aminoglycosides

Aminoglycosides including **gentamicin** are bactericidal and active against some Gram-positive and many Gram-negative organisms including *Pseudomonas aeruginosa*. Aminoglycosides are not absorbed from the gut and must therefore be given by injection for systemic infections. Excretion is mainly by the kidney and accumulation occurs in renal impairment.

Use of gentamicin should be restricted to trained health personnel and care must be taken to ensure correct dosage and duration of treatment are not exceeded, because most adverse effects are dose related. The most important adverse effects are ototoxicity and nephrotoxicity and they are most common in the elderly and in patients with renal impairment. These groups and, if possible, all patients should be monitored for ototoxicity by audiometry. If there is impairment of renal function the dose interval must be increased; in severe renal impairment, the dose should also be reduced. Plasma concentration monitoring avoids both excessive and subtherapeutic concentrations and can prevent toxicity and ensure efficacy. If possible plasma concentrations should be monitored in all patients, but **must** be measured in infants, the elderly, in obesity, in cystic fibrosis, in high-dosage regimens, in renal impairment, or if treatment lasts for longer than 7 days.

For most infections, doses of up to 5 mg/kg daily in divided doses are used if renal function is normal; higher doses are used occasionally for serious infections. Loading and maintenance doses are based on the patient's weight and renal function (for example, using a nomogram) with adjustments based on plasma gentamicin concentration.

Gentamicin

Gentamicin is a representative aminoglycoside antibiotic. Various drugs can serve as alternatives

Injection, gentamicin (as sulfate) 10 mg/ml, 2-ml vial; 40 mg/ml, 2-ml vial

Uses: pneumonia; cholecystitis; peritonitis; septicaemia; acute pyelonephritis; prostatitis; skin infections; pelvic inflammatory disease; endocarditis; meningitis; listeriosis; tularaemia; brucellosis; plague; surgical prophylaxis; eye (section 21.1)

Contraindications: myasthenia gravis

Precautions: renal impairment (Appendix 4), infants and elderly (dosage adjustment and monitor renal, auditory, and vestibular function, and plasma-gentamicin concentrations); avoid prolonged use; see notes above; pregnancy (Appendix 2); **interactions:** Appendix 1

Dosage:

Infections due to susceptible organisms, *by intramuscular injection or by slow intravenous injection* (over at least 3 minutes) *or by intravenous infusion*, ADULT 2–5 mg/kg daily in divided doses every 8 hours; CHILD up to 2 weeks, 3 mg/kg every 12 hours; 2 weeks–12 years, 2 mg/kg every 8 hours

Streptococcal and enterococcal endocarditis (as part of combination therapy), *by intravenous injection* (over at least 3 minutes), ADULT 80 mg twice daily

Surgical prophylaxis, *by intravenous injection*, ADULT 5 mg/kg as a single dose at induction (with clindamycin)

NOTE. One hour (peak) concentrations should not exceed 10 mg/litre; pre-dose (trough) concentration should be less than 2 mg/litre

DILUTION AND ADMINISTRATION. According to manufacturer's directions

Adverse effects: vestibular and auditory damage, nephrotoxicity; rarely, hypomagnesaemia on prolonged therapy; antibiotic-associated colitis; also, nausea, vomiting, rash

6.2.2.6 Metronidazole

Metronidazole has high activity against anaerobic bacteria and protozoa (see also section 6.4.1).

Metronidazole

Metronidazole is a representative antibacterial and antiprotozoal agent. Various drugs can serve as alternatives

Tablets, metronidazole 200 mg, 250 mg, 400 mg, and 500 mg

Oral suspension, metronidazole (as benzoate) 200 mg/5 ml

Intravenous infusion, metronidazole 5 mg/ml, 100-ml bag

Suppositories, metronidazole 0.5 g, 1 g

Uses: anaerobic bacterial infections, including gingivitis, pelvic inflammatory disease, tetanus, peritonitis, brain abscess, necrotizing pneumonia, antibiotic-associated colitis, leg ulcers and pressure sores and surgical prophylaxis; bacterial vaginosis; tissue nematode infections (6.1.1.3); trichomonal vaginitis, amoebiasis, and giardiasis (section 6.4.1); *Helicobacter pylori* eradication (section 17.1)

Contraindications: chronic alcohol dependence

Precautions: disulfiram-like reaction with alcohol; hepatic impairment and hepatic encephalopathy (Appendix 5); pregnancy (Appendix 2); breastfeeding (Appendix 3); clinical and laboratory monitoring in courses lasting longer than 10 days; **interactions:** Appendix 1

Dosage:

Anaerobic infections (usually treated for 7 days), *by mouth*, ADULT 800 mg initially then 400 mg every 8 hours *or* 500 mg every 8 hours; CHILD 7.5 mg/kg every 8 hours; *by intravenous infusion*, ADULT 500 mg every 8 hours; CHILD 7.5 mg/kg every 8 hours

Surgical prophylaxis, *by mouth*, ADULT 400 mg every 8 hours started 24 hours before surgery, then continued postoperatively, *by intravenous infusion* (see below) or *by rectum* (see below); CHILD 7.5 mg/kg every 8 hours

Surgical prophylaxis, *by rectum*, ADULT 1 g 2 hours before surgery then 1 g every 8 hours; CHILD 5–10 years, 500 mg 2 hours before surgery then 500 mg every 8 hours

Surgical prophylaxis *by intravenous infusion* (if rectal administration inappropriate), ADULT 500 mg shortly before surgery then every 8 hours until oral administration can be started; CHILD 7.5 mg/kg every 8 hours

Bacterial vaginosis, *by mouth*, ADULT 2 g as a single dose *or* 400–500 mg twice daily for 5–7 days

Leg ulcers and pressure sores, *by mouth*, ADULT 400 mg every 8 hours for 7 days

Acute ulcerative gingivitis, *by mouth*, 200–250 mg every 8 hours for 3 days; CHILD 1–3 years, 50 mg every 8 hours for 3 days; 3–7 years, 100 mg every 12 hours for 3 days; 7–10 years, 100 mg every 8 hours for 3 days

Acute dental infections, *by mouth*, ADULT 200 mg every 8 hours for 3–7 days

Antibiotic-associated colitis, *by mouth*, 400 mg 3 times daily

PATIENT ADVICE. Metronidazole tablets should be swallowed whole with water, during or after a meal; metronidazole suspension should be taken one hour before a meal

Adverse effects: nausea, vomiting, unpleasant metallic taste, furred tongue and gastrointestinal disturbances; rarely, headache, drowsiness, dizziness, ataxia, darkening of urine, erythema multiforme, pruritus, urticaria, angioedema, and anaphylaxis; abnormal liver function tests, hepatitis, jaundice, thrombocytopenia, aplastic anaemia, myalgia, arthralgia; peripheral neuropathy, epileptiform seizures, leukopenia, on prolonged or high dosage regimens

6.2.2.7   Nitrofurantoin

Nitrofurantoin is bactericidal *in vitro* to most Gram-positive and Gram-negative urinary-tract pathogens and it is used to treat acute and recurrent urinary-tract infections. It is also used prophylactically.

Nitrofurantoin

Tablets, nitrofurantoin 100 mg

Uses: urinary-tract infections

Contraindications: impaired renal function (Appendix 4); infants less than 3 months; G6PD-deficiency including breastfeeding of affected infants (Appendix 3); pregnancy, at term (Appendix 2); porphyria

Precautions: pulmonary disorders or hepatic impairment (Appendix 5); monitor lung and liver function on long-term therapy (discontinue if lung function deteriorates); neurological or allergic disorders; anaemia; diabetes mellitus; elderly and debilitated; vitamin B and folate deficiency; false positive urinary glucose (if testing for reducing substances); urine may be coloured yellow or brown

Dosage:

Acute uncomplicated urinary-tract infections, *by mouth*, ADULT 100 mg every 12 hours *or* 50 mg every 6 hours with food for 7 days; CHILD over 3 months, 3 mg/kg daily in 4 divided doses

Severe recurrent urinary-tract infection, *by mouth*, ADULT 100 mg every 6 hours with food for 7 days (dose reduced to 200 mg daily in divided doses, if severe nausea)

Prophylaxis of urinary-tract infections (see Precautions), *by mouth*, ADULT 50–100 mg at night; CHILD over 3 months, 1 mg/kg at night

Adverse effects: dose-related gastrointestinal disorders; nausea; hypersensitivity reactions including urticaria, rash, pruritus, angioedema; anaphylaxis reported; rarely, cholestatic jaundice, hepatitis, exfoliative dermatitis; erythema multiforme, pancreatitis, arthralgia; blood disorders; pulmonary reactions (discontinue treatment); peripheral neuropathy; benign intracranial hypertension; transient alopecia

---

6.2.2.8   Spectinomycin

Spectinomycin is active against Gram-negative organisms including *Neiserria gonorrhoea*. It is not suitable for the treatment of syphilis and patients being treated for gonorrhoea should be observed for evidence of syphilis. It should be used only when alternative therapies are inappropriate.

Spectinomycin

Injection (Powder for solution for injection), spectinomycin (as hydrochloride), 2-g vial

Uses: uncomplicated and disseminated gonorrhoea (see notes above); adult and neonatal gonococcal conjunctivitis; chancroid

Precautions: renal impairment; pregnancy and breastfeeding

Dosage:

Uncomplicated gonococcal infections and chancroid, *by deep intramuscular injection*, ADULT 2 g as a single dose (may be increased to 4 g as a single dose divided between 2 injection sites in difficult to treat cases and where there is known antibiotic resistance)

Disseminated gonococcal infections, *by deep intramuscular injection*, ADULT 2 g twice daily for 7 days

Neonatal gonococcal conjunctivitis, *by deep intramuscular injection*, neonate 25 mg/kg (maximum 75 mg) as a single dose

RECONSTITUTION AND ADMINISTRATION. According to manufacturer's directions

Adverse effects: nausea, dizziness, fever, urticaria; rarely, anaphylaxis; pain at injection site

6.2.2.9 Sulfonamides and trimethoprim

The usefulness of sulfonamides is limited by an increasing incidence of bacterial resistance. For many indications they have been replaced by antibiotics that are more active and safer. **Sulfadiazine** is used in the prevention of rheumatic fever recurrence. **Sulfamethoxazole** is used in combination with **trimethoprim** because of their synergistic activity. In some countries, indications for the use of this combination have been restricted. The treatment of *Pneumocystis carinii* infections must only be undertaken with specialist supervision where there are appropriate monitoring facilities (section 6.4.5). **Trimethoprim** is also used alone for respiratory-tract infections and, in particular, for urinary-tract infections.

Sulfadiazine

Sulfadiazine is a representative sulfonamide antibacterial. Various drugs can serve as alternatives

Tablets, sulfadiazine 500 mg

Uses: prevention of recurrences of rheumatic fever; toxoplasmosis (section 6.4.5)

Contraindications: hypersensitivity to sulfonamides; renal failure (Appendix 4) or liver failure; porphyria

Precautions: hepatic and renal impairment; maintain adequate fluid intake (to avoid crystalluria); avoid in blood disorders (unless under specialist supervision); monitor blood counts and discontinue immediately if blood disorder develops; rashes—discontinue immediately; elderly; asthma; G6PD deficiency; pregnancy (Appendix 2); breastfeeding (Appendix 3); avoid in infants under 6 weeks; **interactions:** Appendix 1

Dosage:

Prevention of recurrences of rheumatic fever, *by mouth*, ADULT 1 g daily; CHILD 500 mg daily

Adverse effects: nausea, vomiting, diarrhoea, headache; hypersensitivity reactions including rashes, pruritus, photosensitivity reactions, exfoliative dermatitis, and erythema nodosum; rarely, erythema multiforme and toxic epidermal necrolysis; crystalluria—resulting in haematuria, oliguria, anuria; blood disorders including granulocytopenia, agranulocytosis, aplastic anaemia, purpura—discontinue immediately; also reported, liver damage, pancreatitis, antibiotic-associated colitis, eosinophilia, cough and shortness of breath, pulmonary infiltrates, aseptic meningitis, depression, convulsions, ataxia, tinnitus, and electrolyte disturbances

---

Sulfamethoxazole with trimethoprim

Sulfamethoxazole with trimethoprim is a representative antibacterial drug combination. Various drugs can serve as alternatives

Tablets, sulfamethoxazole 100 mg with trimethoprim 20 mg; sulfamethoxazole 400 mg with trimethoprim 80 mg; sulfamethoxazole 800 mg with trimethoprim 160 mg

Oral suspension, sulfamethoxazole 200 mg with trimethoprim 40 mg/5 ml

Injection (Solution for dilution for infusion), sulfamethoxazole 80 mg with trimethoprim 16 mg/ml, 5-ml and 10-ml ampoules

Uses: urinary-tract infections; respiratory-tract infections including bronchitis, pneumonia, infections in cystic fibrosis; melioidosis; listeriosis; brucellosis; granuloma inguinale; otitis media; skin infections; *Pneumocystis carinii* pneumonia (section 6.4.5)

Contraindications: hypersensitivity to sulfonamides or trimethoprim; severe renal and hepatic failure; porphyria

Precautions: renal or hepatic impairment (Appendices 4 and 5); maintain adequate fluid intake (to avoid crystalluria); avoid in blood disorders (unless under specialist supervision); monitor blood counts and discontinue immediately if blood disorder develops; rash—discontinue immediately; elderly; asthma; G6PD deficiency; folate deficiency; pregnancy (Appendix 2); breastfeeding (Appendix 3); avoid in infants under 6 weeks; **interactions:** Appendix 1

Dosage:

Severe infections due to susceptible organisms, *by mouth or by intravenous infusion*, ADULT sulfamethoxazole 800 mg with trimethoprim 160 mg every 12 hours, increased to sulfamethoxazole 1.2 g with trimethoprim 240 mg, every 12 hours in more severe infections; *by mouth*, CHILD 6 weeks–5 months, sulfamethoxazole 100 mg with trimethoprim 20 mg every 12 hours; 6 months–5 years, sulfamethoxazole 200 mg with trimethoprim 40 mg every 12 hours; 6–12 years, sulfamethox-

azole 400 mg with trimethoprim 80 mg every 12 hours; *by intravenous infusion*, CHILD sulfamethoxazole 30 mg/kg daily with trimethoprim 6 mg/kg daily in 2 divided doses
DILUTION AND ADMINISTRATION. According to manufacturer's directions

Adverse effects: nausea, vomiting, diarrhoea, headache; hypersensitivity reactions including rashes, pruritus, photosensitivity reactions, exfoliative dermatitis, and erythema nodosum; rarely, erythema multiforme and toxic epidermal necrolysis; crystalluria—resulting in haematuria, oliguria, anuria; blood disorders including granulocytopenia, agranulocytosis, aplastic anaemia, purpura—discontinue immediately; also reported, liver damage, pancreatitis, antibiotic-associated colitis, eosinophilia, cough and shortness of breath, pulmonary infiltrates, aseptic meningitis, depression, convulsions, ataxia, tinnitus, and electrolyte disturbances; megaloblastic anaemia due to trimethoprim

---

Trimethoprim

Tablets, trimethoprim 100 mg, 200 mg
Injection (Solution for injection), trimethoprim (as lactate) 20 mg/ml, 5-ml ampoule

Uses: urinary-tract infections; bronchitis

Contraindications: blood disorders; severe renal impairment; porphyria

Precautions: renal impairment (Appendix 4); pregnancy (Appendix 2); breastfeeding (Appendix 3); predisposition to folate deficiency; blood counts on long-term therapy (but practical value not proven); neonates (specialist supervision required); **interactions:** Appendix 1

Dosage:

Acute infections, *by mouth*, ADULT 200 mg every 12 hours; CHILD 6 weeks–5 months, 25 mg twice daily; 6 months–5 years, 50 mg twice daily; 6–12 years, 100 mg twice daily

Acute infections, *by slow intravenous injection or by intravenous infusion*, ADULT 150–250 mg every 12 hours; CHILD under 12 years, 6–9 mg/kg daily in 2–3 divided doses

Chronic infections and prophylaxis, *by mouth*, ADULT 100 mg at night; CHILD 1–2 mg/kg at night
DILUTION AND ADMINISTRATION. According to manufacturer's directions

Adverse effects: rashes, pruritus; depression of haematopoiesis; gastrointestinal disturbances including nausea and vomiting; rarely exfoliative dermatitis and toxic epidermal necrolysis; aseptic meningitis

6.2.2.10 Clindamycin

Clindamycin is a bacteriostatic antibacterial with activity against Gram-positive aerobes and a wide range of anaerobes. However, its use is limited because of adverse effects. Antibiotic-associated colitis can occur with a wide range of antibacterials, but occurs most frequently with clindamycin. It may be fatal and is most common in women and the elderly; it can develop during or after treatment with clindamycin. Patients should discontinue treatment immediately if diarrhoea develops. Clindamycin is recommended for the treatment of staphylococcal bone and joint infections and for intra-abdominal sepsis. It is also used for endocarditis prophylaxis when a penicillin is not appropriate.

Clindamycin

Clindamycin is a complementary drug when penicillin is not appropriate

Capsules, clindamycin (as hydrochloride) 150 mg

Injection (Solution for injection), clindamycin (as phosphate) 150 mg/ml, 2-ml ampoule

Uses: staphylococcal bone and joint infections; peritonitis; endocarditis prophylaxis

Contraindications: diarrhoeal states

Precautions: discontinue immediately if diarrhoea or colitis develop; hepatic impairment (Appendix 5); renal impairment (Appendix 4); monitor liver and renal function on prolonged therapy and in neonates and infants; elderly; females; pregnancy (Appendix 2); breastfeeding (Appendix 3); avoid rapid intravenous administration; **interactions:** Appendix 1

Dosage:

Osteomyelitis or peritonitis, *by mouth*, ADULT 150–300 mg every 6 hours; up to 450 mg every 6 hours in severe infections; CHILD 3–6 mg/kg every 6 hours; *by deep intramuscular injection or by intravenous infusion*, ADULT 0.6–2.7 g daily in 2–4 divided doses, increased up to 4.8 g daily in life-threatening infections; single doses over 600 mg by intravenous infusion only; single doses by intravenous infusion not to exceed 1.2 g; NEONATES 15–20 mg/kg daily; CHILD over 1 month, 15–40 mg/kg daily in 3–4 divided doses; severe infections, at least 300 mg daily, regardless of weight

Endocarditis prophylaxis (for procedures under local or no anaesthetic), *by mouth*, ADULT 600 mg, 1 hour before procedure

Endocarditis prophylaxis (for procedures under general anaesthetic), *by intravenous infusion*, ADULT 300 mg over at least 10 minutes, at induction or 15 minutes before procedure, then 150 mg 6 hours later by mouth or infusion

PATIENT ADVICE. Patients should discontinue immediately and contact doctor if diarrhoea develops; capsules should be swallowed with a glass of water

DILUTION AND ADMINISTRATION. According to manufacturer's directions

Adverse effects: diarrhoea (discontinue treatment); nausea, vomiting, abdominal discomfort, antibiotic-associated colitis; rashes, urticaria, and rarely anaphylaxis; erythema multiforme, exfoliative and vesiculobullous dermatitis; jaundice and altered liver function tests; neutropenia, eosinophilia, agranulocytosis, and thrombocytopenia; pain, induration, and abscess after intramuscular injection; thrombophlebitis after intravenous injection

6.2.2.11 Vancomycin

Vancomycin is not significantly absorbed from the gastro-intestinal tract and must be given intravenously for systemic infections which cannot be treated with other effective, less toxic antimicrobials. It is used to treat serious infections due to Gram-positive cocci including methicillin-resistant staphylococcal infections, brain abscess, staphylococcal meningitis and septicaemia.

Vancomycin

Vancomycin is available for restricted use

Infusion (Powder for solution for infusion), vancomycin (as hydrochloride) 500-mg vial

Uses: methicillin-resistant staphylococcal pneumonia; staphylococcal meningitis; endocarditis prophylaxis (with gentamicin)

Precautions: avoid rapid infusion (risk of anaphylactoid reactions, see Adverse effects); rotate infusion sites; renal impairment (Appendix 4); elderly; history of deafness—avoid; blood counts, urinalysis, and renal function tests in all patients—use only in hospital setting; monitor auditory function and plasma-vancomycin concentrations in elderly or in renal impairment; pregnancy (Appendix 2); breastfeeding (Appendix 3); **interactions:** Appendix 1

Dosage:

Serious staphylococcal infections, *by intravenous infusion*, ADULT 500 mg over at least 60 minutes every 6 hours *or* 1 g over at least 100 minutes every 12 hours; NEONATE up to 1 week, 15 mg/kg initially, then 10 mg/kg every 12 hours; INFANT 1–4 weeks, 15 mg/kg initially, then 10 mg/kg every 8 hours; CHILD over 1 month, 10 mg/kg every 6 hours

Endocarditis prophylaxis (for procedures under general anaesthetic), *by intravenous infusion*, ADULT 1 g over at least 100 minutes then gentamicin 120 mg at induction or 15 minutes before procedure

RECONSTITUTION AND ADMINISTRATION. According to the manufacturer's directions

NOTE. Plasma concentration monitoring required; peak plasma concentration (measured 2 hours after infusion) should not exceed 30 mg/litre; pre-dose (trough) concentration should not exceed 10 mg/litre

Adverse effects: nephrotoxicity including renal failure and interstitial nephritis; ototoxicity (discontinue if tinnitus occurs); blood disorders; nausea, chills, fever, eosinophilia, anaphylaxis, rashes, including exfoliative dermatitis, Stevens-Johnson syndrome, and vasculitis; phlebitis; on rapid infusion, severe hypotension (with shock, cardiac arrest), wheezing, dyspnoea, urticaria, pruritus, flushing of the upper body ('red man' syndrome), pain and muscle spasm of back and chest

---

6.2.3 Antileprosy drugs

Leprosy is a chronic mycobacterial infection due to *Mycobacterium leprae*, which is a slow-growing intracellular bacillus that infiltrates the skin, peripheral nerves, the nasal and other mucosa, and the eyes; it affects people of all ages and both sexes. The incubation period between infection and appearance of leprosy is normally between 2 to 10 years, but may be up to 20 years. It is transmitted from person-to-person when bacilli are shed from the nose; most individuals have natural immunity and symptoms are suppressed. For treatment purposes patients may be classified as having paucibacillary (PB) or multibacillary (MB) leprosy. The 2 forms may be distinguished by skin smears, but facilities are not always available to process them and their reliability is often doubtful. In practice, most leprosy programmes classify and choose a regimen based on number of skin lesions; these are PB single-lesion leprosy (1 lesion), PB leprosy (2–5 skin lesions) and MB leprosy (more than 5 skin lesions).

Combination therapy has become essential to prevent the emergence of resistance. **Rifampicin** is now combined with **dapsone** to treat PB leprosy and **rifampicin** and **clofazimine** are now combined with **dapsone** to treat MB leprosy. The WHO Action Programme for the Elimination of Leprosy currently provides oral multidrug therapy (MDT) in blister packs which ensure better patient adherence. More recently, a single dose of combination therapy has been recommended to cure patients with single-skin-lesion leprosy. Any patient with a positive skin smear should be treated with the MDT regimen for MB leprosy. The regimen for PB leprosy should never be given to a patient with MB leprosy. If diagnosis in a particular patient is not possible the MDT regimen for MB leprosy must be used.

Lepra reactions are episodes of sudden increase in the activity of leprosy and are often accompanied by neuritis; reactions must always be treated promptly to prevent permanent nerve damage and disability. Leprosy multidrug therapy should continue during a lepra reaction without interruption. This reduces the frequency and severity of lepra reactions.

Type I lepra reactions, or reversal reactions, are delayed hypersensitivity reactions and may occur in either PB or MB leprosy. If there is no nerve damage, type I reactions may be treated with analgesics such as acetylsalicylic acid or paracetamol. If there is nerve involvement corticosteroids, such as oral prednisolone should be used in addition to analgesics.

The type II lepra reaction, also known as erythema nodosum leprosum (ENL), is an antibody response to dead leprosy bacteria and occurs only in MB leprosy. Therapy for type II reactions may include analgesics, such as acetylsalicylic acid or paracetamol, and corticosteroids, such as oral prednisolone. In patients not responding to corticosteroids, clofazimine may be used. Thalidomide is rarely useful and in any case it should be avoided in women of childbearing age since it is a proven teratogen. If this is not possible, it is imperative that pregnancy is excluded before this treatment is initiated. Severe type II lepra reactions should be treated under medical supervision in hospital.

If a patient does not respond to lepra reaction treatment within 6 weeks or seems to become worse, the patient must be sent immediately to the nearest specialist centre. Neuritis may occur during or independently of lepra reactions. It can be successfully treated with a 12-week course of oral prednisolone; if patients do not respond, specialist centre treatment is required.

TREATMENT REGIMENS. Single doses of rifampicin 600 mg, ofloxacin 400 mg and minocycline 100 mg in combination are recommended for the treatment of single-lesion paucibacillary (PB) leprosy in adults. Children aged 5 to 14 years may be given half the adult single dose; appropriate dose adjustments are required for younger children. Although minocycline and ofloxacin are not recommended for use in children or ofloxacin for adolescents, field trials with single-dose regimens of these drugs for the treatment of single-lesion PB leprosy have not shown adverse effects.

The recommended regimen for paucibacillary leprosy in adults (50–70 kg) is rifampicin 600 mg once monthly under supervision and dapsone 100 mg daily, self-administered. Children aged 10–14 years may be given rifampicin 450 mg once monthly under supervision and dapsone 50 mg daily. Appropriate dose adjustments are required for younger children. For example, dapsone 25 mg daily and rifampicin 300 mg once a month under supervision. Treatment is continued for 6 months for PB leprosy.

The recommended regimen for multibacillary (MB) leprosy in adults (50–70 kg) is rifampicin 600 mg and clofazimine 300 mg, both given once a month under supervision together with clofazimine 50 mg and dapsone 100 mg, both daily. Children aged 10–14 years may be given rifampicin 450 mg and clofazimine 150 mg, both once a month under supervision together with clofazimine 50 mg every other day and dapsone 50 mg daily. Appropriate dosage adjustments are required for younger children. For example, dapsone 25 mg daily, clofazimine 50 mg twice a week, and clofazimine 100 mg and rifampicin 300 mg once a month under supervision. Treatment is continued for 12 months for MB leprosy.

For patients who cannot take rifampicin because of allergy, other diseases, or rifampicin-resistant leprosy, and for patients who refuse to take clofazimine, there are alternative regimens which incorporate ofloxacin and minocycline.

Clofazimine
Capsules, clofazimine 50 mg, 100 mg

Uses: multibacillary (MB) leprosy; type II lepra reactions

Precautions: pre-existing gastrointestinal symptoms (reduce dose, increase dose interval or discontinue if symptoms develop during treatment); liver and renal impairment; pregnancy and breastfeeding; may discolour soft contact lenses

Dosage:

Multibacillary leprosy (in combination with dapsone and rifampicin, see notes above), *by mouth*, ADULT 50 mg once daily and 300 mg once a month, under supervision; CHILD 10–14 years 50 mg on alternate days and 150 mg once a month under supervision; CHILD under 10 years, see notes above; continue treatment for 12 months

Type II lepra reaction (erythema nodosum leprosum; see notes above), *by mouth*, ADULT and CHILD 200–300 mg daily in 2 or 3 divided doses; 4–6 weeks treatment may be required before effect is seen

Adverse effects: reversible discoloration of skin, hair, cornea, conjunctiva, tears, sweat, sputum, faeces, and urine; dose-related gastrointestinal symptoms including pain, nausea, vomiting and diarrhoea; severe mucosal and submucosal oedema, with prolonged treatment with high doses—may be severe enough to cause subacute small-bowel obstruction (see also Precautions)

Dapsone

Tablets, dapsone 25 mg, 50 mg, 100 mg

Uses: paucibacillary (PB) and multibacillary (MB) leprosy

Contraindications: hypersensitivity to sulfones; severe anaemia

Precautions: anaemia (treat severe anaemia before therapy, and monitor blood counts during treatment); G6PD deficiency (including breastfeeding affected infants); pregnancy (Appendix 2); breastfeeding (Appendix 3); porphyria; **interactions:** Appendix 1

BLOOD DISORDERS. On long-term treatment patients and their carers should be told how to recognize blood disorders and advised to seek immediate medical attention if symptoms such as fever, sore throat, rash, mouth ulcers, purpura, bruising or bleeding develop

Dosage:

Paucibacillary leprosy (in combination with rifampicin, see notes above), *by mouth*, ADULT 100 mg daily; CHILD 10–14 years 50 mg daily; CHILD under 10 years, see notes above; continue treatment for 6 months

Multibacillary leprosy (in combination with rifampicin and clofazimine, see notes above), ADULT 100 mg daily; CHILD 10–14 years 50 mg daily; CHILD under 10 years, see notes above; continue treatment for 12 months

Adverse effects: haemolysis and methaemoglobinaemia; allergic dermatitis (rarely including toxic epidermal necrolysis and the Stevens-Johnson syndrome); rarely, hepatitis and agranulocytosis; 'dapsone syndrome' resembling mononucleosis—rare hypersensitivity reaction with symptoms including rash, fever, jaundice, and eosinophilia; gastrointestinal irritation; headache, nervousness, insomnia, blurred vision, paraesthesia, reversible peripheral neuropathy, and psychoses reported

Rifampicin

Tablets, rifampicin 150 mg, 300 mg
Capsules, rifampicin 150 mg, 300 mg

Uses: paucibacillary leprosy; multibacillary leprosy; tuberculosis (section 6.2.4)

Contraindications: hypersensitivity to rifamycins; jaundice

Precautions: reduce dose in hepatic impairment (Appendix 5); liver function tests and blood counts required in liver disorders, elderly, and on prolonged therapy; renal impairment (if dose above 600 mg daily); pregnancy (Appendix 2); breastfeeding (Appendix 3); porphyria; discolours soft contact lenses; **important:** advise patients on oral contraceptives to use additional means; **interactions:** Appendix 1

NOTE. Resumption of rifampicin treatment after a long interval may cause serious immunological reactions, resulting in renal impairment, haemolysis, or thrombocytopenia—discontinue permanently if serious adverse effects occur

LIVER DISORDERS. Patients or their carers should be told how to recognize signs of liver disorders and advised to discontinue treatment and seek immediate medical attention if symptoms such as persistent nausea, vomiting, malaise or jaundice develop

Dosage:

Single-lesion paucibacillary leprosy (in combination with ofloxacin and minocycline; see notes above), *by mouth,* ADULT 600 mg as a single dose; CHILD 5–14 years 300 mg as a single dose; CHILD under 5 years, see notes above

Paucibacillary leprosy (in combination with dapsone; see notes above), *by mouth,* ADULT 600 mg once a month under supervision; CHILD 10–14 years 450 mg once a month under supervision; CHILD under 10 years, see notes above; continue treatment for 6 months

Multibacillary leprosy (in combination with dapsone and clofazimine; see notes above), *by mouth,* ADULT 600 mg once a month under supervision; CHILD 10–14 years 450 mg once a month under supervision; CHILD under 10 years, see notes above; continue treatment for 12 months

PATIENT ADVICE. Take dose at least 30 minutes before a meal, since absorption is reduced by food

Adverse effects: severe gastrointestinal disturbances including anorexia, nausea, vomiting, and diarrhoea (antibiotic-associated colitis reported); rashes, fever, influenza-like syndrome and respiratory symptoms, collapse, shock, haemolytic anaemia, acute renal failure, and thrombocytopenic purpura—more frequent with intermittent therapy; alterations of liver function—jaundice and potentially fatal hepatitis (dose-related; do not exceed maximum daily dose of 600 mg); urine, tears, saliva, and sputum coloured orange-red

Minocycline

Tablets, minocycline (as hydrochloride) 50 mg, 100 mg [not included on WHO Model List 11th revision]

Uses: single-lesion paucibacillary leprosy

Contraindications: pregnancy (Appendix 2); systemic lupus erythematosus

Precautions: hepatic impairment—monitor liver function before use (Appendix 5); avoid exposure to sunlight—photosensitivity reaction; children (see notes above); breast-feeding (Appendix 3); **interactions:** Appendix 1

SKILLED TASKS. May impair ability to perform skilled tasks, for example operating machinery, driving

Dosage:

Single-lesion paucibacillary leprosy (in combination with rifampicin and ofloxacin; see notes above), *by mouth,* ADULT 100 mg as a single dose; CHILD 5–14 years 50 mg as a single dose; CHILD under 5 years, see notes above

Adverse effects: dizziness and vertigo (more common in women); nausea, vomiting, and diarrhoea; headache and visual disturbances—may indicate intracranial hypertension; hepatotoxicity, pancreatitis, and antibiotic-associated colitis reported; severe exfoliative rashes; pigmentation (sometimes irreversible); discoloration of conjunctiva, tears, and sweat; systemic lupus erythematosus and liver damage reported

Ofloxacin

Tablets, ofloxacin 200 mg, 400 mg [not included on WHO Model List 11th revision]

Uses: single-lesion paucibacillary leprosy

Precautions: epilepsy or history of CNS disorders; renal impairment (Appendix 4); hepatic impairment (Appendix 5); avoid exposure to sunlight—photosensitivity reactions; pregnancy (Appendix 2); breastfeeding (Appendix 3); children and adolescents (arthropathy in weight-bearing joints in young *animals*; see also notes above); **interactions:** Appendix 1

SKILLED TASKS. May impair ability to perform skilled tasks, for example operating machinery or driving

Dosage:

Single-lesion paucibacillary leprosy (in combination with rifampicin and minocycline; see notes above), *by mouth,* ADULT 400 mg as a single dose; CHILD 5–14 years 200 mg as a single dose; CHILD under 5, see notes above

Adverse effects: convulsions in patients with or without history of convulsions; nausea, vomiting, abdominal pain, diarrhoea; headache, visual disturbances, sleep disorders and other CNS disturbances; psychotic reactions—discontinue treatment; rashes (rarely Stevens-Johnson syndrome and toxic epidermal necrolysis), pruritus, and fever

6.2.4   Antituberculosis drugs

Tuberculosis is a chronic infectious disease caused primarily by
Mycobacterium tuberculosis or sometimes *M. bovis*. Infection
is usually due to inhalation of infected droplet nuclei with the
lung generally being the first organ affected, but the primary
infection is usually asymptomatic. Infection and inflammatory
responses resolve with the development of acquired immunity.
Surviving bacteria may become dormant or in susceptible
patients, progress to active primary disease; dormant organisms
may produce disease and this often occurs if immune status is
altered.

Tuberculosis is the most prevalent infectious disease of adults
and causes 26% of avoidable adult deaths in the developing
world. More than 80% of tuberculosis cases are pulmonary
(PTB). At least 30% of patients who are infected with HIV will
also develop active tuberculosis. The increase in resistant strains
and poor compliance which may contribute to resistance and
treatment failure has led to the development of regimens with
directly supervised treatment. Directly Observed Treatment,
Short-course (DOTS) therapy which lasts for 6 or 8 months,
given under direct observation is one of the most important
components of the WHO strategy against tuberculosis.
Simplified drug regimens and intermittent therapy have been
introduced to improve compliance. WHO does not generally
recommend twice weekly regimens. If a patient receiving a
twice weekly regimen misses a dose of tablets, the missed dose
represents a bigger fraction of the total number of treatment
doses than if the patient was receiving a three times weekly or
daily dose regimen. Therefore, there is a greater risk of
treatment failure with twice weekly regimens. Fixed dose
combination tablets incorporating 2 or more drugs are also used
to improve compliance and decrease inadvertent medication
errors.

Modern short-course therapy is usually in 2 phases. The initial
phase (2 months) involves the concurrent use of at least 3 drugs
to reduce the bacterial population rapidly and prevent drug-
resistant bacteria emerging. The second continuation phase (4–6
months) involves fewer drugs and is used to eliminate any
remaining bacteria and prevent recurrence. Direct observation
of therapy is considered essential to ensure compliance in the
initial phase and also useful in the continuation phase if patients
are receiving rifampicin. The six antituberculosis drugs,
isoniazid, **rifampicin**, **pyrazinamide**, **streptomycin**, (which
are bactericidal) **ethambutol** and **thioacetazone** (which are
bacteriostatic) are used in various combinations as part of WHO
recommended treatment regimens. In supervised regimens
change of drug regimen should be considered only if the
patient fails to respond after 5 months of DOTS.

Isoniazid, rifampicin, and pyrazinamide are components of all antituberculosis drug regimens currently recommended by WHO. Unsupervised and alternative regimens as set out in the following tables may be administered as specified.

> Additional reserve antituberculosis drugs for the treatment of drug-resistant tuberculosis should be used in specialized centres only with WHO-recommended TB control strategy, DOTS, and treatment programmes.

Worldwide, an important predisposing cause of immunosuppression leading to tuberculosis is human immunodeficiency virus (HIV) infection; it increases susceptibility to primary infection and increases the reactivation rate of tuberculosis. Preventative antituberculosis therapy of such persons is recommended.

Chemoprophylaxis with isoniazid can prevent the development of clinically apparent disease in persons in close contact with infectious patients, and in other persons at high risk particularly those who are immunodeficient.

Where the disease remains highly prevalent routine immunization of infants within the first year of age with BCG vaccine is cost-effective. However, there is no evidence that BCG will protect children older than 15 years of age. Infants born to HIV-positive mothers should be vaccinated during the first year of life, provided they have no clinical signs suggestive of HIV.

The **tuberculin test** has limited diagnostic value. A positive tuberculin test indicates previous exposure to mycobacterial antigens through infection with one of the tubercle bacilli, or BCG vaccination. The tuberculin test does not distinguish between tuberculosis and other mycobacterial infection, between active and quiescent disease, or between acquired infection and seroconversion induced by BCG vaccination.

Recommended 6-month treatment regimens for tuberculosis[a]

Drug	Initial phase (2 months)	Continuation phase (4 months)
Isoniazid	5 mg/kg daily	5 mg/kg daily
Rifampicin	10 mg/kg daily	10 mg/kg daily
Pyrazinamide	25 mg/kg daily	
together with		
Streptomycin	15 mg/kg daily	
or		
Ethambutol	15 mg/kg daily	
Isoniazid	10 mg/kg 3 times weekly	10 mg/kg 3 times weekly
Rifampicin	10 mg/kg 3 times weekly	10 mg/kg 3 times weekly
Pyrazinamide	35 mg/kg 3 times weekly	
together with		
Streptomycin	15 mg/kg 3 times weekly	
or		
Ethambutol	30 mg/kg 3 times weekly[c]	

Recommended 8-month treatment regimen for tuberculosis[a]

Drug	Initial phase (2 months)	Continuation phase (6 months)
Isoniazid	5 mg/kg daily	5 mg/kg daily
Rifampicin	10 mg/kg daily	
Pyrazinamide	30 mg/kg daily	
Thioacetazone		2.5 mg/kg daily
together with		
Streptomycin	15 mg/kg daily	
or		
Ethambutol	25 mg/kg daily[b]	

[a] Unless otherwise indicated, doses are suitable for both adults and children
[b] 15 mg/kg for children
[c] Not suitable for children

Possible alternative treatment regimens for each treatment category

TB treatment category	TB patients	Initial phase (daily)	Continuation phase (daily or 3 times per week)
I	New smear-positive PTB; new smear-nega-tive PTB with extensive parenchyma involve-ment; new cases of severe forms of extra-pulmonary TB.	2 EHRZ (SHRZ) 2 EHRZ (SHRZ) 2 EHRZ (SHRZ)	6 HE 4 HR 4 H_3R_3
II	Sputum smear-positive relapse; treatment fail-ure; treatment after interruption.	2 SHRZE/1 HRZE 2 SHRZE/1 HRZE	$5H_3R_3E_3$ 5 HRE
III	New smear-negative PTB (other than cate-gory I); new less severe forms of extra-pulmon-ary TB.	2 HRZ 2 HRZ 2 HRZ	6 HE 4 HR 4 H_3R_3
IV	Chronic case (still spu-tum positive after supervised re-treat-ment)	NOT APPLICABLE (Refer to WHO guidelines for use of second-line drugs in specialized centres).	

NOTE. Some authorities recommend a 7-month continuation phase with daily isoniazid and rifampicin (7HR) for Category 1 patients with the following forms of TB: TB meningitis, miliary TB, spinal TB with neurological signs. H = isoniazid, R = rifampicin, Z = pyrazinamide, E = ethambutol, S = streptomycin.

A regimen consists of 2 phases, the initial phase and the continuation phase. The number before a phase is the duration of that phase in months. The number in subscript after a letter is the number of doses of that drug per week. If there is no number in subscript after a letter, then treatment with that drug is daily. An alternative drug (or drugs) appears as a letter (or letters) in parentheses.

Ethambutol hydrochloride

Tablets, ethambutol hydrochloride 100 mg, 400 mg

Uses: tuberculosis, in combination with other drugs (see notes and tables above)

Contraindications: optic neuritis; children under 5 years—unable to report symptomatic visual disturbances; severe renal impairment

Precautions: visual disturbances—ocular examination recommended before and during treatment (see note below); reduce dose in renal impairment (Appendix 4) and monitor plasma concentration; elderly; pregnancy; breastfeeding (Appendix 3)

NOTE. Patients should report visual disturbances immediately and discontinue treatment; children who are incapable of reporting symptomatic visual changes accurately should be given alternative therapy, as should, if possible, any patient who cannot understand warnings about visual adverse effects

Dosage:

Tuberculosis (initial phase of combination therapy; see notes and tables above), *by mouth*, ADULT 15 mg/kg daily *or* 30 mg/kg 3 times a week; CHILD 15 mg/kg daily

Adverse effects: optic neuritis—reduced visual acuity and red/green colour blindness (early changes usually reversible, prompt withdrawal may prevent blindness); peripheral neuritis—especially in legs; gout; rarely, rash, pruritus, urticaria, thrombocytopenia

---

Ethambutol hydrochloride with isoniazid

Tablets, ethambutol hydrochloride 400 mg with isoniazid 150 mg

Uses: tuberculosis, in combination with other drugs (see notes and tables above)

Contraindications: preparation not suitable for use in children; see Ethambutol Hydrochloride and Isoniazid

Precautions: see Ethambutol Hydrochloride and Isoniazid

Dosage:

Tuberculosis, continuation phase of 8-month regimen in place of thioacetazone with isoniazid (see notes and tables), *by mouth*, ADULT ethambutol hydrochloride 800 mg and isoniazid 300 mg daily

Adverse effects: see Ethambutol Hydrochloride and Isoniazid

Isoniazid

Tablets, isoniazid 100 mg, 300 mg
Injection (Solution for injection), isoniazid 25 mg/ml, 2-ml ampoule

Uses: tuberculosis treatment, in combination with other drugs (see notes and tables above); tuberculosis prophylaxis

Contraindications: drug-induced hepatic disease

Precautions: hepatic impairment (monitor hepatic function; Appendix 5); malnutrition, chronic alcohol dependence, chronic renal failure (Appendix 4), diabetes mellitus, and HIV infection—prophylactic pyridoxine 10 mg daily required because risk of peripheral neuritis; epilepsy; slow acetylator status (increased risk of adverse effects); history of psychosis; pregnancy; breastfeeding (Appendix 3); porphyria; **interactions:** Appendix 1

LIVER DISORDERS. Patients or their carers should be told how to recognize signs of liver disorder, and advised to discontinue treatment and seek immediate medical attention if symptoms such as nausea, vomiting, malaise or jaundice develop

Dosage:

Tuberculosis, treatment (combination therapy; see also notes and tables), *by mouth*, ADULT and CHILD 5 mg/kg (4–6 mg/kg) daily (maximum, 300 mg daily), *or* 10 mg/kg 3 times weekly

Tuberculosis, treatment in critically ill patients unable to take oral therapy (combination therapy), *by intramuscular injection*, ADULT 200–300 mg as single daily dose; CHILD 10–20 mg/kg daily

Tuberculosis, prophylaxis, *by mouth*, ADULT 300 mg daily for at least 6 months; CHILD 5 mg/kg daily for at least 6 months

PATIENT ADVICE. Isoniazid should be taken on an empty stomach; if taken with food to reduce gastrointestinal irritation, oral absorption and bioavailability may be impaired

Adverse effects: gastrointestinal disorders including nausea and vomiting, diarrhoea and pain; hypersensitivity reactions including fever, rashes, joint pain, erythema multiforme, purpura usually during first weeks of treatment; peripheral neuropathy; optic neuritis, toxic psychoses, and convulsions; hepatitis (especially over age of 35 years and regular users of alcohol)—withdraw treatment; also reported, systemic lupus erythematosus-like syndrome, pellagra, hyperglycaemia and gynaecomastia

---

Pyrazinamide
Tablets, pyrazinamide 400 mg, 500 mg

Uses: tuberculosis, in combination with other drugs (see notes and tables above)

Contraindications: severe hepatic impairment; porphyria

Precautions: hepatic impairment (monitor hepatic function; Appendix 5); renal impairment; diabetes mellitus (monitor blood glucose—may change suddenly); gout; breastfeeding (Appendix 3)

LIVER DISORDERS. Patients or their carers should be told how to recognize signs of liver disorder, and advised to discontinue treatment and seek immediate medical attention if symptoms such as persistent nausea, vomiting, malaise or jaundice develop

Dosage:

Tuberculosis (initial phase of combination therapy; see notes and tables above), *by mouth*, ADULT and CHILD 25 mg/kg daily *or* 35 mg/kg 3 times weekly

Adverse effects: hepatotoxicity including fever, anorexia, hepatomegaly, jaundice, liver failure; nausea, vomiting; arthralgia; gout; sideroblastic anaemia; urticaria; skin flushing

Rifampicin

Capsules, rifampicin 150 mg, 300 mg

Uses: tuberculosis, in combination with other drugs (see notes and tables above); leprosy (section 6.2.3)

Contraindications: hypersensitivity to rifamycins; jaundice

Precautions: reduce dose in hepatic impairment (Appendix 5); liver function tests and blood counts required in liver disorders, elderly, and on prolonged therapy; renal impairment (if dose above 600 mg daily); pregnancy (Appendix 2); breastfeeding (Appendix 3); porphyria; discolours soft contact lenses; **important:** advise patients on oral contraceptives to use additional means; **interactions:** Appendix 1

NOTE. Resumption of rifampicin treatment after a long interval may cause serious immunological reactions, resulting in renal impairment, haemolysis, or thrombocytopenia—discontinue permanently if serious adverse effects occur

LIVER DISORDERS. Patients or their carers should be told how to recognize signs of liver disorders and advised to discontinue treatment and seek immediate medical attention if symptoms such as persistent nausea, vomiting, malaise or jaundice develop

Dosage:

Tuberculosis (combination therapy; see notes and tables above), *by mouth*, ADULT and CHILD 10 mg/kg daily *or* 3 times weekly (maximum dose, 600 mg daily)

PATIENT ADVICE. Take dose at least 30 minutes before a meal, as absorption is reduced when taken with food

Adverse effects: severe gastrointestinal disturbances including anorexia, nausea, vomiting, and diarrhoea (antibiotic-associated colitis reported); rashes, fever, influenza-like syndrome and respiratory symptoms, collapse, shock, haemolytic anaemia, acute renal failure, and thrombocytopenic purpura—more frequent with intermittent therapy; alterations of liver function—jaundice and potentially fatal hepatitis (dose related; do not exceed maximum dose of 600 mg daily); urine, tears, saliva, and sputum coloured orange-red

Rifampicin with isoniazid

Tablets, rifampicin 60 mg with isoniazid 30 mg; rifampicin 150 mg with isoniazid 75 mg; rifampicin 300 mg with isoniazid 150 mg; rifampicin 60 mg with isoniazid 60 mg; rifampicin 150 mg with isoniazid 150 mg

Uses: tuberculosis (see notes and tables above)

Contraindications: see under Rifampicin and Isoniazid

Precautions: preparation not suitable for use in children; see under Rifampicin and Isoniazid

Dosage:

Tuberculosis, 6-month regimen (combination therapy; see notes and tables), *by mouth*, ADULT 10 mg/kg (rifampicin) and 5 mg/kg (isoniazid) daily

Tuberculosis, 6-month regimen (combination therapy; see notes and tables), *by mouth*, ADULT 10 mg/kg (rifampicin) and 10 mg/kg (isoniazid) 3 times a week

Adverse effects: see under Rifampicin and Isoniazid

Rifampicin with isoniazid and pyrazinamide

Tablets, rifampicin 60 mg, isoniazid 30 mg, and pyrazinamide 150 mg; rifampicin 150 mg, isoniazid 75 mg, and pyrazinamide 400 mg; rifampicin 150 mg, isoniazid 150 mg, and pyrazinamide 500 mg

Uses: tuberculosis, in combination with other drugs (see notes and tables above)

Contraindications: preparation not suitable for use in children; see Rifampicin, Isoniazid, and Pyrazinamide

Precautions: see Rifampicin, Isoniazid, and Pyrazinamide

Dosage:

Tuberculosis, initial phase of 6-month treatment regimens (see notes and tables above), *by mouth*, ADULT rifampicin 10 mg/kg, isoniazid 5 mg/kg, and pyrazinamide 25 mg/kg daily *or* rifampicin 10 mg/kg, isoniazid 10 mg/kg, and pyrazinamide 35 mg/kg 3 times a week

Adverse effects: see Rifampicin, Isoniazid, and Pyrazinamide

Rifampicin with isoniazid, pyrazinamide and ethambutol hydrochloride

Tablets, rifampicin 150 mg, isoniazid 75 mg, pyrazinamide 400 mg, and ethambutol hydrochloride 275 mg

Uses: tuberculosis (see notes and tables above)

Contraindications: preparation not suitable for use in children; see Rifampicin, Isoniazid, Pyrazinamide, and Ethambutol Hydrochloride

Precautions: see Rifampicin, Isoniazid, Pyrazinamide, and Ethambutol Hydrochloride

Dosage:

Tuberculosis, induction phase of 6-month regimen (see notes and tables above), *by mouth*, ADULT rifampicin 10 mg/kg, isoniazid 5 mg/kg, pyrazinamide 25 mg/kg, and ethambutol hydrochloride 15 mg/kg daily

Adverse effects: see Rifampicin, Isoniazid, Pyrazinamide, and Ethambutol Hydrochloride

Streptomycin

Injection (Powder for solution for injection), streptomycin (as sulfate) 1-g vial

Uses: tuberculosis, in combination with other drugs (see notes and tables above)

Contraindications: hearing disorders; myasthenia gravis; pregnancy (Appendix 2)

Precautions: children—painful injection, avoid use if possible; renal impairment (Appendix 4), infants, and elderly (dosage adjustment and monitor renal, auditory, and vestibular function, and plasma streptomycin concentrations); **interactions:** Appendix 1

Dosage:

Tuberculosis (initial phase of combination therapy; see notes and tables above), *by deep intramuscular injection*, ADULT and CHILD 15 mg/kg daily *or* 3 times a week (patients over 60 years or those weighing less than 50 kg may not tolerate doses above 500–750 mg daily)

RECONSTITUTION AND ADMINISTRATION. According to manufacturer's directions

NOTE. One hour (peak) concentration should be 15–40 mg/litre; pre-dose (trough) concentration should be less than 5 mg/litre (less than 1 mg/litre in renal impairment or those over 50 years)

Adverse effects: vestibular and auditory damage, nephrotoxicity; hypersensitivity reactions—withdraw treatment; paraesthesia of mouth; rarely, hypomagnesaemia on prolonged therapy; antibiotic-associated colitis; also, nausea, vomiting, rash; rarely, haemolytic anaemia, aplastic anaemia, agranulocytosis, thrombocytopenia; pain and abscess at injection site

Thioacetazone with isoniazid

Thioacetazone with isoniazid is a complementary drug combination

Tablets, thioacetazone 50 mg with isoniazid 100 mg; thioacetazone 150 mg with isoniazid 300 mg

Uses: tuberculosis, in combination with other drugs (see notes and tables above)

Contraindications: see Isoniazid; hepatic impairment; renal impairment; HIV infection—thioacetazone associated with high incidence of serious, sometimes fatal cutaneous hypersensitivity reactions, including exfoliative dermatitis

Precautions: see Isoniazid; determine efficacy and toxicity of thioacetazone—geographical differences; hypersensitivity reactions—withdraw treatment; **interactions:** Appendix 1

Dosage:

Tuberculosis, continuation phase of 8-month regimen (see notes and tables above), *by mouth*, ADULT and CHILD thioacetazone 2.5 mg/kg daily and isoniazid 5 mg/kg daily

Adverse effects: see Isoniazid; thioacetazone causes the following—nausea, vomiting, diarrhoea; hypersensitivity reactions including conjunctivitis, vertigo, rashes; fatal exfoliative dermatitis, acute hepatic failure reported; also, agranulocytosis, thrombocytopenia and aplastic anaemia

BCG vaccine

Injection (Powder for solution for injection), live bacteria of a strain derived from the bacillus of Calmette and Guerin

Uses: for active immunization against tuberculosis; see also section 19.3.1.1

Contraindications: see section 19.3.1; generalized oedema; hypogammaglobulinaemia and immunodeficiency due to antimetabolites, irradiation, corticosteroids; HIV positive—except asymptomatic children in areas of high tuberculosis risk; malignant disease; antimycobacterial treatment

Precautions: see section 19.3.1; pregnancy (Appendix 2); eczema, scabies—vaccine site must be lesion-free; **interactions:** Appendix 1

Dosage:

Immunization against tuberculosis, *by intradermal injection*, INFANTS up to 3 months, 0.05 ml; ADULT and CHILD over 3 months 0.1 ml

RECONSTITUTION AND ADMINISTRATION. According to manufacturer's directions

Adverse effects: lymphadenitis and keloid formation; osteitis and localized necrotic ulceration; rarely, disseminated BCG infection in immunodeficient patients; rarely, anaphylaxis

---

Tuberculin purified protein derivative (tuberculin PPD)
Injection, tuberculin purified protein derivative 10 units/ml, 100 units/ml

Uses: test for hypersensitivity to tuberculoprotein

Contraindications: should not be used within 3 weeks of receiving a live viral vaccine

Precautions: elderly; malnutrition, viral or bacterial infections (including HIV and severe tuberculosis), malignant disease, corticosteroid or immunosuppressant therapy—diminished sensitivity to tuberculin; avoid contact with open cuts, abraded or diseased skin, eyes or mouth

Dosage:

Test for hypersensitivity to tuberculoprotein, *by intradermal injection*, ADULT and CHILD 5 or 10 units (1 unit may be used in hypersensitive patients or if tuberculosis is suspected)

ADMINISTRATION. According to manufacturer's directions

Adverse effects: occasionally nausea, headache, malaise, rash; immediate local reactions (more common in atopic patients); rarely, vesicular or ulcerating local reactions, regional adenopathy and fever

---

6.3   Antifungal drugs

Fungal infections can be superficial or systemic. Superficial infections affect only the skin, hair, nails or mucous membranes whereas systemic fungal infections affect the body as a whole.

Systemic fungal infections are sometimes caused by inhalation, ingestion or inoculation of primary pathogens, and sometimes by opportunistic invasion of commensals in patients with lowered host resistance. They are increasing in prevalence not only because of the pandemic of HIV infection, but also because of the rise in illicit intravenous drug use in many countries, and greater use of broad spectrum antibiotics and invasive medical procedures. In immunodeficient patients systemic fungal infections are often disseminated.

Amphotericin B is a lipophilic polyene antibiotic; it is fungistatic against a broad spectrum of pathogenic fungi, including *Candida* spp., *Aspergillus* spp., *Cryptococcus neoformans*, *Histoplasma capsulatum*, *Blastomyces dermatitidis*, *Coccidioides immitis*, *Paracoccidioides brasiliensis*, *Mucor*,

Absidia and *Phicopes* spp.; it is active against algal *Prototheca* spp. and against the *Leishmania protozoa*. It is used in conjunction with flucytosine to treat cryptococcal meningitis and systemic candidosis .

Amphotericin B has to be administered parenterally as there is little or no absorption from the gastrointestinal tract; amphotericin B is liable to cause nephrotoxicity. Duration of therapy varies with the initial severity of the infection and the clinical response of the patient. In some infections a satisfactory response is only obtained after several months of continuous treatment. Intrathecal infusion has been used successfully in patients with meningeal coccidioidomycosis.

Griseofulvin is a fungistatic antibiotic derived from *Penicillium griseofulvum* with selective activity against the dermatophytes causing ringworm, *Microsporum canis*, *Trichophyton rubrum* and *T. verrucosum*. It has no activity against pityriasis versicolor or candida infections. Griseofulvin is deposited selectively in keratin precursor cells of skin, hair and nails where it disrupts the mitotic apparatus of fungal cells thus preventing fungal invasion of newly-formed cells. It is unsuitable for prophylactic use. Close attention should be given to hygiene and to possible reservoirs of reinfection in clothing, footware and bedding.

Fluconazole, an orally active synthetic imidazole derivative, possesses fungistatic activity against dermatophytes, yeasts and other pathogenic fungi. It is widely used in the treatment of serious gastrointestinal and systemic mycoses as well as in the management of superficial infections. Fluconazole is also used to prevent fungal infections in immunocompromised patients.

Flucytosine is a synthetic fluorinated pyrimidine with a narrow spectrum of antifungal activity, particularly against *Cryptococcus* and *Candida* spp. In susceptible fungi, it is converted to fluorouracil by cytosine deaminase. Flucytosine is myelosuppressive and plasma concentrations above 75 micrograms/ml are associated with myelotoxicity.

Nystatin, a polyene antifungal antibiotic derived from *Streptomyces noursei*, is effective against infections caused by a wide range of yeasts and yeast-like fungi. It is used for the prophylaxis and treatment of candidosis .

Potassium iodide aqueous oral solution is a clear liquid with a characteristic, strong salty taste. It is effective against sporotrichosis and subcutaneous phycomycosis, which are fungal infections caused by *Sporothrix schenckii* and *Basidiobolus haptosporus* respectively. In subcutaneous sporotrichosis, amphotericin B is often effective in patients unable to tolerate iodides. Itraconazole, by mouth has been tried as an alternative to potassium iodide in both cutaneous and extracutaneous sporotrichosis. In phycomycosis, fluconazole may be effective.

Amphotericin B

Injection (powder for solution for injection), amphotericin b 50-mg vial

Uses: life-threatening fungal infections including histoplasmosis, coccidioidomycosis, paracoccidioidomycosis, blastomycosis, aspergillosis, cryptococcosis, mucormycosis, sporotrichosis, and candidosis; leishmaniasis (section 6.4.2)

Precautions: close medical supervision throughout treatment and initial test dose required (see note, below); renal impairment (Appendix 4); hepatic and renal function tests; blood counts and plasma electrolyte monitoring; corticosteroids (avoid, except to control reactions); pregnancy (Appendix 2); breastfeeding (Appendix 3); avoid rapid infusion (risk of arrhythmias); **interactions:** Appendix 1

ANAPHYLAXIS. Anaphylaxis occurs rarely with intravenous amphotericin B and a test dose is advisable before the first infusion. The patient should be observed for about 30 minutes after the test dose

Dosage:

Systemic fungal infections, *by intravenous infusion*, ADULT and CHILD initial test dose of 1 mg over 20–30 minutes, then 250 micrograms/kg daily, gradually increased up to 1 mg/kg daily or in severe infection, up to 1.5 mg/kg daily or on alternate days

NOTE. Prolonged treatment usually necessary; if interrupted for longer than 7 days, recommence at 250 micrograms/kg daily and increase gradually

RECONSTITUTION AND ADMINISTRATION. According to manufacturer's directions

Adverse effects: fever, headache, anorexia, weight loss, nausea and vomiting, malaise, diarrhoea, muscle and joint pain, dyspepsia, and epigastric pain; renal function disturbances including hypokalaemia, hypomagnesaemia and renal toxicity; blood disorders; cardiovascular toxicity (including arrhythmias); neurological disorders (including peripheral neuropathy); abnormal liver function (discontinue treatment); rash; anaphylactoid reactions (see above); pain and thrombophlebitis at injection site

Griseofulvin

Tablets, griseofulvin 125 mg, 250 mg
Capsules, griseofulvin 250 mg

Uses: fungal infections of the skin, scalp, hair and nails where topical treatment has failed or is inappropriate

Contraindications: severe liver disease (Appendix 5); pregnancy (avoid pregnancy during and for 1 month after treatment; men should not father children within 6 months of treatment; Appendix 2); porphyria; systemic lupus erythematosus and related disorders

Precautions: pre-existing hepatic insufficiency (closely monitor hepatic function throughout treatment); blood disorders (monitor blood count weekly during first month of treatment); breastfeeding; **interactions:** Appendix 1

SKILLED TASKS. May impair ability to perform skilled tasks, for example operating machinery, driving

Dosage:

Superficial fungal infections, *by mouth*, ADULT 0.5–1 g (but not less than 10 mg/kg) daily with food in single or divided doses; CHILD 10 mg/kg daily with food in single or divided doses

NOTE. Duration of treatment depends on the infection and thickness of keratin at site of infection; at least 4 weeks for skin and hair, at least 6 weeks for scalp ringworm and in severe infection, up to 3 months; 6 months for fingernails and 12 months or more for toenails

Adverse effects: headache, nausea, vomiting, diarrhoea, rashes, dizziness, fatigue reported; dry mouth and angular stomatitis; leukopenia, agranulocytosis; proteinuria reported; photosensitivity; lupus erythematosus, toxic epidermal necrolysis, erythema multiforme; serum sickness, angioedema; peripheral neuropathy; confusion and impaired coordination

---

Fluconazole

Fluconazole is a representative azole antifungal. Various drugs can serve as alternatives

Capsules, fluconazole 50 mg

Oral suspension (Powder for oral suspension), fluconazole 50 mg/5 ml

Infusion (Solution for infusion), fluconazole 2 mg/ml, 25-ml bottle, 100-ml bottle

Uses: systemic mycoses including histoplasmosis, non-meningeal coccidioidomycosis, paracoccidioidomycosis and blastomycosis; treatment and, in AIDS and other immunosuppressed patients, prophylaxis of cryptococcal meningitis; oesophageal and oropharyngeal candidosis, vaginal candidosis and systemic candidosis

Precautions: renal impairment (Appendix 4); pregnancy (Appendix 2); breastfeeding (Appendix 3); raised liver enzymes (review need for treatment; risk of hepatic necrosis; Appendix 5); **interactions:** Appendix 1

Dosage:

Systemic mycoses, *by mouth or by intravenous infusion*, ADULT 200 mg daily for at least 6 months; CHILD over 2 years 3–6 mg/kg daily for at least 6 months

Cryptococcal meningitis (following amphotericin B induction therapy), *by mouth or by intravenous infusion*, ADULT 800 mg daily for 2 days, then 400 mg daily for 8 weeks; CHILD 6–12 mg/kg daily (every 72 hours in NEONATES up to 2 weeks old, every 48 hours in NEONATES 2–4 weeks old)

Prevention of relapse of cryptococcal meningitis in AIDS patients after completion of primary therapy, *by mouth or by intravenous infusion*, ADULT 100–200 mg daily

Systemic candidosis (in patients unable to tolerate amphotericin B), *by mouth or by intravenous infusion*, ADULT 400 mg as initial dose, then 200 mg daily for at least 4 weeks; CHILD 6–12 mg/kg daily (every 72 hours in NEONATES up to 2 weeks old, and every 48 hours in NEONATES 2–4 weeks old)

Oesophageal and oropharyngeal candidosis, *by mouth or by intravenous infusion*, ADULT 200 mg as an initial dose, then 100 mg daily until symptoms resolved; up to 400 mg daily in very resistant infections; CHILD 3–6 mg/kg on the first day, then 3 mg/kg daily (every 72 hours in NEONATES up to 2 weeks old, every 48 hours in NEONATES 2–4 weeks old)

Vaginal candidosis, *by mouth*, ADULT 150 mg as a single dose

Adverse effects: nausea, vomiting, abdominal distension and discomfort; headache; elevation of liver enzymes, infrequently (see Precautions above); rash (withdraw treatment); angioedema, anaphylaxis, bullous lesions, toxic epidermal necrolysis and Stevens-Johnson syndrome reported (skin reactions more common in AIDS); rarely, thrombocytopenia

---

Nystatin

Tablets, nystatin 100 000 units, 500 000 units
Oral suspension, nystatin 100 000 units/ml
Lozenge, nystatin 100 000 units
Pessaries, nystatin 100 000 units

Uses: oral, oesophageal, intestinal, vaginal, and cutaneous candidosis

Precautions: pregnancy and breastfeeding (Appendices 2 and 3)

Dosage:

Oral candidosis, *by mouth*, ADULT and CHILD, 100 000 units after food 4 times daily

Intestinal and oesophageal candidosis, *by mouth*, ADULT 500 000 units 4 times daily; CHILD 100 000 units 4 times daily; continue for 48 hours after clinical cure

Vaginal candidosis, *vaginal administration*, ADULT insert 1–2 pessaries at night for at least 2 weeks

Adverse effects: nausea, vomiting, diarrhoea at high doses; oral irritation and sensitization; rash and rarely, Stevens-Johnson syndrome

---

Flucytosine

Flucytosine is a complementary drug
Capsules, flucytosine 250 mg
Infusion (Solution for infusion), flucytosine 10 mg/ml, 250-ml infusion

Uses: adjunct to amphotericin B (or fluconazole) in cryptococcal meningitis; adjunct to amphotericin B in systemic candidosis

Precautions: elderly; renal impairment (Appendix 4); also use with amphotericin B (both nephrotoxic); liver- and kidney function tests and blood counts required (weekly in renal impairment or in blood disorders); pregnancy (Appendix 2); breastfeeding (Appendix 3); **interactions:** Appendix 1

Dosage:

Systemic candidosis and cryptococcosis, *by intravenous infusion* (over 20–40 minutes), ADULT and CHILD 200 mg/kg daily in 4 divided doses, for usually no more than 7 days (at least 4 months in cryptococcal meningitis); extremely sensitive organisms, 100–150 mg/kg daily in 4 divided doses

Systemic candidosis, initial treatment or after intravenous therapy, *by mouth*, ADULT and CHILD 50–150 mg/kg daily in 4 divided doses

NOTE. For plasma concentration monitoring blood should be taken shortly before starting next infusion (or before next dose by mouth); plasma concentration for optimum response 25–50 mg/litre—should not be allowed to exceed 80 mg/litre

Adverse effects: rash, nausea, vomiting and diarrhoea; alterations in liver function tests; less frequently, confusion, hallucinations, convulsions, headache, sedation, vertigo; blood disorders including leukopenia, potentially fatal thrombocytopenia and aplastic anaemia

---

Potassium iodide

Potassium iodide is a complementary drug

Oral solution, potassium iodide 1 g/ml (saturated solution)

Uses: sporotrichosis; subcutaneous phycomycosis; thyrotoxicosis (section 18.8)

Contraindications: hypersensitivity to iodides; pregnancy (Appendix 2); breastfeeding (Appendix 3); acute bronchitis or active tuberculosis

Precautions: Addison disease; cardiac disease; hyperthyroidism; myotonia congenita; renal impairment

Dosage:

Sporotrichosis and subcutaneous phycomycosis, *by mouth*, ADULT initially 1 ml 3 times daily, increased by 1 ml daily, depending on tolerance, to 10 ml daily; continue treatment for at least 4 weeks after resolution or stabilization of lesions

NOTE. If signs of iodism occur, suspend treatment temporarily and restart after a few days at lower dosage

Adverse effects: goitre, hypothroidism, hyperthyroidism; iodism characterized by metallic taste, increased salivation, coryza and irritation and swelling of the eyes (resulting from prolonged administration); also gastrointestinal disturbances and diarrhoea; pulmonary oedema, bronchitis; depression, insomnia, impotence, headache reported

---

6.4 Antiprotozoal drugs

6.4.1 Antiamoebic, antigiardial and antitrichomonal drugs

AMOEBIASIS. Amoebic dysentery is caused by *Entamoeba histolytica*. It is transmitted by the faeco-oral route and infection is usually caused by ingestion of cysts from contaminated food and drink. Asymptomatic carriers are common in endemic areas. In non-endemic areas, symptomless carriers should be treated with a luminal amoebicide which will reduce the risk of transmission and protect the patient from invasive amoebiasis. **Diloxanide furoate** is most widely used, but other compounds, including **clefamide**, **etofamide**, and **teclozan**, are also effective. Treatment with diloxanide furoate is regarded as successful if stools are free of *E. histolytica* for one month. Several specimens should be examined in evaluating response to treatment.

Symptomatic (invasive) amoebiasis may be classified as intestinal or extra-intestinal. Intestinal amoebiasis is either amoebic dysentery or non-dysenteric amoebic colitis. Extra-intestinal amoebiasis most commonly involves the liver, but may involve the skin, genito-urinary tract, lung and brain. Invasive amoebiasis is more likely in malnutrition, immunosuppression and pregnancy. Amoebic dysentery may take a fulminating course in late pregnancy and the puerperium; treatment with **metronidazole** may be life saving. In less severe infection, metronidazole should, if possible, be avoided in the first trimester. All patients with invasive amoebiasis require treatment with a systemically active compound such as **metronidazole**, **ornidazole** and **tinidazole** followed by a luminal amoebicide in order to eliminate any surviving organisms in the colon. Combined preparations are useful.

In severe cases of amoebic dysentery, tetracycline given in combination with a systemic amoebicide lessens the risk of superinfection, intestinal perforation and peritonitis. Hepatic abscesses should be lanced by needle aspiration.

GIARDIASIS. Giardiasis is caused by *Giardia intestinalis* and is acquired by oral ingestion of *Giardia* cysts. Giardiasis can be treated with **tinidazole** in a single dose or with another 5-nitroimidazole such as **metronidazole**; both are highly effective and should be offered when practicable to all infected patients. Family and institutional contacts should also be treated. Larger epidemics are difficult to eradicate because of the high proportion of symptomless carriers and because excreted cysts can survive for long periods outside the human host.

TRICHOMONIASIS. Trichomoniasis is an infection of the genito-urinary tract caused by *Trichomonas vaginalis* and transmission is usually sexual. In women it causes vaginitis although some are asymptomatic. It is usually asymptomatic in men but may cause urethritis. Patients and their sexual partners should be treated with **metronidazole** or other nitroimidazole.

Diloxanide furoate

Diloxanide furoate is a representative amoebicide. Various drugs can serve as alternatives

Tablets, diloxanide furoate 500 mg

Uses: amoebiasis (asymptomatic carriers in non-endemic areas; eradication of residual luminal amoebae after treatment of invasive disease with other drugs)

Precautions: pregnancy (defer treatment until after first trimester, Appendix 2); breastfeeding (Appendix 3)

Dosage:

Amoebiasis (see above), *by mouth*, ADULT 500 mg 3 times daily for 10 days; CHILD over 25 kg, 20 mg/kg daily in 3 divided doses for 10 days; course may be repeated if necessary

Adverse effects: flatulence; occasionally, vomiting, pruritus and urticaria

---

Metronidazole

Metronidazole is a representative antibacterial and antiprotozoal agent. Various drugs can serve as alternatives

Tablets, metronidazole 200 mg, 250 mg, 400 mg, 500 mg
Oral suspension, metronidazole (as benzoate) 200 mg/5 ml
Intravenous infusion, metronidazole 5 mg/ml, 100-ml bag

Uses: invasive amoebiasis and giardiasis; trichomoniasis; tissue nematode infections (section 6.1.1.3); bacterial infections (section 6.2.2.6); *Helicobacter pylori* eradication (section 17.1)

Contraindications: chronic alcohol dependence

Precautions: disulfiram-like reaction with alcohol; hepatic impairment and hepatic encephalopathy (Appendix 5); pregnancy (Appendix 2; see also notes above); breastfeeding (Appendix 3); clinical and laboratory monitoring in courses lasting longer than 10 days; **interactions:** Appendix 1

Dosage:

Invasive amoebiasis, *by mouth*, ADULT and CHILD 30 mg/kg daily in 3 divided doses for 8–10 days; subsequent course of luminal amoebicide (see notes above)

Invasive amoebiasis (if oral administration not possible), *by intravenous infusion*, ADULT and CHILD 30 mg/kg daily in 3 divided doses (until patient able to complete course with oral drugs); subsequent course of luminal amoebicide (see notes above)

Giardiasis, *by mouth*, ADULT 2 g once daily for 3 days; CHILD 15 mg/kg daily in divided doses for 5–10 days

Urogenital trichomoniasis, *by mouth*, ADULT 2 g as a single dose; sexual partners should be treated concomitantly

NOTE. In amoebiasis and giardiasis, various dosage regimens are used and definitive recommendations should be based on local experience

PATIENT ADVICE. Metronidazole tablets should be swallowed whole with water, during or after a meal; metronidazole suspension should be taken one hour before a meal

Adverse effects: nausea, vomiting, unpleasant metallic taste, furred tongue and gastrointestinal disturbances; rarely headache, drowsiness, dizziness, ataxia, darkening of urine, erythema multiforme, pruritus, urticaria, angioedema, and anaphylaxis; abnormal liver function tests, hepatitis, jaundice, thrombocytopenia, aplastic anaemia, myalgia, arthralgia; peripheral neuropathy, epileptiform seizures, leukopenia, on prolonged or high dosage regimens

6.4.2   Antileishmanial drugs

Leishmaniasis is caused by the protozoa *Leishmania*. It can be categorized as visceral, cutaneous or mucocutaneous. It may be a self-limiting localized skin lesion but may range from this to disseminated progressive disease. In endemic areas there is usually a reservoir of disease in a mammalian host and the usual vectors are sandflies.

VISCERAL LEISHMANIASIS. It is caused by parasites of the *Leishmania donovani* complex, and is usually responsive initially to the **pentavalent antimony compounds, meglumine antimoniate** or **sodium stibogluconate**. Both dosage and duration of treatment need to be adjusted according to the clinical response. Patients are considered to be clinically cured when no parasites are detected in splenic or bone marrow aspirates. However, biopsies should be repeated after 3 and 12 months since relapse is frequent. Antimonials combined with **allopurinol, pentamidine isetionate** and **amphotericin B** have been used with success in patients in relapse who have become unresponsive to antimonials alone.

CUTANEOUS LEISHMANIASIS. It comprises two conditions. The Old World variety is caused by *L. tropica, L. major, L. infantum* and *L. aethiopica*. The New World variety is caused by *L. amazonensis, L. mexicana, L. peruviana, L. guyanensis, L. panamensis* and *L. braziliensis*. These conditions are character-ized by a cell-mediated reaction of varying intensity at the site of inoculation. The New World variety tends to be more severe and slower to heal. Infections caused by *L. major, L. mexicana, L. tropica* and *L. peruviana*, are responsive to intralesional injections of antimonial compounds. Mild lesions can often be left to heal spontaneously. However, it is preferable to treat *L. tropica* infections with a view to reducing transmission since humans seem to be the only host. When the lesion is inflamed or ulcerated or when obstruction of lymphatic drainage or destruction of cartilage creates a risk of serious disfigurement or disability, antimonials should be administered systemically as well as locally. Infections due to *L. braziliensis* and the less common *L. panamensis* should be treated with antimonials because of the risk of mucosal involvement. *L. aethiopica* is less responsive at conventional doses and the sores should be left to heal spontaneously if there is no evidence of diffuse cutaneous involvement. *L. guyanensis* infections should be treated with pentamidine.

MUCOCUTANEOUS LEISHMANIASIS. It is caused by *L. braziliensis* and *L. panamensis*. In this form of the disease the primary lesions do not heal and spread to the mucosa may occur. It usually responds to antimonials and, when relapses occur, more extended courses of treatment are often successful. Patients who still fail to respond should receive **amphotericin B** or **pentamidine isetionate**, although neither treatment is highly satisfactory. Because of resistance to antimonials, *L. aethiopica* infections should be treated with pentamidine from the outset until complete healing occurs.

Emergency use of corticosteroids may be needed to control pharyngeal or tracheal oedema produced by severe inflammation resulting from antigens liberated from dead parasites during the early phase of treatment.

Antibiotics may also be needed to treat secondary infections, and plastic surgery offers the only means of ameliorating disfiguring scars.

DIFFUSE CUTANEOUS LEISHMANIASIS. It usually occurs following infection with *L. aethiopica* or *L. mexicana* and is usually treated with **antimonial compounds**, but relapses must be expected and repeated courses of **pentamidine isetionate** may be needed until clinical immunity becomes established.

Pentavalent antimony compounds

Meglumine antimoniate is a representative pentavalent antimony compound used to treat leishmaniasis; sodium stibogluconate can serve as an alternative

Injection (Solution for injection), pentavalent antimony (as meglumine antimoniate) 85 mg/ml, 5-ml ampoule; pentavalent antimony (as sodium stibogluconate) 100 mg/ml, 100-ml bottle

Uses: leishmaniasis (see notes above)

Contraindications: severe kidney disorders; breastfeeding

Precautions: provide protein-rich diet throughout treatment and, if possible, correct iron and other nutritional deficiencies; renal and hepatic impairment (Appendices 4 and 5); monitor cardiac, renal and hepatic function—reduce dose or withdraw treatment if abnormalities occur; pregnancy—in potentially fatal visceral leishmaniasis, treat without delay; intravenous injections must be given slowly over 5 minutes (to reduce risk of local thrombosis) and stopped if coughing or substernal pain; mucocutaneous disease (see below); treat intercurrent infection (for example pneumonia)

MUCOCUTANEOUS DISEASE. Successful treatment of mucocutaneous leishmaniasis may induce severe inflammation around lesions (may be life-threatening if pharyngeal or tracheal involvement)—may require corticosteroids

Dosage:
NOTE. Doses are expressed in terms of pentavalent antimony

Visceral leishmaniasis, *by intramuscular injection*, ADULT and CHILD 20 mg/kg daily for a minimum of 20 days; if relapse, retreat immediately with same daily dosage

Cutaneous leishmaniasis (except *L. aethiopica*, *L. braziliensis*, *L. amazonensis*), *by intralesional injection*, ADULT and CHILD 1–3 ml into base of lesion; if no apparent response, may be repeated once or twice at intervals of 1–2 days; *by intramuscular injection*, ADULT and CHILD 10–20 mg/kg daily until a few days after clinical cure and negative slit-skin smear; relapse is unusual

Cutaneous leishmaniasis (*L. braziliensis*), *by intramuscular injection*, ADULT and CHILD 20 mg/kg daily, until lesion has healed and for at least 4 weeks; relapse may occur due to inadequate dosage or interrupted treatment; relapse after full course of treatment requires treatment with pentamidine (see below)

Mucocutaneous leishmaniasis (*L. braziliensis*), *by intramuscular injection*, ADULT and CHILD 20 mg/kg daily until slit-skin smears are negative and for at least 4 weeks; if inadequate response or signs of toxicity, 10–15 mg/kg every 12 hours for same period; if relapse, retreat for at least twice as long; if unresponsive to treatment, treat with pentamidine or amphotericin B (see below)

Diffuse cutaneous leishmaniasis (*L. amazonensis*), *by intramuscular injection*, ADULT and CHILD 20 mg/kg daily for several months after clinical improvement occurs; relapse must be expected until immunity develops

ADMINISTRATION. Meglumine antimoniate may be given by deep intramuscular injection. Sodium stibogluconate may be given by intramuscular injection or by slow intravenous injection (over at least 5 minutes). Both may be administered intralesionally

Adverse effects: anorexia, nausea, vomiting, abdominal pain, ECG changes (possibly requiring dose reduction or withdrawal), headache, lethargy, myalgia; raised liver enzymes; renal function impairment; coughing and substernal pain (see Precautions); rarely anaphylaxis, fever, sweating, flushing, vertigo, bleeding from nose or gum, jaundice, rash; pain and thrombosis on intravenous administration; pain on intramuscular injection

---

Pentamidine isetionate

Injection (Powder for solution for injection), pentamidine isetionate 200-mg vial, 300-mg vial

Uses: leishmaniasis (see notes, above); African trypanosomiasis (section 6.4.4.1); *Pneumocystis carinii* pneumonia (section 6.4.5)

Contraindications: severe renal impairment

Precautions: risk of severe hypotension following administration (establish baseline blood pressure and administer with patient lying down); monitor blood pressure during administration and treatment period; hypotension or hypertension; hypoglycaemia or hyperglycaemia; hepatic impairment; leukopenia, thrombocytopenia, anaemia; immunodeficiency—if acute deterioration in bone marrow, renal or pancreatic function, interrupt or discontinue treatment; renal impairment (Appendix 4); pregnancy—in potentially fatal visceral leishmaniasis, treat without delay (Appendix 2); breastfeeding (Appendix 3); carry out laboratory monitoring according to manufacturer's literature

Dosage:

Visceral leishmaniasis (unresponsive to or intolerant of pentavalent antimony compounds), *by deep intramuscular injection or by intravenous infusion*, ADULT and CHILD 4 mg/kg 3 times a week for 5–25 weeks or longer, until two consecutive splenic aspirates taken 14 days apart are negative

Cutaneous leishmaniasis (*L. aethiopica*, *L. guyanensis*), *by deep intramuscular injection or by intravenous infusion*, ADULT and CHILD 3–4 mg/kg once or twice a week until the lesion is no longer visible; relapse is unusual

Diffuse cutaneous leishmaniasis (*L. aethiopica*), *by deep intramuscular injection or by intravenous infusion*, ADULT and CHILD 3–4 mg/kg once a week, continued for at least 4 months after parasites no longer detectable in slit-skin smears; relapse frequent during first few months until immunity established

Mucocutaneous leishmanisais (*L. braziliensis*, *L. aethiopica*), *by deep intramuscular injection or by intravenous infusion*, ADULT and CHILD 4 mg/kg 3 times a week for 5–25 weeks or longer, until lesion no longer visible

RECONSTITUTION AND ADMINISTRATION. According to manufacturer's directions.

NOTE. Pentamidine isetionate is toxic; care required to protect personnel during handling and administration.

Deep intramuscular injection is the WHO preferred route of administration

Adverse effects: nephrotoxicity; acute hypotension—with dizziness, headache, breathlessness, tachycardia and syncope following rapid intravenous injection; hypoglycaemia—may be followed by hyperglycaemia and type I diabetes mellitus; pancreatitis; also hypocalcaemia, gastrointestinal disturbances, confusion, hallucinations, arrhythmias; thrombocytopenia, leukopenia, abnormal liver function tests; anaemia; hyperkalaemia; rash, Stevens-Johnson syndrome, reported; pain, local induration, sterile abscess and muscle necrosis at injection site

---

Amphotericin B

Amphotericin b is a complementary drug for the treatment of leishmaniasis
Injection (Powder for solution for injection), amphotericin B 50-mg vial

Uses: visceral and mucocutaneous leishmaniasis unresponsive to pentavalent antimony compounds; fungal infections (section 6.3)

Precautions: close medical supervision throughout treatment and initial test dose required (see note below); renal impairment (Appendix 4); hepatic and renal function tests; blood counts and plasma electrolyte monitoring; corticoster-

oids (avoid except to control reactions); pregnancy
(Appendix 2); breastfeeding (Appendix 3); avoid rapid
infusion (risk of arrhythmias); **interactions:** Appendix 1

ANAPHYLAXIS. Anaphylaxis occurs rarely with intravenous amphotericin B
and a test dose is advisable before the first infusion. The patient should be
observed for about 30 minutes after the test dose

Dosage:
Visceral and mucocutaneous leishmaniasis (unresponsive to
pentavalent antimony compounds), *by intravenous infusion,*
ADULT initial test dose of 1 mg over 20–30 minutes, then, 5–
10 mg, increased by 5–10 mg daily up to maximum of 0.5–
1 mg/kg, which is then administered on alternate days (total
cumulative dose of 1–3 g usually required)

RECONSTITUTION AND ADMINISTRATION. According to manufacturer's
directions

Adverse effects: fever, headache, anorexia, weight loss, nausea
and vomiting, malaise, diarrhoea, muscle and joint pain,
dyspepsia, and epigastric pain; renal function disturbances
including hypokalaemia, hypomagnesaemia and renal toxicity; blood disorders; cardiovascular toxicity (including
arrhythmias); neurological disorders (including peripheral
neuropathy); abnormal liver function (discontinue treatment);
rash; anaphylactoid reactions (see above); pain and thrombophlebitis at injection site

6.4.3   Antimalarial drugs

Human malaria, which is transmitted by anopheline mosquitoes
(and rarely by congenital transmission, transfusion of infected
blood or use of contaminated syringes among drug addicts), is
caused by four species of plasmodial parasites. *Plasmodium
vivax* is the most extensively distributed and causes much
debilitating disease. *P. falciparum* is also widespread, and
causes the most severe infections which are responsible for
nearly all malaria-related deaths. *P. ovale* is mainly confined to
Africa and is less prevalent, while *P. malariae*, which causes the
least severe but most persistent infections, also occurs widely.

Certain tissue forms of *P. vivax* and *P. ovale* which persist in
the liver for many months and even years are responsible for the
relapses characteristic of malaria. Such latent forms are not
generated by *P. falciparum* or *P. malariae*. Recrudescence of
these infections results from persistent blood forms in
inadequately treated or untreated patients.

Treatment of malaria

Blood schizontocides are the mainstay of the treatment of acute
malaria and some are used for prophylaxis. They include the 4-
aminoquinolines (**chloroquine**), the related arylaminoalcohols
(**mefloquine** and **quinine**), and **artemisinin** and its derivatives
(**artemether** and **artesunate**). They suppress malaria by
destroying the asexual blood forms of the parasites but, because
they are not active against intrahepatic forms, they do not
eliminate infections by *P. vivax* and *P. ovale*.

Some antimetabolites act synergistically when given in combination. For example, **pyrimethamine** in combination with a sulfonamide or sulfone (**sulfadoxine**) and some antibiotics (particularly tetracyclines for example **doxycycline**) are blood schizontocides. Because they act more slowly, these substances are of little value when used alone. The tetracyclines are used primarily as adjuncts to quinine where multiple-drug-resistant *P. falciparum* is prevalent.

Chloroquine, a rapidly acting schizontocide, is well tolerated, safe and inexpensive. It should be used to treat malaria wherever the parasites remain susceptible. *P. malariae* and *P. ovale* remain fully sensitive to chloroquine. However, widespread chloroquine-resistant strains of *P. falciparum* have been reported in south-east Asia, parts of the Indian subcontinent, South America, Africa and Oceania and also strains of *P. vivax* resistant to chloroquine in Papua New Guinea and Indonesia.

A 3-day course by mouth is sufficient to eliminate susceptible *P. falciparum* infections, since effective plasma concentrations are sustained for several weeks.

Parenteral administration may be used when there is no expectation of resistance in cases of severe and complicated malaria, when the patient is unable to take oral medication and when neither quinine nor quinidine are available. The intravenous route is preferred, but it is essential to administer by slow intravenous infusion. Rapid administration (or high dose) can result in cardiovascular toxicity and other potentially fatal symptoms of acute overdose. The intramuscular and subcutaneous routes may be used if facilities for administration by intravenous infusion are not available.

If subsequent relapse occurs in *P. ovale* and *P. vivax* infections **primaquine** should be administered, after a second course of chloroquine, to eliminate the intrahepatic infection.

The combination of **pyrimethamine with sulfadoxine** is recommended for therapeutic use only in areas of high chloroquine resistance. A single dose of pyrimethamine with sulfadoxine is usually sufficient to eliminate infection; quinine should also be given for 3 days in patients in whom quinine may accelerate reduction of parasitaemia and in those patients with risk of fulminating disease. However, resistance to these combinations is now widespread, particularly in south-east Asia and South America and, occurs at low prevalence in east and central Africa. Because sulfonamides can induce hypersensitivity in pregnant women and possible kernicterus in the newborn, quinine should be used, whenever possible, to treat chloroquine-resistant malaria during pregnancy (see note on quinine).

Mefloquine remains effective except in certain areas of resistance in Thailand, Myanmar and Cambodia. No parenteral preparations are currently available, and it is thus suitable only for patients who can take drugs by mouth. It is generally well tolerated, although, some adverse effects have been reported (see notes). However, because of the danger of the emergence of mefloquine-resistant strains of *P. falciparum* and because of its potential toxicity, it should be used only following either microscopic or careful clinical diagnosis of *P. falciparum* infections that are known or strongly suspected to be resistant to chloroquine or sulfadoxine with pyrimethamine.

Quinine, given orally, should be reserved for *P. falciparum* infections likely to be unresponsive to other drugs. Resistance to quinine was, until recently, rare, but the prevalence of resistant strains is now increasing in parts of south-east Asia and South America. Doxycycline, which is an effective oral schizontocide should be given in combination with quinine except in pregnant women and children under 8 years.

In multi-drug resistant malaria, preparations of **artemisinin** or its derivatives (**artemether** or **artesunate**) offer the only prospect of cure. They should not be used in the first trimester of pregnancy. For the treatment of multiresistant falciparum malaria oral **artesunate** may be an effective antimalarial. It should always be given in combination with mefloquine. Parenteral artemether or artesunate, whose use is restricted, are effective alternatives to quinine for the treatment of severe falciparum malaria and are preferred in areas where decreased efficacy of quinine has been documented. To ensure radical cure following parenteral treatment with artemether or oral treatment with artesunate, a full therapeutic dose of mefloquine should be given. A fixed-dose oral formulation of **artemether with lumefantrine** has recently become available and is recommended for the treatment of uncomplicated falciparum malaria in areas with significant resistance. The combination is not for use in pregnancy or breastfeeding.

Trials are ongoing to determine the safety and efficacy of artemisinin with other antimalarials.

Prophylaxis against malaria

No drug regimen gives assured protection to everybody, and indiscriminate use of existing antimalarials increases the risk of inducing resistance.

Chloroquine, which is usually well tolerated at the required dosage, is preferred where *P. falciparum* remains fully sensitive. The recommended prophylactic regimen (see below) has been employed effectively even in areas of marginal resistance. However, it must be started 1 week before exposure, and be maintained in pregnant women until after delivery and for at least 4 weeks after the last risk of exposure in the case of non-immune individuals. This is sufficient to ensure elimination of *P. falciparum* and *P. malariae*, but not of *P. vivax* and *P. ovale*, whose residual hepatic forms survive.

Mefloquine may be used for prophylaxis in areas of high risk or where multiple-drug resistance has been reported. The recommended prophylactic regimen (see notes below) should be started 1 week before exposure and continued for 4 weeks after last exposure. Mefloquine should not be used for prophylaxis during pregnancy. Its therapeutic use has been shown to be safe during the second and third trimesters. However, it should be used in early pregnancy only if alternative drugs are either not available or unlikely to be effective and when it is impracticable for the woman to leave the endemic area.

Proguanil, a predominantly tissue schizontocide with little blood schizontocidal activity, is a causal prophylactic agent since it is active against pre-erythrocytic intrahepatic forms, particularly of *P. falciparum*. The latent persistent liver forms of *P. ovale* and *P. vivax* are unresponsive. However, there is evidence that it may be effective against *P. vivax* only immediately after the initial infection. *P. falciparum* resistance to proguanil or related compounds may occur in malaria endemic areas and particularly where it has been employed in mass prophylaxis. Proguanil is used for prophylaxis with chloroquine in areas where there is resistance to chloroquine but a low risk of infection as it may give some protection against *P. falciparum* and may alleviate symptoms if an attack occurs. Proguanil and chloroquine may also be used prophylactically in areas of high risk or multi-drug resistance as a second choice where mefloquine is not appropriate.

There is no evidence that proguanil is harmful in prophylactic doses during pregnancy. Because of the vulnerablility of pregnant women to falciparum malaria, it should be used at full prophylactic dosage wherever the disease is prevalent and likely to be responsive to proguanil, if chloroquine is not available or with chloroquine, if the latter alone is unlikely to be effective.

Artemether

Artemether is a restricted drug used for the treatment of malaria
Oily injection (Solution for injection) artemether 80 mg/ml, 1-ml ampoule

Uses: treatment of severe *P. falciparum* malaria in areas where evidence that quinine is ineffective

Contraindications: first trimester of pregnancy

Dosage:

Treatment of severe *P. falciparum* malaria (in areas of quinine resistance), *by intramuscular injection*, ADULT and CHILD over 6 months, loading dose of 3.2 mg/kg, then 1.6 mg/kg daily until patient can tolerate oral medication or to maximum of 7 days; this is followed by a single dose of mefloquine 15 mg/kg (or occasionally, if necessary 25 mg/kg) to effect a radical cure
ADMINISTRATION. Since small volumes are required for children, a 1-ml syringe should be used to ensure correct dosage

Adverse effects: headache, nausea, vomiting, abdominal pain, diarrhoea; dizziness, tinnitus, neutropenia, elevated liver enzyme values; cardiotoxicity (after high doses); neurotoxicity—in *animal* studies

Artemether with lumefantrine

Tablets, artemether 20 mg with lumefantrine 120 mg

Uses: treatment of acute uncomplicated malaria due to *Plasmodium falciparum* or mixed infections including *P. falciparum* in areas with significant drug resistance

Contraindications: pregnancy; breastfeeding (Appendix 3); family history of sudden death, congenital prolongation of QTc interval (also see Precautions)

Precautions: ECG required before and during treatment in cardiac disorders including bradycardia, heart failure, history of arrhythmias, QT interval prolongation, electrolyte disturbances, concomitant administration of drugs that prolong QT interval; monitor patients unable to take food (greater risk of recrudescence); severe renal impairment or hepatic impairment; **interactions:** Appendix 1

Dosage:

Treatment of uncomplicated falciparum malaria, *by mouth*, ADULT and CHILD over 12 years and body weight over 35 kg, initially 4 tablets followed by 5 doses of 4 tablets each after 8, 24, 36, 48 and 60 hours (total 24 tablets over 60 hours); CHILD body weight 10–14 kg, initially 1 tablet followed by 5 doses of 1 tablet each after 8, 24, 36, 48 and 60 hours (total 6 tablets over 60 hours); body weight 15–24 kg, initially 2 tablets followed by 5 doses of 2 tablets each after 8, 24, 36, 48 and 60 hours (total 12 tablets over 60 hours); body weight 25–34 kg, initially 3 tablets followed by 5 doses of 3 tablets each after 8, 24, 36, 48 and 60 hours (total 18 tablets over 60 hours)

PATIENT ADVICE. Take tablets with food; repeat dose if vomiting occurs within 1 hour of administration

Adverse effects: abdominal pain, anorexia, diarrhoea, nausea and vomiting; headache, dizziness, sleep disorders; palpitations; arthralgia, myalgia; cough; asthenia, fatigue; pruritus, rash

Artesunate

Artesunate is a restricted drug used for the treatment of malaria

Tablets, artesunate 50 mg

Uses: treatment of uncomplicated *P. falciparum* malaria in areas of multiple-drug resistance

Contraindications: first trimester of pregnancy

Precautions: risk of recurrence if used alone in non-immune patients

Dosage:

Treatment of uncomplicated malaria (in areas of multiple-drug resistance), *by mouth*, ADULT and CHILD over 6 months, 4 mg/kg daily for 3 days; a single dose of mefloquine 15 mg/kg (or occasionally 25 mg/kg, if necessary) is given on day 2 or 3 to effect a radical cure; if artesunate used alone, treat for 7 days

Adverse effects: headache, nausea, vomiting, abdominal pain, diarrhoea, dizziness, tinnitus, neutropenia, elevated liver enzyme values; ECG abnormalities, including prolongation of QT interval; temporary suppression of reticulocyte response and induction of blackwater fever, reported; neurotoxicity—in *animal* studies

Chloroquine

Chloroquine is a representative antimalarial. Various drugs can serve as alternatives

Tablets, chloroquine base (as phosphate or sulfate) 100 mg, 150 mg

Oral syrup, chloroquine base (as phosphate or sulfate) 50 mg/5 ml

Injection (Solution for injection), chloroquine base (as phosphate or sulfate) 40 mg/ml, 5-ml ampoule

Uses: treatment of acute malaria caused by *P. malariae* and susceptible *P. falciparum*; *P. vivax* and *P. ovale* (followed by primaquine to eliminate intrahepatic forms); prophylaxis of malaria for pregnant women and non-immune individuals at risk; rheumatic disorders (section 2.4)

Precautions: if patient continues to deteriorate after chloroquine—suspect resistance and administer quinine intravenously as emergency measure; hepatic impairment; renal impairment (Appendix 4); pregnancy (but in malaria, benefit considered to outweigh risk; Appendix 2); breastfeeding (Appendix 3); may exacerbate psoriasis; neurological disorders (avoid for prophylaxis if history of epilepsy); may aggravate myasthenia gravis; severe gastrointestinal disorders; G6PD deficiency; avoid concurrent therapy with hepatotoxic drugs; **interactions:** Appendix 1

Dosage:

NOTE. All doses are in terms of the base

Treatment of malaria, *by mouth*, ADULT and CHILD 10 mg/kg followed by 5 mg/kg 6–8 hours later; then 5 mg/kg daily on next 2 days (*or* 10 mg/kg for 2 days, followed by 5 mg/kg daily on day 3); total dose, 25 mg/kg over 3 days

PATIENT ADVICE. Oral chloroquine should be taken after meals to minimize nausea and vomiting; if part or all a dose is vomited, the same amount must be immediately readministered

Treatment of malaria (in patients unable to take chloroquine by mouth), *by very slow intravenous infusion* (over at least 8 hours), ADULT and CHILD 10 mg/kg as an initial dose, then 2 further infusions of 5 mg/kg at 8-hour intervals (as soon as patient is able to take chloroquine by mouth, discontinue infusions and complete the course with oral preparations total dose, 25 mg/kg over 3 days); *by intramuscular or by subcutaneous injection* (when intravenous infusion facilities not available) ADULT and CHILD 2.5 mg/kg every 4 hours *or* 3.5 mg/kg every 6 hours (until total dose of 25 mg/kg administered)

Prophylaxis of malaria, *by mouth*, ADULT 300 mg once a week; CHILD 5 mg/kg once a week

PATIENT ADVICE. Warn travellers about importance of avoiding mosquito bites, importance of taking prophylaxis regularly, and importance of immediate visit to doctor if ill within 1 year and especially within 3 months of return

DILUTION AND ADMINISTRATION. According to manufacturer's directions. Avoid rapid parenteral administration (risk of toxic plasma concentrations and fatal cardiovascular collapse)

Adverse effects: headache, gastrointestinal disturbances; also convulsions; visual disturbances (retinopathy associated with long-term, high dose therapy or inappropriate self-medication); depigmentation or loss of hair; rashes; pruritus—may become intolerable; bone-marrow suppression; atrioventricular block (may be result of inappropriate self-medication); porphyria and psoriasis in susceptible individuals

Doxycycline

Doxycycline is a representative antimalarial tetracycline. Various drugs can serve as alternatives

Doxycycline is a complementary drug for the treatment of malaria

Capsules, doxycycline (as hydrochloride) 100 mg

Uses: supplement to quinine in treatment of multiple-drug resistant *P. falciparum* malaria (where quinine resistance, in cases of hypersensitivity to sulfonamides); short-term prophylaxis of multiple-drug resistant *P. falciparum* malaria; bacterial infections (section 6.2.2.3)

Contraindications: pregnancy (Appendix 2); children under 8 years; porphyria; systemic lupus erythematosus

Precautions: avoid exposure to sunlight or sunlamps—photosensitivity reported; hepatic impairment (Appendix 5); breast-feeding (Appendix 3); **interactions:** Appendix 1

Dosage:

Supplement to malaria treatment (see notes above), *by mouth*, ADULT and CHILD over 8 years, 100 mg twice daily for 7–10 days

Short-term prophylaxis of malaria, *by mouth*, ADULT 100 mg daily for up to 8 weeks; CHILD over 8 years, 1.5 mg/kg daily for up to 8 weeks; doxycycline should be started on the day before exposure and continued for 4 weeks after last risk of exposure

PATIENT ADVICE. Capsules should be swallowed whole with plenty of fluid while sitting or standing to prevent oesophageal irritation. May be given with food or milk, to counter gastric irritation

Adverse effects: gastrointestinal disturbances; erythema (discontinue treatment); photosensitivity; headache and visual disturbances; hepatotoxicity, pancreatitis and antibiotic-associated colitis reported; staining of growing teeth and occasional dental hypoplasia

Mefloquine

Mefloquine is a complementary drug for the treatment of malaria

Tablets, mefloquine (as hydrochloride) 250 mg

Uses: treatment of uncomplicated malaria due to multiple-resistant *P. falciparum*; treatment of severe and complicated malaria, after quinine; adjunct to treatment with artemisinin and derivatives; prophylaxis of malaria for travellers to areas where high risk of multiple-resistant *P. falciparum*

Contraindications: prophylaxis in first trimester of pregnancy (Appendix 2); history of neuropsychiatric disorders or convulsions; hypersensitivity to quinine

Precautions: exclude pregnancy before starting prophylaxis (see also Contraindications); cardiac conduction disorders; avoid for prophylaxis in severe hepatic impairment (Appendix 5) and in epilepsy; not recommended for infants under 3 months (5 kg); breastfeeding (Appendix 3); **interactions:** Appendix 1

SKILLED TASKS. May impair ability to perform skilled tasks, for example operating machinery, driving; effects may persist for up to 3 weeks

Dosage:
NOTE. All doses are in terms of the base

Treatment of malaria, *by mouth*, ADULT and CHILD 15 mg/kg (up to maximum of 1 g) as a single dose

Prophylaxis of malaria, *by mouth*, ADULT 250 mg once a week; CHILD over 15 kg, 5 mg/kg once a week; prophylaxis should start at least 1 week before departure and continue for 4 weeks after last exposure

Adverse effects: nausea, vomiting, diarrhoea, abdominal pain, anorexia, headache, dizziness (can be severe), loss of balance, somnolence, insomnia and abnormal dreams; neurological and psychiatric disturbances including sensory and motor neuropathies, tremor, ataxia, visual disturbances, tinnitus, vestibular disorders; convulsions, anxiety, depression, confusion, hallucinations, panic attacks, emotional instability, aggression, agitation and psychoses; circulatory disorders, tachycardia, bradycardia, cardiac conduction disorders; muscle weakness, myalgia, arthralgia; rash, urticaria, pruritus, alopecia; disturbances in liver function tests, leukopenia, leucocytosis, thrombocytopenia; rarely, Stevens-Johnson syndrome, atrioventricular block and encephalopathy

Primaquine
Tablets, primaquine (as phosphate) 7.5 mg, 15 mg

Uses: elimination of intrahepatic forms of *P. vivax* and *P. ovale* (after standard chloroquine therapy); elimination of gametocytes of *P. falciparum* (after routine therapy with a blood schizontocide)

Contraindications: pregnancy (treatment with primaquine should be delayed until after delivery; Appendix 2); breastfeeding (Appendix 3); conditions that predispose to granulocytopenia (including active rheumatoid arthritis and lupus erythematosus)

Precautions: monitor blood count; if methaemoglobinaemia or haemolysis occurs, withdraw treatment and consult physician; G6PD deficiency (exclude before radical treatment for *P. vivax* and *P. ovale*, but not before single dose gametocytocidal treatment)

Dosage:
NOTE. All doses are in terms of the base

Radical treatment of *P. vivax* and *P. ovale* malaria (after standard chloroquine therapy), *by mouth*, ADULT 250 micrograms/kg daily (*or* 15 mg daily) for 14 days; CHILD 250 micrograms/kg daily for 14 days; in G6PD deficiency, ADULT 750 micrograms/kg once a week for 8 weeks; CHILD 500–750 micrograms/kg once a week for 8 weeks

Gametocytocidal treatment of *P. falciparum* (after routine blood schizontocide therapy), *by mouth*, ADULT and CHILD 500–750 micrograms/kg as a single dose

Adverse effects: anorexia, nausea and vomiting, abdominal pain; acute haemolytic anaemia (frequently in G6PD deficiency); rarely, methaemoglobinaemia, haemoglobinuria, agranulocytosis, granulocytopenia and leukopenia

---

Proguanil hydrochloride
Tablets, proguanil hydrochloride 100 mg

Uses: with chloroquine, prophylaxis of malaria in areas of low resistance

Contraindications: use in areas of known resistance to either proguanil or pyrimethamine

Precautions: renal impairment (Appendix 4); pregnancy (folate supplements required, Appendix 2); breastfeeding (Appendix 3); **interactions:** Appendix 1

Dosage:

Prophylaxis of malaria, *by mouth*, ADULT 200 mg daily, after food; CHILD under 1 year, 25 mg daily; CHILD 1–4 years, 50 mg daily; CHILD 5–8 years, 100 mg daily; CHILD 9–14 years, 150 mg daily

PATIENT ADVICE. Warn travellers about the importance of avoiding mosquito bites, importance of taking prophylaxis regularly, and importance of immediate visit to doctor if ill within 1 year and especially within 3 months of return

Adverse effects: mild gastric intolerance, diarrhoea; occasional mouth ulcers and stomatitis; skin reactions and hair loss reported

---

Pyrimethamine with sulfadoxine
Pyrimethamine with sulfadoxine is a representative antimalarial drug combination. Various drugs can serve as alternatives

Pyrimethamine with sulfadoxine are complementary drugs for the treatment of malaria

Tablets, pyrimethamine 25 mg with sulfadoxine 500 mg

Uses: treatment of malaria due to susceptible *P. falciparum* in areas of high chloroquine resistance and in patients who have not responded to chloroquine; additionally quinine may be given for 3 days (see notes above)

Contraindications: hypersensitivity to sulfonamides or pyrimethamine; severe hepatic or renal impairment (except where no alternative treatment available)

Precautions: avoid in blood disorders—unless specialist supervision; discontinue immediately if blood disorder occurs; rash, sore throat, mouth ulcers, or shortness of breath—withdraw treatment; G6PD deficiency; pregnancy (Appendix 2); breastfeeding (Appendix 3); **interactions:** Appendix 1

Dosage:

Treatment of malaria due to susceptible *P. falciparum* (see notes above), *by mouth*, ADULT pyrimethamine 75 mg with sulfadoxine 1.5 g (3 tablets) as a single dose; CHILD 5–10 kg, half tablet; 11–20 kg, 1 tablet; 21–30 kg, 1½ tablets; 31–45 kg, 2 tablets, as a single dose

Adverse effects: rashes, pruritus, slight hair loss; rarely Stevens-Johnson syndrome and toxic epidermal necrolysis; gastrointestinal disturbances including nausea, vomiting, stomatitis; rarely, hepatitis, leukopenia, thrombocytopenia, megaloblastic anaemia and purpura—withdraw treatment; fatigue, headache, fever, polyneuritis, also reported; pulmonary infiltrates such as eosinophilic or allergic alveolitis—if symptoms of cough or shortness of breath—withdraw treatment

---

Quinine

Quinine is a representative antimalarial. Various drugs can serve as alternatives

Tablets, quinine sulfate 300 mg; quinine bisulfate 300 mg

Injection (Solution for dilution for infusion), quinine dihydrochloride 300 mg/ml, 2-ml ampoule

Uses: multiple-drug resistant *P. falciparum* malaria

Contraindications: haemoglobinuria; optic neuritis; tinnitus

Precautions: atrial fibrillation, conduction defects, heart block; monitor for signs of cardiac toxicity and blood glucose levels (with intravenous use); pregnancy (but appropriate for treatment of malaria, Appendix 2); renal impairment (Appendix 4); G6PD deficiency; may aggravate myasthenia gravis; **interactions:** Appendix 1

Dosage:

NOTE. Quinine (anhydrous base) 100 mg ≡ quinine bisulfate 169 mg ≡ quinine dihydrochloride 122 mg ≡ quinine sulfate 121 mg

Quinine bisulfate 300 mg tablets provide *less* quinine than 300 mg of the sulfate or dihydrochloride

Treatment of multiple-drug resistant *P. falciparum* malaria, *by mouth*, ADULT 600 mg (quinine sulfate) every 8 hours for 3, 7, or 10 days; CHILD 10 mg/kg (quinine sulfate) every 8 hours for 3, 7, or 10 days; duration of treatment depends on local susceptibility of *P. falciparum* and whether or not additional antimalarials also used

PATIENT ADVICE. If all or part of a dose is vomited within one hour, the same amount must be readministered immediately

---

Treatment of multiple-drug resistant *P. falciparum* malaria (in patients unable to take quinine by mouth), *by slow intravenous infusion* (over 4 hours), ADULT 20 mg/kg (quinine dihydrochloride) followed by 10 mg/kg (quinine dihydrochloride) every 8 hours; CHILD 20 mg/kg (quinine dihydrochloride) followed by 10 mg/kg (quinine dihydrochloride) every 12 hours; initial dose should be halved in patients who have received quinine, quinidine or mefloquine during the previous 12–24 hours

DILUTION AND ADMINISTRATION. According to manufacturer's directions; intravenous injection of quinine is so hazardous that it has been superceded by infusion; where facilities for intravenous infusion are unavailable, an appropriate dilution may be administered by intramuscular injection

Adverse effects: cinchonism (tinnitus, headache, blurred vision, altered auditory acuity, nausea, diarrhoea, hot and flushed skin, rashes, confusion); hypersensitivity reactions including angioedema; rarely haemorrhage and asthma; hypoglycaemia (especially after parenteral administration); renal damage (culminating in acute renal failure and anuria); blood disorders; cardiovascular, gastrointestinal and CNS effects; very toxic in overdosage—immediate medical attention required

6.4.4   Antitrypanosomal drugs

6.4.4.1   African trypanosomiasis

African trypanosomiasis, or sleeping sickness, is a protozoan infection transmitted by *Glossina* spp. (tsetse flies). Two subspecies of *Trypanosoma brucei*—*T. brucei gambiense* and *T. brucei rhodesiense*—produce distinctive clinical forms of the disease. The early stage of African trypanosomiasis results from infection of the blood stream and lymph nodes. The late meningoencephalitic stage results from infection of the central nervous system. Signs of the later stage develop within a few weeks in *T. b. rhodesiense* infection but only after several months or years in *T. b. gambiense* infection.

Treatment of early-stage infections of *T. b. rhodesiense* with **suramin sodium** and *T. b. gambiense* with **pentamidine isetionate** can be curative if started before the central nervous system has become involved. In areas where pentamidine resistance occurs, suramin sodium may be used for *T. b. gambiense* infection. **Melarsoprol** is used for confirmed cases of *T. b. gambiense* or *T. b. rhodesiense* with meningoencephalitic involvement. Several treatment regimens for adults and children are currently used in the absence of clear evidence that one is better than another. Most treatment regimens have low starting doses (especially for children and debilitated patients), increasing to a maximum of 3.6 mg/kg daily. It is given in short courses of 3–4 days with an interval of 7–10 days between courses. A severe febrile reaction may occur after the first injection, especially if patients have a large number of trypanosomes in their blood; therefore, suramin or pentamidine are often given before starting melarsoprol treatments. An increasing number of melarsoprol treatment failures have been reported in the last years in several countries. **Eflornithine** is an alternative drug which has been shown to be both effective and considerably less toxic than melarsoprol in patients with meningoencephalopathy resulting from *T. b. gambiense* trypanosomiasis.

Melarsoprol

Injection (Solution for injection), melarsoprol 3.6% in propylene glycol

Uses: treatment of meningoencephalitic stage of *T. b. gambiense* or *T. b. rhodesiense* infections

Contraindications: pregnancy; avoid use during influenza epidemics

Precautions: hospitalization and close medical supervision required throughout treatment; episodes of reactive encephalopathy (may require treatment suspension); treat intercurrent infections such as pneumonia and malaria before malarsoprol administration; malnutrition (if possible, correct with protein-rich diet); G6PD deficiency; leprosy—may precipitate erythema nodosum

Dosage:

Treatment of *T. b. gambiense* and *T. b. rhodesiense* with meningoencephalitic involvement (see notes above and table below), *by slow intravenous injection*, ADULT and CHILD dose gradually increased to maximum of 3.6 mg/kg daily in courses of 3–4 days with intervals of 7–10 days between courses

ADMINISTRATION. Injection very irritant—avoid extravasation. Patients should remain supine and fasting for at least 5 hours after injection

Adverse effects: fatal reactive encephalopathy characterized by headache, tremor, slurred speech, convulsions and ultimately coma (in 3–8% of patients, usually at end of first 3–4 days of treatment); myocardial damage; albuminuria; hypertension; hypersensitivity reactions; agranulocytosis; dose-related renal and hepatic impairment; hyperthermia, urticaria, headache, diarrhoea and vomiting—in late stage of treatment

Pentamidine isetionate

Injection (Powder for solution for injection), pentamidine isetionate 200-mg vial, 300-mg vial

Uses: treatment of haemolymphatic stage of *T. b. gambiense* infection; adjunct to melarsoprol in meningoencephalitic stage of *T. b. gambiense* infection; leishmaniasis (section 6.4.2); *Pneumocystis carinii* pneumonia (section 6.4.5)

Contraindications: severe renal impairment; *T. b. rhodesiense* infection (since primary resistance observed)

Precautions: cerebrospinal fluid examination before treatment (pentamidine not likely to be effective if leukocyte count greater then 5 cells/mm^3, total protein greater then 37 mg/100 ml, or trypanosomes detected in centrifuge deposits); risk of severe hypotension following administration (establish baseline blood pressure and administer with patient lying down); monitor blood pressure during administration and treatment period; hypotension or hypertension; hepatic impairment; hypoglycaemia or hyperglycaemia; leukopenia; thrombocytopenia; anaemia; immunodeficiency—if acute deterioration in bone marrow, renal or pancreatic function, interrupt or discontinue treatment; renal impairment (Appendix 4); pregnancy—should not be withheld, even if evidence of meningoencephalitic involvement, as melarsoprol contraindicated (Appendix 2); breastfeeding (Appendix 3)

Dosage:

Treatment of haemolymphatic stage of *T. b. gambiense* infection, *by intramuscular injection*, ADULT and CHILD 4 mg/kg daily *or* on alternate days for a total of 7–10 doses

Treatment of meningoencephalitic stage of *T. b. gambiense* (prior to melarsoprol), *by intramuscular injection*, ADULT and CHILD 4 mg/kg daily on days one and two

RECONSTITUTION AND ADMINISTRATION. According to manufacturer's directions. Pentamidine isetionate is toxic; care is required to protect personnel during handling and administration

Adverse effects: nephrotoxicity; acute hypotension, hypoglycaemia—may be followed by hyperglycaemia and type I diabetes mellitus; pancreatitis; also hypocalcaemia, gastrointestinal disturbances, confusion, hallucinations, arrhythmias; thrombocytopenia, leukopenia, abnormal liver function tests; anaemia; hyperkalaemia; rash, Stevens-Johnson syndrome reported; pain, local induration, sterile abscess and muscle necrosis at injection site

---

Suramin sodium

Injection (Powder for solution for injection), suramin sodium 1-g vial

Uses: treatment of haemolymphatic stage of *T. b. gambiense* and *T. b. rhodesiense* infections; adjunct to melarsoprol in meningoencephalitic stage of *T. b. gambiense* and *T. b. rhodesiense* infections; onchocerciasis (section 6.1.2.3)

Contraindications: previous anaphylaxis or suramin sensitivity; severe liver or renal function impairment; elderly or debilitated

Precautions: administer only under close medical supervision in hospital and with general condition improved as far as possible before treatment; first dose—possible loss of consciousness (see under Dosage, below); maintain satisfactory food and fluid intake during treatment; urine tests before and weekly during treatment—reduce dose if moderate albuminuria, discontinue immediately if severe albuminuria or casts in urine; pregnancy—should not be withheld, even if evidence of meningoencephalitic involvement, as melarsoprol contraindicated

Dosage:

Treatment of haemolymphatic *T. b. gambiense* and *T. b. rhodesiense* infections, *by slow intravenous injection*, ADULT and CHILD 5 mg/kg on day 1, 10 mg/kg on day 3 and 20 mg/kg on days 5, 11, 17, 23 and 30

Treatment of meningoencephalitic *T. b. gambiense* and *T. b. rhodesiense* infections (prior to melarsoprol), *by slow intravenous injection*, ADULT and CHILD 5 mg/kg on day 1, 10 mg/kg on day 3 and in some regimens, 20 mg/kg on day 5

RECONSTITUTION OF INJECTION. Reconstitute in water for injections to produce a final concentration of 10%

FIRST (TEST) DOSE. Administer first dose with particular caution; wait at least 1 minute after injecting the first few microlitres; inject next 0.5 ml over 30 seconds and wait one minute; inject the remainder over several minutes

Adverse effects: rarely, immediate and potentially fatal reaction with nausea, vomiting, shock and loss of consciousness during first dose—see First (Test) Dose, above; albuminuria; abdominal pain; severe diarrhoea; stomal ulceration; exfoliative dermatitis; fever; tiredness; anorexia; malaise; polyuria; thirst; raised liver enzyme values; paraesthesia and hyperaesthesia of palms and soles

---

Eflornithine hydrochloride

Eflornithine hydrochloride is a complementary drug

Infusion (Solution for dilution for infusion), eflornithine hydrochloride 200 mg/ml, 100-ml ampoule

Uses: treatment of haemolymphatic and meningoencephalitic stages of *T. b. gambiense* infection

Contraindications: pregnancy; breastfeeding

Precautions: hospitalization and close supervision throughout treatment; blood and lymph node aspirates examined daily until trypanosome negative for two consecutive days, then weekly during treatment; examination for leukocytes, total protein content and trypanosome presence in CSF after course of treatment and at intervals for following 24 months; renal impairment (Appendix 4)

Dosage:

Treatment of *T. b. gambiense* infections, *by intravenous infusion*, ADULT 100 mg/kg over 45 minutes, every 6 hours for at least 14 days; if relapse occurs, repeat course of treatment

DILUTION AND ADMINISTRATION. According to manufacturer's directions

Adverse effects: diarrhoea, anaemia, leukopenia, thrombocytopenia and convulsions; impaired hearing reported; vomiting, anorexia, alopecia, abdominal pain, headache, facial oedema, eosinophilia and dizziness—less common and reversible on treatment withdrawal

Treatment schedules (adults and children) for African trypanosomiasis with meningoencephalitic involvement[1]

Day	Drug	Dose (mg/kg)
For *T. b. rhodesiense* infection, as used in Kenya and Zambia		
1	suramin	5.00
3	suramin	10.00
5	suramin	20.00
7	melarsoprol	0.36
8	melarsoprol	0.72
9	melarsoprol	1.10
16	melarsoprol	1.40
17	melarsoprol	1.80
18	melarsoprol	1.80
25	melarsoprol	2.20
26	melarsoprol	2.90
27	melarsoprol	3.60
34	melarsoprol	3.60
35	melarsoprol	3.60
36	melarsoprol	3.60
For *T. b rhodesiense* infection, as used in Uganda and the United Republic of Tanzania		
1	suramin	5.00
3	suramin	10.00
5	melarsoprol	1.80
6	melarsoprol	2.20
7	melarsoprol	2.56
14	melarsoprol	2.56
15	melarsoprol	2.90
16	melarsoprol	3.26
23	melarsoprol	3.60
24	melarsoprol	3.60
25	melarsoprol	3.60
For *T. b. gambiense* infection, as used in Côte d' Ivoire		
1	pentamidine i.m	4.00
2	pentamidine i.m	4.00
4	melarsoprol	1.20
5	melarsoprol	2.40
6	melarsoprol	3.60
17	melarsoprol	1.20
18	melarsoprol	2.40
19	melarsoprol	3.60
20	melarsoprol	3.60
30	melarsoprol	1.20
31	melarsoprol	2.40
32	melarsoprol	3.60
33	melarsoprol	3.60

[1] All doses i.v. unless otherwise stated

6.4.4.2 American trypanosomiasis

American trypanosomiasis (Chagas disease) is caused by the protozoan parasite *Trypanosoma cruzi* which are carried by reduviid or triatomine bugs which feed on human blood. The acute febrile phase of the disease frequently passes unrecognized. Occasionally, however, infection follows a fulminating course terminating in a fatal myocarditis and meningoencephalitis. In about half of the surviving cases, and after a latent interval ranging from 10 to more than 20 years, chronic myopathy degeneration results in arrhythmias, cardiac enlargement and less, frequently, oesophageal and colonic dilatation. At this stage, only symptomatic treatment is of benefit.

At present the only therapeutic agents of value are **benznidazole** and **nifurtimox**. Both suppress parasitaemia and are efficacious during the early stages of infection.

Safe use of both drugs in pregnancy has not been established and treatment should be deferred until after the first trimester. They should be instituted immediately to avoid the risk of congenital transmission.

Studies are in progress to determine whether benznidazole and nifurtimox have any influence on the later manifestations of the disease. Symptomatic treatment may be necessary in advanced cases.

Benznidazole

Tablets, benznidazole 100 mg

Uses: acute American trypanosomiasis (Chagas disease)

Contraindications: early pregnancy

Precautions: hepatic, renal or haematological insufficiency—require close medical supervision; monitor blood count, especially leukocytes, throughout treatment

Dosage:

Acute American trypanosomiasis (Chagas disease), *by mouth*, ADULT 5–7 mg/kg daily in two divided doses for 60 days; CHILD up to 12 years 10 mg/kg daily in two divided doses for 60 days

Adverse effects: rashes—if severe and accompanied by fever and purpura, discontinue treatment; nausea, vomiting and abdominal pain; dose-related paraesthesia and peripheral neuritis—discontinue treatment; leukopenia and rarely, agranulocytosis

Nifurtimox

Tablets, nifurtimox 30 mg, 120 mg, 250 mg

Uses: acute American trypanosomiasis (Chagas disease)

Contraindications: early pregnancy

Precautions: history of convulsions or psychiatric disease—requires close medical supervision; avoid alcohol—to reduce incidence and severity of adverse effects; co-administer aluminium hydroxide to reduce gastrointestinal irritation

Dosage:

Acute American trypanosomiasis (Chagas disease), *by mouth*, ADULT 8–10 mg/kg daily in 3 divided doses for 90 days; CHILD 15–20 mg/kg daily in 4 divided doses for 90 days

Adverse effects: anorexia, loss of weight, nausea, vomiting, gastric pain, insomnia, headache, vertigo, excitability, myalgia, arthralgia, convulsions—dose-related, reduce dose; peripheral neuritis—may require discontinuation; rashes and other allergic reactions

6.4.5 Antipneumocystosis and antitoxoplasmosis drugs

PNEUMOCYSTOSIS. *Pneumocystis carinii* is classified as a protozoan although there is evidence to suggest that it is probably a fungus. *Pneumocystis carinii* pneumonia is probably acquired by the airborne route. In otherwise healthy persons it rarely produces signs of infection. However, it is a frequent cause of opportunistic infection in immunosuppressed, debilitated or malnourished patients; it is the commonest cause of pneumonia in AIDS and the most frequent immediate cause of death in these patients.

Sulfamethoxazole with **trimethoprim** is the treatment of choice for *Pneumocystis carinii* pneumonia and is also used for prophylaxis in high-risk patients; **pentamidine isetionate** is used in patients unresponsive to or intolerant of sulfamethoxazole with trimethoprim.

The treatment of *Pneumocystis carinii* infections must only be undertaken with specialist supervision where there are appropriate monitoring facilities.

TOXOPLASMOSIS. Toxoplasmosis is caused by infection with the protozoan parasite *Toxoplasma gondii*. Most infections are self-limiting and do not require treatment. However, in immunodeficiency, primary infection may result in encephalitis, myocarditis or pneumonitis; impairment of immunity (such as occurs in AIDS) in a previously infected person, may result in encephalitis or meningoencephalitis. Congenital transmission may occur if there is a primary infection in early pregnancy or if the mother is immunodeficient. Such cases often result in spontaneous abortion, fetal death or severe congenital disease. Ocular toxoplasmosis causes chorioretinitis and is often the result of a childhood infection that becomes apparent in adulthood.

The treatment of choice for toxoplasmosis is **pyrimethamine** with **sulfadiazine**; a folate supplement is also given to counteract the megaloblastic anaemia associated with these drugs.

Sulfamethoxazole with trimethoprim

Tablets, sulfamethoxazole 400 mg with trimethoprim 80 mg; sulfamethoxazole 800 mg with trimethoprim 160 mg

Oral suspension, sulfamethoxazole 200 mg with trimethoprim 40 mg/5 ml

Injection (Solution for dilution for infusion), sulfamethoxazole 80 mg with trimethoprim 16 mg/ml, 5-ml and 10-ml ampoules

Uses: *Pneumocystis carinii* pneumonia; bacterial infections (section 6.2.2.9)

Contraindications: hypersensitivity to sulfonamides or tri-methoprim; severe hepatic or renal failure; porphyria

Precautions: renal and hepatic impairment (Appendices 4 and 5); maintain adequate fluid intake (to avoid crystalluria; avoid in blood disorders (unless under specialist supervision); monitor blood counts and discontinue immediately if blood disorder develops; rash—discontinue immediately; elderly; asthma; G6PD deficiency; folate deficiency; pregnancy (Appendix 2); breastfeeding (Appendix 3); **interactions:** Appendix 1

Dosage:

Treatment of *Pneumocystis carinii* pneumonia (see notes above), *by mouth or by intravenous infusion*, ADULT and CHILD sulfamethoxazole up to 100 mg/kg daily with trimethoprim up to 20 mg/kg daily in 2–4 divided doses for 14–21 days

Prophylaxis of *Pneumocystis carinii* pneumonia (see notes above), *by mouth*, ADULT and CHILD sulfamethoxazole 25 mg/kg with trimethoprim 5 mg/kg in 2 divided doses on alternate days (3 times a week)

DILUTION AND ADMINISTRATION. According to manufacturer's directions

Adverse effects: nausea, vomiting, diarrhoea, headache; hypersensitivity reactions including rashes, pruritus, photo-sensitivity reactions, exfoliative dermatitis and erythema nodosum; rarely, erythema multiforme and toxic epidermal necrolysis; crystalluria—resulting in haematuria, oliguria, anuria; blood disorders including granulocytopenia, agranulo-cytosis, aplastic anaemia, purpura—discontinue immediately; also reported, liver damage, pancreatitis, antibiotic-associated colitis, eosinophilia, cough and shortness of breath, pulm-onary infiltrates, aseptic meningitis, depression, convulsions, ataxia, tinnitus, and electrolyte disturbances; megaloblastic anaemia due to trimethoprim

---

Pentamidine isetionate

Injection (Powder for solution for injection), pentamidine isetionate 200-mg vial, 300-mg vial

Nebulizer solution, pentamidine isetionate 300-mg bottle

Uses: *Pneumocystis carinii* pneumonia; leishmaniasis (section 6.4.2); African trypanosomiasis (section 6.4.4.1)

Contraindications: severe renal impairment

Precautions: risk of severe hypotension following administra-tion (establish baseline blood pressure and administer with patient lying down); monitor blood pressure during admin-istration and treatment period; hypotension or hypertension; hypoglycaemia or hyperglycaemia; hepatic impairment; renal impairment (Appendix 4); leukopenia, thrombocytopenia, anaemia; immunodeficiency—if acute deterioration in bone marrow, renal or pancreatic function, interrupt or discontinue treatment; pregnancy—in potentially fatal *P. carinii* pneu-monia, treat without delay (Appendix 2); breastfeeding (Appendix 3); carry out laboratory monitoring according to manufacturer's literature

Dosage:

Treatment of *P. carinii* pneumonia (see notes above), *by slow intravenous infusion or by deep intramuscular injection*, ADULT and CHILD 4 mg/kg daily for at least 14 days

Prophylaxis of *P.carinii* pneumonia (see notes above), *by slow intravenous infusion*, ADULT and CHILD 4 mg/kg once every 4 weeks *or by inhalation of nebulized solution*, ADULT 300 mg as a single dose once every 4 weeks; CHILD 4 mg/kg as a single dose once every 4 weeks

RECONSTITUTION AND ADMINISTRATION. According to manufacturer's directions. Pentamidine isetionate is toxic; care is required to protect personnel during handling and administration

Adverse effects: nephrotoxicity; acute hypotension—with dizziness, headache, breathlessness, tachycardia and syncope following rapid intravenous injection; hypoglycaemia—may be followed by hyperglycaemia and type I diabetes mellitus; pancreatitis; also hypocalcaemia, gastrointestinal disturbances, confusion, hallucinations, arrhythmias; thrombocytopenia, leukopenia, abnormal liver function tests; anaemia; hyperkalaemia; rash, Stevens-Johnson syndrome reported; pain, local induration, sterile abscess and muscle necrosis at injection site

Pyrimethamine

Tablets, pyrimethamine 25 mg, 50 mg

Uses: toxoplasmosis (with sulfadiazine); malaria (with sulfadoxine) (section 6.4.3)

Contraindications: hepatic and renal impairment

Precautions: pregnancy (avoid in first trimester but give in later pregnancy if danger of congenital transmission; Appendix 2); breastfeeding (Appendix 3); blood counts required with prolonged treatment; folate supplements throughout treatment; **interactions:** Appendix 1

Dosage:

Toxoplasmosis (in second and third trimesters of pregnancy), *by mouth*, ADULT 25 mg daily for 3–4 weeks

Toxoplasmosis in neonates, *by mouth*, NEONATE 1 mg/kg daily; duration of treatment depends on whether neonate has overt disease—continue for 6 months, or is without overt disease but, born to mother infected during pregnancy—treat for 4 weeks, followed by further courses if infection confirmed

Toxoplasmosis in immunodeficiency, *by mouth*, ADULT 200 mg in divided doses on first day, then 75–100 mg daily for at least 6 weeks, followed by a suppressive dose of 25–50 mg daily

Chorioretinitis, *by mouth*, ADULT 75 mg daily for 3 days then 25 mg daily for 4 weeks; in unresponsive patients, 50 mg daily for a further 4 weeks

NOTE. For the treatment of toxoplasmosis, pyrimethamine must always be taken with sulfadiazine (see below)

Adverse effects: depression of haematopoiesis with high doses; megaloblastic anaemia; rashes; insomnia; gastrointestinal disturbances

Sulfadiazine

Tablets, sulfadiazine 500 mg

Uses: toxoplasmosis (with pyrimethamine); rheumatic fever (section 6.2.2.9)

Contraindications: hypersensitivity to sulfonamides; severe renal failure (Appendix 4) or severe hepatic impairment; porphyria

Precautions: hepatic and renal impairment; maintain adequate fluid intake (to avoid crystalluria); avoid in blood disorders (unless under specialist supervision); monitor blood counts and discontinue immediately if blood disorder develops; rashes—discontinue immediately; elderly; asthma; G6PD deficiency; pregnancy—avoid in first trimester, but may be given thereafter if danger of congenital transmission (Appendix 2); breastfeeding (Appendix 3); **interactions:** Appendix 1

Dosage:

Toxoplasmosis (in second and third trimesters of pregnancy), *by mouth*, ADULT 3 g daily in 4 divided doses

Toxoplasmosis in neonates, *by mouth*, NEONATE 85 mg/kg daily in 2 divided doses; duration of treatment depends on whether the neonate has overt disease—continue for 6 months, or is without overt disease but born to mother infected during pregnancy—treat for 4 weeks, followed by further courses, if infection confirmed

Toxoplasmosis in immunodeficiency, *by mouth*, ADULT 4–6 g daily in 4 divided doses for at least 6 weeks, followed by a suppressive dose of 2–4 g daily

Chorioretinitis, *by mouth*, ADULT 2 g daily in 4 divided doses

NOTE. For the treatment of toxoplasmosis, sulfadiazine must always be taken with pyrimethamine (see above)

Adverse effects: nausea, vomiting, diarrhoea, headache; hypersensitivity reactions including rashes, pruritus, photosensitivity reactions, exfoliative dermatitis, and erythema nodosum; rarely, erythema multiforme and toxic epidermal necrolysis; crystalluria—resulting in haematuria, oliguria, anuria; blood disorders including granulocytopenia, agranulocytosis, aplastic anaemia, purpura—discontinue immediately; also reported, liver damage, pancreatitis, antibiotic-associated colitis, eosinophilia, cough and shortness of breath, pulmonary infiltrates, aseptic meningitis, depression, convulsions, ataxia, tinnitus, and electrolyte disturbances

6.5 Antiviral drugs

6.5.1 Herpes and cytomegalovirus infections

HERPES SIMPLEX VIRUS (HSV). **Aciclovir** is active against herpes viruses but does not eradicate them. It is only effective if started at onset of infection; it is also used for prevention of recurrence in the immunocompromised. Genital lesions, oesophagitis and proctitis may be treated with oral aciclovir. HSV encephalitis or pneumonitis should be treated with intravenous aciclovir.

HERPES ZOSTER VIRUS. While most HIV positive patients with zoster experience only one self-limiting course, some will experience repeated episodes. Treatment should be reserved for debilitating disease and when there is high risk of serious complications, such as in advanced HIV disease. Aciclovir is the treatment of choice and it can be administered in high oral dose or in the case of lack of response to oral therapy or CNS involvement, it should be given intravenously.

CYTOMEGALOVIRUS (CMV). Parenteral antiviral **ganciclovir** arrests retinochoroiditis and enteritis caused by CMV in HIV infected patients. Maintenance therapy with oral ganciclovir should be given to prevent relapse of retinitis. Alternative therapy with intravenous **foscarnet** can be used if necessary.

Aciclovir

Tablets, aciclovir 200 mg, 400 mg, 800 mg

Oral suspension, aciclovir 200 mg/5 ml

Infusion (Powder for solution for infusion), aciclovir (as sodium salt) 250-mg vial, 500-mg vial

Uses: treatment of primary genital herpes; disseminated varicella-zoster in immunocompromised patients; herpes simplex encephalitis

Precautions: maintain adequate hydration; renal impairment (Appendix 4); pregnancy (Appendix 2); breastfeeding (Appendix 3)

Dosage:

Treatment of primary genital herpes, *by mouth,* ADULT 200–400 mg 5 times daily for 5–7 days; occasionally up to 800 mg 5 times daily

Prevention of recurrence of genital herpes, *by mouth,* ADULT 400 mg twice daily

Disseminated varicella-zoster in immunocompromised patients, *by intravenous infusion,* ADULT 10 mg/kg 3 times daily for 7 days

Herpes simplex encephalitis, *by intravenous infusion,* ADULT 10 mg/kg 3 times daily for 10 days

RECONSTITUTION AND ADMINISTRATION. According to manufacturer's directions

Adverse effects: rashes; nausea and vomiting, rises in bilirubin and liver enzymes, increases in blood urea and creatinine, decreases in haematological indices, headache, dizziness, fatigue; on intravenous infusion, local inflammation (rarely ulceration), confusion, hallucinations, agitation, tremors, somnolence, psychosis, convulsions and coma

6.5.2   Antiretroviral drugs

Antiretroviral drugs do not cure HIV (human immunodeficiency virus) infection; they only temporarily suppress viral replication and improve symptoms. Patients receiving these drugs require careful monitoring by appropriately trained health professionals in an adequately resourced setting. Rigorous promotion of measures to prevent new infections remains essential and its need is not diminished by the availability of antiretroviral drugs. Effective therapy requires the simultaneous use of 3 or 4 drugs; alternative regimens are necessary to meet specific requirements at start-up, to substitute for first-line regimens in cases of intolerance, or to replace failing regimens. The use of a 3- or 4-drug combination as specified in the WHO treatment guidelines is recommended. The use of fixed-dose preparations for these combinations is also recommended if the pharmaceutical quality is assured and interchangeability with the single products is demonstrated as specified by the relevant drug regulatory authority.

Selection of 2 or 3 protease inhibitors from the Model List will need to be determined by each country after consideration of local treatment guidelines and experience, as well as comparative costs of available products. Low-dose ritonavir is used in combination with indinavir, lopinavir or saquinavir as a 'booster'; ritonavir is not recommended as a drug in its own right.

PRINCIPLES OF TREATMENT. Treatment is aimed at reducing the plasma viral load as much as possible and for as long as possible; it should be started before the immune system is irreversibly damaged. The need for early drug treatment should, however, be balanced against the development of toxicity. Commitment to treatment and strict adherence over many years are required; the regimen chosen should take into account convenience and the patient's tolerance of it. The development of resistance is reduced by using a combination of 3 or 4 drugs; such combinations should have additive or synergistic activity while ensuring that their toxicity is not additive. Testing for resistance to antiviral drugs, particularly in therapeutic failure, should be considered.

Women of childbearing age receiving antiretroviral therapy must have available effective contraceptive methods to prevent unintended pregnancy. Women who are taking non-nucleoside reverse transcriptase inhibitors or protease inhibitors which can lower blood concentration of hormonal oral contraceptives, should be advised to use additional or alternative contraceptives.

DRUGS USED TO TREAT HIV INFECTION. **Zidovudine**, a nucleoside reverse transcriptase inhibitor (or 'nucleoside analogue'), was the first anti-HIV drug to be introduced. Other nucleoside reverse transcriptase inhibitors include **abacavir**, **didanosine**, **lamivudine**, **stavudine**, and zalcitabine.

The protease inhibitors include amprenavir, **indinavir**, **lopinavir**, **nelfinavir**, **ritonavir** and **saquinavir**. Ritonavir in low doses is used in combination with indinavir, lopinavir or saquinavir as a booster. The small amount of ritonavir in such combinations has no intrinsic antiviral activity but it increases the antiviral activity of the other protease inhibitors by reducing their metabolism. Indinavir, nelfinavir, ritonavir and possibly saquinavir inhibit the cytochrome P450 enzyme system and therefore have a potential for significant drug interactions. Protease inhibitors are associated with lipodystrophy and metabolic effects (see below).

The non-nucleoside reverse transcriptase inhibitors include **efavirenz** and **nevirapine**. They interact with a number of drugs metabolized in the liver; the doses of protease inhibitors may need to be increased when they are given with efavirenz or nevirapine. Nevirapine is associated with a high incidence of rash (including Stevens-Johnson syndrome) and occasionally fatal hepatitis. Rash is also associated with efavirenz but it is usually milder. Efavirenz treatment has also been associated with an increased plasma cholesterol concentration.

INITIATION OF TREATMENT. The time for initiating antiviral treatment is determined by the clinical stage of the HIV infection as indicated by symptoms, and where available, by the CD4-cell count or total lymphocyte count; the plasma viral load, if available, is also a valuable guide for staging the disease (see Monitoring, below).

Recommended initial treatment with a combination of drugs ('highly active antiretroviral therapy', HAART) includes:

2 nucleoside reverse transcriptase inhibitors (section 6.5.2.1)

plus

a non-nucleoside reverse transcriptase inhibitor (section 6.5.2.2)

or a third nucleoside reverse transcriptase inhibitor (section 6.5.2.1)

or a protease inhibitor which may be combined with ritonavir as booster (section 6.5.2.3).

MONITORING. In resource-limited settings the basic clinical assessment before initiating antiretroviral therapy includes documentation of past medical history, identification of current and past HIV-related illnesses, identification of co-existing medical conditions that may influence the choice of therapy (for example, pregnancy or tuberculosis) as well as current symptoms and physical signs.

The *absolute minimum laboratory tests* before initiating antiretroviral therapy are an HIV antibody test (in patients over 18 months of age) and a haemoglobin or haematocrit measurement.

Additional basic testing should include:

- white blood cell count;
- differential cell count (to identify a decline in neutrophils and the possibility of neutropenia);
- total lymphocyte count;
- serum alanine or aspartate aminotransferase concentration to assess the possibility of hepatitis co-infection and to monitor for hepatotoxicity;
- serum creatinine and/or blood urea nitrogen to assess baseline renal function;
- serum glucose;
- pregnancy tests for women.

Desirable supplemental tests include measurement of bilirubin, amylase and serum lipids. CD4-cell determinations are, of course, very desirable and efforts should be made to make these widely available. Viral load testing is currently considered optional because of constraints on resources.

CHANGING THERAPY. Deterioration of the condition (including clinical and virological changes) usually calls for replacement of the failing drugs. Intolerance to adverse effects and drug-induced organ dysfunction usually require change in therapy.

The choice of an alternative regimen depends on factors such as the response to previous treatment, tolerance and the possibility of cross-resistance. If treatment fails, a new second-line regimen will be needed. If toxicity occurs, either a new second-line regimen is indicated or, if the toxicity is related to an identifiable drug in the regimen, the offending drug can be replaced with another drug that does not have the same adverse effects.

PREGNANCY. Treatment of HIV infection in pregnancy aims to:
- minimize the viral load and disease progression in the mother;
- reduce the risk of toxicity to the fetus (although the teratogenic potential of most antiretroviral drugs is unknown);
- prevent transmission of infection to the neonate.

In pregnant women, it may be desirable to initiate antiretroviral therapy after the first trimester, although for pregnant women who are severely ill, the benefit of early therapy outweighs the potential risk to the fetus. All treatment options require careful assessment by a specialist.

The use of zidovudine, lamivudine, nevirapine, nelfinavir and saquinavir are recommended for women of child-bearing potential or who are pregnant. Efavirenz should be avoided because of its potential teratogenic effect on the fetus in the first trimester. First-line treatment in pregnant women should when possible include zidovudine and lamivudine. Monotherapy with either zidovudine or with nevirapine reduces transmission of infection to the neonate (see also below), but combination antiretroviral therapy maximizes the chance of preventing transmission and represents optimal therapy for the mother. Low-dose ritonavir is required if either indinavir or saquinavir is used in pregnancy because adequate drug concentration is achieved only with ritonavir boosting. Information is lacking on the use of lopinavir with ritonavir in pregnancy.

Lactic acidosis and hepatic steatosis associated with nucleoside reverse transcriptase inhibitors may be more frequent in pregnant women and therefore the combination of stavudine and didanosine should be used in pregnancy only when no alternatives are available. Protease inhibitors have been associated with glucose intolerance and pregnant women should be instructed to recognize symptoms of hyperglycaemia and to seek health care advice if they occur.

Various regimens have been used to specifically prevent the transmission of HIV from mother to the neonate at term. More information is available in *New Data on the Prevention of Mother-to-Child Transmission of HIV and their Policy Implications: Conclusions and Recommendations* (WHO/ RHR/01.28), which reflects an inter-agency consultation held on 11–13 October 2000.

BREASTFEEDING. Antiretroviral drugs may be present in breastmilk, and may reduce viral load in breastmilk and reduce the risk of transmission through breastfeeding. However, the concentration of antiretroviral drugs in breastmilk may not be adequate to prevent viral replication and there is therefore the possibility of promoting the development of drug-resistant virus which could be transmitted to the infant.

Women with HIV infection should be counselled about the risks of breastfeeding and, where possible, they should limit or avoid breastfeeding; in particular, breastfeeding should be avoided where replacement feeding is acceptable, affordable, sustainable, and safe. HIV-infected women should be counselled on infant feeding options and they should be supported in their choice.

POST-EXPOSURE PROPHYLAXIS. Treatment with antiretroviral drugs may be appropriate following occupational exposure to HIV-contaminated material. Immediate expert advice should be sought in such cases; national guidelines on post-exposure prophylaxis for healthcare workers have been developed and local ones may also be available.

LIPODYSTROPHY AND METABOLIC EFFECTS. Combination antiretroviral therapy, including regimens containing a protease inhibitor, is associated with redistribution of body fat in some patients (for example, decreased fat under the skin, increased abdominal fat, 'buffalo humps' and breast enlargement). Protease inhibitors are also associated with metabolic abnormalities such as hyperlipidaemia, insulin resistance, and hyperglycaemia. Clinical examination should include an evaluation of fat distribution; measurement of serum lipids and blood glucose should be considered.

6.5.2.1 Nucleoside reverse transcriptase inhibitors

In some settings it may not be possible to carry out full monitoring described under each drug entry; in such cases the level of monitoring should be determined by local guidelines (see also notes above)

Abacavir
ABC
Tablets, abacavir (as sulfate) 300 mg

Oral solution, abacavir (as sulfate) 100 mg/5 ml

Uses: HIV infection in combination with at least two other antiretroviral drugs

Precautions: hepatic impairment (see below and Appendix 5); renal impairment (Appendix 4); pregnancy (see notes above and Appendix 2); breastfeeding (see notes above)

HYPERSENSITIVITY REACTIONS. Life-threatening hypersensitivity reactions reported—characterized by fever or rash and possibly nausea, vomiting, diarrhoea, abdominal pain, lethargy, malaise, headache, myalgia and renal failure; less frequently mouth ulceration, oedema, hypotension, dyspnoea, sore throat, cough, paraesthesia, arthralgia, conjunctivitis, lymphadeno-pathy, lymphocytopenia and anaphylaxis (hypersensitivity reactions presenting as sore throat, influenza-like illness, cough and breathlessness identified); rarely myolysis; laboratory abnormalities may include raised liver enzymes (see below) and creatine kinase; symptoms usually appear in the first 6 weeks, but may occur at any time; monitor for symptoms every 2 weeks for 2 months; discontinue immediately if any symptom of hypersensitivity develops and do not rechallenge (risk of more severe hypersensitivity reaction); discontinue if hypersensitivity cannot be ruled out, even when other diagnoses possible—if rechallenge necessary it must be carried out in hospital setting; if abacavir is stopped for any reason other than hypersensitivity, exclude hypersensitivity reaction as the cause and rechallenge only if medical assistance is readily available; care needed with concomitant use of drugs which cause skin toxicity

PATIENT ADVICE. Patients should be told the importance of regular dosing (intermittent therapy may increase sensitization), how to recognize signs of hypersensitivity, and advised to seek immediate medical attention if symptoms develop or before re-starting treatment

HEPATIC DISEASE. Potentially life-threatening lactic acidosis and severe hepatomegaly with steatosis reported—caution in liver disease, liver enzyme abnormalities, or risk factors for liver disease (particularly in obese women); suspend or discontinue if deterioration in liver function tests, hepatic steatosis, progressive hepatomegaly or unexplained lactic acidosis

Dosage:

HIV infection (in combination with other antiretroviral drugs), *by mouth*, ADULT 300 mg twice daily; CHILD 3 months–16 years, 8 mg/kg twice daily

Adverse effects: hypersensitivity reactions (see above), nausea, vomiting, diarrhoea, anorexia, lethargy, fatigue, fever, head-ache, pancreatitis, lactic acidosis (see hepatic disease, above)

Didanosine

ddI, DDI

Chewable tablets, didanosine (with calcium and magnesium antacids) 25 mg, 50 mg; 100 mg, 150 mg, 200 mg

Oral solution (Powder for oral solution), didanosine (with calcium and magnesium antacids) 100 mg/sachet, 167 mg/sachet, 250 mg/sachet

Enteric-coated capsules (Gastro-resistant capsules), didanosine 125 mg, 200 mg, 250 mg, 400 mg

NOTE. Antacids in formulation may affect absorption of other drugs—see **interactions:** Appendix 1 (antacids)

Uses: HIV infection in combination with at least two other antiretroviral drugs

Precautions: history of pancreatitis (preferably avoid, other-wise extreme caution, see also below); peripheral neuropathy or hyperuricaemia (see under Adverse effects); history of liver disease (see below); renal and hepatic impairment (see Appendices 4 and 5); pregnancy and breastfeeding (see notes above); dilated retinal examinations recommended (especially in children) every 6 months, or if visual changes occur; **interactions:** Appendix 1

PANCREATITIS. If symptoms of pancreatitis develop or if serum amylase or lipase is raised (even if asymptomatic) suspend treatment until diagnosis of pancreatitis excluded; on return to normal values re-initiate treatment only if essential (using low dose increased gradually if appropriate). Whenever possible avoid concomitant treatment with other drugs known to cause pancreatic toxicity (for example intravenous pentamidine isetionate); monitor closely if concomitant therapy unavoidable. Since significant elevations of triglycerides cause pancreatitis monitor closely if elevated

HEPATIC DISEASE. Potentially life-threatening lactic acidosis and severe hepatomegaly with steatosis reported therefore caution in liver disease, excessive alcohol intake, liver enzyme abnormalities, or risk factors for liver disease (particularly in obese women); suspend or discontinue if deterioration in liver function tests, hepatic steatosis, progressive hepatomegaly or unexplained lactic acidosis

Dosage:

HIV infection (in combination with other antiretroviral drugs), *by mouth*, ADULT body weight under 60 kg 250 mg daily in 1–2 divided doses, over 60 kg body weight 400 mg daily in 1–2 divided doses; CHILD under 3 months, 50 mg/m^2 twice daily; 3 months–13 years, 90 mg/m^2 twice daily *or* 240 mg/m^2 once daily

PATIENT ADVICE. To ensure sufficient antacid from tablets containing antacid, each dose to be taken as 2 tablets (CHILD under 1 year 1 tablet) chewed thoroughly, crushed or dispersed in water; tablets should be taken at least 1 hour before food or on an empty stomach

Adverse effects: pancreatitis (see also under Precautions); peripheral neuropathy especially in advanced HIV infection– suspend (reduced dose may be tolerated when symptoms resolve); hyperuricaemia (suspend treatment if significant elevation); diarrhoea (occasionally serious); also reported, nausea, vomiting, dry mouth, asthenia, headache, hypersensitivity reactions, retinal and optic nerve changes (especially in children), diabetes mellitus, raised liver enzymes (see also under Precautions), liver failure

Lamivudine

3TC
Tablets, lamivudine 150 mg
Oral solution, lamivudine 50 mg/5 ml

Uses: HIV infection in combination with at least two other antiretroviral drugs

Precautions: renal impairment (Appendix 4), hepatic disease (see below); pregnancy and breastfeeding (see notes above); **interactions:** Appendix 1

HEPATIC DISEASE. Potentially life-threatening lactic acidosis and severe hepatomegaly with steatosis reported therefore caution (particularly in obese women) in liver disease, liver enzyme abnormalities, or risk factors for liver disease; suspend or discontinue if deterioration in liver function tests, hepatic steatosis, progressive hepatomegaly or unexplained lactic acidosis. Recurrent hepatitis in patients with chronic hepatitis B may occur on discontinuation of lamivudine

Dosage:

HIV infection (in combination with other antiretroviral drugs), *by mouth*, ADULT 150 mg twice daily *or* 300 mg once daily; INFANT under 1 month, 2 mg/kg twice daily; CHILD 1 month or over, 4 mg/kg twice daily

Adverse effects: nausea, vomiting, diarrhoea, abdominal pain; cough; headache, insomnia; malaise, fever, rash, alopecia, muscle disorders; nasal symptoms; peripheral neuropathy reported; rarely pancreatitis (discontinue); neutropenia, anaemia and thrombocytopenia; lactic acidosis; raised liver enzymes and serum amylase reported

---

Stavudine
d4T
Capsules, stavudine 15 mg, 20 mg, 30 mg, 40 mg
Oral solution (Powder for oral solution), stavudine 5 mg/5 ml

Uses: HIV infection in combination with at least two other antiretroviral drugs

Precautions: history of peripheral neuropathy (see below); history of pancreatitis or concomitant use with other drugs associated with pancreatitis; hepatic disease (see below); renal impairment (Appendix 4); pregnancy and breastfeeding (see notes above); **interactions:** Appendix 1

PERIPHERAL NEUROPATHY. Suspend if peripheral neuropathy develops— characterized by persistent numbness, tingling or pain in feet or hands; if symptoms resolve satisfactorily on withdrawal, resume treatment at half previous dose

HEPATIC DISEASE. Potentially life-threatening lactic acidosis and severe hepatomegaly with steatosis reported therefore caution in liver disease, liver enzyme abnormalities, or risk factors for liver disease (particularly in obese women); suspend or discontinue if deterioration in liver function tests, hepatic steatosis, progressive hepatomegaly or unexplained lactic acidosis

Dosage:

HIV infection (in combination with other antiretroviral drugs), *by mouth*, ADULT body weight under 60 kg, 30 mg twice daily preferably at least 1 hour before food; body weight over 60 kg, 40 mg twice daily; CHILD over 3 months, body weight under 30 kg, 1 mg/kg twice daily; body weight over 30 kg, 30 mg twice daily

Adverse effects: peripheral neuropathy (dose-related, see above); pancreatitis; nausea, vomiting, diarrhoea, constipation, anorexia, abdominal discomfort; chest pain; dyspnoea; headache, dizziness, insomnia, mood changes; asthenia, musculoskeletal pain; influenza-like symptoms, rash and other allergic reactions; lymphadenopathy; neoplasms; elevated liver enzymes (see hepatic disease, above) and serum amylase; neutropenia, thrombocytopenia

---

Zidovudine
Azidothymidine, AZT, ZDV
NOTE. The abbreviation AZT which has sometimes been used for zidovudine has also been used for another drug
Capsules, zidovudine 100 mg, 250 mg

Tablets, zidovudine 300 mg

Syrup (Oral solution), zidovudine 50 mg/5 ml

Infusion (Concentrate for solution for infusion), zidovudine 10 mg/ml, 20-ml vial

Uses: HIV infection in combination with at least two other antiretroviral drugs; monotherapy for prevention of maternal-fetal HIV transmission (but see notes above under Pregnancy)

Contraindications: abnormally low neutrophil counts or haemoglobin (consult product literature); neonates either with hyperbilirubinaemia requiring treatment other than photo-therapy or with raised transaminase (consult product litera-ture)

Precautions: haematological toxicity; vitamin B_{12} deficiency (increased risk of neutropenia); reduce dose or interrupt treatment according to product literature if anaemia or myelosuppression; renal impairment (Appendix 4); hepatic impairment (see below and Appendix 5); risk of lactic acidosis, (see below); elderly; pregnancy and breastfeeding (see notes above); **interactions:** Appendix 1

HEPATIC DISEASE. Potentially life-threatening lactic acidosis and severe hepatomegaly with steatosis reported therefore caution in liver disease, liver enzyme abnormalities, or risk factors for liver disease (particularly in obese women), suspend or discontinue if deterioration in liver function tests, hepatic steatosis, progressive hepatomegaly or unexplained lactic acidosis

Dosage:

HIV infection (in combination with other antiretroviral drugs), *by mouth*, ADULT 500–600 mg daily in 2–3 divided doses; INFANT under 4 weeks, 4 mg/kg twice daily; CHILD 4 weeks–13 years 180 mg/m² twice daily

Prevention of maternal-fetal HIV transmission, see notes above under Pregnancy

ADMINISTRATION AND DILUTION. According to manufacturer's directions

Adverse effects: anaemia (may require transfusion), neutrope-nia, and leukopenia (all more frequent with high dose and advanced disease); also include, nausea and vomiting, abdominal pain, dyspepsia, diarrhoea, flatulence, taste disturbance, pancreatitis, liver disorders including fatty change and raised bilirubin and liver enzymes (see hepatic disease, above); chest pain, dyspnoea, cough; influenza-like symptoms, headache, fever, paraesthesia, neuropathy, con-vulsions, dizziness, somnolence, insomnia, anxiety, depres-sion, loss of mental acuity, malaise, anorexia, asthenia, myopathy, myalgia; pancytopenia, thrombocytopenia; gynae-comastia; urinary frequency; rash, pruritus, pigmentation of nail, skin and oral mucosa

6.5.2.2   Non-nucleoside reverse transcriptase inhibitors

In some settings it may not be possible to carry out full monitoring described under each drug entry; in such cases the level of monitoring should be determined by local guidelines (see also notes above)

Efavirenz

EFV, EFZ

Capsules, efavirenz 50 mg, 100 mg, 200 mg

Oral solution, efavirenz 150 mg/5 ml

Uses: HIV infection in combination with at least two other antiretroviral drugs

Contraindications: pregnancy (see notes above and Appendix 2; substitute nevirapine for efavirenz in pregnant women or women for whom effective contraception cannot be assured)

Precautions: hepatic impairment (avoid if severe; Appendix 5); severe renal impairment; breastfeeding (see notes above); elderly; history of mental illness or substance abuse; **interactions:** Appendix 1

RASH. Rash, usually in the first 2 weeks, is the most common adverse effect; discontinue if severe rash with blistering, desquamation, mucosal involvement or fever; if rash mild or moderate, may continue without interruption—rash usually resolves within 1 month

Dosage:

HIV infection (in combination with other antiretroviral drugs), *by mouth*, ADULT 600 mg once daily; CHILD over 3 years, body weight 10–15 kg, 200 mg once daily; body weight 15–19 kg, 250 mg once daily; body weight 20–24 kg, 300 mg once daily; body weight 25–32 kg, 350 mg once daily; body weight 33–39 kg, 400 mg once daily; body weight 40 kg and over, adult dose

Adverse effects: rash including Stevens-Johnson syndrome (see also above); dizziness, headache, insomnia, somnolence, abnormal dreams, fatigue, impaired concentration (administration at bedtime especially in the first 2–4 weeks reduces CNS effects); nausea; less frequently vomiting, diarrhoea, hepatitis, depression, anxiety, psychosis, amnesia, ataxia, stupor, vertigo; also reported raised serum cholesterol, elevated liver enzymes (especially if seropositive for hepatitis B or C), pancreatitis

Nevirapine

NVP

Tablets, nevirapine 200 mg

Oral suspension, nevirapine 50 mg/5 ml

Uses: HIV infection, in combination with at least two other antiretroviral drugs; prevention of mother-to-child transmission in HIV-infected patients (but see notes above under Pregnancy)

Precautions: hepatic impairment (see below and Appendix 5); renal impairment; pregnancy (see notes above); breastfeeding (see notes above); **interactions:** Appendix 1

HEPATIC DISEASE. Potentially life-threatening hepatotoxicity including fatal fulminant hepatitis reported usually occurring in first 8 weeks; monitor liver function before long-term treatment then every 2 weeks for 2 months then after 1 month and then every 3–6 months; discontinue permanently if abnormalities in liver function tests accompanied by hypersensitivity reaction (rash, fever, arthralgia, myalgia, lymphadenopathy, hepatitis, renal impairment, eosinophilia, granulocytopenia); suspend if severe abnormalities in liver function tests but no hypersensitivity reaction—discontinue permanently if significant liver function abnormalities recur; monitor patient closely if mild to moderate abnormalities in liver function tests with no hypersensitivity reaction

RASH. Rash, usually in first 8 weeks, is most common adverse effect; incidence reduced if introduced at low dose and dose increased gradually; discontinue permanently if severe rash or if rash accompanied by blistering, oral lesions, conjunctivitis, swelling, general malaise or hypersensitivity reactions; if rash mild or moderate may continue without interruption but dose should not be increased until rash resolves

PATIENT ADVICE. Patients should be told how to recognize hypersensitivity reactions and advised to seek immediate medical attention if symptoms develop

Dosage:

HIV infection (in combination with other antiretroviral drugs), *by mouth*, ADULT 200 mg once daily for first 14 days then (if no rash present) 200 mg twice daily; INFANT 15–30 days old, 5 mg/kg once daily for 14 days, then (if no rash present) 120 mg/m^2 twice daily for 14 days, then 200 mg/m^2 twice daily; CHILD 1 month–13 years, 120 mg/m^2 twice daily for first 14 days, then (if no rash present) 200 mg/m^2 twice daily

Prevention of mother-to-child transmission of HIV (see also notes above under Pregnancy), *by mouth*, ADULT 200 mg as a single dose at onset of labour; NEONATE 2 mg/kg as a single dose within 72 hours of birth

NOTE. If treatment interrupted for more than 7 days reintroduce with 200 mg daily (INFANT 15–30 days old, 5 mg/kg; CHILD over 1 month, 120 mg/ m^2) and increase dose cautiously

Adverse effects: rash including Stevens-Johnson syndrome and rarely, toxic epidermal necrolysis (see also Precautions above); hepatitis or jaundice reported (see also Precautions above); nausea, vomiting, abdominal pain, diarrhoea, headache, drowsiness, fatigue, fever; hypersensitivity reactions (may involve hepatic reactions and rash, see Precautions above); anaphylaxis, angioedema, urticaria also reported

6.5.2.3 Protease inhibitors

In some settings it may not be possible to carry out full monitoring described under each drug entry; in such cases the level of monitoring should be determined by local guidelines (see also notes above)

Indinavir

IDV

Capsules, indinavir (as sulfate) 200 mg, 333 mg, 400 mg

Uses: HIV infection in combination with two nucleoside reverse transcriptase inhibitors and usually with low-dose ritonavir booster

Precautions: hepatic impairment (Appendix 5); ensure adequate hydration to reduce risk of nephrolithiasis; diabetes mellitus; haemophilia; pregnancy (see notes above and Appendix 2); breastfeeding (see notes above); metabolism of many drugs inhibited if administered concomitantly; **interactions:** Appendix 1

Dosage:

HIV infection (in combination with nucleoside reverse transcriptase inhibitors and low-dose ritonavir booster), *by mouth*, ADULT indinavir 800 mg and ritonavir 100 mg both twice daily

HIV infection (in combination with nucleoside reverse transcriptase inhibitors but without ritonavir booster), *by mouth*, ADULT 800 mg every 8 hours; CHILD and ADOLESCENT 4–17 years, 500 mg/m^2 every 8 hours (maximum 800 mg every 8 hours); CHILD under 4 years, safety and efficacy not established

PATIENT ADVICE. Administer 1 hour before or 2 hours after a meal; may be administered with low-fat, light meal; when given with didanosine, allow 1 hour between the drugs (antacids in didanosine reduce absorption of indinavir)

Adverse effects: nausea, vomiting, diarrhoea, abdominal discomfort, dyspepsia, flatulence, pancreatitis, dry mouth, taste disturbances; headache, dizziness, insomnia; myalgia, myositis, rhabdomyolysis, asthenia, hypoaesthesia, paraesthesia; hyperglycaemia; anaphylactoid reactions, rash (including Stevens-Johnson syndrome), pruritus, dry skin, hyperpigmentation, alopecia, paronychia; interstitial nephritis, nephrolithiasis (may require interruption or discontinuation; more frequent in children), dysuria, haematuria, crystalluria, proteinuria, pyuria (in children); hepatitis, transient hyperbilirubinaemia; blood disorders including neutropenia, haemolytic anaemia; lipodystrophy and metabolic effects, see notes above

Lopinavir with ritonavir

LPV/r

Capsules, lopinavir 133.3 mg and ritonavir 33.3 mg

Oral solution, lopinavir 400 mg and ritonavir 100 mg/5 ml

NOTE. 5 ml oral solution ≡ 3 capsules; where appropriate capsules may be used instead of oral solution; oral solution excipients include propylene glycol and alcohol 42%

Uses: HIV infection in combination with two other antiretroviral drugs

NOTE. Ritonavir increases effect of lopinavir (see notes above); low dose in combination does not have intrinsic antiviral activity

Precautions: hepatic impairment—avoid if severe (Appendix 5); renal impairment (Appendix 4); haemophilia; pregnancy (see notes above and Appendix 2); breastfeeding (see notes above and Appendix 3); diabetes mellitus; oral solution contains propylene glycol—avoid in hepatic and renal impairment, and in pregnancy, increased susceptibility to propylene glycol toxicity in slow metabolizers; **interactions:** Appendix 1

PANCREATITIS. Signs and symptoms suggestive of pancreatitis (including raised serum amylase and lipase) should be evaluated—discontinue if pancreatitis diagnosed

Dosage:

HIV infection (in combination with other antiretroviral drugs), *by mouth*, ADULT and ADOLESCENT with body surface area of 1.3 m^2 or greater, 3 capsules *or* 5 ml twice daily (lopinavir

400 mg and ritonavir 100 mg twice daily); CHILD 6 months–13 years, lopinavir 225 mg/m^2 and ritonavir 57.5 mg/m^2 twice daily (or body weight 7–15 kg lopinavir 12 mg/kg and ritonavir 3 mg/kg twice daily, body weight 15–40 kg lopinavir 10 mg/kg and ritonavir 5 mg/kg twice daily)

NOTE. Increase dose by 33% if used with efavirenz or with nevirapine

PATIENT ADVICE. Each dose to be taken with food

Adverse effects: diarrhoea, nausea, vomiting, colitis, abdominal discomfort, asthenia, headache, insomnia; rash; less frequently, dry mouth, pancreatitis (see also Precautions), dyspepsia, dysphagia, oesophagitis, influenza-like syndrome, appetite changes; hypertension, palpitations, thrombophlebitis, vasculitis, chest pain, dyspnoea, agitation, anxiety, ataxia, hypertonia, confusion, depression, dizziness, dyskinesia, paraesthesia, peripheral neuritis, somnolence; Cushing syndrome, hypothyroidism, sexual dysfunction, anaemia, leukopenia, dehydration, oedema, lactic acidosis; arthralgia, myalgia, abnormal vision, otitis media, taste disturbances, tinnitus; acne, alopecia, dry skin, pruritus, skin discoloration, nail disorders, sweating; lipodystrophy and metabolic effects (see notes above); raised bilirubin and lowered sodium, low platelet and low neutrophil counts also reported in children

Nelfinavir

NFV

Tablets, nelfinavir (as mesilate) 250 mg

Oral powder, nelfinavir (as mesilate) 50 mg/g

Uses: HIV infection in combination with two other antiretroviral drugs

Precautions: hepatic and renal impairment; diabetes mellitus; haemophilia; pregnancy and breastfeeding (see notes above); **interactions:** Appendix 1

Dosage:

HIV infection (in combination with other antiretroviral drugs), *by mouth*, ADULT 1.25 g twice daily *or* 750 mg 3 times daily; CHILD under 1 year, 40–50 mg/kg 3 times daily *or* 65–75 mg/kg twice daily; 1–13 years, 55–65 mg/kg twice daily

PATIENT ADVICE. Administer with or after food; powder may be mixed with water, milk, formula feeds or pudding; it should **not** be mixed with acidic foods or juices owing to its taste

Adverse effects: diarrhoea, nausea, vomiting, flatulence, abdominal pain; rash; reports of elevated creatine kinase, hepatitis, pancreatitis, neutropenia, hypersensitivity reactions including bronchospasm, fever, pruritus and facial oedema, lipodystrophy and metabolic effects, see notes above

Ritonavir

r, RTV

Capsules, ritonavir 100 mg

Oral solution, ritonavir 400 mg/5 ml

Uses: HIV infection, as a booster to increase effect of indinavir, lopinavir or saquinavir and in combination with two other antiretroviral drugs

Contraindications: severe hepatic impairment

Precautions: hepatic impairment; diabetes mellitus; haemophilia; pregnancy and breastfeeding (see notes above); **interactions:** Appendix 1

PANCREATITIS. Signs and symptoms suggestive of pancreatitis (including raised serum amylase and lipase) should be evaluated—discontinue if pancreatitis diagnosed

Dosage:

HIV infection (as a booster with other antiretroviral drugs), *by mouth*, ADULT 100 mg twice daily; CHILD 6 months–13 years 57.5 mg/m^2 twice daily (*or* 3–5 mg/kg twice daily) (maximum 100 mg twice daily)

Adverse effects: nausea, vomiting, diarrhoea (may impair absorption—close monitoring required), abdominal pain, taste disturbances, dyspepsia, anorexia, throat irritation; vasodilatation; headache, circumoral and peripheral paraesthesia, hyperaesthesia, dizziness, sleep disturbances, asthenia, rash, leukopenia; raised liver enzymes, bilirubin, and uric acid; occasionally flatulence, eructation, dry mouth and ulceration, cough, anxiety, fever, pain, myalgia, weight loss, decreased thyroxine, sweating, pruritus, electrolyte disturbances, anaemia, neutropenia, increased prothrombin time; pancreatitis (see also Pancreatitis, above); lipodystrophy and metabolic effects, see notes above

---

Saquinavir

SQV

Capsules (gel-filled), saquinavir 200 mg

Uses: HIV infection in combination with two other antiretroviral drugs and usually with low-dose ritonavir booster

Contraindications: severe hepatic impairment (Appendix 5)

Precautions: hepatic impairment (Appendix 5); renal impairment (Appendix 4); diabetes mellitus; haemophilia; pregnancy and breastfeeding (see notes above); **interactions:** Appendix 1

Dosage:

HIV infection (in combination with nucleoside reverse transcriptase inhibitors and low-dose ritonavir booster), *by mouth*, ADULT saquinavir 1 g and ritonavir 100 mg twice daily

HIV infection (in combination with other antiretroviral drugs but without ritonavir booster), *by mouth*, ADULT 1.2 g every 8 hours after a meal; CHILD under 16 years, safety and efficacy not established

PATIENT ADVICE. Administer with or after food

NOTE. To avoid confusion between the different formulations of saquinavir, prescribers should specify the brand to be dispensed; absorption from gel-filled capsules containing saquinavir is much greater than from capsules containing saquinavir mesilate. Treatment should generally be initiated with gel-filled capsules

Adverse effects: diarrhoea, buccal and mucosal ulceration, abdominal discomfort, nausea, vomiting; headache, peripheral neuropathy, paraesthesia, dizziness, insomnia, mood changes, ataxia, musculoskeletal pain, asthenia; fever, pruritus, rash and other skin eruptions, rarely Stevens-Johnson syndrome; other rare adverse effects include thrombocytopenia and other blood disorders, seizures, liver damage, pancreatitis and nephrolithiasis; reports of elevated creatine kinase, raised liver enzymes and neutropenia when used in combination therapy; lipodystrophy and metabolic effects (see notes above)

6.6 Insect repellents

Diethyltoluamide, an effective insect repellent, is used for the prevention of infections transmitted by insect bites, ticks, harvest mites and fleas. One application offers protection for 4 to 8 hours.

Diethyltoluamide

Cutaneous solution, diethyltoluamide 50%, 75%

Uses: insect repellent against mosquitoes, biting flies, ticks, harvest mites and fleas

Precautions: avoid contact with eyes or mouth, mucous membranes, areas of flexures, wounds, broken or irritated skin

Administration: Apply sparingly to exposed skin and when treatment no longer needed, wash skin thoroughly with soap and water

Adverse effects: systemic toxicity—reported with application of large topical doses, especially in children; occasionally, hypersensitivity reactions

Section 7: Antimigraine drugs

Chronic recurrent headache is associated with many disorders, both somatic and psychogenic. An accurate diagnosis must consequently be made before appropriate treatment can be initiated for migraine. Untreated, migraine attacks last for several hours and sometimes for as long as 3 days.

Migraine headache is frequently accompanied by episodes of gastrointestinal disturbance including nausea and vomiting. The headache may be preceded or accompanied by aura (classical migraine) which is characterised by visual disturbances such as flickering lines and fragmented vision or sensory disturbances such as tingling or numbness; rarely, hemiparesis or impaired consciousness may occur. Migraine without aura (common migraine) is the more common form occurring in about 75% of patients who experience migraine.

Emotional or physical stress, lack of or excess sleep, missed meals, menstruation, alcohol and specific foods including cheese and chocolate are often identified as precipitating factors; oral contraceptives may increase the frequency of attacks. Avoidance of such precipitating factors can be of great benefit in preventing or reducing the frequency of attacks and should be addressed in detail. Women taking combined oral contraceptives who experience an onset or increase in frequency of headaches should be advised of other contraceptive measures.

The two principal strategies of migraine management are treatment of acute attacks and prophylactic treatment.

7.1   Acute migraine attack

Treatment of acute attacks may be non-specific using simple analgesics, or specific using ergotamine. If nausea and vomiting are features of the attack, an antiemetic drug may be given. Treatment is generally by mouth; some drugs are available as suppositories which may be administered if the oral route is not effective (poor oral bioavailability, or absorption from the gut impaired by vomiting) or not practicable (patient unable to take drugs orally).

Simple analgesics including NSAIDs (nonsteroidal anti-inflammatory drugs) can be effective in mild to moderate forms of migraine if taken early in the attack; most migraine headaches respond to **paracetamol**, **acetylsalicylic acid** or an NSAID such as **ibuprofen**. Peristalsis is often reduced during migraine attacks and, if available, a dispersible or effervescent preparation of the drug is preferred because of enhanced absorption compared with a conventional tablet. The risk of Reye syndrome due to acetylsalicylic acid in children under the age of 12 years can be avoided by giving paracetamol instead.

Ergotamine should be considered only when attacks are unresponsive to non-opioid analgesics. It is poorly absorbed when taken orally or sublingually. Rectal suppositories may offer an advantage when other routes of administration are unsatisfactory. To be fully effective ergotamine must be taken in adequate amounts as early as possible during each attack. Adverse effects limit how much ergotamine can be used in a single attack and consequently the recommended dosage should never be exceeded, and at least four days should elapse between successive treatments. Even normal dosage can lead to dependence, tolerance to adverse effects and to a withdrawal syndrome on discontinuing the drug. Adverse effects include nausea, vomiting, diarrhoea and vertigo; chronic ergotism is characterized by severe peripheral vasoconstriction which can lead to gangrene in the extremeties. The severity of adverse effects prevents the use of ergotamine for migraine prophylaxis.

An antiemetic such as **metoclopramide**, given as a single dose orally or by intramuscular injection at the onset of a migraine attack, preferably 10–15 minutes before the analgesic or ergotamine, is useful not only in relieving nausea but also in restoring gastric motility, thus improving absorption of the antimigraine drug.

Products which contain barbiturates or codeine are undesirable, particularly in combination with ergotamine, since they may cause physical dependence and withdrawal headaches.

Ergotamine tartrate

> Drug subject to international control under the United Nations Convention against Illicit Traffic in Narcotic Drugs and Psychotropic Substances (1988)

Tablets, ergotamine tartrate 1 mg
Suppositories, ergotamine tartrate 2 mg

Uses: treatment of acute migraine attacks unresponsive to analgesics

Contraindications: pregnancy (Appendix 2) and breastfeeding (Appendix 3); children; peripheral vascular disorders, coronary artery disease, obliterative vascular disease and Raynaud syndrome, severe hypertension, sepsis; severe renal or hepatic dysfunction (Appendices 4 and 5); hyperthyroidism; porphyria

Precautions: elderly; daily rebound headaches indicative of ergotamine dependence; discontinuation after regular normal dosage may result in withdrawal headache; stop medication immediately if numbness or tingling in extremities or anginal pain develops and contact doctor; **interactions:** see Appendix 1

Dosage:

Treatment of acute migraine attack, *by mouth or by rectum*, ADULT 1–2 mg at first sign of attack, maximum 4 mg in 24 hours; do not repeat at intervals of less than 4 days, maximum 8 mg in any one week; not to be used more than twice in any 1 month; CHILD not recommended

Adverse effects: nausea, vomiting, vertigo, abdominal pain, diarrhoea, muscle cramps, increased headache; precordial pain, myocardial ischaemia; rarely myocardial infarction; repeated high dosage may cause ergotism with gangrene and confusion; pleural and peritoneal fibrosis may occur with excessive use

Acetylsalicylic acid

Tablets, acetylsalicylic acid 300 mg, 500 mg
Dispersible tablets, acetylsalicylic acid 300 mg
Suppositories, acetylsalicylic acid 300 mg

Uses: acute migraine attacks; tension headache; also pyrexia, mild to moderate pain and inflammation (section 2.1.1); antiplatelet (section 12.5)

Contraindications: hypersensitivity (including asthma, angioedema, urticaria or rhinitis) to acetylsalicylic acid or any other NSAID; children under 12 years (Reye syndrome); gastrointestinal ulceration; haemophilia; gout

Precautions: asthma, allergic disease; impaired renal or hepatic function (Appendices 4 and 5); pregnancy (Appendix 2); breastfeeding (Appendix 3); elderly; G6PD-deficiency; dehydration; **interactions:** see Appendix 1

Dosage:

Treatment of acute migraine attack, *by mouth* preferably with or after food, ADULT 300–900 mg at first sign of attack, may be repeated every 4–6 hours if necessary; maximum 4 g daily; CHILD contraindicated under 12 years; *by rectum*, ADULT 600–900 mg inserted at first sign of attack, may be repeated every 4 hours if necessary; maximum 3.6 g daily; CHILD contraindicated under 12 years

Adverse effects: generally mild and infrequent but high incidence of gastrointestinal irritation with slight asymptomatic blood loss, increased bleeding time; bronchospasm and skin reactions in hypersensitive patients; see also section 2.1.1

Paracetamol

Tablets, paracetamol 300 mg, 500 mg
Suppositories, paracetamol 250 mg, 500 mg

Uses: acute migraine attacks, tension headache; also mild to moderate pain, pyrexia (section 2.1.2)

Precautions: hepatic impairment (Appendix 5); renal impairment; alcohol dependence; pregnancy and breastfeeding (Appendices 2 and 3); **overdosage:** see section 4.2.1; **interactions:** see Appendix 1

Dosage:

Treatment of acute migraine attack, *by mouth*, ADULT 0.5–1 g at first sign of attack, may be repeated every 4–6 hours if necessary, maximum 4 g daily; CHILD 6–12 years 250–500 mg at first sign of attack, may be repeated every 4–6 hours if necessary, maximum 4 doses in 24 hours; *by rectum*, ADULT and CHILD over 12 years 0.5–1 g at first sign of attack, may be repeated every 4–6 hours if necessary, maximum 4 doses in 24 hours; CHILD 6–12 years 250–500 mg at first sign of attack, may be repeated every 4–6 hours if necessary, maximum 4 doses in 24 hours

Adverse effects: rare, but rashes, blood disorders; acute pancreatitis reported after prolonged use; **important:** liver damage (and less frequently renal damage) following overdosage

---

Ibuprofen

An example of a nonsteroidal anti-inflammatory drug. Various drugs can serve as alternatives

Tablets, ibuprofen 200 mg, 400 mg, 600 mg

Uses: acute migraine attacks, tension headache; also mild to moderate pain and inflammation, pyrexia (section 2.1.3)

Contraindications: hypersensitivity (including asthma, angioedema, urticaria or rhinitis) to acetylsalicylic acid or any other NSAID; active peptic ulceration

Precautions: hepatic or renal impairment (Appendices 4 and 5); cardiac disease; elderly; pregnancy and breastfeeding (Appendices 2 and 3); coagulation defects; allergic disorders; **interactions:** see Appendix 1

Dosage:

Treatment of acute migraine attack, *by mouth* preferably with or after food, ADULT 400–600 mg at first sign of attack, may be repeated every 6–8 hours if necessary, maximum 2.4 g daily; CHILD 8–12 years 200 mg at first sign of attack, may be repeated every 6–8 hours if necessary

Adverse effects: gastrointestinal disturbances including nausea, diarrhoea, dyspepsia, gastric ulceration; hypersensitivity reactions including rash, bronchospasm; headache, dizziness, tinnitus, renal failure; rarely hepatic damage; very rarely exfoliative dermatitis, purpura; prolonged administration, see section 2.1.3

Metoclopramide hydrochloride

Tablets, metoclopramide hydrochloride 10 mg
Injection, metoclopramide hydrochloride 5 mg/ml, 2-ml ampoule

Uses: nausea and vomiting associated with migraine; also nausea and vomiting in gastrointestinal disorders and cytotoxic therapy (section 17.2)

Contraindications: gastrointestinal obstruction, haemorrhage or perforation; epilepsy; phaeochromocytoma

Precautions: hepatic or renal impairment (Appendices 4 and 5); elderly; children and young adults; pregnancy and breastfeeding (Appendices 2 and 3); porphyria; **interactions:** see Appendix 1

Dosage:

Nausea and vomiting of migraine, *by mouth or by intramuscular injection*, ADULT single dose of 10–20 mg at first sign of attack preferably 10–15 minutes before antimigraine drug; ADOLESCENT single dose of 5–10 mg (5 mg if body weight less than 60 kg)

Adverse effects: drowsiness, restlessness, diarrhoea; prolonged
administration, see section 17.2

7.2   Migraine prophylaxis

Prophylactic treatment should be considered for patients in
whom treatment of acute migraine attacks with analgesics or
ergotamine is ineffective, or in whom attacks occur more than
once a month, or for those with less frequent but severe or
prolonged attacks. Prophylaxis can reduce the severity and
frequency of attacks but does not eliminate them completely;
additional symptomatic treatment is still needed. However,
long-term prophylaxis is undesirable and treatment should be
reviewed at 6-monthly intervals. Of the many drugs that have
been advocated beta-adrenoceptor antagonists (beta-blockers)
are most frequently used. **Propranolol,** a non-selective beta-
blocker and other related compounds with similar profile such
as **atenolol** are generally preferred. The potential for beta-
blockers to interact with ergotamine should be borne in mind.
Tricyclic antidepressants, such as **amitriptyline** (section
24.2.1) or calcium-channel blocking drugs such as **verapamil**
(section 12.1) may be of value.

Propranolol hydrochloride

An example of a beta-blocker. Various drugs can serve as alternatives
Tablets, propranolol hydrochloride 20 mg, 40 mg, 80 mg, 160 mg

Uses: prophylaxis of migraine

Contraindications: asthma or history of obstructive airways
disease, uncontrolled heart failure, Prinzmetal angina, marked
bradycardia, hypotension, sick sinus syndrome, second- or
third-degree atrioventricular block, cardiogenic shock, metabolic acidosis, severe peripheral arterial disease; phaeochromocytoma

Precautions: first-degree atrioventricular block; renal impairment (Appendix 4); liver disease (Appendix 5); pregnancy
and breastfeeding (Appendices 2 and 3); portal hypertension;
diabetes mellitus; myasthenia gravis; history of hypersensitivity (increased reaction to allergens, also reduced response
to epinephrine); **interactions:** see Appendix 1

Dosage:

Prophylaxis of migraine, *by mouth* ADULT initially 40 mg 2–3
times daily, increased by same amount at weekly intervals if
necessary; usual range 80–160 mg daily; CHILD under 12 years,
20 mg 2–3 times daily

Adverse effects: bradycardia, heart failure, hypotension,
conduction disorders, bronchospasm, peripheral vasoconstriction, exacerbation of intermittent claudication and
Raynaud phenomenon, gastrointestinal disturbances, fatigue,
sleep disturbances including nightmares; rarely, rash, dry eyes
(reversible), exacerbation of psoriasis

Section 8:
Antineoplastic and immunosuppressive drugs and drugs used in palliative care

8.1   Immunosuppressive drugs

NOTE. WHO advises that adequate resources and specialist supervision are a prerequisite for the introduction of this class of drugs

Immunosuppressive drugs are used in organ transplant recipients to suppress rejection; they are also used as second-line drugs in chronic inflammatory conditions. Treatment should only be initiated by a specialist. Careful monitoring of blood counts is required in patients receiving immunosuppressive drugs and the dose should be adjusted to prevent bone-marrow toxicity. Immunosuppressed patients are particularly prone to atypical infections.

Azathioprine is the most widely used drug in transplant recipients. It is useful when corticosteroid therapy alone has proven inadequate or for other conditions when a reduction in the dose of concurrently administered corticosteroids is required. It is metabolized to mercaptopurine and, as with mercaptopurine, doses need to be reduced when given with allopurinol. The predominant toxic effect is myelosuppression, although hepatic toxicity also occurs.

Ciclosporin is a potent immunosuppressant which is virtually free of myelotoxic effects, but is markedly nephrotoxic. It is particularly useful for the prevention of graft rejection and for the prophylaxis of graft-versus-host disease. The dose is adjusted according to plasma-ciclosporin concentrations and renal function. Dose-related increases in serum creatinine and blood urea nitrogen (BUN) during the first few weeks may necessitate dose reduction.

Corticosteroids such as **prednisolone** (section 8.3) have significant immunosuppressant activity and can also be used to prevent rejection of organ transplants.

Azathioprine

Azathioprine is a representative immunosuppressant. Various drugs can serve as alternatives

Tablets, azathioprine 50 mg

Injection (Powder for solution for injection), azathioprine (as sodium salt), 100-mg vial

Uses: to prevent rejection in transplant recipients; rheumatoid arthritis (section 2.4); inflammatory bowel disease (section 17.4)

Contraindications: hypersensitivity to azathioprine and mercaptopurine; breastfeeding (Appendix 3)

Precautions: monitor for toxicity throughout treatment; full blood counts necessary every week (or more frequently with higher doses and in renal or hepatic impairment) for first 4 weeks of treatment, and at least every 3 months thereafter; reduce dose in elderly; pregnancy (Appendix 2); renal impairment (Appendix 4); liver disease (Appendix 5); **interactions:** Appendix 1

BONE MARROW SUPPRESSION. Patients shold be warned to report immediately any signs or symptoms of bone marrow suppression, for example unexplained bruising or bleeding, infection

Dosage:

Transplant rejection, *by mouth or by intravenous injection* (over at least 1 minute) *or by intravenous infusion,* ADULT up to 5 mg/kg on day of surgery, then reduced to 1–4 mg/kg daily for maintenance

RECONSTITUTION AND ADMINISTRATION. According to manufacturer's directions

NOTE. Intravenous injection is alkaline and very irritant; the intravenous route should therefore **only** be used if oral administration is not possible

Adverse effects: hypersitivity reactions including malaise, dizziness, vomiting, fever, muscular pains, arthralgia, disturbed liver function, cholestatic jaundice, arrhythmias, hypotension or interstitial nephritis call for immediate withdrawal; haematological toxicity includes leukopenia and thrombocytopenia (reversible upon withdrawal) and increased susceptibility to infections; pancreatitis; nausea; pneumonitis

Ciclosporin

Ciclosporin is a representative drug for organ transplantation. Various drugs can serve as alternatives

Capsules, ciclosporin 25 mg

Concentrate for infusion (Concentrate for solution for infusion), ciclosporin 50 mg/ml, 1-ml ampoule

Uses: rejection in kidney, liver, heart or bone-marrow transplantation; graft versus-host disease

Precautions: monitor kidney function (dose dependent increase in serum creatinine and urea during first few weeks may necessitate dose reduction, exclude rejection if kidney transplant, also Appendix 4); monitor liver function (adjust dosage according to bilirubin and liver enzymes, also Appendix 5); monitor blood pressure (discontinue if hypertension cannot be controlled by antihypertensives); monitor serum potassium, particularly if marked renal impairment (and avoid high dietary potassium intake); hyperuricaemia; measure blood lipids before and during treatment; avoid in porphyria; pregnancy (Appendix 2); breastfeeding (Appendix 3); **interactions:** Appendix 1

Dosage:

NOTE. Lower doses are required when ciclosporin is used with other immunosuppressants

Organ transplantation, *by mouth,* ADULT and CHILD over 3 months 10–15 mg/kg 4–12 hours before surgery, then 10–15 mg/kg daily for 1–2 weeks, reducing to 2–6 mg/kg daily for maintenance (adjust dose according to blood concentration and kidney function)

By intravenous infusion over 2–6 hours, one-third of the dose by mouth

Bone marrow transplantation, graft-versus-host disease, *by mouth,* ADULT and CHILD over 3 months 12.5–15 mg/kg daily for 2 weeks, starting on day before surgery, followed by 12.5 mg/kg daily for 3–6 months, then gradually tailed off (may take up to 1 year after transplant)

By intravenous infusion over 2–6 hours, ADULT and CHILD over 3 months 3–5 mg/kg daily for 2 weeks, starting on day before surgery, followed by maintenance by mouth

CONVERSION. Any conversion between brands should be undertaken very carefully, and the manufacturer consulted for further information

DILUTION AND ADMINISTRATION. According to manufacturer's directions

NOTE. Concentrate contains polyethoxylated castor oil, which has been associated with anaphylaxis; observe patient for 30 minutes after starting infusion, and then at frequent intervals

Adverse effects: dose-related and reversible increases in serum creatinine and urea unrelated to tissue rejection; burning sensation in hands and feet during initial therapy; electrolyte disturbances including hyperkalaemia, hypomagnesaemia; hepatic dysfunction; hyperuricaemia; hypercholesterolaemia; hypertension (especially in heart transplant patients); increased incidence of malignancies and lymphoproliferative disorders; increased susceptibility to infections due to immunosuppression; gastrointestinal disturbances; gingival hyperplasia; hirsutism; fatigue; allergic reactions; thrombocytopenia (sometimes with haemolytic uraemic syndrome); also mild anaemia, tremors, convulsions, neuropathy; dysmenorrhoea or amenorrhoea; pancreatitis, myopathy or muscle weakness; cramp; gout; oedema; headache

8.2 Cytotoxic (antineoplastic) drugs

NOTE. WHO advises that adequate resources and specialist supervision are a prerequisite for the introduction of this class of drugs

The treatment of cancer with drugs, radiotherapy and surgery is complex and should only be undertaken by an oncologist. For this reason, the following information is provided merely as a guide. Chemotherapy may be curative or used to alleviate symptoms or to prolong life. Where the condition can no longer be managed with cytotoxic therapy, alternative palliative treatment (section 8.4) should be considered.

For some tumours, single-drug chemotherapy may be adequate, but for many malignancies a combination of drugs provides the best response. Examples of combination therapy include:

- 'CHOP' (cyclophosphamide, doxorubicin, vincristine, prednisolone) for non-Hodgkin disease;
- 'ABVD' (doxorubicin, bleomycin, vinblastine, dacarbazine) for Hodgkin disease;
- 'MOPP' (chlormethine, vincristine, procarbazine, prednisolone) for Hodgkin disease.

Cytotoxic drugs are often combined with other classes of drugs (section 8.3) in the treatment of malignant conditions. Such drugs include hormone agonists and antagonists, corticosteroids and immunostimulant drugs. Combinations are, however, more toxic than single drugs.

The following information covers drugs that have specific anti-tumour activity. However, they are toxic drugs which should be used with great care and monitoring. The specific doses and details of contraindications, precautions and adverse effects for cytotoxic drugs have been omitted from this section since treatment should be **undertaken by specialists** using agreed regimens. Health authorities may wish to formulate their own regimens on the basis of expert advice.

PRECAUTIONS. Treatment with cytotoxic drugs should be initiated only after baseline tests of liver and kidney function have been performed and baseline blood counts established. It may be necessary to modify or delay treatment in certain circumstances. The patient should also be monitored regularly during chemotherapy and cytotoxic drugs withheld if there is significant deterioration in bone-marrow, liver or kidney function.

Many cytotoxic drugs are teratogenic and should not be administered during pregnancy especially in the first trimester. Contraceptive measures are required during therapy and possibly for a period after therapy has ended.

Cytotoxic drugs should be administered with care to avoid undue toxicity to the patient or exposure during handling by the health care provider. Local policies for the handling and reconstitution of cytotoxic drugs should be strictly adhered to; also all waste, including patient's body fluids and excreta (and any material contaminated by them) should be treated as hazardous.

Extravasation of intravenously administered cytotoxic drugs can result in severe pain and necrosis of surrounding tissue. If extravasation occurs, aspiration of the drug should first be attempted, then the affected limb is elevated and warm compresses applied to speed and dilute the infusion or it is localized by applying cold compresses until the inflammation subsides; in severe cases, hydrocortisone cream may be applied topically to the site of inflammation. The manufacturer's literature should also be consulted for more specific information.

ADVERSE EFFECTS. Cytotoxic drugs have a considerable potential to damage normal tissue. Specific adverse effects apply, but a number of effects are common to all cytotoxics such as bone-marrow and immunological suppression. Furthermore, the concomitant use of immunosuppressive drugs will enhance susceptibility to infections. Fever associated with neutropenia or immunosuppression requires immediate treatment with antibiotics.

Nausea and vomiting. Nausea and vomiting following administration of cytotoxic drugs and abdominal radiotherapy are often distressing and may compromise further treatment. Symptoms may be acute (occurring within 24 hours of treatment), delayed (first occurring more than 24 hours after treatment), or anticipatory (occurring before subsequent doses). Delayed and anticipatory symptoms are more difficult to control than acute symptoms and require different management.

Cytotoxic drugs associated with a low risk of emesis include etoposide, fluorouracil, low-dose methotrexate, and the vinca alkaloids; those with an intermediate risk include low-dose cyclophosphamide, doxorubicin, and high-dose methotrexate; and the highest risk is with cisplatin, high-dose cyclophosphamide, and dacarbazine.

For patients at a low risk of emesis, pretreatment with an oral phenothiazine (for example chlorpromazine, section 24.1), continued for up to 24 hours after chemotherapy, is often helpful. For patients at a higher risk dexamethasone 6–10 mg by mouth (section 18.1) may be added before chemotherapy. For patients at a high risk of emesis or when other therapies are ineffective, high doses of intravenous metoclopramide (section 17.2) may be used.

NOTE. High doses of metoclopramide are preferably given by continuous intravenous infusion: an initial dose of 2 to 4 mg/kg is given over 15 to 20 minutes, followed by a maintenance dose of 3 to 5 mg/kg over 8 to 12 hours; the total dose should not exceed 10 mg/kg in 24 hours.

Dexamethasone is the drug of choice for the prevention of delayed symptoms; it is used alone or with metoclopramide.

Good symptom control is the best way to prevent anticipatory symptoms and the addition of diazepam to antiemetic therapy is helpful because of its sedative, anxiolytic and amnesic effects.

Hyperuricaemia. Hyperuricaemia may complicate treatment of conditions such as non-Hodgkin lymphoma and leukaemia. Renal damage may result from the formation of uric acid crystals. Patients should be adequately hydrated and hyperuricaemia may be managed with allopurinol (section 2.3.2) initiated 24 hours before cytotoxic treatment and continued for 7 to 10 days afterwards.

Alopecia. Alopecia is common during treatment with cytotoxic drugs. There is no drug treatment, but the condition often reverses spontaneously once treatment has stopped.

ALKYLATING DRUGS

Alkylating drugs are among the most widely used drugs in cancer chemotherapy. They act by damaging DNA and therefore interfering with cell replication. However, there are two complications. Firstly, they affect gametogenesis and may cause permanent male sterility; in women, the reproductive span may be shortened by the onset of a premature menopause. Secondly, they are associated with a marked increase in the incidence of acute non-lymphocytic leukaemia, in particular when combined with extensive radiation therapy.

Cyclophosphamide requires hepatic activation; it can therefore be given orally and is not vesicant when given intravenously. Like all alkylating drugs its major toxic effects are myelosuppression, alopecia, nausea and vomiting. It can also cause haemorrhagic cystitis; an increased fluid intake for 24 to 48 hours will help to avoid this complication. Cyclophosphamide is used either as part of treatment or as an adjuvant in non-Hodgkin lymphoma, breast cancer, childhood leukaemia, and ovarian cancer. It is also used in several palliative regimens.

Chlorambucil is used to treat chronic lymphocytic leukaemia, non-Hodgkin lymphomas, Hodgkin disease and ovarian cancer. Adverse effects, apart from bone marrow suppression, are uncommon.

Chlormethine (mustine) forms part of the regimen for treatment of advanced Hodgkin disease and malignant lymphomas. Its toxicity includes myelosuppression, severe nausea and vomiting, alopecia and thrombophlebitis due to vesicant effect.

Chlorambucil

Tablets, chlorambucil 2 mg

Uses: chronic lymphocytic leukaemia; some non-Hodgkin lymphomas; Hodgkin disease and ovarian cancer

Contraindications: see notes above and consult specialist literature

Precautions: see notes above and consult specialist literature; renal impairment (Appendix 4); **interactions:** Appendix 1

Dosage:
Consult specialist literature

Adverse effects: see notes above and consult specialist literature

---

Chlormethine hydrochloride

Mustine hydrochloride

Injection (Powder for solution for injection), chlormethine hydrochloride 10-mg vial

Uses: Hodgkin disease; some non-Hodgkin lymphomas; polycythaemia vera; mycosis fungoides; brain tumours, neuroblastoma

Contraindications: see notes above and consult specialist literature

Precautions: see notes above and consult specialist literature; **interactions:** Appendix 1

Dosage:
Consult specialist literature

Adverse effects: see notes above and consult specialist literature

NOTE. Irritant to tissues

Cyclophosphamide

Tablets, cyclophosphamide 25 mg

Injection (Powder for solution for injection), cyclophosphamide 500-mg vial

Uses: malignant lymphomas including non-Hodgkin lymphoma, lymphocytic lymphoma, Burkitt lymphoma; multiple myeloma; leukaemias, mycosis fungoides; neuroblastoma; adenocarcinoma of the ovary; retinoblastoma; breast cancer; severe rheumatoid arthritis (section 2.4)

Contraindications: see notes above and consult specialist literature; pregnancy and breastfeeding (Appendices 2 and 3)

Precautions: see notes above and consult specialist literature; renal and hepatic impairment (Appendices 4 and 5); **interactions:** Appendix 1

Dosage:

Consult specialist literature

Adverse effects: see notes above and consult specialist literature

CYTOTOXIC ANTIBIOTICS

Bleomycin is used in regimens for the treatment of Hodgkin disease and testicular cancer. It has several antineoplastic drug toxicities; it is known to cause dose-related pneumonitis and fibrosis which can be fatal, and is associated with rare acute hypersensitivity reactions. Cutaneous toxicity has also been reported.

Doxorubicin is the most widely used anthracycline antibiotic. It is used for acute leukaemias although other anthracyclines are more commonly used in these circumstances. Doxorubicin also plays a palliative role in the treatment of other malignancies. The primary toxic effects are myelosuppression, alopecia, nausea, vomiting, and dose-related cardiomyopathy. It is also vesicant and can cause severe skin ulceration on extravasation.

Dactinomycin is used to treat paediatric cancers. Its toxicity is similar to that of doxorubicin, but it is not cardiotoxic.

Daunorubicin is used in acute leukaemias. Its toxicity is similar to that of doxorubicin.

Bleomycin

Injection (Powder for solution for injection), bleomycin (as sulfate) 15-USP unit vial

Uses: adjunct to surgery and radiotherapy in palliative treatment of Hodgkin and non-Hodgkin lymphomas; reticulum cell sarcoma and lymphoma; carcinomas of the head, neck, larynx, cervix, penis, skin, vulva, testicles and including embryonal cell carcinoma, choriocarcinoma and teratoma; malignant effusions

Contraindications: see notes above and consult specialist literature

Precautions: see notes above and consult specialist literature; renal impairment (Appendix 4); **interactions:** Appendix 1

Dosage:

Consult specialist literature

NOTE. Doses of bleomycin are expressed in units of the base. As a result of recent labelling changes, 1 USP unit is equivalent to 1000 international units

Adverse effects: see notes above and consult specialist literature

---

Dactinomycin

Actinomycin D

Injection (Powder for solution for injection), dactinomycin 500-microgram vial

Uses: trophoblastic tumours, Wilm tumour, Ewing sarcoma, rhabdomycosarcoma

Contraindications: see notes above and consult specialist literature

Precautions: see notes above and consult specialist literature; **interactions:** Appendix 1

Dosage:

Consult specialist literature

Adverse effects: see notes above and consult specialist literature

NOTE. Irritant to tissues

Daunorubicin

Injection (Powder for solution for injection), daunorubicin (as hydrochloride) 20-mg vial

Uses: acute leukaemias

Contraindications: see notes above and consult specialist literature

Precautions: see notes above and consult specialist literature; renal and hepatic impairment (Appendices 4 and 5); **interactions:** Appendix 1

Dosage:

Consult specialist literature

Adverse effects: see notes above and consult specialist literature

NOTE. Irritant to tissues

Doxorubicin hydrochloride

Doxorubicin hydrochloride is a representative cytotoxic antibiotic. Various drugs can serve as alternatives

Injection (Powder for solution for injection), doxorubicin hydrochloride 10-mg vial, 50-mg vial

Uses: acute leukaemias; carcinomas of the breast, bladder, ovary and thyroid; neuroblastoma; Wilm tumour; non-Hodgkin and Hodgkin lymphomas; soft tissue sarcomas, osteosarcoma

Contraindications: see notes above and consult specialist literature; pregnancy and breastfeeding (Appendices 2 and 3)

Precautions: see notes above and consult specialist literature; hepatic impairment (Appendix 5); **interactions:** Appendix 1

Dosage:

Consult specialist literature

Adverse effects: see notes above and consult specialist literature

NOTE. Irritant to tissues

ANTIMETABOLITES AND ADJUNCTIVE THERAPY

Cytarabine is used in the treatment of acute leukaemia; children may tolerate high doses better than adults. Its effects are highly dependent upon the schedule of administration. It causes myelosuppression, mucositis, and in high doses, central neurotoxicity.

Fluorouracil is primarily used in the adjuvant treatment of colorectal and breast cancer. It is also employed in the palliative treatment of other malignancies. It causes myelosuppression and the palmar-plantar syndrome (erythema and painful desquamation of the hands and feet). When its action is modified by other drugs (such as calcium folinate), its toxicity profile can change; mucositis and diarrhoea may be significant problems. Central neurotoxicity can also occur.

Mercaptopurine is frequently used in the therapy of child-hood leukaemia. It can be administered orally and myelosup-pression and nausea are the only important toxic effects.

Methotrexate is used to treat a variety of malignancies and it plays a major role as an adjuvant for the treatment of breast cancer. Like fluorouracil, methotrexate is myelotoxic, but nausea and vomiting are minimal. It also causes mucositis. Renal impairment reduces methotrexate excretion and can exacerbate toxicity.

Calcium folinate is used to counteract the folate-antagonist action of methotrexate and thus speed recovery from metho-trexate-induced mucositis or myelosuppression. Calcium folin-ate also enhances the effects of fluorouracil when the two are used together for metastatic colorectal cancer.

Cytarabine
Injection (Powder for solution for injection), cytarabine 100-mg vial

Uses: acute lymphoblastic leukaemia; chronic myeloid leuk-aemia; meningeal leukaemia; erythroleukemia; non-Hodgkin lymphoma

Contraindications: see notes above and consult specialist literature

Precautions: see notes above and consult specialist literature; hepatic impairment (Appendix 5); **interactions:** Appendix 1

Dosage:

Consult specialist literature

Adverse effects: see notes above and consult specialist literature

---

Fluorouracil
Injection, fluorouracil 50 mg/ml, 5-ml ampoule

Uses: carcinomas of the colorectum, breast, stomach, pancreas, cervix, prostate, ovary and endometrium; liver tumours; head and neck tumours; actinic keratoses (section 13.5)

Contraindications: see notes above and consult specialist literature

---

Precautions: see notes above and consult specialist literature; **interactions:** Appendix 1

Dosage:

Consult specialist literature

Adverse effects: see notes above and consult specialist literature

---

Mercaptopurine

Tablets, mercaptopurine 50 mg

Uses: acute leukaemias

Contraindications: see notes above and consult specialist literature

Precautions: see notes above and consult specialist literature; renal impairment (Appendix 4); **interactions:** Appendix 1

Dosage:

Consult specialist literature

Adverse effects: see notes above and consult specialist literature

---

Methotrexate

Tablets, methotrexate 2.5 mg
Injection, methotrexate (as sodium salt) 25mg/ml, 2-ml vial

Uses: carcinoma of the breast, head and neck, and lung; trophoblastic tumours; acute lymphoblastic leukaemia, meningeal leukaemia; non-Hodgkin lymphomas; advanced cases of mycosis fungoides; non-metastatic osteosarcoma; severe rheumatoid arthritis (section 2.4)

Contraindications: see notes above and consult specialist literature; pregnancy (Appendix 2)

Precautions: see notes above and consult specialist literature; renal and hepatic impairment (Appendices 4 and 5); **interactions:** Appendix 1

Dosage:

Consult specialist literature

Adverse effects: see notes above and consult specialist literature

---

Calcium folinate

Tablets, folinic acid (as calcium folinate) 15 mg
Injection, folinic acid (as calcium folinate) 3 mg/ml, 10-ml ampoule

Uses: high-dose methotrexate therapy ('folate rescue'); inadvertent overdose of methotrexate; with fluorouracil in the palliative treatment of advanced colorectal cancer

Precautions: not for pernicious anaemia or other megaloblastic anaemias due to vitamin B_{12} deficiency; pregnancy (Appendix 2); breastfeeding; **interactions:** Appendix 1

Dosage:

Antidote to methotrexate (usually started 24 hours after methotrexate), *by intramuscular or intravenous injection or by intravenous infusion*, ADULT and CHILD up to 120 mg in divided doses over 12–24 hours, then 12–15 mg *by intramuscular injection or* 15 mg *by mouth* every 6 hours for 48–72 hours

Methotrexate overdosage (started as soon as possible, preferably within 1 hour of methotrexate), *by intravenous injection or infusion*, ADULT and CHILD, dose equal to or higher than that of methotrexate, at rate not exceeding 160 mg/minute

With fluorouracil in colorectal cancer, consult specialist literature

ADMINISTRATION. According to manufacturer's directions

NOTE. Intrathecal injection of calcium folinate is contraindicated

Adverse effects: allergic reactions; pyrexia after parenteral administration

VINCA ALKALOIDS AND ETOPOSIDE

The vinca alkaloids, **vinblastine** and **vincristine**, are primarily used in the treatment of acute leukaemias. Vinblastine is also used for Hodgkin disease and some solid tumours. Vincristine is also used in the management of non-Hodgkin lymphoma. Both can cause neurotoxicity, but this is more of a problem with vincristine. Myelosuppression is more common with vinblastine.

Etoposide is an important component of the treatment of testicular carcinoma and is used in several regimens for lung cancers. It causes myelosuppression and alopecia and it can cause hypotension during infusion. It does not produce significant nausea and vomiting.

Etoposide

Capsules, etoposide 100 mg

Concentrate for infusion (Concentrate for solution for infusion), etoposide 20 mg/ml, 5-ml vial

Uses: refractory testicular tumours; lung cancer

Contraindications: see notes above and consult specialist literature

Precautions: see notes above and consult specialist literature; hepatic impairment (Appendix 5); **interactions:** Appendix 1

Dosage:

Consult specialist literature

Adverse effects: see notes above and consult specialist literature

NOTE. Irritant to tissues

Vinblastine sulfate

Injection (Powder for solution for injection), vinblastine sulfate 10-mg vial

Uses: disseminated Hodgkin and non-Hodgkin lymphoma; advanced testicular carcinoma, breast carcinoma; palliative treatment of Kaposi sarcoma; trophoblastic tumours; Letterer-Siwe disease

Contraindications: see notes above and consult specialist literature; pregnancy and breastfeeding (Appendices 2 and 3)

Precautions: see notes above and consult specialist literature; hepatic impairment (Appendix 5); **interactions:** Appendix 1

Dosage:

Consult specialist literature

NOTE. Vinblastine is for intravenous administration only. Intrathecal injection causes severe neurotoxicity which is usually fatal

Adverse effects: see notes above and consult specialist literature

NOTE. Irritant to tissues

Vincristine sulfate

Injection (Powder for solution for injection), vincristine sulfate 1-mg vial, 5-mg vial

Uses: acute lymphoblastic leukaemia; neuroblastoma, Wilm tumour, Hodgkin and non-Hodgkin lymphomas; rhabdomyosarcoma, Ewing sarcoma; mycosis fungoides

Contraindications: see notes above and consult specialist literature; pregnancy and breastfeeding (Appendices 2 and 3)

Precautions: see notes above and consult specialist literature; hepatic impairment (Appendix 5); **interactions:** Appendix 1

Dosage:

Consult specialist literature

NOTE. Vincristine is for intravenous administration only. Intrathecal injection causes severe neurotoxicity which is usually fatal

Adverse effects: see notes above and consult specialist literature

NOTE. Irritant to tissues

OTHER ANTINEOPLASTIC DRUGS

The enzyme **asparaginase** is an important component in the management of childhood leukaemia, but is not used in any other malignancy. Its toxicity profile is broad and the drug must be carefully administered because of the risk of anaphylaxis.

Cisplatin is a platinum compound used in the treatment of ovarian and testicular malignancies. It is also a component of regimens used in non-small cell and small cell lung cancer and plays a palliative role in other malignancies. Cisplatin is myelosuppressive and also produces slight alopecia. However, it causes severe dose-related nausea and vomiting. It is also nephrotoxic and neurotoxic. Nephrotoxicity can be reduced by maintaining high urine output during cisplatin administration and immediately afterwards, but neurotoxicity is often dose-limiting.

Dacarbazine, thought to act as an alkylating drug, is a component of a regimen for Hodgkin disease. It is also used in the palliative therapy of metastatic malignant melanoma. Its major toxic effects are myelosuppression, and intense nausea and vomiting.

Levamisole is an anthelminthic with immunostimulating properties; it is used in combination with fluorouracil as adjuvant therapy for colorectal cancer following resection of the tumour. Its major toxic effects are a variety of CNS symptoms, nausea, dermatitis and hypersensitivity reactions.

Procarbazine is used in the treatment of advanced Hodgkin disease. Toxic effects include myelosuppression, nausea, vomiting, CNS symptoms and depression. Procarbazine possesses a weak monoamine oxidase inhibitory effect but dietary restriction is not necessary.

Asparaginase
Crisantaspase
Injection (Powder for solution for injection), asparaginase 10 000-unit vial

Uses: acute lymphoblastic leukaemia

Contraindications: see notes above and consult specialist literature

Precautions: see notes above and consult specialist literature; **interactions:** Appendix 1

Dosage:
Consult specialist literature

Adverse effects: see notes above and consult specialist literature

Cisplatin
Injection (Powder for solution for injection), cisplatin 10-mg vial, 50-mg vial

Uses: metastatic testicular tumours, metastatic ovarian tumours, advanced bladder carcinoma and other solid tumours

Contraindications: see notes above and consult specialist literature

Precautions: see notes above and consult specialist literature; renal impairment (Appendix 4); **interactions:** Appendix 1

Dosage:
Consult specialist literature

Adverse effects: see notes above and consult specialist literature

Dacarbazine
Injection (Powder for solution for injection), dacarbazine 100-mg vial

Uses: metastatic malignant melanoma; Hodgkin disease

Contraindications: see notes above and consult specialist literature; pregnancy (Appendix 2)

Precautions: see notes above and consult specialist literature; renal and hepatic impairment (Appendices 4 and 5); **interactions:** Appendix 1

Dosage:
Consult specialist literature

Adverse effects: see notes above and consult specialist literature

NOTE. Irritant to tissues

Levamisole
Tablets, levamisole (as hydrochloride) 50 mg

Uses: with fluorouracil for the treatment of colorectal carcinoma after complete resection of primary tumour; intestinal nematode infections (section 6.1.1.2)

Contraindications: see notes above and consult specialist literature

Precautions: see notes above and consult specialist literature; **interactions:** consult manufacturer's literature

Dosage:

Consult specialist literature

Adverse effects: see notes above and consult specialist literature

---

Procarbazine

Capsules, procarbazine (as hydrochloride) 50 mg

Uses: part of MOPP regimen in Hodgkin and non-Hodgkin lymphomas

Contraindications: see notes above and consult specialist literature

Precautions: see notes above and consult specialist literature; renal and hepatic impairment (Appendices 4 and 5); **interactions:** Appendix 1

Dosage:

Consult specialist literature

Adverse effects: see notes above and consult specialist literature

---

8.3   Hormones and antihormones

The corticosteroids **prednisolone, dexamethasone** and **hydrocortisone** are synthetic hormones given at pharmacological doses particularly for haematological malignancies. Although there is no evidence for therapeutic superiority, prednisolone is commonly used; it is an important component of curative regimens for lymphomas and childhood leukaemias and elsewhere it has a palliative role. However, chronic use leads to the development of a cushingoid syndrome.

Tamoxifen is an estrogen-receptor antagonist. Its important role in breast cancer is use after surgery and for palliative management in patients with advanced disease. When given at recommended doses, it has few adverse effects, although, it can induce uterine endometrial malignancies.

Diethylstilbestrol, a synthetic estrogen, is used to manipulate the hormonal environment in patients with hormone-sensitive tumours (for example breast and testes). It has few significant adverse effects in women but in men it causes gynaecomastia, and, more importantly, increases the risk of cardiovascular disease. For breast cancer diethylstilbestrol has been superseded by tamoxifen but it can be used for its anti-androgen effect in prostate cancer as an adjunct or for palliation.

Prednisolone

Prednisolone is a representative corticosteroid. Various drugs can serve as alternatives

Tablets, prednisolone 5 mg

Injection (Powder for solution for injection), prednisolone (as sodium phosphate or sodium succinate), 20-mg vial, 25-mg vial

Uses: with antineoplastic drugs for acute lymphoblastic and chronic lymphocytic leukaemia, Hodgkin disease, and non-Hodgkin lymphoma; inflammatory and allergic reactions (sections 3.1 and 18.1); eye (section 21.2)

Contraindications: untreated bacterial, viral, and fungal infections; avoid live virus vaccines

Precautions: monitor body weight, blood pressure, fluid and electrolyte balance, and blood glucose concentration throughout treatment; adrenal suppression during and for some months after withdrawal—intercurrent infection or surgery may require increased dose of corticosteroid (or temporary reintroduction if already withdrawn); quiescent amoebiasis, strongyloidiasis, or tuberculosis possibly reactivated; increased severity of viral infections, particularly chickenpox and measles—passive immunization with immunoglobulin required; hypertension, recent myocardial infarction, congestive heart failure; renal impairment; hepatic impairment (Appendix 5); diabetes mellitus; osteoporosis; glaucoma; severe psychosis, epilepsy; peptic ulcer; pregnancy (Appendix 2); breastfeeding (Appendix 3); **interactions:** Appendix 1

Dosage:

Leukaemia and lymphomas, *by mouth,* ADULT initially up to 100 mg daily, then gradually reduced if possible to 20–40 mg daily; CHILD up to 1 year, initially up to 25 mg, then 5–10 mg; 2–7 years, initially up to 50 mg, then 10–20 mg; 8–12 years, up to 75 mg, then 15–30 mg

By intramuscular injection, ADULT up to 100 mg 1–2 times weekly

By intravenous injection, ADULT up to 60 mg daily

Adverse effects: gastrointestinal effects including dyspepsia, oesophageal ulceration, development of or aggravation of peptic ulcers, abdominal distension, acute pancreatitis; increased appetite and weight gain; adrenal suppression with high doses, leading to cushingoid symptoms (moon face, acne, bruising, abdominal striae, truncal obesity, muscle wasting); menstrual irregularities and amenorrhoea; hypertension; osteoporosis, with resultant vertebral collapse and long-bone fractures; avascular osteonecrosis; ophthalmic effects including glaucoma, subcapsular cataracts, exacerbation of viral or fungal eye infections; diabetes mellitus; thromboembolism; delayed tissue healing; myopathy, muscle weakness of arms and legs; depression, psychosis, epilepsy; raised intracranial pressure; hypersensitivity reactions

Tamoxifen

Tablets, tamoxifen (as citrate) 10 mg, 20 mg

Uses: adjuvant treatment of estrogen-receptor-positive breast cancer; metastatic breast cancer

Contraindications: pregnancy (exclude before treatment and advise non-hormonal contraception if appropriate, see also Appendix 2); breastfeeding (Appendix 3)

Precautions: monitor for endometrial changes (increased incidence of hyperplasia, polyps, and cancer); cystic ovarian swellings in premenopausal women; increased risk of thromboembolism when used with antineoplastic drugs; avoid in porphyia; **interactions:** Appendix 1

Dosage:

Breast cancer, *by mouth,* ADULT 20 mg daily

Adverse effects: hot flushes; endometrial changes (symptoms such as vaginal bleeding and other menstrual irregularities, vaginal discharge, pelvic pain require immediate investigation); increased pain and hypercalcaemia with bony metastases; tumour flare; nausea and vomiting; liver enzyme changes (rarely cholestasis, hepatitis, hepatic necrosis); thromboembolic events; decreased platelet count; oedema; alopecia; rash; headache; visual disturbances including corneal changes, cataracts, retinopathy; rarely hypersensitivity reactions including angioedema, Stevens-Johnson syndrome, bullous pemphigoid

8.4 Drugs used in palliative care

NOTE. The WHO Expert Committee on Essential Drugs recommends that all the drugs mentioned in Cancer Pain Relief: with a Guide to Opioid Availability, 2nd edition. Geneva: WHO 1996 be considered essential. These drugs are included in the relevant sections of the model list according to their therapeutic use, for example analgesics.

Palliative care includes both pain relief and the symptomatic relief of conditions including dyspnoea, restlessness and confusion, anorexia, constipation, pruritus, nausea and vomiting, and insomnia. Health authorities should be encouraged to develop their own palliative care services.

Pain relief can be achieved with drugs and neurosurgical, pyschological and behavioural approaches adapted to individual patient needs. If carried out correctly, most patients with cancer pain can obtain effective relief. Pain is best treated with a combination of drug and non-drug measures. Some types of pain respond well to a combination of a non-opioid and an opioid. With others, relief is obtained by combining a corticosteroid and an opioid. Neuropathic pains often show little response to non-opioid and opioid analgesics, but may be eased by tricyclic antidepressants and anticonvulsants. Cancer patients often have many fears and anxieties, and may become depressed. Very anxious or deeply depressed patients may need an appropriate psychotropic drug in addition to an analgesic. If this fact is not appreciated, the pain may remain intractable.

In the majority of patients, cancer pain can be relieved with analgesics:

- **by mouth**: if possible analgesics should be given by mouth. Rectal suppositories are useful in patients with dysphagia, uncontrolled

vomiting or gastrointestinal obstruction. Continuous subcutaneous
infusion offers an alternative route.

- **by the clock**: analgesics are more effective in preventing pain than in the
relief of established pain, therefore doses should be given at fixed time
intervals and titrated against the patient's pain; if pain occurs between
doses, a rescue dose should be given, and the next dose increased.
- **by the ladder**: the first step is to give a non-opioid analgesic such as
acetylsalicylic acid, paracetamol or **ibuprofen**, if necessary with an
adjuvant drug. If this does not relieve the pain, an opioid for mild to
moderate pain such as **codeine** should be added. When this combination
fails to relieve pain, an opioid for moderate to severe pain such as
morphine should be substituted.
- **for the individual**: there are no standard doses for opioid drugs. The
range for oral morphine is from as little as 5 mg to more than 100 mg
every 4 hours.
- **with attention to detail**: the first and last doses of the day should be
linked to the patient's waking time and bedtime. Ideally the drug regimen
should be written out in full for the patient and his or her family. The
patient should be warned about possible adverse effects.

Drugs for neuropathic pain

Neuropathic pain only responds partially to opioids and a
corticosteroid is often required, particularly in the case of nerve
compression. Alternatively neuropathic pain often responds to a
tricyclic antidepressant, such as **amitriptyline**, anticonvulsants
such as **carbamazepine** or **valproate**, or a local anaesthetic
such as intravenous **lidocaine**.

Adjuvant therapy

These drugs may be necessary for one of three reasons:
- to treat the adverse effects of the analgesics (for example antiemetics
such as **metclopramide** and laxatives with opioids)
- to enhance pain relief (for example a corticosteroid such as **prednisolone**
in nerve compression pain)
- to treat concomitant psychological disturbances such as insomnia,
anxiety and depression.

Section 9:
Antiparkinson drugs

9.1   Drugs used in parkinsonism

The use of pharmacotherapy will depend upon the degree of incapacity of the patient and is generally not justified until symptoms compromise working ability and social relationships; although levodopa is used in the early stages in some patients. Close supervision is then needed to ensure that treatment regimens are tolerated and that appropriate changes are made to the regimen as the disease progresses.

The most effective form of therapy is a combination of **levodopa** and a peripheral dopa-decarboxylase inhibitor, such as **carbidopa**. The response to levodopa with carbidopa is a compromise between increased mobility and adverse effects. Dyskinesias may be dose limiting and increasingly frequent with increased duration of treatment. Many factors including tolerance and progression of the disease may result in complications after 2 to 5 years of treatment. 'End-of-dose' deterioration occurs when there is a reduced duration of benefit from a dose, resulting in disability and dystonias. The 'on-off' phenomenon is characterized by sudden swings from mobility to episodes of akinesia, tremor and rigidity lasting from a few minutes to several hours. Amelioration of these effects can sometimes be achieved by administering levodopa in a sustained-release preparation or in a greater number of fractionated doses throughout the day. Supplementary use of amantadine, bromocriptine or selegiline can be of value either to enhance the effect of levodopa or to reduce 'end-of-dose' fluctuations and 'on-off' effects. Psychiatric symptoms inducing disruption of sleep, vivid dreams and hallucinations are characteristic adverse effects that may occur at any time, especially in the elderly, and may require dose reduction or withdrawal of levodopa.

Anticholinergic (more correctly termed antimuscarinic) drugs such as **biperiden** are usually sufficient in drug-induced pseudo-parkinsonism. They are also used as adjunctive therapy in other forms of parkinsonism where the primary need is to stimulate dopaminergic activity in the striatal system.

Levodopa with carbidopa

Carbidopa is a representative peripheral dopa decarboxylase inhibitor. Various drugs can serve as alternatives

Tablets, levodopa 100 mg with carbidopa 10 mg, levodopa 250 mg with carbidopa 25 mg

Uses: all forms of parkinsonism other than drug-induced

Contraindications: concurrent use of monoamine oxidase inhibitors; angle-closure glaucoma; confirmed or suspected malignant melanoma

Precautions: pulmonary disease, peptic ulceration, cardiovascular disease (including previous myocardial infarction); diabetes mellitus, osteomalacia, open-angle glaucoma, psychiatric illness (avoid if severe); close supervision of patients is necessary with monitoring of hepatic, haematological, cardiovascular and renal function in long-term therapy; elderly: avoid rapid dose increases; avoid abrupt withdrawals; pregnancy (toxicity in *animals*) (Appendix 2), breastfeeding (Appendix 3); **interactions:** Appendix 1

Dosage:

Parkinsonism, *by mouth*, ADULT expressed in terms of levodopa, initially 100 mg (with carbidopa 10 mg) twice daily, increased by 100 mg (with carbidopa 10 mg) every few days as necessary, to a maximum of levodopa 1.5 g

ADMINISTRATION. Optimum daily dose must be determined for each patient by careful monitoring and be taken after meals

Adverse effects: nausea, anorexia and vomiting, particularly at the start of treatment; postural hypotension at the start of treatment, particularly in elderly and those receiving anti-hypertensives; confusion, vivid dreams, dizziness, tachy-cardia, arrhythmias; reddish discoloration of body fluids; drowsiness, headache, flushing, gastrointestinal bleeding, peripheral neuropathy; taste disturbances, pruritis, rash, liver enzyme changes; psychiatric symptoms including psychosis, depression, hallucinations, delusions and neurological disturbances including dyskinesias may be dose-limiting; painful dystonic spasms ('end-of-dose' effects) and ('on-off' effects) after prolonged treatment (see notes above); neuroleptic malignant syndrome, on sudden withdrawal

---

Biperiden hydrochloride

Biperiden hydrochloride is a representative anticholinergic drug. Various drugs can serve as alternatives
Tablets, biperiden hydrochloride 2 mg

Uses: drug-induced extrapyramidal symptoms (but not tardive dyskinesias) and adjunctive treatment of parkinsonism

Contraindications: angle-closure glaucoma; obstructive uro-pathy; myasthenia gravis; gastrointestinal obstruction

Precautions: elderly; cardiovascular disease, hepatic or renal impairment; avoid abrupt withdrawal; **interactions:** Appendix 1

SKILLED TASKS. May impair ability to perform skilled tasks, for example operating machinery, driving

Dosage:

Drug-induced extrapyramidal symptoms, parkinsonism, *by mouth*, ADULT, initially 1 mg twice daily, increased to 2 mg 3 times daily, gradually increased according to response and tolerance to maximum 16 mg daily

Adverse effects: drowsiness, dry mouth, constipation, blurred vision; hesitancy of micturition, dizziness, tachycardia, arrhythmias, confusion and psychiatric disturbances with high dosage, especially in the elderly, may require withdrawal of treatment

9.2   Drugs used in essential tremor and related disorders

ESSENTIAL TREMOR. It can be treated with beta-blockers such as **propranolol** (120 mg daily) (section 7.2) which may be of value if the tremor results in physical or social disability.

DYSTONIAS. If no identifiable cause is found and the patient does not go into spontaneous remission, a trial of **levodopa** should be given to determine whether the patient has dopamine-responsive dystonia. If there is no response within three months, the drug should be withdrawn and small doses of an anticholinergic drug such as **biperiden** should be given. The dosage may be increased gradually and up to 16 mg daily may be tolerated. In patients who fail to respond to either levodopa or an anticholinergic, other drugs including diazepam, baclofen, carbamazepine or phenothiazines may be of value. Psychological treatments have also been used successfully in the management of dyskinesias.

CHOREA. Choreiform movements can be induced by certain drugs including levodopa, phenytoin and antipsychotic drugs. Huntington disease is the most common of the hereditary choreas. Drug treatment is symptomatic and does not alter the progression of the disease. The aim of therapy is to reduce dopaminergic transmission which results from excessive or enhanced cholinergic activity. Antipsychotic drugs antagonize dopamine and usually lessen the chorea temporarily. Tetrabenazine, the dopamine-depleting drug is currently under investigation.

TICS. Tics which resemble choreiform movements are commonly associated with anxiety. However, in the more complex multiple tic disorder, Tourette syndrome, treatment with antipsychotic drugs may be required.

TARDIVE DYSKINESIA. It is associated with chronic administration of antipsychotic drugs. It is characterized by involuntary, repetitive, choreiform movement of the cheek, mouth and fingers. The first step of treatment should always be discontinuation of the antipsychotic drug or dosage reduction if the underlying psychotic disorder permits. In some cases the disorder may be irreversible and if the symptoms are very disabling small dosages of reserpine may be tried.

Section 10: Drugs affecting the blood

10.1 Antianaemia drugs

IRON-DEFICIENCY ANAEMIA. Anaemia has many different aetiologies. It occurs when the haemoglobin concentration falls below the normal range for the age and sex of the individual. It is essential that a correct diagnosis is made before initiating therapy.

Any serious underlying cause of iron-deficiency anaemia, including gastric erosion and colonic carcinoma, should be excluded before giving iron replacement. Prophylaxis with iron salts in pregnancy should be given to women who have additional factors for iron-deficiency; low-dose iron and folic acid preparations are used for the prophylaxis of megaloblastic anaemia in pregnancy.

Ferrous salts should be given orally wherever possible. They differ only marginally in efficiency of absorption and thus the choice of preparation is usually decided by incidence of adverse effects and cost. The oral dose of elemental iron for treatment of iron-deficiency anaemia in adults should be 100–200 mg daily with meals.

The approximate elemental iron content of various ferrous salts is ferrous fumarate 200 mg (65 mg iron), ferrous gluconate 300 mg (35 mg iron), ferrous succinate 100 mg (35 mg iron), ferrous sulfate 300 mg (60 mg iron), and dried ferrous sulfate 200 mg (65 mg iron).

Iron intake in the evening has been reported to improve its absorption. Iron intake with meals may reduce bioavailability but improve tolerability and adherence.

If adverse effects arise with one salt, dosage can be reduced or a change made to an alternative iron salt. The haemoglobin concentration should rise by about 100–200 mg/100 ml per day or 2 g/100 ml over 3–4 weeks. After the haemoglobin has risen to normal, treatment should be continued for a further three months in an attempt to replenish the iron stores. Gastrointestinal irritation may occur. Nausea and epigastric pain are dose-related. Oral iron may exacerbate diarrhoea in patients with inflammatory bowel disease but care is also needed in patients with intestinal strictures and diverticulae. Iron as **iron dextran** should be given parenterally only if the patient has severe gastrointestinal adverse effects with oral preparations, continuing severe blood loss or malabsorption. Parenteral iron may cause more harm than benefit. Provided that the oral iron preparation is taken reliably and is absorbed, then the haemoglobin response is not significantly faster with the parenteral route than the oral route.

MEGALOBLASTIC ANAEMIAS. These are due to the lack of either vitamin B_{12} (hydroxocobalamin) or folate or both. The clinical features of folate-deficient megaloblastic anaemia are similar to those of vitamin B_{12} deficiency except that the accompanying severe neuropathy does not occur; it is essential to determine which deficiency is present and the underlying cause is established in every case. **Hydroxocobalamin** is the form of vitamin B_{12} used for treatment of vitamin B_{12} deficiency whether due to dietary deficiency or malabsorption including pernicious anaemia (due to a lack of intrinsic factor essential for B_{12} absorption). Folate deficiency due to poor nutrition, pregnancy, antiepileptics or malabsorption is treated with **folic acid** but this should never be administered without vitamin B_{12} in undiagnosed megaloblastic anaemia because of the risk of precipitating neurological changes due to vitamin B_{12} deficiency.

Preparations containing a **ferrous salt and folic acid** are used for the prevention of megaloblastic anaemia in pregnancy. The low doses of folic acid in these preparations are inadequate for the treatment of megaloblastic anaemias.

PREVENTION OF NEURAL TUBE DEFECTS. **Folic acid** 5 mg is given to prevent the recurrence of neural tube defect in women who wish to become pregnant (or are at risk of becoming pregnant). To prevent first occurrence of neural tube defect women of childbearing age should be advised to take folic acid as a medicinal or food supplement at a dose of 400 micrograms daily before conception and continue until the twelfth week of pregnancy.

Ferrous salts

Tablets, dried ferrous sulfate 200 mg (65 mg iron); ferrous sulfate 300 mg (60 mg iron); ferrous fumarate 210 mg (68 mg iron); ferrous gluconate 300 mg (35 mg iron)

Uses: iron-deficiency anaemia

Contraindications: haemosiderosis, haemochromatosis; any form of anaemia not caused by iron deficiency; patients receiving repeated blood transfusions; parenteral iron therapy

Precautions: should not be administered for longer than 6 months; pregnancy; peptic ulcer, regional enteritis, ulcerative colitis, intestinal strictures, diverticulae; **overdosage:** see section 4.2.4; **interactions:** Appendix 1

Dosage:

Iron-deficiency anaemia, *by mouth*, ADULT elemental iron 100–200 mg daily in divided doses

Adverse effects: constipation, diarrhoea, dark stools, nausea, epigastric pain, gastrointestinal irritation; long-term or excessive administration may cause haemosiderosis

Iron dextran

Iron dextran is a representative parenteral iron preparation. Various drugs can serve as alternatives

Injection (Solution for injection), iron dextran (iron 50 mg/ml), 2-ml ampoule

Uses: iron-deficiency anaemia in patients with severe intolerance to oral iron, continuing severe blood loss or malabsorption

Contraindications: history of allergies including asthma; severe hepatic impairment, kidney infection; pregnancy (toxicity in *animals*)

Precautions: test dose should be given at least 1 hour before therapeutic dose and facilities for management of anaphylaxis should be available; **overdosage:** see section 4.2.4

Dosage:

Iron-deficiency anaemia, *by deep intramuscular injection*, ADULT calculated according to body-weight and iron deficit

Adverse effects: pain, swelling, and staining at injection site; nausea, vomiting, taste disturbances, dizziness, hypersensitivity reactions including fatal anaphylaxis reported (see Precautions); delayed reactions including arthralgia, myalgia, regional lymphadenopathy, chills, fever, malaise, headache, and haematuria may occur

---

Folic acid

Tablets, folic acid 1 mg, 5 mg

Injection (Solution for injection), folic acid (as sodium salt) 1 mg/ml, 1-ml ampoule

Uses: treatment of folate-deficiency megaloblastic anaemia; prevention of neural tube defect in pregnancy

Contraindications: should never be given without vitamin B_{12} in undiagnosed megaloblastic anaemia or other vitamin B_{12} deficiency states because risk of precipitating subacute combined degeneration of the spinal cord; folate-dependent malignant disease

Precautions: women receiving antiepileptic therapy need counselling before starting folic acid; **interactions:** Appendix 1

Dosage:

Treatment of folate-deficiency, megaloblastic anaemia, *by mouth*, ADULT 5 mg daily for 4 months; up to 15 mg daily may be necessary in malabsorption states

Prevention of first occurrence of neural tube defect, *by mouth*, ADULT 400–500 micrograms daily before conception and during the first twelve weeks of pregnancy

Prevention of recurrence of neural tube defect, *by mouth*, ADULT 5 mg daily (reduced to 4 mg daily, if suitable preparation available) from at least 4 weeks before conception until twelfth week of pregnancy

NOTE. Patients unable to take folic acid *by mouth*, may be given the same dose as sodium salt *by deep intramuscular injection*

Ferrous salt with folic acid

Tablets, dried ferrous sulfate 325 mg (105 mg iron), folic acid 350 micrograms; dried ferrous sulfate 160 mg (50 mg iron), folic acid 400 micrograms; ferrous fumarate 322 mg (105 mg iron), folic acid 350 micrograms

Uses: prevention of iron and folic acid deficiencies in pregnancy

---

Precautions: low doses of folic acid in the combination preparations above are inadequate for treatment of megaloblastic anaemia; **overdosage:** see section 4.2.4; **interactions:** Appendix 1

Dosage:
Prevention of iron and folic acid deficiencies in pregnancy, *by mouth* ADULT the equivalent of about 100 mg elemental iron with 350–400 micrograms folic acid daily throughout pregnancy

Adverse effects: see Ferrous salts

Hydroxocobalamin
Injection (Solution for injection), hydroxocobalamin 1 mg/ml, 1-ml ampoule

Uses: megaloblastic anaemia due to vitamin B_{12} deficiency

Precautions: except in emergencies, should not be given before diagnosis confirmed; monitor serum potassium levels—arrhythmias secondary to hypokalaemia in early therapy

Dosage:
Megaloblastic anaemia without neurological involvement, *by intramuscular injection*, ADULT and CHILD initially 0.25–1 mg on alternate days for 1–2 weeks, then 250 micrograms weekly until blood count is within normal range, thereafter 1 mg every 2–3 months

Megaloblastic anaemia with neurological involvement, *by intramuscular injection*, ADULT and CHILD initially 1 mg on alternate days until no further improvement occurs, then 1 mg every 2 months

Prophylaxis of macrocytic anaemias, *by intramuscular injection*, ADULT and CHILD 1 mg every 2–3 months

Tobacco amblyopia and Leber optic atrophy, *by intramuscular injection*, ADULT and CHILD 1 mg daily for 2 weeks, then 1 mg twice weekly until no further improvement, then 1 mg every 1–3 months

Adverse effects: itching, exanthema, fever, chills, hot flushes, nausea, dizziness; rarely acneiform and bullous eruptions, anaphylaxis

---

10.2 Drugs affecting coagulation

Anticoagulants are used to prevent thrombus formation or extension of an existing thrombus in the slower-moving venous side of the circulation, where the thrombus consists of a fibrin web enmeshed with platelets and red cells. They are therefore used widely in the prevention and treatment of deep-vein thrombosis in the legs, prophylaxis of embolization in rheumatic heart disease and atrial fibrillation and to prevent thrombi forming on prosthetic heart valves.

Heparin is a parenteral anticoagulant that initiates anticoagulation rapidly but has a short duration of action. The low molecular weight heparins have a longer duration of action.

For the treatment of deep venous thrombosis and pulmonary embolism heparin is given as an intravenous loading dose followed by continuous intravenous infusion (using an infusion pump) or by intermittent subcutaneous injection. An oral anticoagulant is started at the same time as heparin. The heparin needs to be continued for at least 3 days, until the oral anticoagulant has taken effect. Laboratory monitoring is essential, on a daily basis. Heparin is also used in regimens for the management of myocardial infarction, the management of unstable angina, acute peripheral arterial occlusion and in dialysis.

In patients undergoing general surgery, low-dose heparin by subcutaneous injection is used to prevent postoperative deep-vein thrombosis and pulmonary embolism in high risk patients (those with obesity, malignant disease, history of deep-vein thrombosis or pulmonary embolism, patients over 40 years, those with an established thrombophilic disorder or those undergoing large or complicated surgery). It is also of value in high-risk medical patients, for example obesity, heart failure, when confined to bed.

If haemorrhage occurs it is usually sufficient to withdraw heparin, but if rapid reversal of the effects of heparin is required, **protamine sulfate** is a specific antidote.

Oral anticoagulants take at least 48 to 72 hours for the anticoagulant effect to develop fully; if an immediate effect is needed, heparin must be given concomitantly. **Warfarin** is indicated in deep-vein thrombosis, pulmonary embolism and patients with atrial fibrillation who are at risk of embolization; oral anticoagulants should not be used in cerebral thrombosis or peripheral arterial occlusion as first-line therapy. The main adverse effect of oral anticoagulants is haemorrhage. Prothrombin time should be checked on a daily basis initially then at longer intervals depending on response.

If severe haemorrhage occurs, stop warfarin and give **phytomenadione** (vitamin K) by slow intravenous injection.

ANTICOAGULANTS IN PREGNANCY. Oral anticoagulants are teratogenic and should not be given in the first trimester of pregnancy. Women at risk of pregnancy should be warned of this danger since stopping warfarin before the sixth week of gestation may largely avoid the risk of fetal abnormality. Oral anticoagulants cross the placenta with the risk of placental or fetal haemorrhage, especially during the last few weeks of pregnancy and at delivery. Therefore, if at all possible, oral anticoagulants should be avoided in pregnancy, especially in the first and third trimester. Difficult decisions may have to be made, particularly in women with prosthetic heart valves or with a history of recurrent venous thrombosis or pulmonary embolism.

HAEMOPHILIA. **Desmopressin** by injection may aid haemostasis and be useful in mild forms of haemophilia. For minor procedures including dental surgery, they may circumvent the need for factor VIII. For the use of factor VIII and factor IX in haemophilia, see section 11.2.

Heparin sodium

Injection (Solution for injection), heparin sodium 1000 units/ml, 1-ml ampoule; 5000 units/ml, 1-ml ampoule; 25 000 units/ml, 1-ml ampoule

Uses: treatment and prophylaxis of deep-vein thrombosis and pulmonary embolism

Contraindications: hypersensitivity to heparin; haemophilia and other haemorrhagic disorders, thrombocytopenia, peptic ulcer, recent cerebral haemorrhage, severe hypertension, severe liver or renal disease, after major trauma or recent surgery (especially to eye or nervous system)

Precautions: hepatic impairment (Appendix 5) and renal failure (Appendix 4); hypersensitivity to low molecular weight heparins; spinal or epidural anaesthesia—risk of spinal haematoma; pregnancy (Appendix 2); diabetes mellitus, acidosis, concomitant potassium-sparing drugs—increased risk of hyperkalaemia; **interactions:** Appendix 1

Dosage:

Treatment of deep-vein thrombosis and pulmonary embolism: *by intravenous injection*, ADULT loading dose of 5000 units (10 000 units in severe pulmonary embolism) followed *by continuous intravenous infusion* of 15–25 units/kg/hour *or by subcutaneous injection* of 15 000 units every 12 hours; laboratory monitoring is essential, preferably on a daily basis and dose adjusted accordingly; *by intravenous injection*, SMALL ADULT and CHILD, lower loading dose, then *by continuous intravenous infusion*, 15–25 units/kg/hour *or by subcutaneous injection*, 250 units/kg every 12 hours

Prophylaxis in general surgery, *by subcutaneous injection*, ADULT 5000 units 2 hours before surgery, then every 8–12 hours for 7 days or until patient is ambulant (monitoring not needed); during pregnancy (with monitoring) 5000–10 000 units every 12 hours (**important:** not intended to cover prosthetic heart valve management in pregnancy, which requires specialist management)

Adverse effects: immune-mediated thrombocytopenia usually developing 6 to 10 days after commencement of therapy (requires immediate withdrawal of heparin); haemorrhage, skin necrosis, hypersensitivity reactions including urticaria, angioedema and anaphylaxis, osteoporosis after prolonged use and rarely alopecia

---

Warfarin sodium

Warfarin is a representative oral anticoagulant. Various drugs can serve as alternatives

Tablets, warfarin sodium 1 mg, 2 mg, 5 mg

Uses: prophylaxis of embolization in rheumatic heart disease and atrial fibrillation; prophylaxis after insertion of prosthetic heart valve; prophylaxis and treatment of venous thrombosis and pulmonary embolism; transient ischaemic attacks

Contraindications: pregnancy (see notes above and Appendix 2); peptic ulcer, severe hypertension, bacterial endocarditis

Precautions: hepatic impairment (Appendix 5) or renal failure (Appendix 4), recent surgery, breastfeeding (Appendix 3); **interactions:** Appendix 1

Dosage:

NOTE. Wherever possible, the base-line prothrombin time should be determined before the initial dose is given

Prophylaxis and treatment of thromboembolic disorders, *by mouth,* ADULT usual induction dose is 10 mg daily for 2 days, according to the individual patient; the subsequent dose depends upon the prothrombin time; the usual daily maintenance dose is 3 to 9 mg taken at the same time each day

Adverse effects: haemorrhage; hypersensitivity, rash, alopecia, diarrhoea, unexplained drop in haematocrit, 'purple toes', skin necrosis, jaundice, hepatic dysfunction, nausea, vomiting and pancreatitis

Reversal of anticoagulation

Protamine sulfate

Injection (Solution for injection), protamine sulfate 10 mg/ml, 5-ml ampoule

Uses: antidote to overdosage with heparin

Precautions: if used in excess protamine has an anticoagulant effect; allergic reactions increased in persons at risk including previous treatment with protamine or protamine insulin, fish allergies, men who are infertile or who have had a vasectomy

Dosage:

Heparin overdose, *by intravenous injection* over approximately 10 minutes, 1 mg neutralizes 80–100 units heparin when given within 15 minutes; if longer time, less protamine needed as heparin is rapidly excreted

Adverse effects: nausea, vomiting, lassitude, flushing, hypotension, bradycardia, dyspnoea, allergic reactions

Phytomenadione

Tablets, phytomenadione 10 mg

Injection (Solution for injection), phytomenadione 10 mg/ml, 5-ml ampoule

Uses: antagonist to warfarin; prophylaxis against haemorrhagic disease of the newborn

Precautions: reduce dose in elderly; hepatic impairment; not an antidote to heparin; pregnancy (Appendix 2); **interactions:** Appendix 1

Dosage:

Warfarin-induced hypoprothrombinaemia; no bleeding or minor bleeding, *by slow intravenous injection*, ADULT 500 micrograms *or by mouth*, ADULT 5 mg; less severe haemorrhage, *by mouth or by intramuscular injection*, ADULT 10–20 mg; severe haemorrhage, ADULT, *by slow intravenous injection*, 2.5–25 mg, very rarely up to 50 mg

Haemorrhagic disease of the newborn, treatment, *by intravenous or intramuscular injection*, NEONATE 1 mg with further doses if necessary at 8-hour intervals; prophylaxis, *by intramuscular injection*, NEONATE 0.5–1 mg as single dose *or by mouth*, 2 mg followed by a second dose after 4–7 days and for breast-fed babies a third dose after 1 month

Adverse effects: hypersensitivity reactions including flushing, dyspnoea, bronchospasm, dizziness, hypotension and respiratory or circulatory collapse which may be due to polyethoxylated castor oil surfactant in some injection formulations rather than due to phytomenadione

---

Desmopressin acetate

Injection (Solution for injection), desmopressin acetate 4 micrograms/ml, 1-ml ampoule

Uses: management of mild to moderate haemophilia

Contraindications: cardiac insufficiency and other conditions treated with diuretics

Precautions: renal failure (Appendix 4) and hypertension; elderly; cystic fibrosis; pregnancy (Appendix 2); breastfeeding (Appendix 3)

Dosage:

To increase levels of factor VIII before surgery or treatment of bleeding episodes in mild to moderate haemophilia, *by slow intravenous infusion* (over 15–30 minutes), ADULT 300–400 nanograms/kg

DILUTION AND ADMINISTRATION. According to manufacturer's directions

Adverse effects: fluid retention and hyponatraemia; abdominal pain, headache, nausea, vomiting, epistaxis

Section 11: Blood products and plasma substitutes

11.1 Plasma substitutes

Dextran 70 and **polygeline** are macromolecular substances which are slowly metabolized; they may be used to expand and maintain blood volume in shock arising from conditions such as burns or septicaemia. They are rarely needed when shock is due to sodium and water depletion as, in these circumstances, the shock responds to water and electrolyte repletion.

Plasma substitutes should not be used to maintain plasma volume in conditions such as burns or peritonitis where there is loss of plasma protein, water and electrolytes over periods of several days. In these situations, plasma or plasma protein fractions containing large amounts of albumin should be given.

Plasma substitutes may be used as an immediate short-term measure to treat massive haemorrhage until blood is available. Dextran may interfere with blood group cross-matching or biochemical measurements and these should be carried out before the infusion is begun.

Dextran 70

Dextran is a representative plasma substitute. Various preparations can serve as alternatives

Infusion (Solution for infusion), dextran 70 6% in glucose intravenous infusion 5% or sodium chloride intravenous infusion 0.9%

Uses: short-term blood volume expansion

Contraindications: severe congestive heart failure, renal failure; bleeding disorders such as thrombocytopenia and hypofibrinogenaemia

Precautions: cardiac disease or renal impairment; monitor urine output; avoid haematocrit falling below 25–30%; can interfere with blood group cross-matching and biochemical tests—take samples before start of infusion; monitor for hypersensitivity reactions

Dosage:

Short-term blood volume expansion, *by rapid intravenous infusion,* 500–1000 ml initially, followed by 500 ml if necessary; total dosage should not exceed 20 ml/kg during the initial 24 hours

Adverse effects: urticarial and other hypersensitivity reactions—rarely severe anaphylactoid reactions

---

Polygeline

Polygeline is a representative partially degraded gelatin. Various preparations can serve as alternatives

Infusion (Solution for infusion), polygeline 3.5% with electrolytes, 500-ml bottle

Uses: correction of low blood volume

Contraindications: severe congestive heart failure; renal failure

---

Precautions: blood samples for cross-matching should be taken before infusion; haemorrhagic diathesis; congestive heart failure, renal impairment, hypertension, oesophageal varices; **interactions:** Appendix 1

Dosage:

Correction of low blood volume, *by intravenous infusion*, initially 500–1000 ml of a 3.5% solution

Adverse effects: urticarial and other hypersensitivity reactions—rarely severe anaphylactoid reactions

---

11.2 Plasma fractions for specific use

Factor VIII is essential for blood clotting and the maintenance of effective haemostasis; von Willebrand factor is a mediator in platelet aggregation and also acts as a carrier for factor VIII. Blood coagulation factors VII, IX, and X are essential for the conversion of factor II (prothrombin) to thrombin. Deficiency in any of these factors results in haemophilia. Bleeding episodes in haemophilia require prompt treatment with replacement therapy. **Factor VIII**, used for the treatment of haemophilia A, is a sterile freeze-dried powder containing the blood coagulation factor VIII fraction prepared from pooled human venous plasma. Standard factor VIII preparations also contain von Willebrand factor and may be used to treat von Willebrand disease. Highly purified preparations, including recombinant factor VIII, are available; they are indicated for the treatment of haemophilia A but do not contain sufficient von Willebrand factor for use in the management of von Willebrand disease. **Factor IX Complex** is a sterile freeze-dried concentrate of blood coagulation factors II, VII, IX and X derived from fresh venous plasma. Factor IX complex which is used for the treatment of haemophilia B may also be used for the treatment of bleeding due to deficencies of factor II, VII, and X. High purity preparations of factor IX which do not contain clinically effective amounts of factor II, VII, and X are available. A recombinant factor IX preparation is also available.

All plasma fractions should comply with standard requirements (WHO. Requirements for the collection, processing and quality control of blood, blood components and plasma derivatives: forty-third report of the WHO expert committee, WHO Tec Rep Ser *840* 1994).

Factor VIII concentrate

Factor VIII concentrate is a representative coagulation factor preparation. Various preparations can serve as alternatives
Infusion (Powder for solution for infusion), factor VIII 250–1500 units

Uses: control of haemorrhage in haemophilia A

Precautions: intravascular haemolysis after large or frequently repeated doses in patients with blood groups A, B, or AB (less likely with high potency, highly purified concentrates)

Dosage:
Haemophilia A, *by slow intravenous infusion*, ADULT and CHILD according to patient's needs
Adverse effects: allergic reactions including chills, fever

Factor IX Complex (coagulation factors II, VII, IX, X) concentrate

Factor IX complex concentrate is a representative coagulation factor preparation. Various preparations can serve as alternatives

Infusion (Powder for solution for infusion), factor II, VII, IX, and X 500–1500 units

Uses: replacement therapy for factor IX deficiency in haemophilia

Contraindications: disseminated intravascular coagulation

Precautions: risk of thrombosis (probably less risk with highly purified preparations)

Dosage:
Haemophilia B, *by slow intravenous infusion*, ADULT and CHILD according to patient's needs and specific preparation used

Treatment of bleeding due to deficiencies in factor II, VII or X, *by slow intravenous infusion*, ADULT and CHILD according to patient's needs

Adverse effects: allergic reactions including chills, fever

Section 12:
Cardiovascular drugs

12.1 Antianginal drugs

The three main types of angina are:

- *stable angina* (angina of effort), where atherosclerosis restricts blood flow in the coronary vessels; attacks are usually caused by exertion and relieved by rest
- *unstable angina* (acute coronary insufficiency), which is considered to be an intermediate stage between stable angina and myocardial infarction
- *Prinzmetal angina* (variant angina), caused by coronary vasospasm, in which attacks occur at rest.

Management depends on the type of angina and may include drug treatment, coronary artery bypass surgery, or percutaneous transluminal coronary angioplasty.

Stable angina

Drugs are used both for the relief of acute pain and for prophylaxis to reduce further attacks; they include organic nitrates, beta-adrenoceptor antagonists (beta-blockers), and calcium-channel blockers.

NITRATES. Organic nitrates have a vasodilating effect; they are sometimes used alone, especially in elderly patients with infrequent symptoms. Tolerance leading to reduced antianginal effect is often seen in patients taking prolonged-action nitrate formulations. Evidence suggests that patients should have a 'nitrate-free' interval to prevent the development of tolerance. Adverse effects such as flushing, headache, and postural hypotension may limit nitrate therapy but tolerance to these effects also soon develops. The short-acting sublingual formulation of **glyceryl trinitrate** is used both for prevention of angina before exercise or other stress and for rapid treatment of chest pain. A sublingual tablet of **isosorbide dinitrate** is more stable in storage than glyceryl trinitrate and is useful in patients who require nitrates infrequently; it has a slower onset of action, but effects persist for several hours.

BETA-BLOCKERS. Beta-adrenoceptor antagonists (beta-blockers), such as **atenolol**, block beta-adrenergic receptors in the heart, and thereby decrease heart rate and myocardial contractility and oxygen consumption, particularly during exercise. Beta-blockers are first-line therapy for patients with effort-induced chronic stable angina; they improve exercise tolerance, relieve symptoms, reduce the severity and frequency of angina attacks, and increase the anginal threshold.

Beta-blockers should be withdrawn gradually to avoid precipitating an attack; they should not be used alone in patients with underlying coronary vasospasm (Prinzmetal angina).

Beta-blockers may precipitate asthma and should not be used in patients with asthma or a history of obstructive airways disease. Some, including atenolol, have less effect on beta$_2$ (bronchial) receptors and are therefore relatively cardioselective. Although they have less effect on airways resistance they are not free of this effect and should be avoided.

Beta-blockers slow the heart and may induce myocardial depression, rarely precipitating heart failure. They should not be given to patients who have incipient ventricular failure, second- or third-degree atrioventricular block, or peripheral vascular disease.

Beta-blockers should be used with caution in diabetics since they may mask the symptoms of hypoglycaemia, such as rapid heart rate. Beta-blockers taken together with insulin may precipitate severe hypoglycaemia.

CALCIUM-CHANNEL BLOCKERS. A calcium-channel blocker, such as **verapamil,** is used as an alternative to a beta-blocker to treat stable angina. Calcium-channel blockers interfere with the inward movement of calcium ions through the slow channels in heart and vascular smooth muscle cell membranes, leading to relaxation of vascular smooth muscle. Myocardial contractility may be reduced, the formation and propagation of electrical impulses within the heart may be depressed and coronary or systemic vascular tone may be diminished. Calcium-channel blockers are used to improve exercise tolerance in patients with chronic stable angina due to coronary atherosclerosis or with abnormally small coronary arteries and limited vasodilator reserve.

Calcium-channel blockers can also be used in patients with unstable angina with a vasospastic origin, such as Prinzmetal angina, and in patients in whom alterations in cardiac tone may influence the angina threshold.

Unstable angina
Unstable angina requires prompt aggressive treatment to prevent progression to myocardial infarction.

Initial treatment is with acetylsalicylic acid to inhibit platelet aggregation, followed by heparin. Nitrates and beta-blockers are given to relieve ischaemia; if beta-blockers are contraindicated, verapamil is an alternative, provided left ventricular function is adequate.

Prinzmetal angina
Treatment is similar to that for unstable angina, except that a calcium-channel blocker is used instead of a beta-blocker.

Atenolol
Atenolol is a representative beta-adrenoceptor antagonist. Various drugs can serve as alternatives

Tablets, atenolol 50 mg, 100 mg

Injection (Solution for injection), atenolol 500 micrograms/ml, 10-ml ampoule [not included on WHO Model List 11th revision]

Uses: angina and myocardial infarction; arrhythmias (section 12.2); hypertension (section 12.3); migraine prophylaxis (section 7.2)

Contraindications: asthma or history of obstructive airways disease (unless no alternative, then with extreme caution and under specialist supervision); uncontrolled heart failure,

Prinzmetal angina, marked bradycardia, hypotension, sick sinus syndrome, second- and third-degree atrioventricular block, cardiogenic shock; metabolic acidosis; severe peripheral arterial disease; phaeochromocytoma (unless used with alpha-blocker)

Precautions: avoid abrupt withdrawal in angina; may precipitate or worsen heart failure; pregnancy (Appendix 2); breastfeeding (Appendix 3); first-degree atrioventricular block; liver function deteriorates in portal hypertension; reduce dose in renal impairment (Appendix 4); diabetes mellitus (small decrease in glucose tolerance, masking of symptoms of hypoglycaemia); history of hypersensitivity (increased reaction to allergens, also reduced response to epinephrine); myasthenia gravis; **interactions:** Appendix 1

Dosage:

Angina, *by mouth,* ADULT 50 mg once daily, increased if necessary to 50 mg twice daily or 100 mg once daily

Myocardial infarction (early intervention within 12 hours), *by intravenous injection* at a rate of 1 mg/minute, ADULT 5–10 mg, then *by mouth* 50 mg after 15 minutes, followed by 50 mg after 12 hours, then 100 mg daily

Adverse effects: gastrointestinal disturbances (nausea, vomiting, diarrhoea, constipation, abdominal cramp); fatigue; cold hands and feet; exacerbation of intermittent claudication and Raynaud phenomenon; bronchospasm; bradycardia, heart failure, conduction disorders, hypotension; sleep disturbances, including nightmares; depression, confusion, convulsions; hypo- or hyperglycaemia; exacerbation of psoriasis; rare reports of rashes and dry eyes (oculomucocutaneous syndrome—reversible on withdrawal)

Glyceryl trinitrate

Sublingual tablets, glyceryl trinitrate 500 micrograms

NOTE. Glyceryl trinitrate tablets are unstable. They should therefore be dispensed in glass or stainless steel containers, and closed with a foil-lined cap which contains no wadding. No more than 100 tablets should be dispensed at one time, and any unused tablets should be discarded 8 weeks after opening the container

Uses: prophylaxis and treatment of angina

Contraindications: hypersensitivity to nitrates; hypotension; hypovolaemia; hypertrophic obstructive cardiomyopathy, aortic stenosis, cardiac tamponade, constrictive pericarditis, mitral stenosis; marked anaemia; head trauma; cerebral haemorrhage; angle-closure glaucoma

Precautions: severe hepatic or renal impairment; hypothyroidism; malnutrition; hypothermia; recent history of myocardial infarction; **interactions:** Appendix 1

Dosage:

Angina, *sublingually,* ADULT 0.5–1 mg, repeated as required

Adverse effects: throbbing headache; flushing; dizziness, postural hypotension; tachycardia (paradoxical bradycardia also reported)

Isosorbide dinitrate

Isosorbide dinitrate is a representative nitrate vasodilator. Various drugs can serve as alternatives

Sublingual tablets, isosorbide dinitrate 5 mg

Sustained-release (prolonged-release) tablets or capsules, isosorbide dinitrate 20 mg, 40 mg [not included on WHO Model List 11th revision]

Uses: prophylaxis and treatment of angina; heart failure (section 12.4)

Contraindications: hypersensitivity to nitrates; hypotension; hypovolaemia; hypertrophic obstructive cardiomyopathy, aortic stenosis, cardiac tamponade, constrictive pericarditis, mitral stenosis; marked anaemia; head trauma; cerebral haemorrhage; angle-closure glaucoma

Precautions: severe hepatic or renal impairment; hypothyroidism; malnutrition; hypothermia; recent history of myocardial infarction; **interactions:** Appendix 1

TOLERANCE. Patients taking isosorbide dinitrate for the long-term management of angina may often develop tolerance to the antianginal effect; this can be avoided by giving the second of 2 daily doses of longer-acting oral presentations after an 8-hour rather than a 12-hour interval, thus ensuring a nitrate-free interval each day

Dosage:

Angina (acute attack), *sublingually,* ADULT 5–10 mg, repeated as required

Angina prophylaxis, *by mouth,* ADULT 30–120 mg daily in divided doses (see advice on Tolerance above)

Adverse effects: throbbing headache; flushing; dizziness, postural hypotension; tachycardia (paradoxical bradycardia also reported)

Verapamil hydrochloride

Verapamil is a representative calcium-channel blocker. Various drugs can serve as alternatives

Tablets, verapamil hydrochloride 40 mg, 80 mg

NOTE. Sustained-release (prolonged-release) tablets are available. A proposal to include such a product in a national list of essential drugs should be supported by adequate documentation

Uses: angina, including stable, unstable, and Prinzmetal; arrhythmias (section 12.2)

Contraindications: hypotension, bradycardia, second- and third-degree atrioventricular block, sinoatrial block, sick sinus syndrome; cardiogenic shock; history of heart failure or significantly impaired left ventricular function (even if controlled by therapy); atrial flutter or fibrillation complicating Wolff-Parkinson-White syndrome; porphyria

Precautions: first-degree atrioventricular block; acute phase of myocardial infarction (avoid if bradycardia, hypotension, left ventricular failure); hepatic impairment (Appendix 5); children (specialist advice only); pregnancy (Appendix 2); breastfeeding (Appendix 3); avoid grapefruit juice; **interactions:** Appendix 1

Dosage:

Angina, *by mouth,* ADULT 80–120 mg 3 times daily (120 mg 3 times daily usually required in Prinzmetal angina)

Adverse effects: constipation; less commonly nausea, vomiting, flushing, headache, dizziness, fatigue, ankle oedema; reversible impairment of liver function; allergic reactions (erythema, pruritus, urticaria, angioedema, Stevens-Johnson syndrome); myalgia, arthralgia, paraesthesia, erythromelalgia; increased prolactin concentration; gynaecomastia and gingival hyperplasia on long-term treatment; with high doses, hypotension, heart failure, bradycardia, heart block, and asystole (due to negative inotropic effect)

12.2 Antiarrhythmic drugs

Treatment of arrhythmias requires precise diagnosis of the type of arrhythmia. Antiarrhythmic drugs must be used cautiously since they have a narrow therapeutic index; ECG monitoring is often advised.

When two or more antiarrhythmic drugs are used together, their negative inotropic effects tend to be additive, particularly if myocardial function is impaired. Also, most drugs that are effective in treating arrhythmias can provoke them in some circumstances; this arrhythmogenic effect is often enhanced by hypokalaemia.

Atrial fibrillation

Oral administration of **digoxin** is usually effective in slowing the increased ventricular rate in atrial fibrillation. Intravenous digoxin is occasionally required if the ventricular rate needs rapid control. If adequate control at rest or during exercise cannot be achieved readily with digoxin, a **beta-adrenoceptor antagonist** (beta-blocker) or **verapamil** may be added; both should be used with caution if ventricular function is impaired. Anticoagulants are indicated especially in valvular or myocardial disease, and in the elderly. **Warfarin** is preferred to acetylsalicylic acid in preventing emboli. If atrial fibrillation began within the past 48 hours and there does not appear to be a danger of producing systemic thromboembolism, antiarrhythmic drugs, such as **procainamide** or **quinidine**, may be used to terminate atrial fibrillation or to maintain sinus rhythm after cardioversion.

Atrial flutter

Digoxin will slow the ventricular rate. Reversion to sinus rhythm is best achieved by direct current electrical shock. If the arrhythmia is long-standing, treatment with anticoagulants should be considered before cardioversion to prevent emboli. Intravenous **verapamil** reduces ventricular fibrillation during paroxysmal (sudden onset and intermittent) attacks of atrial flutter. An initial intravenous dose may be followed by oral treatment; hypotension may occur with high doses. It should not be used for tachyarrhythmias where the QRS complex is wide unless a supraventricular origin has been established beyond doubt. If the flutter cannot be restored to sinus rhythm, antiarrhythmics such as **quinidine** can be used.

Paroxysmal supraventricular tachycardia

In most patients this remits spontaneously or can revert to sinus rhythm by reflex vagal stimulation. Failing this, intravenous injection of a beta-adrenoceptor antagonist (beta-blocker) or verapamil may be effective. These drugs should **never** be administered concomitantly because of the risk of hypotension and asystole.

Ventricular tachycardia

Very rapid ventricular fibrillation causes profound circulatory collapse and must be treated immediately with direct current shock. In more stable patients intravenous **lidocaine** or **procainamide** may be used. After sinus rhythm is restored, drug therapy to prevent recurrence of ventricular tachycardia should be considered; a beta-adrenoceptor antagonist (beta-blocker) or verapamil may be effective.

Torsades de pointes is a special form of ventricular tachycardia associated with prolongation of the QT interval. Initial treatment with intravenous infusion of magnesium sulfate is usually effective, followed by temporary pacing; alternatively, isoprenaline infusion may be given with extreme caution until pacing can be instituted. Isoprenaline is an inotropic sympathomimetic; it increases the heart rate and therefore shortens the QT interval, but given alone may induce arrhythmias.

Bradyarrhythmias

Sinus bradycardia (less than 50 beats/minute) associated with acute myocardial infarction may be treated with atropine. Temporary pacing may be required in unresponsive patients. Drugs are of limited value for increasing the sinus rate long term in the presence of intrinsic sinus node disease and permanent pacing is usually required.

Cardiac arrest

In cardiac arrest, **epinephrine** (adrenaline) is given by intravenous injection in a dose of 1 mg (10 ml of 1 in 10 000 solution) as part of the procedure for cardiopulmonary resuscitation.

Atenolol

Atenolol is a representative beta-adrenoceptor antagonist. Various drugs can serve as alternatives

Tablets, atenolol 50 mg, 100 mg

Uses: arrhythmias; angina (section 12.1); hypertension (section 12.3); migraine prophylaxis (section 7.2)

Contraindications: asthma or history of obstructive airways disease (unless no alternative, then with extreme caution and under specialist supervision); uncontrolled heart failure, Prinzmetal angina, marked bradycardia, hypotension, sick sinus syndrome, second- and third-degree atrioventricular block, cardiogenic shock; metabolic acidosis; severe peripheral arterial disease; phaeochromocytoma (unless used with alpha-blocker)

Precautions: avoid abrupt withdrawal in angina; may precipitate or worsen heart failure; pregnancy (Appendix 2); breastfeeding (Appendix 3); first-degree atrioventricular block; liver function deteriorates in portal hypertension; reduce dose in renal impairment (Appendix 4); diabetes mellitus (small decrease in glucose tolerance, masking of symptoms of hypoglycaemia); history of hypersensitivity (increased reaction to allergens, also reduced response to epinephrine); myasthenia gravis; **interactions:** Appendix 1

Dosage:

Arrhythmias, *by mouth,* ADULT 50 mg once daily, increased if necessary to 50 mg twice daily *or* 100 mg once daily

Adverse effects: gastrointestinal disturbances (nausea, vomiting, diarrhoea, constipation, abdominal cramp); fatigue; cold hands and feet; exacerbation of intermittent claudication and Raynaud phenomenon; bronchospasm; bradycardia, heart failure, conduction disorders, hypotension; sleep disturbances, including nightmares; depression, confusion, convulsions; hypo- or hyperglycaemia; exacerbation of psoriasis; rare reports of rashes and dry eyes (oculomucocutaneous syndrome—reversible on withdrawal)

Digoxin
Tablets, digoxin 62.5 micrograms, 250 micrograms
Oral solution, digoxin 50 micrograms/ml
Injection (Solution for injection), digoxin 250 micrograms/ml, 2-ml ampoule

Uses: supraventricular arrhythmias, particularly atrial fibrillation; heart failure (section 12.4)

Contraindications: hypertrophic obstructive cardiomyopathy (unless also severe heart failure); Wolff-Parkinson-White syndrome or other accessory pathway, particularly if accompanied by atrial fibrillation; intermittent complete heart block; second-degree atrioventricular block

Precautions: recent myocardial infarction; sick sinus syndrome; severe pulmonary disease; thyroid disease; elderly (reduce dose); renal impairment (Appendix 4); avoid hypokalaemia; avoid rapid intravenous administration (nausea and risk of arrhythmias); pregnancy (Appendix 2); breastfeeding (Appendix 3); **interactions:** Appendix 1

Dosage:

Atrial fibrillation, *by mouth,* ADULT 1–1.5 mg in divided doses over 24 hours for rapid digitalization *or* 250 micrograms 1–2 times daily if digitalization less urgent; maintenance 62.5–500 micrograms daily (higher dose may be divided), according to renal function and heart rate response; usual range 125–250 micrograms daily (lower dose more appropriate in elderly)

Emergency control of atrial fibrillation, *by intravenous infusion*, ADULT 250–500 micrograms over 10–20 minutes, repeated at intervals of 4–8 hours according to response to total loading dose of 0.5–1 mg

NOTE. Infusion dose may need to be reduced if digoxin or other cardiac glycoside given in previous 2 weeks

Adverse effects: usually associated with excessive dosage and include anorexia, nausea, vomiting, diarrhoea, abdominal pain; visual disturbances, headache, fatigue, drowsiness, confusion, delirium, hallucinations, depression; arrhythmias, heart block; rarely rash, intestinal ischaemia; gynaecomastia on long-term use; thrombocytopenia reported

---

Epinephrine (adrenaline)

Epinephrine is a complementary antiarrhythmic for use in rare disorders or in exceptional circumstances

Injection (Solution for injection), epinephrine hydrochloride 100 micrograms/ml (1 in 10 000), 10-ml ampoule

Uses: cardiac arrest; anaphylaxis (section 3.1)

Precautions: heart disease, hypertension, arrhythmias, cerebrovascular disease; hyperthyroidism, diabetes mellitus; angle-closure glaucoma; second stage of labour; **interactions:** Appendix 1

Dosage:

Caution: different dilutions of epinephrine injection are used for different routes of administration

Cardiac arrest, *by intravenous injection* through a central line using epinephrine injection 1 in 10 000, ADULT 1 mg (10 ml), repeated at 3-minute intervals if necessary

NOTE. If central line not in place, same dose is given via peripheral vein, then flushed through with 20 ml sodium chloride 0.9% injection (to expedite entry into circulation)

Adverse effects: anxiety, tremor, tachycardia, headache, cold extremities; nausea, vomiting, sweating, weakness, dizziness, hyperglycaemia also reported; in overdosage arrhythmias, cerebral haemorrhage, pulmonary oedema

---

Isoprenaline

Isoprenaline is a complementary antiarrhythmic for use in rare disorders or in exceptional circumstances

Injection (Solution for injection), isoprenaline hydrochloride 20 micrograms/ml, 10-ml ampoule

Uses: severe bradycardia, unresponsive to atropine; short-term emergency treatment of heart block; ventricular arrhythmias secondary to atrioventricular nodal block

Precautions: ischaemic heart disease, diabetes mellitus or hyperthyroidism; **interactions:** Appendix 1

Dosage:

Cardiac disorders, *by slow intravenous injection,* ADULT 20–60 micrograms (1–3 ml of solution containing 20 micrograms/ml); subsequent doses adjusted according to ventricular rate

Bradycardia, *by intravenous infusion,* ADULT 1–4 micrograms/minute

Heart block (acute Stokes-Adams attack), *by intravenous infusion,* ADULT 4–8 micrograms/minute

DILUTION AND ADMINISTRATION. According to manufacturer's directions

Adverse effects: arrhythmias, hypotension, sweating, tremor, headache, palpitations, tachycardia, nervousness, excitability, insomnia

Lidocaine hydrochloride
Injection, lidocaine hydrochloride 20 mg/ml, 5-ml ampoule

Uses: ventricular arrhythmias (especially after myocardial infarction); local anaesthesia (section 1.2)

Contraindications: sino-atrial disorder, any grade of atrioventricular block or any other type of conduction disturbances, severe myocardial depression, acute porphyria or hypovolaemia

Precautions: lower dosage in congestive heart failure, bradycardia, hepatic impairment (Appendix 5), marked hypoxia, severe respiratory depression, following cardiac surgery and in elderly; **interactions:** Appendix 1

Dosage:

Ventricular arrhythmias, *by intravenous injection,* ADULT, loading dose of 50–100 mg (*or* 1–1.5 mg/kg) at a rate of 25–50 mg/minute, followed immediately by *intravenous infusion* of 1–4 mg/minute, with ECG monitoring of all patients (reduce infusion dose if required for longer than 24 hours)

Adverse effects: dizziness, paraesthesia, drowsiness, confusion, apnoea, respiratory depression, coma, seizures, and convulsions, hypotension, arrhythmias, heart block, cardiovascular collapse and bradycardia (may lead to cardiac arrest); nystagmus often an early sign of lidocaine overdosage

Procainamide hydrochloride
Procainamide hydrochloride is a representative antiarrhythmic drug. Various drugs can serve as alternatives

It is also a complementary drug for use when drugs in the main list are known to be ineffective or inappropriate for a given patient

Tablets, procainamide hydrochloride 250 mg, 500 mg
Injection (Solution for injection), procainamide hydrochloride 100 mg/ml, 10-ml ampoule

Uses: severe ventricular arrhythmias, especially those resistant to lidocaine or those appearing after myocardial infarction; atrial tachycardia, atrial fibrillation; maintenance of sinus rhythm after cardioversion of atrial fibrillation

Contraindications: asymptomatic ventricular premature contractions, torsades de pointes, systemic lupus erythematosus, heart block, heart failure, hypotension

Precautions: elderly, renal and hepatic impairment (Appendices 4 and 5), asthma, myasthenia gravis, pregnancy; breastfeeding (Appendix 3); initiate only under specialist supervision; **interactions:** Appendix 1

Dosage:

Ventricular arrhythmias, *by mouth*, ADULT up to 50 mg/kg daily in divided doses every 3–6 hours, preferably controlled by monitoring plasma-procainamide concentration (therapeutic concentration usually within range 3–10 micrograms/ml)

Atrial arrhythmias, higher doses may be required

Ventricular arrhythmias, *by slow intravenous injection,* ADULT 100 mg at rate not exceeding 50 mg/minute, with ECG monitoring; may be repeated at 5-minute intervals until arrhythmia controlled; maximum 1 g

Ventricular arrhythmias, *by intravenous infusion,* ADULT 500–600 mg over 25–30 minutes with ECG monitoring, reduced to maintenance dose of 2–6 mg/minute; if further treatment by mouth required, allow interval of 3–4 hours after infusion

Adverse effects: nausea, vomiting, diarrhoea, anorexia, rashes, pruritus, urticaria, flushing, fever, myocardial depression, heart failure, and angioedema, depression, dizziness, and psychosis; blood disorders include leukopenia, haemolytic anaemia and agranulocytosis after prolonged treatment; lupus erythematosus-like syndrome; high plasma procainamide concentration may impair cardiac conduction

---

Quinidine sulfate

Quinidine is a representative antiarrhythmic drug. Various drugs can serve as alternatives

It is also a complementary drug for use when drugs in the main list cannot be made available

Tablets, quinidine sulfate 200 mg

Uses: suppression of supraventricular arrhythmias and ventricular arrhythmias; maintenance of sinus rhythm after cardioversion of atrial fibrillation

Contraindications: complete heart block

Precautions: partial heart block or uncompensated heart failure; myasthenia gravis; acute infections or fever (symptoms may mask hypersensitivity reaction to quinidine); breastfeeding (Appendix 3); **interactions:** Appendix 1

Dosage:

Initial test dose of 200 mg to detect hypersensitivity to quinidine

Arrhythmias, *by mouth,* ADULT 200–400 mg 3–4 times daily; increased if necessary in supraventricular tachycardia to 600 mg every 2–4 hours (maximum 3–4 g daily); frequent ECG monitoring required

Adverse effects: hypersensitivity reactions, nausea, vomiting, diarrhoea, rashes, anaphylaxis, purpura, pruritus, urticaria, fever, thrombocytopenia, agranulocytosis after prolonged treatment, psychosis, angioedema, hepatotoxicity, respiratory difficulties; cardiac effects include myocardial depression, heart failure, ventricular arrhythmias and hypotension; cinchonism including tinnitus, impaired hearing, vertigo, headache, visual disturbances, abdominal pain, and confusion; lupus erythematosus-like syndrome

Verapamil hydrochloride

Tablets, verapamil hydrochloride 40 mg, 80 mg

NOTE. Sustained-release (prolonged-release) tablets are available. A proposal to include such a product in a national list of essential drugs should be supported by adequate documentation

Injection (Solution for injection), verapamil hydrochloride 2.5 mg/ml, 2-ml ampoule

Uses: supraventricular arrhythmias; angina (section 12.1)

Contraindications: hypotension, bradycardia, second- and third-degree atrioventricular block, sinoatrial block, sick sinus syndrome; cardiogenic shock; history of heart failure or significantly impaired left ventricular function (even if controlled by therapy); atrial flutter or fibrillation complicating Wolff-Parkinson-White syndrome; porphyria

Precautions: first-degree atrioventricular block; acute phase of myocardial infarction (avoid if bradycardia, hypotension, left ventricular failure); hepatic impairment (Appendix 5); children (specialist advice only); pregnancy (Appendix 2); breastfeeding (Appendix 3); avoid grapefruit juice; **interactions:** Appendix 1

VERAPAMIL AND BETA-BLOCKERS. Both verapamil and beta-blockers have cardiodepressant activity, and their use together may lead to bradycardia, heart block and left ventricular failure, particularly in patients with myocardial insufficiency. Treatment with beta-blockers should be discontinued at least 24 hours before intravenous administration of verapamil; they should only be given together by mouth if myocardial function is well preserved

Dosage:

Supraventricular arrhythmias, *by mouth,* ADULT 40–120 mg 3 times daily

Supraventricular arrhythmias, *by intravenous injection,* ADULT 5–10 mg over 2 minutes (preferably with ECG monitoring); ELDERLY 5–10 mg over 3 minutes; in paroxysmal tachyarrhythmias, further 5 mg may be given after 5–10 minutes if required

Adverse effects: constipation; less commonly nausea, vomiting, flushing, headache, dizziness, fatigue, ankle oedema; reversible impairment of liver function; allergic reactions (erythema, pruritus, urticaria, angioedema, Stevens-Johnson syndrome); myalgia, arthralgia, paraesthesia, erythromelalgia; increased prolactin concentration; gynaecomastia and gingival hyperplasia on long-term treatment; with high doses, hypotension, heart failure, bradycardia, heart block, and asystole (due to negative inotropic effect)

12.3 Antihypertensive drugs

Management of hypertension

Since treatment for hypertension is often life-long, it is important to integrate the treatment of hypertension into an overall programme of management of associated risk factors and conditions, particularly in elderly patients who often have multiple associated disorders. Mild hypertension is defined as 140–159 mmHg systolic blood pressure and 90–99 mmHg diastolic blood pressure, moderate hypertension 160–180 mmHg systolic and 100–109 mmHg diastolic and severe hypertension more than 180 mmHg systolic and more than 110 mmHg diastolic. The goal of treatment is to obtain the maximum tolerated reduction in blood pressure.

Lifestyle changes should introduced for all patients; they include weight reduction, reduction in alcohol intake, reduction of dietary sodium, stopping tobacco smoking, and reduction in saturated fat intake. The patient should eat a healthy nutritious diet including adequate fruit and vegetables and should exercise regularly. These measures alone may be sufficient in mild hypertension, but patients with moderate to severe hypertension will also require specific antihypertensive therapy.

Drug treatment of hypertension

Five classes of drug are used for first-line treatment of hypertension: diuretics, beta-adrenoceptor antagonists (beta-blockers), angiotensin-converting enzyme (ACE) inhibitors, calcium-channel blockers and alpha-adrenoceptor blocking drugs (alpha-blockers). All five classes are effective in reducing blood pressure; thiazide diuretics and beta-blockers have been shown to reduce mortality due to cardiovascular complications of hypertension. Other classes of drugs may be used in certain situations.

Thiazide diuretics, such as **hydrochlorothiazide** (see also section 16.1), have been used as first-line antihypertensive therapy, and are particularly indicated in the elderly. They have few adverse effects in low doses, but in large doses they may cause a variety of unwanted metabolic effects (principally potassium depletion), reduced glucose tolerance, ventricular ectopic beats and impotence; they should be avoided in gout. These effects can be reduced by keeping the dose as low as possible; higher doses do not produce an increased reduction in blood pressure. Thiazides are inexpensive and, when used in combination, can enhance the effectiveness of many other classes of antihypertensive drug.

Beta-adrenoceptor antagonists (beta-blockers) such as **atenolol** are effective in all grades of hypertension, and are particularly useful in angina and following myocardial infarction; they should be avoided in asthma, chronic obstructive pulmonary disease, and heart block.

Angiotensin-converting enzyme inhibitors (ACE inhibitors) such as **captopril** are effective and well tolerated by most patients. They can be used in heart failure, left ventricular dysfunction and diabetic nephropathy, but should be avoided in renovascular disease and in pregnancy. The most common adverse affect is a dry persistent cough.

Calcium-channel blockers such as **nifedipine** are effective antihypertensives, particularly for isolated systolic hypertension, and in the elderly when thiazides cannot be used.

Short-acting formulations of nifedipine should be avoided as they may evoke reflex tachycardia and cause large variations in blood pressure.

Alpha-adrenoceptor blocking drugs (alpha-blockers) such as **prazosin** are effective in lowering blood pressure but remain too expensive to be considered as first-line therapy in many countries. They are particularly useful in prostatism, but should be avoided in urinary incontinence. They are usually used in combination with other antihypertensives; the first dose being given at bedtime, as profound hypotension may occur.

Drugs acting on the central nervous system are also effective antihypertensive drugs. In particular, **methyldopa** is effective in the treatment of hypertension in pregnancy, and may also be used in asthma and heart failure. **Reserpine** is also used because of its effectiveness and low cost. It should be used in combination with diuretics and prescribed in much lower doses than were formerly used.

Combining antihypertensive drugs often produces a beneficial additive effect.

Hypertension in pregnancy

This is defined as a sustained diastolic blood pressure of 90 mmHg or more. Drug therapy for chronic hypertension during pregnancy remains controversial. If diastolic blood pressure is greater than 95 mmHg, **methyldopa** is the safest drug. Beta-blockers should be used with caution in early pregnancy, since they may retard fetal growth; they are effective and safe in the third trimester. ACE inhibitors are contra-indicated in pregnancy since they may damage fetal and neonatal blood pressure control and renal function. Women who are taking these drugs and become pregnant should have their antihypertensive therapy changed immediately.

Pre-eclampsia and eclampsia. If pre-eclampsia or severe hypertension occurs beyond the 36th week of pregnancy, delivery is the treatment of choice. For acute severe hypertension in pre-eclampsia or eclampsia, intravenous **hydralazine** can be used. **Magnesium sulfate** (section 22.1) is the treatment of choice to prevent eclamptic convulsions.

Hypertensive emergencies

In situations where immediate reduction of blood pressure is essential and treatment by mouth is not possible, intravenous infusion of **sodium nitroprusside** is effective. Over-rapid reduction in blood pressure is hazardous and can lead to reduced organ perfusion and cerebral infarction.

Atenolol

Atenolol is a representative beta-adrenoceptor antagonist. Various drugs can serve as alternatives

Tablets, atenolol 50 mg, 100 mg

Uses: hypertension; angina (section 12.1); arrhythmias (section 12.2); migraine prophylaxis (section 7.2)

Contraindications: asthma or history of obstructive airways disease (unless no alternative, then with extreme caution and under specialist supervision); uncontrolled heart failure, Prinzmetal angina, marked bradycardia, hypotension, sick sinus syndrome, second- or third-degree atrioventricular block, cardiogenic shock; metabolic acidosis; severe peripheral arterial disease; phaeochromocytoma (unless used with alpha-blocker)

Precautions: avoid abrupt withdrawal in angina; may precipitate or worsen heart failure; pregnancy (Appendix 2); breastfeeding (Appendix 3); first-degree atrioventricular block; liver function deteriorates in portal hypertension; reduce dose in renal impairment (Appendix 4); diabetes mellitus (small decrease in glucose tolerance, masking of symptoms of hypoglycaemia); history of hypersensitivity (increased reaction to allergens, also reduced response to epinephrine); myasthenia gravis; **interactions:** Appendix 1

Dosage:

Hypertension, *by mouth,* ADULT 50 mg once daily (higher doses rarely necessary)

Adverse effects: gastrointestinal disturbances (nausea, vomiting, diarrhoea, constipation, abdominal cramp); fatigue; cold hands and feet; exacerbation of intermittent claudication and Raynaud phenomenon; bronchospasm; bradycardia, heart failure, conduction disorders, hypotension; sleep disturbances, including nightmares; depression, confusion, convulsions; hypo- or hyperglycaemia; exacerbation of psoriasis; rare reports of rashes and dry eyes (oculomucocutaneous syndrome—reversible on withdrawal)

Captopril

Captopril is a representative angiotensin-converting enzyme inhibitor. Various drugs can serve as alternatives

Tablets, captopril 25 mg

Uses: hypertension; heart failure (section 12.4)

Contraindications: hypersensitivity to ACE inhibitors (including angioedema); known or suspected renovascular disease; aortic stenosis, outflow tract obstruction; pregnancy (Appendix 2); porphyria

Precautions: use with diuretics; hypotension with first doses, especially in patients on diuretics, on a low-sodium diet, on dialysis, if dehydrated, or with heart failure; peripheral vascular disease or generalized atherosclerosis (risk of clinically silent renovascular disease); monitor renal function before and during treatment; renal impairment (reduce dose, see also Appendix 4); possibly increased risk of agranulocytosis in collagen vascular disease; history of idiopathic or hereditary angioedema (use with care or avoid); breastfeeding (Appendix 3); **interactions:** Appendix 1

USE WITH DIURETICS. Risk of very rapid falls in blood pressure in volume-depleted patients; diuretic should be discontinued, or dose significantly reduced, 2–3 days before starting captopril (may not be possible in heart failure—risk of pulmonary oedema); if diuretic cannot be stopped, medical supervision advised for first 2 hours after administration or until blood pressure has stabilized

ANAPHYLACTOID REACTIONS. Avoid captopril during dialysis with high-flux polyacrilonitrile membranes and during low-density lipoprotein apheresis with dextran sulfate; also withhold before desensitization with wasp or bee venom

Dosage:

Hypertension (used alone), *by mouth*, ADULT initially 12.5 mg twice daily (ELDERLY initially 6.25 mg twice daily, with first dose at bedtime); usual maintenance dose 25 mg twice daily; maximum 50 mg twice daily (rarely 3 times daily in severe hypertension)

Hypertension, with diuretic, *by mouth*, ADULT initially 6.25 mg daily (first dose at bedtime); usual maintenance dose 25 mg twice daily; maximum 50 mg twice daily (rarely 3 times daily in severe hypertension)

Adverse effects: profound hypotension, renal impairment; angioedema (onset may be delayed), rash (possibly associated with pruritus and urticaria); persistent dry cough and upper respiratory-tract symptoms such as sinusitis, rhinitis, sore throat; pancreatitis, gastrointestinal disturbances including nausea, vomiting, dyspepsia, diarrhoea and constipation; altered liver function tests, cholestatic jaundice, hepatitis; blood disorders including thrombocytopenia, leukopenia, neutropenia, and haemolytic anaemia reported; also headache, dizziness, fatigue, malaise, taste disturbance, paraesthesia, bronchospasm, fever, serositis, vasculitis, myalgia, arthralgia, positive antinuclear antibody, raised erythrocyte sedimentation rate, eosinophilia, leukocytosis, and photosensitivity

---

Hydralazine hydrochloride

Hydralazine hydrochloride is a representative vasodilator antihypertensive drug. Various drugs can serve as alternatives

Tablets, hydralazine hydrochloride 25 mg, 50 mg

Injection, (Powder for solution for injection), hydralazine hydrochloride, 20-mg ampoule

Uses: in combination therapy in moderate to severe hypertension, hypertensive crises; hypertension associated with pregnancy (including pre-eclampsia or eclampsia); heart failure (section 12.4)

Contraindications: idiopathic systemic lupus erythematosus, severe tachycardia, high output heart failure, myocardial insufficiency due to mechanical obstruction, cor pulmonale, dissecting aortic aneurysm, or porphyria

Precautions: hepatic impairment (Appendix 5); renal impairment (reduce dose, Appendix 4); coronary artery disease (may provoke angina, avoid after myocardial infarction until stabilized); cerebrovascular disease; check acetylator status before increasing dose above 100 mg daily; test for anti-nuclear factor and for proteinuria every 6 months; pregnancy (Appendix 2); breastfeeding (Appendix 3); occasionally over-rapid blood pressure reduction even with low parenteral doses; **interactions:** Appendix 1

Dosage:

Hypertension, *by mouth*, ADULT 25 mg twice daily, increased if necessary to maximum 50 mg twice daily

Hypertensive crises (including during pregnancy), *by slow intravenous injection,* ADULT 5–10 mg diluted with sodium chloride 0.9%; if necessary may be repeated after 20–30 minutes

Hypertensive crises (including during pregnancy), *by intra-venous infusion,* ADULT initially 200–300 micrograms/minute; maintenance usually 50–150 micrograms/minute

RECONSTITUTION AND ADMINISTRATION. According to manufacturer's directions

Adverse effects: tachycardia, palpitations, postural hypo-tension; fluid retention; gastrointestinal disturbances includ-ing anorexia, nausea, vomiting, diarrhoea, rarely constipation; dizziness, flushing, headache; abnormal liver function, jaundice; systemic lupus erythematosus-like syndrome, particularly in women and slow acetylators; nasal congestion, agitation, anxiety, polyneuritis, peripheral neuritis, rash, fever, paraesthesia, arthralgia, myalgia, increased lacrimation, dyspnoea; raised plasma creatinine, proteinuria, haematuria; blood disorders including haemolytic anaemia, leukopenia, thrombocytopenia

---

Hydrochlorothiazide

Hydrochlorothiazide is a representative thiazide diuretic. Various drugs can serve as alternatives

Tablets, hydrochlorothiazide 25 mg

Uses: alone in mild hypertension, and in combination with other drugs in moderate to severe hypertension; heart failure (section 12.4); oedema (section 16.1)

Contraindications: severe kidney or severe hepatic impair-ment; hyponatraemia, hypercalcaemia, refractory hypokal-aemia, symptomatic hyperuricaemia; Addison disease

Precautions: renal and hepatic impairment (Appendices 4 and 5); pregnancy and breastfeeding (Appendices 2 and 3); elderly (reduce dose); may cause hypokalaemia; may aggravate diabetes mellitus and gout; may exacerbate systemic lupus erythematosus; porphyria; **interactions:** Appendix 1

Dosage:

Hypertension, *by mouth*, ADULT 12.5–25 mg daily; ELDERLY initially 12.5 mg daily

Adverse effects: fluid and electrolyte imbalance leading to dry mouth, thirst, gastrointestinal disturbances (including nausea, vomiting), weakness, lethargy, drowsiness, seizures, head-ache, muscle pains or cramps, hypotension (including postural hypotension), oliguria, arrhythmias; hypokalaemia, hypomagnesaemia, hyponatraemia, hypochloraemic alkalosis, hypercalcaemia; hyperglycaemia, hyperuricaemia, gout; rashes, photosensitivity; altered plasma lipid concentration; rarely impotence (reversible); blood disorders (including neutropenia, thrombocytopenia); pancreatitis, intrahepatic cholestasis; acute renal failure; hypersensitivity reactions (pneumonitis, pulmonary oedema, severe skin reactions)

Methyldopa
Tablets, methyldopa 250 mg

Uses: hypertension, including hypertension in pregnancy

Contraindications: depression; active liver disease; phaeochromocytoma, porphyria

Precautions: history of hepatic impairment (Appendix 5); renal impairment (Appendix 4); blood counts and liver-function tests advised; history of depression; positive direct Coomb test in up to 20% of patients (affects blood cross-matching); interference with laboratory tests; pregnancy and breastfeeding (Appendices 2 and 3); **interactions:** Appendix 1

SKILLED TASKS. May impair ability to perform skilled tasks, for example operating machinery, driving

Dosage:

Hypertension, *by mouth,* ADULT initially 250 mg 2–3 times daily; if necessary, gradually increased at intervals of 2 or more days; maximum 3 g daily

ELDERLY initially 125 mg twice daily, gradually increased to maximum 2 g daily

Adverse effects: tend to be transient and reversible, including sedation, dizziness, lightheadedness, postural hypotension, weakness, fatigue, headache, fluid retention and oedema, sexual dysfunction; impaired concentration and memory, depression, mild psychosis, disturbed sleep and nightmares; drug fever, influenza-like syndrome; nausea, vomiting, constipation, diarrhoea, dry mouth, stomatitis, sialadenitis; liver function impairment, hepatitis, jaundice, rarely fatal hepatic necrosis; bone-marrow depression, haemolytic anaemia, leukopenia, thrombocytopenia, eosinophilia; Parkinsonism; rash (including toxic epidermal necrolysis); nasal congestion; black or sore tongue; bradycardia, exacerbation of angina; myalgia, arthralgia, paraesthesia, Bell palsy; pancreatitis; hypersensitivity reactions including lupus erythematosus-like syndrome, myocarditis, pericarditis; gynaecomastia, hyperprolactinaemia, amenorrhoea; urine darkens on standing

Nifedipine

Nifedipine is a representative dihydropyridine calcium-channel blocker. Various drugs can serve as alternatives

Sustained-release tablets, nifedipine 10 mg

NOTE. Sustained-release (prolonged-release) tablets are available. A proposal to include such a product in a national list should be supported by adequate documentation

Uses: hypertension

Contraindications: cardiogenic shock; advanced aortic stenosis; within 1 month of myocardial infarction; unstable or acute attacks of angina; porphyria

Precautions: stop if ischaemic pain occurs or existing pain worsens shortly after starting treatment; poor cardiac reserve; heart failure or significantly impaired left ventricular function; reduce dose in hepatic impairment (Appendix 5); diabetes mellitus; may inhibit labour; pregnancy (Appendix 2); breastfeeding (Appendix 3); avoid grapefruit juice (may affect metabolism); **interactions:** Appendix 1

Dosage:

Hypertension, *by mouth* (as sustained-release tablets), ADULT usual range 20–100 mg daily in 1–2 divided doses, according to manufacturer's directions

NOTE. Prescribers should be aware that different formulations of sustained-release tablets may not have the same clinical effect; if possible, the patient should be maintained on the same brand

Short-acting formulations of nifedipine should be avoided in hypertension, particularly in patients who also have angina, since their use may be associated with large variations in blood pressure and reflex tachycardia, possibly leading to myocardial or cerebrovascular ischaemia

Adverse effects: headache, flushing, dizziness, lethargy; tachycardia, palpitations; gravitational oedema (only partly responsive to diuretics); rash (erythema multiforme reported), pruritus, urticaria; nausea, constipation or diarrhoea; increased frequency of micturition; eye pain, visual disturbances; gum hyperplasia; paraesthesia, myalgia, tremor; impotence, gynaecomastia; depression; telangiectasis; cholestasis, jaundice

Prazosin

Prazosin is a complementary antihypertensive drug; it should not be used as first-line therapy

Tablets, prazosin (as hydrochloride), 500 micrograms, 1 mg

Uses: hypertension usually in combination with thiazide or beta-blocker

Contraindications: congestive heart failure due to mechanical obstruction such as aortic or mitral valve stenosis, pulmonary embolism, or restrictive pericardial disease

Precautions: elderly, renal impairment (Appendix 4), hepatic impairment (Appendix 5); angina; pregnancy (Appendix 2); breastfeeding (Appendix 3); **interactions:** Appendix 1

SKILLED TASKS. May impair ability to perform skilled tasks, for example operating machinery, driving

Dosage:

Hypertension, *by mouth,* ADULT initially 500 micrograms 2–3 times daily (first dose taken on retiring to bed to avoid collapse); increased to 1 mg 2–3 times daily after 3–7 days; if necessary further increased to maximum 20 mg daily in divided doses

Adverse effects: postural hypotension (may be severe and produce syncope after initial dose, possibly preceded by tachycardia); nausea, vomiting, diarrhoea, constipation; dizziness, vertigo, headache, weakness, lack of energy, depression, nervousness, drowsiness, sleep disturbances, hallucinations; nasal congestion, epistaxis; reddened sclera, blurred vision; dry mouth; paraesthesia, tinnitus, dyspnoea, diaphoresis; rash, arthralgia, pruritus; palpitations, chest pain; oedema; increased urinary frequency, urinary incontinence; priapism, impotence; abnormal liver enzyme values, pancreatitis

---

Reserpine

Reserpine is a representative centrally acting antihypertensive. Various drugs can serve as alternatives

Tablets, reserpine 100 micrograms, 250 micrograms

Injection (Solution for injection), reserpine 1 mg/ml, 1-ml ampoule

Uses: hypertension in combination with a thiazide diuretic; hypertensive crisis (if more effective drugs not available)

Contraindications: history of depression, history of ulcerative colitis or peptic ulcer, phaeochromocytoma; Parkinson disease

Precautions: reduce dose in elderly or severely debilitated patients; arrhythmias, myocardial infarction, impaired respiratory function or impaired renal function; may interfere with laboratory tests; stop reserpine 7–14 days before starting electroconvulsive therapy; **interactions:** Appendix 1

Dosage:

Hypertension, *by mouth,* ADULT initially 100 micrograms once daily, gradually increased to 250 micrograms once daily; maximum daily dose of 500 micrograms should not be exceeded

Hypertensive crisis (but see notes above), *by intramuscular injection,* ADULT 0.5–1 mg, followed if necessary by 2–4 mg every 3 hours

Adverse effects: dizziness, nasal congestion, headache, oedema (may progress to congestive heart failure), drowsiness, lethargy, fatigue, nightmares, depression, increased gastrointestinal motility, diarrhoea, abdominal cramps, increased gastric acid secretion, flushing, bradycardia, hypotension, coma, convulsions, respiratory depression, hypothermia, cyanosis, respiratory distress, anorexia; lethargy in infant if used in mother prior to delivery; peptic ulcers and depression common at high doses

Sodium nitroprusside

Sodium nitroprusside is a representative vasodilator antihypertensive. It is a complementary drug for the treatment of hypertensive crisis

Infusion (Powder for solution for infusion), sodium nitroprusside, 50-mg ampoule

Uses: hypertensive crisis (when treatment by mouth not possible)

Contraindications: severe hepatic impairment; compensatory hypertension; severe vitamin B_{12} deficiency; Leber optic atrophy

Precautions: impaired pulmonary function; hypothyroidism; renal impairment (Appendix 4); ischaemic heart disease, impaired cerebral circulation; hyponatraemia; raised intracranial pressure; elderly; hypothermia; monitor blood pressure and blood-cyanide concentration, also blood-thiocyanate concentration if given for more than 3 days; avoid sudden withdrawal (reduce infusion over 15–30 minutes to avoid rebound effects); pregnancy; breastfeeding; **interactions:** Appendix 1

Dosage:

Hypertensive crisis, *by intravenous infusion*, ADULT initially 0.3 micrograms/kg/minute; usual maintenance dose 0.5–6 micrograms/kg/minute; maximum dose 8 micrograms/kg/minute; stop infusion if no response after 10 minutes at maximum dose

Lower doses in patients already being treated with antihypertensives

RECONSTITUTION AND ADMINISTRATION. According to manufacturer's directions

Adverse effects: severe hypotension; effects associated with over-rapid reduction in blood pressure include headache, dizziness; retching, abdominal pain; perspiration; palpitations, apprehension, retrosternal discomfort; rarely reduced platelet count, acute transient phlebitis

Adverse effects associated with excessive concentration of cyanide metabolite include tachycardia, sweating, hyperventilation, arrhythmias, marked metabolic acidosis (discontinue infusion and give antidote, section 4.2.7)

12.4 Drugs used in heart failure

Treatment of heart failure aims to relieve symptoms, improve exercise tolerance, reduce incidence of acute exacerbations, and reduce mortality. Drugs used to treat heart failure due to left ventricular systolic dysfunction include ACE inhibitors, diuretics, cardiac glycosides and vasodilators. In addition, measures such as weight reduction, moderate salt restriction, and appropriate exercise should be introduced.

The primary treatment of heart failure is with angiotensin-converting enzyme inhibitors (ACE inhibitors) such as **captopril** which can be used in all stages of chronic heart failure to prevent further deterioration and progression of heart disease.

A thiazide diuretic such as **hydrochlorothiazide** is used in the management of mild to moderate heart failure when the patient has mild fluid retention and severe pulmonary oedema is not present; however thiazides are ineffective if renal function is poor. In these patients, and in more severe fluid retention, a loop diuretic such as **furosemide** (section 16.2) is required. In severe fluid retention, intravenous furosemide produces relief of breathlessness and reduces preload sooner than would be expected from the time of onset of diuresis. Hypokalaemia may develop, but is less likely with the shorter-acting loop diuretics than with the thiazides; care is needed to avoid hypotension.

A combination of a thiazide and a loop diuretic may be required to treat refractory oedema. The combination often produces a synergistic effect on solute and water excretion, which relieves symptoms in the diuretic-resistant heart failure patient. However, the combination may produce excessive intravascular volume depletion and electrolyte disturbances including potentially life-threatening hypokalaemia.

Digoxin, a cardiac glycoside, increases the strength of cardiac muscle contractions and increases cardiac output. In mild heart failure, digoxin inhibits the sympathetic nervous system and produces arterial vasodilation. It produces symptomatic improvement, increases exercise tolerance, and reduces the risk of clinical deterioration. It is considered for patients with atrial fibrillation and those who do not respond to ACE inhibitors.

Vasodilators are used in heart failure to reduce systemic vascular resistance. **Isosorbide dinitrate** (section 12.1) produces mainly venous dilatation, which reduces left ventricular preload, leading to a reduction in pulmonary congestion and dyspnoea. **Hydralazine** (section 12.3) produces mainly arterial vasodilation, which reduces left ventricular afterload, and increases stroke volume and cardiac output. Isosorbide dinitrate and hydralazine can be used in combination when an ACE inhibitor cannot be used.

Dopamine, an inotropic sympathomimetic, may be given for short periods in the treatment of severe heart failure. Dosage is critical; at low doses it stimulates myocardial contractility and increases cardiac output and renal perfusion, however higher doses (more than 5 micrograms/kg per minute) cause vasoconstriction, with a worsening of heart failure.

Captopril

Captopril is a representative angiotensin-converting enzyme inhibitor. Various drugs can serve as alternatives

Tablets, captopril 25 mg

Uses: heart failure (with a diuretic); prophylaxis after myocardial infarction; hypertension (section 12.3)

Contraindications: hypersensitivity to ACE inhibitors (including angioedema); known or suspected renovascular disease; aortic stenosis, outflow tract obstruction; pregnancy (Appendix 2); porphyria

Precautions: use with diuretics; hypotension with first doses, especially in patients on diuretics, on a low-sodium diet, on dialysis, if dehydrated, or with heart failure; peripheral vascular disease or generalized atherosclerosis (risk of clinically silent renovascular disease); monitor renal function before and during treatment; renal impairment (reduce dose, see also Appendix 4); possibly increased risk of agranulocytosis in collagen vascular disease; history of idiopathic or hereditary angioedema (use with care or avoid); breastfeeding (Appendix 3); **interactions:** Appendix 1

USE WITH DIURETICS. Risk of very rapid falls in blood pressure in volume-depleted patients; diuretic should be discontinued, or dose significantly reduced, 2–3 days before starting captopril (may not be possible in heart failure—risk of pulmonary oedema); if diuretic cannot be stopped, medical supervision advised for first 2 hours after administration or until blood pressure has stabilized

ANAPHYLACTOID REACTIONS. Avoid captopril during dialysis with high-flux polyacrilonitrile membranes and during low-density lipoprotein apheresis with dextran sulfate; also withhold before desensitization with wasp or bee venom

Dosage:

Heart failure (adjunct), *by mouth,* ADULT, initially 6.25–12.5 mg under close medical supervision; usual maintenance dose 25 mg 2–3 times daily; usual maximum 150 mg daily

Prophylaxis after myocardial infarction (in clinically stable patients), *by mouth,* ADULT initially 6.25 mg, gradually increased over several weeks to 150 mg daily in divided doses

Adverse effects: profound hypotension, renal impairment; angioedema (onset may be delayed), rash (possibly associated with pruritus and urticaria); persistent dry cough and upper respiratory-tract symptoms such as sinusitis, rhinitis, sore throat; pancreatitis, gastrointestinal disturbances including nausea, vomiting, dyspepsia, diarrhoea and constipation; altered liver function tests, cholestatic jaundice, hepatitis; blood disorders including thrombocytopenia, leukopenia, neutropenia, and haemolytic anaemia reported; also headache, dizziness, fatigue, malaise, taste disturbance, paraesthesia, bronchospasm, fever, serositis, vasculitis, myalgia, arthralgia, positive antinuclear antibody, raised erythrocyte sedimentation rate, eosinophilia, leukocytosis, and photosensitivity

---

Digoxin

Tablets, digoxin 62.5 micrograms, 250 micrograms
Oral solution, digoxin 50 micrograms/ml
Injection (Solution for injection), digoxin 250 micrograms/ml, 2-ml ampoule

Uses: heart failure; arrhythmias (section 12.2)

Contraindications: hypertrophic obstructive cardiomyopathy (unless also severe heart failure); Wolff-Parkinson-White syndrome or other accessory pathway, particularly if accompanied by atrial fibrillation; intermittent complete heart block; second-degree atrioventricular block

Precautions: recent myocardial infarction; sick sinus syndrome; severe pulmonary disease; thyroid disease; elderly (reduce dose); renal impairment (Appendix 4); avoid hypokalaemia; avoid rapid intravenous administration (nausea and risk of arrhythmias); pregnancy (Appendix 2); breastfeeding (Appendix 3); **interactions:** Appendix 1

Dosage:

Heart failure, *by mouth,* ADULT 1–1.5 mg in divided doses over 24 hours for rapid digitalization *or* 250 micrograms 1–2 times daily if digitalization less urgent; maintenance 62.5–500 micrograms daily (higher dose may be divided), according to renal function and heart rate response; usual range 125–250 micrograms daily (lower dose more appropriate in elderly)

Emergency loading dose, *by intravenous infusion,* ADULT 250–500 micrograms over 10–20 minutes, repeated at intervals of 4–8 hours according to response to total loading dose of 0.5–1 mg

NOTE. Infusion dose may need to be reduced if digoxin or other cardiac glycoside given in previous 2 weeks

Adverse effects: usually associated with excessive dosage and include anorexia, nausea, vomiting, diarrhoea, abdominal pain; visual disturbances, headache, fatigue, drowsiness, confusion, delirium, hallucinations, depression; arrhythmias, heart block; rarely rash, intestinal ischaemia; gynaecomastia on long-term use; thrombocytopenia reported

Dopamine hydrochloride

Concentrate for infusion (Concentrate for solution for infusion), dopamine hydrochloride 40 mg/ml, 5-ml ampoule

Uses: cardiogenic shock in myocardial infarction or cardiac surgery

Contraindications: tachyarrhythmia, ventricular fibrillation; ischaemic heart disease; phaeochromocytoma; hyperthyroidism

Precautions: correct hypovolaemia before, and maintain blood volume during treatment; correct hypoxia, hypercapnia, and metabolic acidosis before or at same time as starting treatment; low dose in shock due to myocardial infarction; history of peripheral vascular disease (increased risk of ischaemia of extremities); elderly; **interactions:** Appendix 1

Dosage:

Cardiogenic shock, *by intravenous infusion* into large vein, ADULT initially 2–5 micrograms/kg/minute; gradually increased by 5–10 micrograms/kg/minute according to blood pressure, cardiac output and urine output; seriously ill patients up to 20–50 micrograms/kg/minute

DILUTION AND ADMINISTRATION. According to manufacturer's directions

Adverse effects: nausea and vomiting; peripheral vasoconstriction; hypotension with dizziness, fainting, flushing; tachycardia, ectopic beats, palpitations, anginal pain; headache, dyspnoea; hypertension particularly in overdosage

Hydrochlorothiazide

Hydrochlorothiazide is a representative thiazide diuretic. Various drugs can serve as alternatives

Tablets, hydrochlorothiazide 25 mg, 50 mg

Uses: heart failure; hypertension (section 12.3); oedema (section 16.1)

Contraindications: severe kidney or severe hepatic impairment; hyponatraemia, hypercalcaemia, refractory hypokalaemia, symptomatic hyperuricaemia; Addison disease

Precautions: renal and hepatic impairment (Appendices 4 and 5); pregnancy and breastfeeding (Appendices 2 and 3); elderly (reduce dose); may cause hypokalaemia; may aggravate diabetes mellitus and gout; may exacerbate systemic lupus erythematosus; porphyria; **interactions:** Appendix 1

Dosage:

Heart failure, *by mouth,* ADULT initially 25 mg daily on rising, increasing to 50 mg daily if necessary; ELDERLY initially 12.5 mg daily

Adverse effects: fluid and electrolyte imbalance leading to dry mouth, thirst, gastrointestinal disturbances (including nausea, vomiting), weakness, lethargy, drowsiness, seizures, headache, muscle pains or cramps, hypotension (including postural hypotension), oliguria, arrhythmias; hypokalaemia, hypomagnesaemia, hyponatraemia, hypochloraemic alkalosis, hypercalcaemia; hyperglycaemia, hyperuricaemia, gout; rashes, photosensitivity; altered plasma lipid concentration; rarely impotence (reversible); blood disorders (including neutropenia, thrombocytopenia); pancreatitis, intrahepatic cholestasis; acute renal failure; hypersensitivity reactions (pneumonitis, pulmonary oedema, severe skin reactions)

12.5 Antithrombotic drugs and myocardial infarction

Anticoagulants prevent thrombus formation or the extension of an existing thrombus. For further details see section 10.2 (drugs affecting coagulation).

Antiplatelet drugs also help to inhibit thrombus formation by decreasing platelet aggregation.

Thrombolytics (fibrinolytics) such as **streptokinase** are used to break up thrombi; they are used to treat acute myocardial infarction, extensive deep vein thrombosis, major pulmonary embolism and acute arterial occlusion.

Myocardial infarction

Management of myocardial infarction includes two phases:
- initial management of the acute attack
- long-term management, including prevention of further attacks

Initial management

Oxygen (section 1.1.3) should be given to all patients, except those with severe chronic obstructive airways disease.

Pain and anxiety are relieved by slow intravenous injection of an opioid analgesic such as **morphine** (section 2.2). **Metoclopramide** (section 17.2) may also be given by intramuscular injection to prevent and treat nausea and vomiting caused by morphine.

Acetylsalicylic acid 150–300 mg by mouth (preferably chewed or dispersed in water) is given immediately for its antiplatelet effect.

Thrombolytic drugs such as **streptokinase** help to restore perfusion and thus relieve myocardial ischaemia; they should ideally be given within 1 hour of infarction (use after 12 hours requires specialist advice).

Nitrates (section 12.1) may also be given to relieve ischaemic pain.

Early administration of beta-blockers such as **atenolol** (section 12.1) have been shown to reduce both early mortality and the recurrence rate of myocardial infarction; initial intravenous administration is followed by long-term oral treatment (unless the patient has contraindications).

ACE inhibitors (section 12.4) have also been shown to be beneficial in initial management (unless patient has contraindications) when given within 24 hours, and if possible continued for 5–6 weeks.

If arrhythmias occur, they should be treated aggressively, but the likelihood decreases rapidly over the first 24 hours after infarction. Ventricular fibrillation should be treated immediately with a defibrillator; if this is ineffective alone, the antiarrhythmic drug **lidocaine** (section 12.2) should be given.

Long-term management

Acetylsalicylic acid should be given to all patients in a dose of 75–150 mg daily by mouth, unless it is contraindicated. The prolonged antiplatelet effect has been shown to reduce the rate of reinfarction.

Treatment with **beta-blockers** should be continued for at least 1 year, and possibly for up to 3 years.

ACE inhibitors such as **captopril** (section 12.4) should also be used since they reduce mortality, particularly in patients with left ventricular dysfunction.

Nitrates (section 12.1) may be required for patients with angina.

The use of **statins** (section 12.6) may also be considered in patients with high risk of recurrence.

Stroke

Stroke (cerebrovascular accident) may be ischaemic or haemorrhagic; precise diagnosis is essential, as management for the two types of stroke is quite different.

Primary prevention of both types of stroke includes reduction of high blood pressure, stopping smoking, weight reduction, and cholesterol reduction. Atrial fibrillation, acute myocardial infarction, and valvular disease may produce embolism and ischaemic stroke. Prophylaxis in these patients includes oral anticoagulants such as warfarin (section 10.2) and antiplatelet drugs such as acetylsalicylic acid. Treatment of acute ischaemic stroke includes use of **acetylsalicylic acid**, anticoagulants such as heparin, and of thrombolytics, such as streptokinase. Streptokinase must be used with extreme caution due to risk of bleeding. Long-term therapy with acetylsalicylic acid reduces the risk of having another stroke.

Antiplatelet and thrombolytic drugs are not used in the management of haemorrhagic stroke, as they may exacerbate bleeding. The main treatment is to normalize blood pressure.

Acetylsalicylic acid is normally given for at least one year after coronary artery bypass surgery. It is also given to patients with prosthetic heart valves who have had cerebral embolism despite warfarin treatment.

Acetylsalicylic acid

Tablets, acetylsalicylic acid 100 mg

Uses: prophylaxis of cerebrovascular disease or myocardial infarction; pyrexia, pain, inflammation (section 2.1.1); migraine (section 7.1)

Contraindications: hypersensitivity (including asthma, angioedema, urticaria or rhinitis) to acetylsalicylic acid or any other NSAID; children under 12 years (risk of Reye syndrome); active peptic ulceration; haemophilia and other bleeding disorders

Precautions: asthma; uncontrolled hypertension; pregnancy (Appendix 2); breastfeeding (Appendix 3); see also section 2.1.1; **interactions:** Appendix 1

Dosage:

Prophylaxis of cerebrovascular disease or myocardial infarction, *by mouth*, ADULT 75–300 mg daily

Adverse effects: bronchospasm; gastrointestinal haemorrhage (rarely major), also other haemorrhage (for example subconjunctival); see also section 2.1.1

Streptokinase

Streptokinase is a complementary drug; it is used in the management of myocardial infarction and thromboembolism

Powder for infusion (Powder for solution for infusion), streptokinase 100 000-unit vial, 750 000-unit vial

Uses: life-threatening deep-vein thrombosis, pulmonary embolism, acute arterial thromboembolism; thrombosed arteriovenous shunts; acute myocardial infarction

Contraindications: recent haemorrhage, surgery (including dental), parturition, trauma; heavy vaginal bleeding; haemorrhagic stroke, history of cerebrovascular disease (especially recent or if residual disability); coma; severe hypertension;

coagulation defects; bleeding diatheses, aortic dissection; risk of gastrointestinal bleeding such as recent history of peptic ulcer, oesophageal varices, ulcerative colitis; acute pancreatitis; sever liver disease; acute pulmonary disease with cavitation; previous allergic reactions

Precautions: risk of bleeding from any invasive procedure, including injection; external chest compression; pregnancy (Appendix 2); abdominal aneurysm or where thrombolysis may give rise to embolic complications such as enlarged left atrium with atrial fibrillation (risk of dissolution of clot and subsequent embolization); diabetic retinopathy (small risk of retinal haemorrhage); recent or concurrent anticoagulant treatment

Dosage:

Thrombosis, *by intravenous infusion,* ADULT 250 000 units over 30 minutes, followed by 100 000 units every hour for 12–72 hours according to condition with monitoring of clotting parameters

Myocardial infarction, *by intravenous infusion,* ADULT 1 500 000 units over 60 minutes

Thrombosed arteriovenous shunts, consult manufacturer's literature

Adverse effects: nausea and vomiting; bleeding, usually limited to site of injection but internal bleeding including intracranial haemorrhage may occur (if serious bleeding occurs, discontinue infusion—coagulation factors may be required); hypotension, arrhythmias (particularly in myocardial infarction); allergic reactions including rash, flushing, uveitis, anaphylaxis; fever, chills, back or abdominal pain; Guillain-Barre syndrome reported rarely

12.6 Lipid-regulating drugs

The primary aim of therapy is to reduce progression of atherosclerosis and to improve survival in patients with established cardiovascular disease, to reduce premature cardiac morbidity and mortality in people at high risk of cardiovascular events and to prevent pancreatitis due to hypertriglyceridaemia. Before starting drug therapy dietary measures, reduction of blood pressure and cessation of smoking should be tried. The WHO Expert Committee on Essential Drugs recognizes the value of lipid-lowering drugs in treating patients with hyperlipidaemia. Beta-hydroxy-beta-methylglutaryl-coenzyme A (HMG Co A) reductase inhibitors, often referred to as 'statins', are potent and effective lipid-lowering drugs with a good tolerability profile. Several of these drugs have been shown to reduce the incidence of fatal and non-fatal myocardial infarction, stroke and mortality (all causes), as well as the need for coronary bypass surgery. All remain very costly, but may be cost-effective for secondary prevention of cardiovascular disease as well as for primary prevention in some very high-risk patients. Since no single drug has been shown to be significantly more effective or less expensive than others in the group, none is included in the model list; the choice of drug for use in patients at highest risk should be decided at national level.

Section 13: Dermatological Drugs (topical)

13.1 Antifungal drugs

RINGWORM. **Benzoic acid** and **methylrosanilinium chloride** (gentian violet) solution are inexpensive and effective fungistatic compounds for the treatment of dermatophyte infections such as ringworm. Minor skin lesions due to ringworm can be cleared with repeated applications of **compound benzoic acid** ointment (Whitfield ointment), which combines the fungistatic action of benzoic acid with the keratolytic action of salicylic acid. However, the most effective topical treatment for dermatophyte infections is a cream containing an imidazole such as **miconazole**, which is effective for long-established lesions but is more expensive than compound benzoic acid ointment. Extensive and generalized infections of the skin, nails and scalp should be treated systemically for several weeks with **griseofulvin** or **fluconazole** (see section 6.3).

Scalp ringworm (tinea capitis) typically appears as a patch of scaling alopecia, or a swollen inflammatory area (tinea kerion). Mild forms may remit spontaneously at puberty. Inflamed lesions should be treated systemically with **griseofulvin**. Application of **miconazole** cream may accelerate healing of scaly lesions.

Ringworm on the body (tinea corporis) can also be cleared with **compound benzoic acid** ointment or a topical imidazole such as **miconazole**. In resistant cases a 4-week course of oral **griseofulvin** is required.

Foot ringworm (tinea pedis or athlete's foot) is usually treated topically. **Compound benzoic acid** ointment should be applied twice daily to all infected areas and all toe clefts for at least 4 weeks. Systemic therapy with griseofulvin or fluconazole may be required if the foot is extensively infected. Tinea pedis commonly recurs and may be treated with miconazole cream. Severe weeping lesions respond to frequent soaking in solutions of 1:10 000 **potassium permanganate**, and systemic antifungals may also be needed.

Nail infections (onychomycosis, tinea unguium) are difficult to treat; fingernails may require 6 months treatment with oral griseofulvin and toenails may require 12 months or more of this treatment. Approximately 60% of nail infections either do not respond or relapse after treatment with griseofulvin.

Ringworm of the groin (tinea cruris) is usually limited to the skin of the inner thigh in contact with the scrotum. Flexural eczema, often superinfected with candida or bacteria, occurs in the same site. The latter is frequently treated with combined antifungal/corticosteroid preparations, but must not be treated with a corticosteroid alone, which will worsen the condition. An imidazole cream such as **miconazole** applied daily for 2 weeks is usually effective. Lesions unresponsive to topical preparations can usually be cleared with a 4-week course of **griseofulvin**.

CANDIDOSIS. Candida can infect the oral cavity, the vagina or the skin. Cutaneous lesions tend to occur in patients with diabetes mellitus and some chronic debilitating conditions, including hypoparathyroidism and various congenital disorders of the immune system. The most severe infections of candida are now seen in patients with HIV infection.

Cutaneous candidosis usually responds to **miconazole** cream as a twice daily application. Chronic candida paronychia, which can result ultimately in nail dystrophy, is more difficult to cure. Treatment should be based on determination of the underlying cause and its reduction or elimination; hands and folds of the nail must be kept dry and daily application of an imidazole cream for several months may be required, ensuring penetration of the cleft between the nail plate and the swollen skin around the nail.

PITYRIASIS VERSICOLOR. Pityriasis (tinea) versicolor is caused by a commensal yeast. Application of **sodium thiosulfate** twice daily for 4 weeks is usually curative although areas of depigmentation on darker skins remain after completion of treatment. Relapses can be frequent, however, probably because much of the infected area may appear normal and be left untreated. Better results have been reported with topical applications of **miconazole** or **selenium sulfide**.

Benzoic acid with salicylic acid
Ointment, benzoic acid 6%, salicylic acid 3%

Uses: mild dermatophyte infections, particularly tinea pedis and tinea corporis

Administration: Apply twice daily until the infected skin is shed (usually at least 4 weeks)

Adverse effects: occasionally localized, mild inflammatory reaction

---

Miconazole nitrate
Miconazole is a representative topical antifungal. Various drugs can serve as alternatives
Cream, miconazole nitrate 2%

Uses: superficial fungal infections due to dermatophytes and yeasts, and secondary infections caused by Gram-positive cocci, including ringworm, intertrigo, candida napkin rash, paronychia, and pityriasis versicolor

Administration: Apply twice daily to clean dry lesions, continuing for at least 10 days after the condition has cleared

Adverse effects: occasional local irritation and burning, also contact dermatitis; discontinue if sensitization occurs

---

Selenium sulfide
Selenium sulfide is a complementary drug for use in rare disorders or in exceptional circumstances
Lotion, selenium sulfide 2.5% [not included on WHO Model List 11th revision]

Detergent-based suspension (shampoo), selenium sulfide 2.5%

Uses: pityriasis versicolor (lotion), seborrhoeic dermatitis (detergent-based suspension)

Contraindications: children under 5 years

Precautions: do not apply to damaged skin (risk of systemic toxicity); avoid contact with eyes; do not use within 48 hours of applying any type of hair colouring or permanent waving preparations

Administration: Pityriasis versicolor, apply lotion with a small amount of water to the entire affected area and rinse off after 10 minutes; repeat after 3 and 6 days

Seborrhoeic dermatitis, massage 5–10 ml of shampoo into wet hair and leave for 2–3 minutes before rinsing thoroughly; repeat twice weekly for 2 weeks, then once weekly for 2 weeks, and then only when needed

NOTE. To minimise absorption, rinse hair thoroughly after use and remove all traces from skin (including nails)

Adverse effects: local irritation, hair discoloration or loss; absorption may result in systemic toxicity including tremors, weakness, lethargy, pain in lower abdomen, occasional vomiting (symptoms usually resolve within 10 days)

Sodium thiosulfate
Cutaneous solution, sodium thiosulfate 15%

Uses: pityriasis versicolor; cyanide poisoning (section 4.2.7)

Administration: Apply twice daily for 4 weeks

13.2 Anti-infective (antibacterial) drugs

Staphylococcal infections of the skin such as impetigo, folliculitis, and furunculi and streptococcal infections such as cellulitis and erysipelas are very common where the climate is hot and humid, where standards of hygiene are compromised, and in immunodeficient patients.

In all skin infections, an important part of treatment is cleansing and thorough drying. Washing with soap and water will often help to prevent infection. Light localized infections can often be treated effectively with an antiseptic solution such as **chlorhexidine** (section 15.1). Superficial crusts should be gently washed with soap and water or a weak solution of **aluminium acetate** (section 13.4) or a 0.01% solution of **potassium permanganate**. Infected burns should be treated with **silver sulfadiazine**, which is bactericidal against both Gram-positive and Gram-negative organisms.

An ointment containing 2% mupirocin, which is active against Gram-positive bacteria, is of value, particularly in impetigo. To prevent the development of resistance, mupirocin should not be used for more than 10 days. Topical preparations containing **neomycin** and **bacitracin** are also widely used but these carry a risk of sensitization particularly with continued or repeated use.

Topical use of preparations containing antimicrobials which are widely used systemically should be avoided. These include penicillins, sulfonamides, streptomycin and gentamicin, which should be reserved for the systemic treatment of infections because of the possibility of inducing sensitivity and favouring the emergence of resistant organisms. Only widespread superficial or deep-seated infections associated with fever require treatment with a systemic antibiotic (sections 6.2.1 and 6.2.2). Whenever possible, the choice of an antimicrobial should be based on the results of sensitivity tests.

Methylrosanilinium chloride

Gentian violet; Crystal violet
Methylrosanilinium chloride is a representative topical anti-infective drug. Various drugs can serve as alternatives
Cutaneous solution, methylrosanilinium chloride 0.5%

Uses: superficial fungal and bacterial infections

Contraindications: excoriated or ulcerated lesions, broken skin, mucous membranes

Administration: Apply 2 or 3 times daily for 2–3 days

Adverse effects: severe irritation (discontinue treatment); temporary staining of skin, permanent staining of fabrics; *animal* carcinogenicity (restricted use in some countries)

Potassium permanganate

Cutaneous solution, potassium permanganate 1:10 000 (0.01% solution)
NOTE. Potassium permanganate is sometimes supplied as an aqueous stock solution of 1 in 1000 (0.1%) for dilution before use

Uses: wet dressings to assist healing of suppurating superficial wounds, tropical ulcers, tinea pedis, pemphigus, impetigo

Contraindications: avoid occlusive dressings

Precautions: irritant to mucous membranes

Administration: Suppurating superficial wounds and tropical ulcers, wet dressings of 1:10 000 (0.01%) solution, changed 2 or 3 times daily; tropical ulcers also require treatment for 2–4 weeks with procaine benzylpenicillin (section 6.2.1.1)

Tinea pedis, soak severe weeping lesions in 1:10 000 (0.01%) solution every 8 hours

Pemphigus, soak compresses in 1:10 000 (0.01%) solution and apply every 4 hours

Impetigo, superficial crusts should be gently separated with a 1:10 000 (0.01%) solution

Adverse effects: local irritation; skin and fabrics stained brown

Neomycin with bacitracin

Bacitracin is a representative topical antibacterial. Various drugs can serve as alternatives
Ointment, neomycin sulfate 5 mg, bacitracin zinc 500 units/g

Uses: superficial bacterial infections of the skin due to staphylococci and streptococci

Precautions: avoid application to substantial areas of skin or to broken skin (risk of significant systemic absorption); overgrowth of resistant organisms on prolonged use

Administration: Apply thin layer 3 times daily

Adverse effects: sensitization, especially to neomycin, causing reddening and scaling; anaphylaxis reported rarely; systemic absorption leading to irreversible ototoxicity, particularly in renal impairment

---

Silver sulfadiazine
Cream, silver sulfadiazine 1%

Uses: prophylaxis and treatment of infection in burns

Contraindications: hypersensitivity to sulfonamides; pregnancy (Appendix 2); neonates

Precautions: renal or hepatic impairment; G6PD deficiency; breastfeeding (Appendix 3)

Administration: Apply using aseptic technique daily (more frequently if volume of exudate is large) whilst there is a possibility of infection, or until healing is complete

Adverse effects: allergic reactions include rashes, burning and itching; argyria and sulfonamide-induced systemic toxicity, including blood disorders following application to large areas or prolonged use; transient leukopenia reported

---

13.3 Anti-inflammatory and antipruritic drugs

CONTACT DERMATITIS. Contact dermatitis can result from an allergic or irritant skin reaction. Removal of the substance provoking the reaction is the first step in treating this condition. Mild cases of contact dermatitis can be treated with topical **hydrocortisone** which suppresses inflammation. A short course of oral prednisolone or a topical corticosteroid such as **betamethasone** should be considered for more severe cases and for suppression of severe acute reactions associated with blistering, exudation and oedema. Soaking in clean water or mild saline solution is recommended in the acute stages of severe dermatitis.

PRURITUS. Pruritus or itching is a common symptom of many skin diseases. However, contact with certain substances, conditions that dry the skin, stress, and extremes of temperature may also be a cause. Thus, an important part of treatment is to eliminate or minimize the reason for the irritation.

Corticosteroids, such as hydrocortisone or betamethasone applied topically, can give relief. Soothing baths, or the application of calamine lotion or an emollient cream may also be helpful. Systemic antihistamines, such as oral chlorphenamine (section 3.1), may relieve generalized pruritus.

ATOPIC DERMATITIS. Atopic dermatitis (or eczema) is a common skin disorder, which mainly occurs in infants and children; it is associated with intense itching, with areas of red skin. Pruritus may be partially relieved by applying astringent **aluminium acetate** (section 13.4) lotion to exudative lesions and emollients to lichenified plaques. Topical **hydrocortisone** should be applied in short courses of 1–2 weeks to treat even mild areas of involvement. The use of **betamethasone** should be considered in the treatment of persistent localized dermatitis in adults. Topical antihistamines are not effective and should be avoided because of the risk of sensitization. However, a sedative antihistamine can be given at night to calm pruritus and facilitate sleep (see section 3.1). A secondary infection, often involving *Staphylococcus aureus*, may be responsible for exacerbations; in such cases, an oral antibiotic such as erythromycin can be given for 7–10 days (section 6.2.2.4).

SEBORRHOEIC DERMATITIS. Use of a keratolytic shampoo and exposure to ultraviolet light reduce both the inflammation and the scaling resulting from seborrhoeic dermatitis of the scalp (dandruff). The shampoo should be massaged into the scalp, immediately rinsed off and then reapplied until a foam is produced, leaving the second application in contact with the scalp for at least 5 minutes. **Selenium sulfide**, which has both antifungal and keratolytic properties, is widely used in many proprietary shampoos. A combination of sulfur and salicylic acid, which has an additional antimicrobial action, is also effective.

ICHTHYOSIS. In ichthyosis, emollients such as aqueous creams and emulsifying creams should be applied daily (or more frequently in severe cases) to affected skin. The addition of a keratolytic, such as **salicylic acid** 5% can be helpful.

LICHEN PLANUS. Lichen planus is a chronic, papular, pruritic skin eruption that occurs typically in middle age and later life; the condition is often mild and may need no treatment. In more severe cases, when the underlying cause cannot be identified, a topical corticosteroid offers the only prospect of remission.

PITYRIASIS ROSEA. In pityriasis rosea, a common self-limiting dermatosis that is probably of infective origin, **calamine lotion** helps to relieve pruritus in most cases. If it does not, topical application of **hydrocortisone** in a concentration not exceeding 1% is worth trying.

Calamine

Calamine is a representative topical antipruritic. Various drugs can serve as alternatives

Lotion (cutaneous suspension), calamine 8% (USP), 15%(BP)

Uses: mild pruritus

Administration: Apply liberally 3–4 times daily

CORTICOSTEROIDS

Betamethasone

Betamethasone is a representative potent topical corticosteroid. Various drugs can serve as alternatives

Cream, betamethasone (as valerate) 0.1%

Ointment, betamethasone (as valerate) 0.1%

Uses: severe inflammatory skin conditions inluding contact dermatitis, atopic dermatitis (eczema), seborrhoeic dermatitis, lichen planus, psoriasis and intractable pruritus

Contraindications: untreated skin infections or broken skin, rosacea, acne, perioral dermatitis

Precautions: children (avoid prolonged use); adrenal suppression if used on a large area of the body or for a long time, particularly with an occlusive dressing or on broken skin; avoid use on the face for more than 7 days; secondary infection requires treatment with an appropriate antimicrobial

Administration: ADULTS and CHILDREN over 2 years of age, apply small quantity to the affected area 1–2 times daily until improvement occur, then less frequently

Adverse effects: exacerbation of local infection; local atrophic changes particularly on the face and in skinfolds, characterized by thinning of the dermis, depigmentation, dilatation of superficial blood vessels and formation of striae; perioral dermatitis; acne at site of application; suppression of the hypothalamic-pituitary-adrenal axis with prolonged or widespread use (particularly under occlusion)

Hydrocortisone acetate

Hydrocortisone acetate is a representative mild topical corticosteroid. Various drugs can serve as alternatives

Cream, hydrocortisone acetate 1%

Ointment, hydrocortisone acetate 1%

Uses: contact dermatitis, atopic dermatitis (eczema), lichen planus; intractable pruritus and phototoxic reactions, including polymorphic light eruptions and actinic prurigo; short-term treatment of psoriasis of the face, scalp, palms and soles

Contraindications: untreated skin infections or broken skin; rosacea, acne, perioral dermatitis

Precautions: children (avoid prolonged use); occlusive dressings increase penetration into keratinized lesions (use occlusive dressings only at night and for no longer than 2 days; avoid use on weeping lesions); secondary infection requires treatment with an appropriate antimicrobial

Administration: Apply a small quantity to the affected area 1–2 times daily until improvement occurs, then less frequently

Adverse effects: exacerbation of local infection; atrophic changes (see under Betamethasone) less likely with mild corticosteroids, but infants and children particularly susceptible

13.4 Astringents

Aluminum acetate is a topical astringent used as an antiseptic for various skin conditions including suppurating superficial wounds and tropical ulcers, and the lesions produced by pemphigus and impetigo. **Potassium permanganate** (section 13.2) may be used in the same way.

Aluminium acetate

Solution for dilution (Concentrate for cutaneous solution), aluminium acetate 13%

Uses: wet dressings to assist healing of suppurating superficial wounds, tropical ulcers and eczematous skin lesions; removal of adherent crusts

Precautions: avoid use of plastic or rubber occlusive dressings

Administration: Suppurating superficial wounds and tropical ulcers, apply dressings soaked in 0.65% (1:20) solution for 30–120 minutes daily, changing dressings every 5–15 minutes; tropical ulcers also require treatment with procaine benzylpenicillin for 2–4 weeks (section 6.2.1.1)

Pemphigus, apply dressings soaked in 5% (1:2.6) solution every 4 hours

Impetigo, apply dressings soaked in 0.65% (1:20) solution until superficial crusts can be separated

13.5 Drugs affecting skin differentiation and proliferation

ACNE VULGARIS. Acne is a disorder of the pilosebaceous follicles and typically first appears during puberty when androgenic stimulation triggers excessive production of sebum. *Mild acne* is characterized by comedones and a few pustules which heal without scarring, and usually responds to topical therapy alone. In *moderate acne*, where there are more extensive pustules causing mild scarring, oral antibiotics such as a tetracycline or erythromycin (section 6.2.2.4) are commonly used. In *severe acne*, widespread pustules are accompanied by nodular abscesses and cysts, requiring treatment with estrogens, antiandrogens, or retinoids. Since scarring of the skin resulting from severe nodular acne causes major distress, acne should always be treated as soon as possible. Exposure to substances suspected of causing or aggravating the condition should be avoided. Systemic treatment must be continued for several months before a response can be anticipated. During this time, topical preparations should be applied to the affected areas to prevent the development of new lesions.

Benzoyl peroxide is a keratolytic drug with bacteriostatic activity against *Propionibacterium acnes*; treatment is usually started at a lower strength and increased as tolerance develops to the initial irritant reaction.

Preparations containing **sulfur**, which is bactericidal and promotes desquamation, are often used, and may be combined with salicylic acid, which is a keratolytic agent.

Topical antibiotics such as clindamycin are widely used in inflammatory acne. However, treatment must be maintained for 2 to 3 months before any benefit is seen and this prolonged course carries the risk of selection and spread of antibiotic-resistant organisms.

Benzoyl peroxide

Cream, benzoyl peroxide 5%
Lotion (cutaneous suspension), benzoyl peroxide 5%

Uses: mild to moderate acne and as an adjunct to oral therapy in more severe cases

Precautions: avoid contact with eyes, mouth, and mucous membranes; avoid use of occlusive dressings

Administration: Initially apply to clean skin on alternate days, increasing frequency to 1–2 times daily as tolerance to irritant effect develops

Adverse effects: initial irritation common but subsides with continued use; rarely, contact sensitivity occurs, occasionally even 1 application can cause severe irritation; may bleach fabrics, hair and skin

PSORIASIS. Psoriasis, which affects people of all ages in all countries, is one of the most common chronic dermatoses in industrialized countries, and is characterized by epidermal thickening and scaling. Considerable local variations in its prevalence have been variously attributed to genetic, climatic, nutritional and ecological factors. Various biological events may trigger psoriasis, such as streptococcal or viral infection, an emotional crisis or pregnancy. Psoriasis vulgaris (chronic plaque psoriasis) is the most common form of the condition, usually affecting extensor surfaces of the limbs and the scalp. Guttate psoriasis, commonly seen in children, is often caused by a streptococcal infection; lesions may disappear following antimicrobial treatment. The condition is also known to resolve spontaneously but more commonly transforms into chronic plaque psoriasis. No treatment is known to assure remission, although sunlight often clears lesions.

Dithranol restores the normal rate of epidermal cell proliferation and keratinization, and localized psoriasis vulgaris can frequently be cleared by daily applications for a period of 2 to 4 weeks. A short contact method of application causes little, if any, irritation or staining of normal skin, and is particularly useful for outpatient management. There is a risk of severe conjunctivitis if dithranol enters the eye.

Crude coal tar is also effective in the treatment of psoriasis. Some preparations additionally contain salicylic acid as a keratolytic. Good results are often obtained when daily applications or baths are combined with exposure to ultraviolet light or sunlight.

Emollients containing low concentrations of **salicylic acid** (1–2%) are a useful adjunct to treatment, particularly where there is thick scaling. A cream containing **urea** 10%, which has moisturizing, keratolytic and antimitotic properties, may prove more effective than an emollient.

Topical corticosteroids such as hydrocortisone or betamethasone are widely used in mild or moderate psoriasis. However, when extensive areas of the body surface are involved or when there is erythrodermic psoriasis, sufficient may be absorbed to cause adrenal suppression; also rebound often occurs after stopping treatment, resulting in a more unstable form of psoriasis.

Coal tar
Solution (cutaneous solution), coal tar 5%

Uses: chronic psoriasis, either alone or in combination with exposure to ultraviolet light

Contraindications: inflamed, broken or infected skin

Precautions: skin protection possibly required to reduce photosensitivity reactions

Administration: Apply 1–4 times daily, preferably starting with lower strength preparation

Coal tar bath, use 100 ml in bath of tepid water and soak for 10–20 minutes; use once daily to once every 3 days for at least 10 baths; often alternated with ultraviolet (UVB) rays, allowing at least 24 hours between exposure and treatment with coal tar

Adverse effects: irritation, photosensitivity reactions; rarely hypersensitivity; skin, hair and fabrics discoloured

---

Dithranol
Ointment, dithranol 0.1–2%

Uses: moderately severe psoriasis

Contraindications: hypersensitivity; avoid use on face, acute eruptions, excessively inflamed areas

Precautions: irritant—avoid contact with eyes and healthy skin

Administration: Initiate under medical supervision: starting with 0.1%, carefully apply to lesions only, leave in contact for 30 minutes, then wash off thoroughly; repeat application daily, gradually increasing strength to 2% and contact time to 60 minutes at weekly intervals; wash hands thoroughly after use

Adverse effects: local irritation; discontinue use if excessive erythema or spread of lesions; conjunctivitis following contact with eyes; staining of skin, hair, and fabrics

ACTINIC KERATOSES. The lesions of actinic keratoses are distributed primarily over sun-exposed areas. Horny growths, which are often covered by light brown scales, are usually asymptomatic but can be disfiguring. They respond to light cautery and cryosurgery or topical application of **fluorouracil** over a three-week period. Simple emollients may be satisfactory for people with many lesions.

Fluorouracil
Cream, fluorouracil 5%

Uses: actinic keratoses; genital warts unresponsive to podophyllum resin; malignant disease (section 8.2)

Contraindications: haemorrhagic ulcerated tissue

Precautions: avoid mucous membranes and eyes; since UV light intensifies the inflammatory reaction, avoid prolonged exposure to sunlight

Administration: Apply thinly 1–2 times daily until marked inflammatory response occurs (usually 3–4 weeks); healing may require further 2 months after completion of treatment
NOTE. Avoid use of metal applicator

Adverse effects: local inflammatory and allergic reactions; rarely erythema multiforme; photosensitivity reactions during and for up to 2 months after treatment

---

Urea
Cream, urea 10%

Uses: hydrating agent and keratolytic for dry, scaling and itching skin conditions

Precautions: avoid application to face or broken skin; avoid contact with eyes

Administration: Apply twice daily, preferably to damp skin

Adverse effects: transient stinging and local irritation

WARTS. Warts most commonly affect the hands, feet (plantar warts, verrucas), and anogenital region (condylomata acuminata); all are caused by the human papilloma virus. They may regress spontaneously at any time within months or years of their first appearance; however, particularly in immunosuppressed patients, they may spread and be difficult to cure. Many common, plane and plantar warts can reasonably be left untreated, but painful or unsightly lesions generally respond to application of preparations containing **salicylic acid.** Where available, cryotherapy using liquid nitrogen applied with a cotton-tip or a spray is highly effective; however, freezing the skin can produce temporary or permanent depigmentation (particularly on dark skin), and should be used with caution.

Anogenital warts are usually transmitted by sexual contact; they should always be treated, although they frequently recur, because of the increased risk of cervical cancer. **Podophyllum resin,** a caustic antimitotic agent, may be applied to small external lesions. The risk of extensive local necrosis and of systemic toxicity exclude the use of podophyllum resin on larger surfaces. When available podophyllotoxin is a less toxic alternative. Where podophyllum is contraindicated or ineffective surgical removal, electrocautery, cryosurgery and laser therapy are possible options. Topical application of **fluoro-uracil** has been reported to be of value in resistant cases but the treatment is expensive and efficacy is still under investigation.

Podophyllum resin

An example of an application to treat warts. Various drugs can serve as alternatives

Solution (cutaneous solution), podophyllum resin 10–25%

Uses: external anogenital warts; plantar warts

Contraindications: pregnancy (Appendix 2); breastfeeding; children

Precautions: avoid use on large areas, mucous membranes; irritant to eyes; avoid contact with normal skin

Administration: Medical supervision required; apply carefully to warts, avoiding contact with normal tissue; rinse off after 1–4 hours; may be repeated at weekly intervals but no more than 4 times in all; only few warts to be treated at any one time

Adverse effects: systemic effects resulting from cutaneous absorption include nausea, vomiting, abdominal pain and diarrhoea; also transient leukopenia and thrombocytopenia; delayed neurotoxicity including visual and auditory hallucinations, delusions, disorientation, confusion and delirium following excessive application

---

Salicylic acid

Topical solution (cutaneous solution), salicylic acid 5%
Ointment, salicylic acid 1–6%

Uses: hyperkeratotic conditions

Contraindications: broken or inflamed skin; children under 2 years

Precautions: avoid contact with eyes, mouth, and mucous membranes; avoid application to large areas

Administration: Apply once daily, starting with lower strength preparations; gradually increase strength until satisfactory response obtained

Adverse effects: local irritation, dermatitis; salicylism on excessive application or treatment of large areas, particularly in children

---

13.6 Scabicides and pediculicides

SCABIES. Scabies is caused by a mite, *Sarcoptes scabiei,* that burrows into the skin. It is readily transmitted from person to person, therefore the entire household must be treated at the same time to prevent reinfection. It is not necessary to take a bath before treatment with an acaricide, but all clothing and bedding should be washed to prevent reinfection.

Benzyl benzoate is an inexpensive scabicide. It must be applied to all skin surfaces, from the scalp to the soles of the feet, avoiding contact with the eyes; it is too irritant for use on children. **Permethrin** is less irritant and more effective than benzyl benzoate, but also more expensive; it may be used on children. Young infants can be treated with a cream containing precipitated **sulfur** 6–10% applied once daily for one week.

PEDICULOSIS. Pediculosis of the head and body is caused by *Pediculus humanus capitis* and *Pediculus humanus corporis* respectively; pubic lice (crab lice) infestations are caused by *Pthirus pubis*, which may also affect the eye lashes and brows. All are transmitted by person to person contact, and may also contaminate clothing and bedding. All members of the affected household (and sexual contacts) must be treated at the same time, and clothing and bedding should be washed or exposed to the air; in head lice infestations, hair brushes and combs should also be disinfected.

Head and body lice are readily treated with **permethrin**; **malathion** is effective against pubic lice. **Benzyl benzoate** may be used for all lice infestations.

Benzyl benzoate

Benzyl benzoate is a representative parasiticide. Various drugs can serve as alternatives

Lotion (cutaneous suspension), benzyl benzoate 25%

Uses: scabies; head, body and pubic lice

Precautions: do not use on inflamed or broken skin; avoid contact with eyes and mucous membranes; not recommended for children; breastfeeding (withhold during treatment)

Administration: Scabies, ADULT, apply over whole body, repeat without bathing on following day, then wash off after further 24 hours

Pediculosis, ADULT, apply to affected area and wash off 24 hours later; further applications possibly needed after 7 and 14 days

Adverse effects: local irritation, particularly in children

Permethrin

Cream, permethrin 5%
Lotion (cutaneous suspension), permethrin 1%

Uses: scabies; head and body lice

Precautions: do not use on inflamed or broken skin; avoid contact with eyes; breastfeeding (withhold during treatment)

Administration: Scabies and body lice, apply cream over whole body, and wash off after 8–12 hours

Head lice, apply lotion to clean damp hair, and rinse off after 10 minutes

Adverse effects: local irritation; rarely rashes and oedema

13.7 Ultraviolet blocking agents

Exposure of skin to sunlight is beneficial in moderation since ultraviolet light is vital for the synthesis of vitamin D. Excessive exposure is hazardous, however, particularly in light-skinned persons who tan poorly, and in patients with pathological or drug-induced photosensitivity. Photodamage is first evident as acute sunburn and, in the longer term, as premature ageing of the skin. Excessive exposure to sunlight predisposes to the development of malignant and pre-malignant skin lesions including actinic keratoses, squamous cell carcinoma, basal cell carcinoma and malignant melanoma, and also exacerbates cutaneous porphyrias, systemic lupus erythematosus, rosacea, and possible herpes labialis.

The best protection is to reduce exposure and thereby avoid sunburn either by the use of protective clothing or, when this is not practicable, by regular use of sunscreen products with a sun protection factor (SPF) rating of at least 15.

The major categories of chemical sunscreens include cinnamates, which are UVB absorbers, and dibenzoylmethanes, which are UVA absorbers. Physical sunscreens, such as titanium dioxide, are opaque and reflect ultraviolet light. Many sunscreen products combine sunscreens from different groups in order to widen the range of protection. An example of a broad-spectrum topical sun protection product which protects from both UVA and UVB contains octyl methoxycinnamate (2-ethylhexyl-p-methoxycinnamate) 3%, avobenzone (butyl-methoxydibenzoylmethane) 2%, and titanium dioxide 2%, formulated in an acrylate polymer or an oily basis.

Section 14: Diagnostics

14.1   Ophthalmic drugs

For general information on the use of eye drops, see section 21.

Fluorescein sodium is used in ocular diagnostic procedures and for locating damaged areas of the cornea due to injury or disease.

Tropicamide is a short-acting relatively weak mydriatic that dilates the pupil and paralyses the ciliary muscle. It facilitates the examination of the fundus of the eye.

Fluorescein sodium
Eye drops, solution, fluorescein sodium 1%

Uses: detection of lesions and foreign bodies in the eye

Contraindications: avoid use with soft contact lenses

Precautions: SKILLED TASKS. Transient blurring of vision—advise patient not to operate machinery or drive until vision is clear

Dosage:
Detection of lesions and foreign bodies in eye, *by ocular instillation,* ADULT and CHILD instil sufficient solution dropwise to stain damaged area

---

Tropicamide
Tropicamide is a representative mydriatic. Various drugs can serve as alternatives

Eye drops, solution, tropicamide 0.5%

Uses: dilatation of the pupil to examine the fundus

Precautions: patients aged over 60 years and hypermetropic (long-sighted)—may precipitate acute angle-closure glaucoma; darkly pigmented iris, more resistant to pupillary dilatation—exercise caution to avoid overdosage
SKILLED TASKS. Avoid operating machinery or driving for 1–2 hours after mydriasis

Dosage:
Dilatation of pupil to examine the fundus, *by ocular instillation,* ADULT and CHILD 1 or 2 drops, 15–20 minutes before examination of eye

Adverse effects: transient stinging and raised intraocular pressure; on prolonged administration—local irritation, hyperaemia, oedema and conjunctivitis

14.2   Radiocontrast media

Radiographic contrast media are needed for delineating soft tissue structures such as blood vessels, stomach, bowel loops and body cavities not otherwise visualized by standard X-ray examination. The contrast media in this group containing heavy atoms (metal or iodine) absorb a significantly different amount of X-rays than the surrounding soft tissue, thereby making the examined structures visible on radiographs.

Barium sulfate is a metal salt which is used to delineate the gastrointestinal tract. It is not absorbed by the body and does not interfere with stomach or bowel secretion or produce misleading radiographic artefacts. Barium sulfate may be used in either single or double contrast techniques or computer-assisted axial tomography. For double contrast examination gas can be introduced into the gastrointestinal tract by using suspensions of barium sulfate containing carbon dioxide or by using separate gas producing preparations. Air administered by a gastrointestinal tube can be used as an alternative to carbon dioxide to achieve a double contrast effect.

Diatrizoates (meglumine diatrizoate and sodium diatrizoate) are iodinated ionic monomeric organic compounds. Both salts have been used alone in diagnostic radiography but a mixture of both is often preferred to minimize adverse effects and to improve the quality of the examination. Diatrizoates are mainly used for urography and for computer-assisted axial tomography examinations. Owing to their high osmolality and the resulting hypertonic solutions, they are associated with a high incidence of adverse effects. Radiodensity depends on iodine concentration, and osmolality depends on number of particles in a given weight of solvent. The osmolality for a given radiodensity can be reduced by using an ionic dimeric medium such as **meglumine iotroxate** which contains twice the number of iodine atoms in a molecule or by using a non-ionic medium such as **iohexol** that does not dissociate into cation and anion. Low osmolality media such as iohexol are associated with a reduction in some adverse effects (see below), but they are generally more expensive. **Iopanoic acid** is an oral iodinated ionic monomeric organic compound. It is absorbed from the gastrointestinal tract, excreted into the bile and concentrated in the gallbladder thus making it ideal for cholecystography. **Propyliodone** is an iodinated organic compound which is used for the examination of the bronchial tract. **Meglumine iotroxate** is excreted into the bile after intravenous administration and used for cholangiography.

HYPERSENSITIVITY. Anaphylactoid reactions to iodinated radiocontrast media are more common with high osmolality compounds. Patients with a history of asthma or allergy, drug hypersensitivity, adrenal suppression, heart disease, previous reaction to contrast media, and those receiving beta-adrenoceptor antagonists (beta-blockers) or interleukin-2 are at increased risk. Non-ionic media are preferred for these patients and beta-blockers should be discontinued if possible.

Barium sulfate
Oral suspension (or Rectal suspension), barium sulfate 30 to 200% w/v

Uses: radiographic examination of the gastrointestinal tract (see notes above)

Contraindications: intestinal obstruction or conditions predisposing to obstruction such as pyloric stenosis; intestinal perforation or conditions with risk of perforation, such as acute ulcerative colitis, diverticulitis, or after rectal or colonic biopsy, sigmoidoscopy or radiotherapy

---

Precautions: adequate hydration after procedure to prevent severe constipation

Dosage:

Radiographic examination of gastrointestinal tract, ADULT and CHILD, route and dosage depend on procedure and preparation used (consult manufacturer's literature)

ADMINISTRATION. Only by specialist radiographers, according to manufacturer's directions

Adverse effects: constipation or diarrhoea, abdominal cramps and bleeding; perforation of bowel resulting in peritonitis, adhesions, granulomas and high mortality rate; electrocardiographical changes—may occur with rectal administration; pneumonitis or granuloma formation—following accidental aspiration into lungs

---

Diatrizoates

Diatrizoates are representative iodinated ionic monomeric contrast media. Various media can serve as alternatives

Injection (Solution for injection), iodine (as sodium and/or meglumine diatrizoate) 140–420 mg/ml, 20-ml ampoules

Uses: urography, venography, operative cholangiography, splenoportography, arthrography, diskography

Contraindications: hypersensitivity to iodine-containing compounds

Precautions: history of allergy, atopy or asthma; severe hepatic impairment; renal impairment (Appendix 4); dehydration—correct fluid and electrolyte balance before administration; multiple myeloma (risk if dehydrated, may precipitate fatal renal failure); cardiac disease, hypertension, phaeochromocytoma, sickle-cell disease, hyperthyroidism, elderly, debilitated or children—increased risk of adverse effects; pregnancy; breastfeeding; may interfere with thyroid-function tests; biguanides (withdraw 48 hours before administration; restart when renal function stabilized); **important:** because of risk of hypersensitivity reactions, adequate resuscitation facilities must be immediately available when radiographic procedures are carried out

Dosage:

Diagnostic radiography, ADULT and CHILD, route and dosage depend on procedure and preparation used (consult manufacturer's literature)

ADMINISTRATION. Only by specialist radiographers, according to manufacturer's directions

Adverse effects: nausea, vomiting, metallic taste, flushing, sensations of heat, weakness, dizziness, headache, coughing, rhinitis, sweating, sneezing, lacrimation, visual disturbances, pruritus, salivary gland enlargement, pallor, cardiac disorders, haemodynamic disturbances and hypotension; rarely, convulsions, paralysis, coma, rigors, arrhythmias, pulmonary oedema, circulatory failure and cardiac arrest; occasionally anaphylactoid or hypersensitivity reactions; hyperthyroidism; pain on injection; extravasation may result in tissue damage, thrombophlebitis, thrombosis, venospasm and embolism

---

Iohexol

Iohexol is a representative iodinated non-ionic contrast medium. Various media can serve as alternatives

Injection (Solution for injection), iodine (as iohexol) 140–350 mg/ml, 5-ml, 10-ml, and 20-ml ampoules

Uses: urography, venography, angiography, ventriculography, operative cholangiography, splenoportography, arthrography, diskography; computer-assisted axial tomography

Contraindications: hypersensitivity to iodine-containing compounds

Precautions: history of allergy, atopy or asthma; severe hepatic impairment; renal impairment (Appendix 4); dehydration—correct fluid and electrolyte balance before administration; multiple myeloma (risk if dehydrated, may precipitate fatal renal failure); cardiac disease, hypertension, phaeochromocytoma, sickle-cell disease, hyperthyroidism, elderly, debilitated or children—increased risk of adverse effects; pregnancy; breastfeeding; may interfere with thyroid-function tests; biguanides (withdraw 48 hours before administration; restart when renal function stabilized; **important:** because of risk of hypersensitivity reactions, adequate resuscitation facilities must be immediately available when radiographic procedures are carried out

Dosage:

Diagnostic radiography, ADULT and CHILD, route and dosage depend on procedure and preparation used (consult manufacturer's literature)

ADMINISTRATION. Only by specialist radiographers, according to manufacturer's directions

Adverse effects: (see also notes above); nausea, vomiting, metallic taste, flushing, sensations of heat, weakness, dizziness, headache, coughing, rhinitis, sweating, sneezing, lacrimation, visual disturbances, pruritus, salivary gland enlargement, pallor, cardiac disorders, haemodynamic disturbances and hypotension; rarely, convulsions, paralysis, coma, rigors, arrhythmias, pulmonary oedema, circulatory failure and cardiac arrest; occasionally anaphylactoid or hypersensitivity reactions; hyperthyroidism; pain on injection; extravasation may result in tissue damage, thrombophlebitis, thrombosis, venospasm and embolism

---

Iopanoic acid

Iopanoic acid is a representative iodinated ionic monomeric contrast medium. Various media can serve as alternatives

Tablets, iopanoic acid 500 mg

Uses: examination of the gallbladder and biliary tract

Contraindications: severe renal disease and hepatic disease (Appendices 4 and 5); jaundice caused by biliary-tract obstruction; impaired absorption due to acute gastrointestinal disorders

Precautions: hypersensitivity to iodine-containing compounds or other contrast media; severe hyperthyroidism, hyperuricaemia or cholangitis; may interfere with thyroid-function tests; **important:** because of risk of hypersensitivity reactions, adequate resuscitation facilities must be immediately available when radiographic procedures are carried out

Dosage:

Examination of gallbladder and biliary tract, *by mouth*, ADULT 3 g with plenty of water 10–14 hours before examination; if examination needs to be repeated, a further 3 g on the same day; alternatively, repeat examination carried out after 5–7 days with single 6-g dose (maximum dose; 6 g over 24 hours; avoid doses over 3 g in renal impairment)

ADMINISTRATION. Only by specialist radiographers, according to manufacturer's directions

Adverse effects: nausea and vomiting, abdominal pain and diarrhoea; mild stinging on micturition, rashes and flushing; acute renal failure, thrombocytopenia and hypersensitivity reactions reported; also uricosuric and anticholinesterase effects

---

Meglumine iotroxate

Meglumine iotroxate is a representative iodinated ionic dimeric contrast medium. Various media can serve as alternatives. It is a complementary drug

Injection (Solution for injection), iodine 50 mg/ml (as meglumine iotroxate 105 mg/ml), 100-ml bottle

Uses: examination of the gallbladder and biliary tract

Contraindications: hypersensitivity to iodine-containing compounds

Precautions: history of allergy, atopy or asthma; severe hepatic impairment; renal impairment (Appendix 4); dehydration—correct fluid and electrolyte balance before administration; multiple myeloma (risk if dehydrated, may precipitate fatal renal failure); cardiac disease, hypertension, phaeochromocytoma, sickle-cell disease, hyperthyroidism, elderly, debilitated or children—increased risk of adverse effects; pregnancy; breastfeeding; may interfere with thyroid-function tests; biguanides (withdraw 48 hours before administration; restart when renal function stabilized; **important:** because of risk of hypersensitivity reactions, adequate resuscitation facilities must be immediately available when radiographic procedures are carried out

---

Dosage:

Examination of gallbladder and biliary tract, *by intravenous injection*, ADULT 100 ml of meglumine iotroxate 10.5% solution over at least 15 minutes (consult manufacturer's literature)

ADMINISTRATION. Only by specialist radiographers, according to manufacturer's directions

Adverse effects: nausea, vomiting, metallic taste, flushing, sensations of heat, weakness, dizziness, headache, cough, rhinitis, sweating, sneezing, lacrimation, visual disturbances, pruritus, salivary gland enlargement, pallor, cardiac disorders, haemodynamic disturbances and hypotension; rarely, convulsions, paralysis, coma, rigors, arrhythmias, pulmonary oedema, circulatory failure and cardiac arrest; occasionally anaphylactoid or hypersensitivity reactions; hyperthyroidism; pain on injection; extravasation may result in tissue damage, thrombophlebitis, thrombosis, venospasm and embolism

---

Propyliodone

Propyliodone is a representative iodinated organic contrast medium. Various drugs can serve as alternatives

Oily suspension, propyliodone 600 mg/ml, 20-ml ampoule

Uses: examination of the bronchial tree (use only if no other alternative available)

Contraindications: hypersensitivity to iodine-containing compounds; severe heart disease

Precautions: asthma, bronchiectasis, pulmonary emphysema or reduced pulmonary function; use of excessive volume or too rapid administration may result in lobar collapse; may interfere with thyroid-function tests; **important:** because of risk of hypersensitivity reactions, adequate resuscitation facilities must be immediately available when radiographic procedures are carried out

Dosage:

Examination of bronchial tree, *by instillation into the lungs*, ADULT dose (consult manufacturer's literature)

ADMINISTRATION. Only by specialist radiographers, according to manufacturer's directions

Adverse effects: pyrexia, malaise, arthralgia, cough; occasionally, dyspnoea, atelectasis, pneumonia; rarely, hypersensitivity reactions

Section 15:
Disinfectants and
Antiseptics

15.1 Disinfectants and antiseptics

ANTISEPTICS. An antiseptic is a type of disinfectant, which destroys or inhibits growth of micro-organisms on living tissues without causing injurious effects when applied to surfaces of the body or to exposed tissues. Some antiseptics are applied to the unbroken skin or mucous membranes, to burns and to open wounds to prevent sepsis by removing or excluding microbes from these areas. Iodine has been modified for use as an antiseptic. The iodophore, **polyvidone-iodine**, is effective against bacteria, fungi, viruses, protozoa, cysts and spores and significantly reduces surgical wound infections. The solution of polyvidone-iodine releases iodine on contact with the skin. **Chlorhexidine** has a wide spectrum of bactericidal and bacteriostatic activity and is effective against both Gram-positive and Gram-negative bacteria although it is less effective against some species of *Pseudomonas* and *Proteus* and relatively inactive against mycobacteria. It is not active against bacterial spores. Chlorhexidine is incompatible with soaps and other anionic materials, such as bicarbonates, chlorides, and phosphates, forming salts of low solubility which may precipitate out of solution. **Ethanol** has bactericidal activity and is used to disinfect skin prior to injection, venepuncture or surgical procedures.

DISINFECTANTS. A disinfectant is a chemical agent, which destroys or inhibits growth of pathogenic micro-organisms in the non-sporing or vegetative state. Disinfectants do not necessarily kill all organisms but reduce them to a level, which does not harm health or the quality of perishable goods. Disinfectants are applied to inanimate objects and materials such as instruments and surfaces to control and prevent infection. They may also be used to disinfect skin and other tissues prior to surgery (see also Antiseptics, above).

Disinfection of water for purposes other than drinking can be either physical or chemical. Physical methods include boiling, filtration and ultraviolet irradiation. Chemical methods include the addition of **chlorine releasing compounds**, such as sodium hypochlorite solution, chloramine T powder, or sodium dichloroisocyanurate (NaDCC) powder or tablets.

Chlorine is a hazardous substance. It is highly corrosive in concentrated solution and splashes can cause burns and damage the eyes. Appropriate precautions must be taken when concentrated chlorine solutions or powders are handled.

The chlorinated phenolic compound, **chloroxylenol**, is effective against a wide range of Gram-positive bacteria. It is less effective against staphylococci and Gram-negative bacteria; it is often ineffective against *Pseudomonas* spp. and inactive against spores.

The aldehyde bactericidal disinfectant, **glutaral**, is strongly active against both Gram-positive and Gram-negative bacteria. It is active against the tuberculosis bacillus, fungi, such as *Candida albicans*, and viruses, such as HIV and hepatitis B. A 2% w/v aqueous alkaline (buffered to pH 8) glutaral solution can be used to sterilize heat-sensitive pre-cleansed instruments and other equipment.

Chlorhexidine gluconate

Chlorhexidine gluconate is a representative disinfectant and antiseptic. Various agents can serve as alternatives

Solution (Concentrate for solution), chlorhexidine gluconate 5%

Uses: antiseptic; disinfection of clean instruments

Precautions: instruments with cemented glass components (avoid preparations containing surface active agents); avoid contact with middle ear, eyes, brain and meninges; not for use in body cavities; alcoholic solutions not suitable before diathermy; syringes and needles treated with chlorhexidine (rinse thoroughly with sterile water or saline before use); inactivated by cork (use glass, plastic or rubber closures); alcohol based solutions are flammable

Administration: Antiseptic (pre-operative skin disinfection and hand washing), *use* 0.5% solution in alcohol (70%)

Antiseptic (wounds, burns and other skin damage), *apply* 0.05% aqueous solution

Disinfection of clean instruments, *immerse* for at least 30 minutes in 0.05% solution containing sodium nitrite 0.1% (to inhibit metal corrosion)

Emergency disinfection of clean instruments, *immerse* for 2 minutes in 0.5% solution in alcohol (70%)

Adverse effects: occasional skin sensitivity and irritation

Chlorine releasing compounds

Chlorine releasing compounds are representative disinfectants. Various agents can serve as alternatives

Powder for solution, chlorine releasing compound, 1 g available chlorine/litre (1000 parts per million; 0.1%)

Uses: disinfection of surfaces, equipment, water

Contraindications: avoid exposure of product to flame; activity diminished in presence of organic material and increasing pH (can cause release of toxic chlorine gas)

Administration: Surface disinfection (minor contamination), *apply* solutions containing 1000 parts per million

Instrument disinfection, *soak* in solution containing 1000 parts per million for a minimum of 15 minutes; to avoid corrosion do not soak for more than 30 minutes; rinse with sterile water

Adverse effects: irritation and burning sensation on skin

Chloroxylenol

Chloroxylenol is a representative disinfectant and antiseptic. Various agents can serve as alternatives

Solution (Concentrate for solution), chloroxylenol 5%

Uses: antiseptic; disinfection of instruments and surfaces

Precautions: aqueous solutions should be freshly prepared; appropriate measures required to prevent contamination during storage or dilution

Administration: Antiseptic (wounds and other skin damage), *apply* a 1 in 20 dilution of 5% concentrate in water

Disinfection of instruments, *use* a 1 in 20 dilution of 5% concentrate in alcohol (70%)

DILUTION AND ADMINISTRATION. According to manufacturer's directions

Adverse effects: skin sensitivity reported

Ethanol

Ethanol is a representative disinfectant. Various agents can serve as alternatives

Cutaneous solution, ethanol 70%

Uses: disinfection of skin prior to injection, venepuncture or surgical procedures

Precautions: flammable; avoid broken skin; patients have suffered severe burns when diathermy has been preceded by application of alcoholic skin disinfectants

Administration: Disinfection of skin, *apply* undiluted solution

Adverse effects: skin dryness and irritation with frequent application

---

Glutaral

Solution, glutaral 2% aqueous alkaline (pH 8) solution

Uses: disinfection and sterilization of instruments and surfaces

Precautions: minimize occupational exposure by adequate skin protection and measures to avoid inhalation of vapour

Administration: Disinfection of clean instruments, *immerse* in undiluted solution for 10–20 minutes; up to 2 hours may be required for certain instruments (for example bronchoscopes with possible mycobacterial contamination); rinse with sterile water or alcohol after disinfection

Sterilization of clean instruments, *immerse* in undiluted solution for up to 10 hours; rinse with sterile water or alcohol after disinfection

Adverse effects: (occupational exposure) nausea, headache, airway obstruction, asthma, rhinitis, eye irritation and dermatitis and skin discoloration

---

Polyvidone-iodine

Polyvidone-iodine is a representative antiseptic. Various agents can serve as alternatives

Cutaneous solution, polyvidone-iodine 10%

Uses: antiseptic; skin disinfection

Contraindications: avoid regular or prolonged use in patients with thyroid disorders or those taking lithium; avoid regular use in neonates; avoid in very low birthweight infants

---

Precautions: pregnancy (Appendix 2); breastfeeding (Appendix 3); renal impairment (Appendix 4)

LARGE OPEN WOUNDS. The application of polyvidone-iodine to large wounds or severe burns may produce systemic adverse effects such as metabolic acidosis, hypernatraemia, and impairment of renal function

Administration: Pre- and post-operative skin disinfection, ADULT and CHILD *apply* undiluted (see also Contraindications above)

Antiseptic (minor wounds and burns), ADULT and CHILD *apply* twice daily (see also Contraindications above)

Adverse effects: irritation of skin and mucous membranes; may interfere with thyroid function tests; systemic effects (see under Precautions)

Section 16: Diuretics

Diuretics increase urinary excretion of water and electrolytes and are used to relieve oedema associated with heart failure, nephrotic syndrome or hepatic cirrhosis. Some diuretics are used at lower doses to reduce raised blood pressure. Osmotic diuretics are mainly used to treat cerebral oedema, and also to lower raised intraocular pressure.

Most diuretics increase urine volume by inhibiting the reabsorption of sodium and chloride ions in the renal tubule; they also modify renal handling of potassium, calcium, magnesium and urate. Osmotic diuretics act differently; they cause an increase in urine volume by an osmotic effect.

Although **loop diuretics** are the most potent their duration of action is relatively short, whilst **thiazide diuretics** are moderately potent but produce diuresis for a longer period. **Potassium-sparing diuretics** are relatively weak. Carbonic anhydrase inhibitors are weak diuretics which are rarely used for their diuretic effect and are principally used to lower intraocular pressure in glaucoma (section 21.4.4).

ELECTROLYTE IMBALANCE. The adverse effects of diuretic therapy are mainly due to the fluid and electrolyte imbalance induced by the drugs. *Hyponatraemia* is an adverse effect of all diuretics. The risk of *hypokalaemia*, which may occur with both thiazide and loop diuretics, depends more on the duration of action than on potency and is thus greater with thiazides than with loop diuretics (when given in equipotent doses). Potassium-sparing diuretics can cause *hyperkalaemia*. Other electrolyte disturbances include *hypercalcaemia* (thiazides), *hypocalcaemia* (loop diuretics) and *hypomagnesaemia* (thiazide and loop diuretics).

Symptoms of fluid and electrolyte imbalance include dry mouth, thirst, gastrointestinal disturbances (including nausea, vomiting), weakness, lethargy, drowsiness, restlessness, seizures, confusion, headache, muscle pains or cramps, hypotension (including postural hypotension), oliguria, arrhythmias.

ELDERLY. The elderly are more susceptible to electrolyte imbalance than younger patients. Treatment should begin with a lower initial dose of the diuretic (commonly about 50% of the adult dose) and then adjusted carefully according to renal function, plasma electrolytes and diuretic response.

16.1 Thiazide diuretics

Thiazide diuretics, such as **hydrochlorothiazide**, are moderately potent and act by inhibiting sodium and chloride reabsorption at the beginning of the distal convoluted tubule. They produce diuresis within 1–2 hours of oral administration and most have a duration of action of 12–24 hours.

Thiazide diuretics are used in the management of oedema associated with mild to moderate congestive heart failure, renal dysfunction or hepatic disease; however, thiazides are not effective in patients with poor renal function (creatinine clearance of less than 30 ml per minute). In severe fluid retention a loop diuretic may be necessary.

In hypertension, a thiazide diuretic is used at a low dose to produce a maximal or near maximal blood-pressure lowering effect with very little biochemical disturbance; the maximum therapeutic effect may not be seen for several weeks. Higher doses should not be used because they do not necessarily increase the hypotensive response but may cause marked changes in plasma potassium, magnesium, uric acid, glucose and lipids. A thiazide diuretic may also be used in combination with another antihypertensive such as a beta-blocker (section 12.3).

Urinary excretion of calcium is reduced by thiazide diuretics and this property is occasionally utilized in the treatment of idiopathic hypercalciuria in patients with calcium-containing calculi. Paradoxically, thiazide diuretics are used in the treatment of diabetes insipidus, since in this disease they reduce urine volume.

Thiazide diuretics, especially in high doses, produce a marked increase in potassium excretion which may cause hypokal-aemia; this is dangerous in patients with severe coronary artery disease and those being treated with cardiac glycosides. In hepatic failure hypokalaemia can precipitate encephalopathy, particularly in alcoholic cirrhosis. Potassium-sparing diuretics are used as a more effective alternative to potassium supple-ments for prevention of hypokalaemia induced by thiazide diuretics; however supplementation with potassium in any form is seldom necessary with the smaller doses of diuretics used to treat hypertension.

Hydrochlorothiazide

An example of a thiazide diuretic. Various drugs can serve as alternatives
Tablets, hydrochlorothiazide, 25 mg, 50 mg

Uses: oedema; diabetes insipidus; hypertension (see also section 12.3); heart failure (section 12.4)

Contraindications: severe kidney or severe hepatic impair-ment; hyponatraemia, hypercalcaemia, refractory hypokal-aemia, symptomatic hyperuricaemia; Addison disease

Precautions: renal and hepatic impairment (Appendices 4 and 5); pregnancy and breastfeeding (Appendices 2 and 3); elderly (reduce dose); may cause hypokalaemia; may aggravate diabetes mellitus and gout; may exacerbate systemic lupus erythematosus; porphyria; **interactions:** see Appendix 1

Dosage:

Hypertension, *by mouth,* ADULT 12.5–25 mg daily; ELDERLY initially 12.5 mg daily

Oedema, *by mouth,* ADULT initially 25 mg daily on rising, increasing to 50 mg daily if necessary; ELDERLY initially 12.5 mg daily

Severe oedema in patients unable to tolerate loop diuretics, *by mouth*, ADULT up to 100 mg *either* daily *or* on alternate days (maximum 100 mg daily)

Nephrogenic diabetes insipidus, *by mouth*, ADULT initially up to 100 mg daily

Adverse effects: hypokalaemia, hypomagnesaemia, hyponatraemia, hypochloraemic alkalosis (for symptoms of fluid and electrolyte imbalance see introductory notes); hypercalcaemia; hyperglycaemia; hyperuricaemia, gout; rash, photosensitivity; altered plasma lipid concentration; rarely impotence (reversible), blood disorders (including neutropenia, thrombocytopenia); pancreatitis, intrahepatic cholestasis and hypersensitivity reactions (including pneumonitis, pulmonary oedema, severe skin reactions) also reported; acute renal failure

16.2 Loop diuretics

Loop diuretics, or high-ceiling diuretics, such as **furosemide**, are the most potent and rapidly produce an intense dose-dependent diuresis of relatively short duration. Oral furosemide produces diuresis within 30–60 minutes of administration, with the maximum diuretic effect in 1–2 hours. The diuretic action lasts for 4–6 hours. Intravenous furosemide produces diuresis within 5 minutes, with the maximum diuretic effect in 20–60 minutes and diuresis complete within 2 hours.

Loop diuretics inhibit reabsorption from the ascending loop of Henlé in the renal tubule and are useful, particularly in situations where rapid and effective diuresis is needed such as reduction of acute pulmonary oedema due to left ventricular failure . They are also used to treat oedema associated with renal and hepatic disorders and are used in high doses in the management of oliguria due to chronic renal insufficiency. Loop diuretics may be effective in patients unresponsive to thiazide diuretics.

Because of their shorter duration of action, the risk of hypokalaemia may be less with loop diuretics than with thiazide diuretics; if required, potassium-sparing diuretics may be used for prevention of hypokalaemia. Loop diuretics may cause hypovolaemia and excessive use can produce severe dehydration with the possibility of circulatory collapse. Furosemide may cause hyperuricaemia and precipitate attacks of gout. Rapid high-dose injection or infusion of furosemide may cause tinnitus and even permanent deafness.

Furosemide

An example of a loop diuretic. Various drugs can serve as alternatives
Tablets, furosemide 40 mg
Injection, furosemide 10 mg/ml, 2-ml ampoule

Uses: oedema; oliguria due to renal failure

Contraindications: renal failure with anuria; precomatose states associated with liver cirrhosis

Precautions: monitor electrolytes particularly potassium and sodium; elderly (reduce dose); pregnancy and breastfeeding (Appendices 2 and 3); correct hypovolaemia before using in oliguria; aggravates diabetes mellitus and gout; renal and hepatic impairment (Appendices 4 and 5); prostatic enlargement; porphyria; **interactions:** see Appendix 1

Dosage:

Oedema, *by mouth,* ADULT initially 40 mg daily on rising; maintenance, 20 mg daily or 40 mg on alternate days; may be increased to 80 mg daily in resistant oedema; CHILD 1–3 mg/kg body weight daily (maximum 40 mg daily)

Acute pulmonary oedema, *by slow intravenous injection,* ADULT 20–50 mg, if necessary increase by 20-mg steps every 2 hours; if effective single dose is more than 50 mg, consider using *slow intravenous infusion* at a rate not exceeding 4 mg/ minute; CHILD 0.5–1.5 mg/kg body weight daily (maximum 20 mg daily)

Oliguria (glomerular filtration rate less than 20 ml/minute), *by slow intravenous infusion* at a rate not exceeding 4 mg/minute, ADULT initially 250 mg over 1 hour; if urine output not satisfactory during hour after first dose, infuse 500 mg over 2 hours then, if no satisfactory response during hour after second dose, infuse 1 g over 4 hours; if no response after third dose, dialysis probably necessary

NOTE. Dose to be diluted in suitable amount of infusion fluid, depending on hydration of patient

Adverse effects: hypokalaemia, hypomagnesaemia, hyponatraemia, hypochloraemic alkalosis (for symptoms of fluid and electrolyte imbalance, see introductory notes), increased calcium excretion, hypovolaemia, hyperglycaemia (but less often than with thiazide diuretics); temporary increase in plasma cholesterol and triglyceride concentration; less commonly hyperuricaemia and gout; rarely rash, photosensitivity, bone marrow depression (withdraw treatment), pancreatitis (with large parenteral doses), tinnitus and deafness (with rapid administration of large parenteral doses and in renal impairment; deafness may be permanent if other ototoxic drugs taken)

16.3 Potassium-sparing diuretics

Potassium-sparing diuretics include **amiloride** and **spironolactone**; they are weak diuretics and reduce potassium excretion and increase sodium excretion in the distal tubule. Amiloride acts about 2 hours after oral administration, reaching a peak in 6–10 hours and persisting for about 24 hours. Spironolactone, which acts by antagonising aldosterone, has a relatively slow onset of action requiring 2–3 days to achieve maximum diuretic effect, and a similar period of 2–3 days for diuresis to cease after discontinuation of treatment.

Amiloride may be used alone, but its principal use is in combination with a thiazide or a loop diuretic to conserve potassium during treatment of congestive heart failure or hepatic cirrhosis with ascites.

Spironolactone is used in the treatment of refractory oedema due to heart failure, hepatic cirrhosis (with or without ascites), nephrotic syndrome and ascites associated with malignancy. It is frequently given with a thiazide or a loop diuretic, helping to conserve potassium in those at risk from hypokalaemia. A low dose of spironolactone is beneficial in severe heart failure in patients who are already taking an ACE inhibitor and a diuretic. Spironolactone is used in the diagnosis and treatment of primary hyperaldosteronism; presumptive evidence for diagnosis is provided by correction of hypokalaemia and of hypertension.

The most dangerous adverse effect of potassium-sparing diuretics, such as amiloride or spironolactone, is hyperkalaemia, which can be life-threatening. These diuretics are thus best avoided or used very carefully in patients who have or may develop hyperkalaemia, such as those with renal failure, patients receiving other potassium-sparing diuretics and patients taking ACE inhibitors or potassium supplements.

Amiloride hydrochloride

An example of a potassium-sparing diuretic. Various drugs can serve as alternatives

Tablets, amiloride hydrochloride 5 mg

Uses: oedema associated with heart failure or hepatic cirrhosis (with ascites), usually with thiazide or loop diuretic

Contraindications: hyperkalaemia; renal failure

Precautions: monitor electrolytes, particularly potassium; renal impairment (Appendix 4); diabetes mellitus; elderly (reduce dose); pregnancy and breastfeeding (Appendices 2 and 3); **interactions:** see Appendix 1

Dosage:

Used alone, *by mouth,* initially 10 mg daily in 1 or 2 divided doses, adjusted according to response (maximum 20 mg daily)

Combined with a thiazide or a loop diuretic, *by mouth*, initially 5 mg daily, increasing to 10 mg if necessary (maximum 20 mg daily)

Adverse effects: hyperkalaemia, hyponatreamia (for symptoms of fluid and electrolyte imbalance see introductory notes), diarrhoea, constipation, anorexia; paraesthesia, dizziness, minor psychiatric or visual disturbances; rash, pruritus; rise in blood urea nitrogen

---

Spironolactone

Tablets, spironolactone, 25 mg

Uses: refractory oedema in congestive heart failure; adjunct to ACE inhibitor and diuretic in severe congestive heart failure; nephrotic syndrome; hepatic cirrhosis with ascites and oedema; ascites associated with malignancy; primary hyperaldosteronism

Contraindications: pregnancy (Appendix 2); breastfeeding; hyperkalaemia; hyponatraemia; severe renal impairment; Addison disease

Precautions: monitor blood urea nitrogen and plasma electrolytes (discontinue if hyperkalaemic); elderly (reduce dose); diabetes mellitus; renal impairment (Appendix 4); hepatic impairment; porphyria; high doses carcinogenic in *rodents*; **interactions:** see Appendix 1

Dosage:

Oedema, *by mouth*, ADULT 100–200 mg daily, increased if necessary to 400 mg daily in resistant oedema; usual maintenance dose 75–200 mg daily; CHILD initially 3 mg/kg body weight daily in divided doses

Primary hyperaldosteronism, *by mouth*, ADULT, diagnosis, 400 mg daily for 3–4 weeks (see notes above); preoperative management, 100–400 mg daily; if not suitable for surgery, lowest effective dose for long-term maintenance

Adjunct in severe heart failure, *by mouth*, ADULT usually 25 mg daily

Adverse effects: hyperkalaemia, hyponatraemia, hyperchloraemic acidosis, dehydration (for symptoms of fluid and electrolyte imbalance see introductory notes); transient increase in blood urea nitrogen; diarrhoea; gynaecomastia, menstrual irregularities; impotence, hirsutism, deepening of voice; rash, ataxia, fever, hepatotoxicity

16.4 Osmotic diuretics

Osmotic diuretics, such as **mannitol**, are administered in sufficiently large doses to raise the osmolarity of plasma and renal tubular fluid. With adequate rehydration, mannitol is mainly used to increase urine flow in patients with acute renal failure. Osmotic diuretics are used to reduce or prevent cerebral oedema, to reduce raised intraocular pressure or to treat disequilibrium syndrome. Mannitol is also used to control intraocular pressure during acute attacks of glaucoma. Reduction of cerebrospinal and intraocular fluid pressure occurs within 15 minutes of the start of infusion and lasts for 3–8 hours after the infusion has been discontinued; diuresis occurs after 1–3 hours.

Circulatory overload due to expansion of extracellular fluid is a serious adverse effect of mannitol; as a consequence, pulmonary oedema can be precipitated in patients with diminished cardiac reserve, and acute water intoxication may occur in patients with inadequate urine flow.

Mannitol

An example of an osmotic diuretic.
Solution for infusion, mannitol 10%, 20%

Uses: cerebral oedema; raised intraocular pressure (emergency treatment or before surgery)

Contraindications: pulmonary oedema; intracranial bleeding (except during craniotomy); severe congestive heart failure; metabolic oedema with abnormal capillary fragility; severe dehydration; renal failure (unless test dose produces diuresis)

Precautions: monitor fluid and electrolyte balance; monitor renal function

Dosage:

Test dose if patient oliguric or renal function is inadequate, *by intravenous infusion,* as a 20% solution, 200 mg/kg body weight infused over 3–5 minutes; repeat test dose if urine output less than 30–50 ml/hour; if response inadequate after second test dose, re-evaluate patient

Raised intracranial or intraocular pressure, *by intravenous infusion,* as a 20% solution infused over 30–60 minutes, 0.25–2 g/kg body weight

Cerebral oedema, *by intravenous infusion,* as a 20% solution infused rapidly, 1 g/kg body weight

Pharmaceutical precautions: solutions containing more than mannitol 15% may crystallize during storage, crystals must be redissolved by warming solution before use and solution must not be used if any crystals remain; intravenous administration sets must have a filter; mannitol should not be administered with whole blood or passed through the same transfusion set as blood

Adverse effects: fluid and electrolyte imbalance (for symptoms see introductory notes); circulatory overload, acidosis; pulmonary oedema particularly in diminished cardiac reserve; chills, fever, chest pain, dizziness, visual disturbances; hypertension; urticaria, hypersensitivity reactions; extravasation may cause oedema, skin necrosis, thrombophlebitis; rarely, acute renal failure (large doses)

Section 17:
Gastrointestinal drugs

17.1 Antacids and other antiulcer drugs

PEPTIC ULCER. Ulcer disease is caused by peptic ulceration that involves the stomach, duodenum, and lower oesophagus. General and inexpensive measures like introducing healthy life-style, stopping smoking and taking antacids should be promoted. The possibilitiy of malignant disease should be considered in all patients over the age of 40 years who are suspected of having an ulcer.

Gastric and duodenal ulcers are healed by 4–6 weeks treatment with H_2-receptor antagonists but there is a high rate of relapse (greater than 70% over 2 years). Prevention of relapse has been revolutionized by an understanding of the role of *Helicobacter pylori* which is causally associated with most peptic ulcers (except those related to NSAID use). Eradication of *H. pylori* reduces the relapse rate to about 10–15%. This is undoubtedly cost-effective compared to the alternatives of long-term maintenance therapy with low dose H_2-receptor antagonists or repeated treatment of recurrent ulcers. Verification of *H. pylori* is recommended, particularly with gastric ulcers, but not necessary before eradication treatment. Eradication regimens are based on a combination of acid-inhibiting drug and antibiotic. The best eradication regimen has not been established. Two eradication regimens are suggested based on their efficacy, simplicity and availability (only adult doses are described). Both regimens are associated with an 80–85% clearance rate. The decision on which regimen to use is a national decision, based on the resources of the country, which must take into account local antibiotic resistance, compliance problems, and the cost implications of various regimens.

TREATMENT:.
Regimen A:
bismuth subsalicylate 107.7 mg orally 6 hourly for 2 weeks
plus
metronidazole 200 mg orally 8 hourly + 400 mg at night for 2 weeks
plus either
tetracycline 500 mg orally 6 hourly for 2 weeks
or
amoxicillin 500 mg orally 6 hourly for 2 weeks

Regimen B:
omeprazole 40 mg orally 24 hourly for 1 week
plus
metronidazole 400 mg orally 8 hourly for 1 week
plus
amoxicillin 500 mg orally 8 hourly for 1 week

NSAID-ASSOCIATED ULCERS. Gastrointestinal bleeding and ulceration may occur with NSAID use. To avoid this, emphasis should be on stopping NSAID use but this is not always possible. NSAID-induced ulcers can be healed by H_2-receptor antagonists although a treatment period of up to 8 weeks may be necessary. In patients who must continue NSAID therapy, prophylaxis by concomitant use of high dose H_2-receptor antagonists is more cost effective if targeted to those at higher risk such as patients with a previous history of peptic ulceration. Omeprazole has been shown to be effective but is more expensive and misoprostol is also effective but is associated with more adverse effects and is expensive.

DYSPEPSIA AND GASTRO-OESOPHAGEAL REFLUX. Dyspepsia, typically as heartburn or food-related discomfort (indigestion) occurs with gastro-oesophageal reflux, gastric and duodenal ulceration and gastric cancer. In most patients dyspepsia is of uncertain origin and there is no identifiable systemic disease. A stepped care approach to treatment is appropriate, with attention first paid to life-style measures such as weight reduction, avoidance of alcohol, cessation of smoking, avoidance of aggravating food, such as fats and elevating the bed head. Antacids are useful and cheap in providing symptom relief in ulcer dyspepsia and gastro-oesophageal reflux and may be of benefit in non-ulcer dyspepsia. The next step is to use H_2-receptor antagonists for more severe symptoms and oesophageal ulceration not responding to the above measures. The extent of oesophageal healing depends on severity of disease and duration of therapy. Effective treatment is important in the presence of severe oesophageal ulceration to prevent longer term outcomes such as oesophageal stricture and carcinoma. Proton pump inhibitors are most effective in erosive ulcerative or stricturing disease.

ZOLLINGER-ELLISON SYNDROME. Management of Zollinger-Ellison syndrome requires high dose H_2-receptor antagonist treatment. The proton pump inhibitors are more effective particularly for cases resistant to other treatment but they are more expensive.

Aluminium hydroxide

Tablets, aluminium hydroxide 500 mg
Oral suspension, aluminium hydroxide 320 mg/5 ml

Uses: ulcer and non-ulcer dyspepsia; gastro-oesophageal reflux; hyperphosphataemia

Contraindications: hypophosphataemia; undiagnosed gastrointestinal or rectal bleeding; appendicitis; porphyria

Precautions: impaired renal function and renal dialysis (Appendix 4); hepatic impairment (Appendix 5); constipation; dehydration; fluid restriction; gastrointestinal disorders associated with decreased bowel motility or obstruction; **interactions:** Appendix 1

Dosage:

Dyspepsia, gastro-oesophageal reflux, *by mouth*, ADULT 1–2 tablets chewed 4 times daily and at bedtime *or* 5–10 ml suspension 4 times daily between meals and at bedtime; CHILD 6–12 years 5 ml up to three times daily

Hyperphosphataemia, *by mouth*, ADULT 2–10 g daily in divided
doses with meals

PATIENT ADVICE. Do not take other medicines within 2–4 hours of aluminium
hydroxide preparations. May be taken with water to reduce constipating
adverse effects

Adverse effects: constipation; intestinal obstruction (large
doses); hypophosphataemia with increased bone resorption,
hypercalciuria and risk of osteomalacia (patients on low
phosphate diet or prolonged therapy); hyperaluminaemia—
resulting in osteomalacia, encephalopathy, dementia, micro-
cytic anaemia (in chronic renal failure treated with aluminium
hydroxide as phosphate-binding agent)

Magnesium hydroxide

Oral suspension, magnesium hydroxide equivalent to magnesium oxide
550 mg/10 ml

Uses: ulcer and non-ulcer dyspepsia; gastro-oesophageal reflux

Contraindications: severe renal impairment

Precautions: renal impairment (Appendix 4); hepatic impairment (Appendix 5); **interactions:** Appendix 1

Dosage:

Dyspepsia, gastro-oesophageal reflux, *by mouth*, ADULT 5–10 ml
repeated according to patient's needs

Adverse effects: diarrhoea; in renal impairment—hypermagnesaemia resulting in loss of deep tendon reflexes and
respiratory depression, with other symptoms including
nausea, vomiting, flushing of skin, thirst, hypotension,
drowsiness, confusion, muscle weakness, bradycardia, coma
and cardiac arrest

Cimetidine

Cimetidine is a representative H_2-receptor antagonist. Various drugs can
serve as alternatives

Tablets, cimetidine 200 mg, 400 mg

Injection (Solution for injection), cimetidine 100 mg/ml, 2-ml ampoule

Uses: benign gastric and duodenal ulceration, stomal ulceration,
gastro-oesophageal reflux, Zollinger-Ellison syndrome, other
conditions where gastric acid reduction is beneficial

Precautions: hepatic impairment (Appendix 5); renal impairment (Appendix 4); pregnancy (Appendix 2); breastfeeding
(Appendix 3); middle aged or older patients and in those
whose symptoms change—may mask gastric cancer; preferably avoid intravenous injection (use intravenous infusion)
particularly in high dosage and in cardiovascular impairment
(risk of arrhythmias); **interactions:** Appendix 1

Dosage:

Benign gastric and duodenal ulceration, *by mouth*, ADULT
400 mg twice daily (with breakfast and at night) *or* 300 mg
with meals and at night *or* 800 mg at night for at least 4 weeks
(duodenal ulcer), 6 weeks (gastric ulcer) and for 8 weeks in
NSAID-associated ulceration; when necessary the dose may
be increased to 400 mg 4 times daily or rarely (as in stress

ulceration) to a maximum of 2.4 g daily in divided doses; INFANT under 1 year, 20 mg/kg daily in divided doses; CHILD over 1 year, 25–30 mg/kg daily in divided doses

Maintenance, *by mouth*, ADULT 400 mg at night *or* 400 mg morning and night

Gastro-oesophageal reflux, *by mouth*, ADULT 400 mg 4 times daily for 4–8 weeks

Zollinger-Ellison syndrome, *by mouth*, ADULT 400 mg 4 times daily (or occasionally more)

Prophylaxis of acid aspiration in obstetrics, *by mouth*, ADULT 400 mg at start of labour, then up to 400 mg every 4 hours, as required (up to maximum of 2.4 g daily)

Prophylaxis of acid aspiration in surgical procedures, *by mouth*, ADULT 400 mg 90–120 minutes before induction of general anaesthesia

Short-bowel syndrome, *by mouth*, ADULT 400 mg twice daily (with breakfast and at bedtime) adjusted according to response

To reduce degradation of pancreatic enzyme supplements, *by mouth*, ADULT 0.8–1.6 g daily in 4 divided doses according to response 1 to $1^1/_2$ hours before meals

NOTE. Cimetidine is usually given by mouth, but parenteral dosing may be substituted for all or part of the recommended oral dose, where oral dosing is impracticable or inappropriate (see also Precautions)

DILUTION AND ADMINISTRATION. According to manufacturer's directions

Adverse effects: gastrointestinal disturbances, altered liver function tests (rarely liver damage), headache, dizziness, rash and tiredness; reversible confusional states, particularly in the elderly and seriously ill; hypersensitivity reactions (fever, arthralgia); bradycardia and atrioventricular block; blood disorders including agranulocytosis and thrombocytopenia; rarely impotence and gynaecomastia

17.2 Antiemetic drugs

Metoclopramide has antiemetic properties and also stimulates upper gastrointestinal motility. Metoclopramide is effective against nausea and vomiting following surgery and chemotherapy and is also effective against radiation-induced nausea and vomiting. Combining metoclopramide with corticosteroids (such as dexamethasone) can improve its antiemetic effect in chemotherapy-induced nausea and vomiting. Metoclopramide may be useful in the management of gastro-oesophageal reflux and gastroparesis, as well as preoperatively in the prevention of aspiration syndromes. It is also used to facilitate intubation of the small bowel during radiographic examinations. Metoclopramide is **not** effective in the prevention or treatment of motion sickness.

Metoclopramide may cause acute dystonic reactions with facial and skeletal muscle spasms and oculogyric crises. These reactions are most common in the young (especially girls and young women) and the elderly; they occur shortly after the start of treatment and subside within 24 hours of drug withdrawal.

Promethazine is a phenothiazine that in addition to D2 dopaminergic blockade has pronounced histamine H_1 and muscarinic receptor blocking properties. It is effective in the prevention and treatment of vertigo and motion sickness. Promethazine may be useful in the prevention and treatment of postoperative and drug-induced nausea and vomiting. It has limited effect on chemotherapy-induced mild to moderate emesis.

Metoclopramide hydrochloride

Tablets, metoclopramide hydrochloride 10 mg
Injection (Solution for injection), metoclopramide hydrochloride 5 mg/ml, 2-ml ampoule

Uses: nausea and vomiting in gastrointestinal disorders and treatment with cytotoxics or radiotherapy; gastro-oesophageal reflux; gastroparesis; premedication and postoperatively; aid to gastrointestinal intubation; nausea and vomiting in migraine (section 7.1)

NOTE. In children (and in some countries, patients under 20 years) use restricted to severe intractable vomiting of known cause, vomiting of radiotherapy and chemotherapy, aid to gastrointestinal intubation, premedication

Contraindications: gastrointestinal obstruction, haemorrhage or perforation; convulsive disorders; phaeochromocytoma

Precautions: elderly, children and young adults; hepatic impairment (Appendix 5); renal impairment (Appendix 4); may mask underlying disorders such as cerebral irritation; avoid for 3–4 days after gastrointestinal surgery; pregnancy (Appendix 2); breastfeeding (Appendix 3); Parkinson disease; depression; porphyria; **interactions:** Appendix 1

Dosage:

Nausea and vomiting, gastro-oesophageal reflux, gastroparesis, *by mouth or by intramuscular injection or by slow intravenous injection*, ADULT 10 mg 3 times daily; YOUNG ADULT 15–19 years (under 60 kg) 5 mg 3 times daily; CHILD up to 1 year (up to 10 kg) 1 mg twice daily, 1–3 years (10–14 kg) 1 mg 2–3 times daily, 3–5 years (15–19 kg) 2 mg 2–3 times daily, 5–9 years (20–29 kg) 2.5 mg 3 times daily, 9–14 years (30 kg and over) 5 mg 3 times daily (usual maximum 500 micrograms/kg daily, particularly for children and young adults)

Premedication, *by slow intravenous injection*, ADULT 10 mg as a single dose

Aid to gastrointestinal intubation, *by mouth or by intramuscular injection or by slow intravenous injection*, ADULT 10–20 mg as a single dose 5–10 minutes before examination; YOUNG ADULT (15–19 years), 10 mg; CHILD under 3 years 1 mg, 3–5 years 2 mg, 5–9 years 2.5 mg, 9–14 years 5 mg

NOTE. High dose metoclopramide with cytotoxic chemotherapy, see section 8.2

Adverse effects: extrapyramidal symptoms (especially in children and young adults; see notes above); tardive dyskinesias on prolonged use; hyperprolactinaemia; drowsiness, restlessness, dizziness, headache, diarrhoea, depression, hypotension and hypertension reported; rarely, neuroleptic malignant syndrome; cardiac conduction abnormalities following intravenous administration

---

Promethazine hydrochloride

Promethazine is a representative phenothiazine antiemetic. Various drugs can serve as alternatives

Tablets, promethazine hydrochloride 10 mg, 25 mg

Elixir (Oral solution), promethazine hydrochloride 5 mg/5 ml

Injection (Solution for injection), promethazine hydrochloride 25 mg/ml, 2-ml ampoule

Uses: nausea, vomiting, labyrinthine disorders, motion sickness; premedication (section 1.3)

Contraindications: porphyria; children under 2 years

Precautions: prostatic hypertrophy; urinary retention; glaucoma; hepatic disease (Appendix 5); epilepsy; elderly and children (more susceptible to adverse effects); pregnancy (Appendix 2); breastfeeding (Appendix 3); **interactions:** Appendix 1

SKILLED TASKS. May impair ability to perform skilled tasks, for example operating machinery, driving

Dosage:

Nausea and vomiting (including postoperative), *by mouth or by intramuscular injection or by slow intravenous injection*, ADULT 12.5 to 25 mg, repeated at intervals of not less than 4 hours (usual maximum, 100 mg in 24 hours)

Motion sickness, prevention, *by mouth*, ADULT 20–25 mg at bedtime on night before travelling, repeated on following morning if necessary; CHILD 2–5 years, 5 mg at night and following morning, if necessary; 5–10 years, 10 mg at night and following morning, if necessary

DILUTION AND ADMINISTRATION. Intravenous injection, according to manfacture's directions

Adverse effects: drowsiness, dizziness, sedation (but paradoxical stimulation may occur, especially with high doses or in children and elderly); headache, psychomotor impairment; urinary retention, dry mouth, blurred vision, gastrointestinal disturbances; hypersensitivity reactions; rashes, photosensitivity reactions; jaundice; blood disorders; cardiovascular adverse effects—after injection; venous thrombosis at site of intravenous injection; pain on intramuscular injection

---

17.3 Antihaemorrhoidal drugs

Haemorrhoids are enlarged or varicose veins of the tissues at the anus or rectal outlet. They are the most frequent cause of rectal bleeding. Anal and perianal pruritus, soreness and excoriation occur commonly in patients suffering from haemorrhoids, fistulas and proctitis. Careful local toilet with attention to any minor faecal soiling, adjustment of the diet to avoid hard stools, the use of bulk-forming materials such as bran and a high residue diet are helpful.

Soothing preparations containing mild astringents such as bismuth subgallate, zinc oxide and hamamelis with lubricants, vasoconstrictors or mild antiseptics, in the form of topical ointments, creams and suppositories, are used to provide symptomatic relief. Local anaesthetics are included in some preparations. Corticosteroids may be combined in such preparations (but should only be used after exclusion of infection).

Local anaesthetic, astringent and anti-inflammatory drug
Ointment or suppository
Uses: short-term symptomatic treatment of hemorrhoids

17.4 Anti-inflammatory drugs

Ulcerative colitis and Crohn disease are inflammatory diseases of the intestinal tract.

ULCERATIVE COLITIS. Acute attacks of ulcerative colitis require treatment with local corticosteroids such as **hydrocortisone** in the form of suppositories or retention enemas. Because of the risk of intestinal perforation, rectal administration of hydrocortisone must be used with extreme caution in patients with severe ulcerative disease and should not be given to such patients without conducting a thorough proctological examination. More extensive disease requires oral corticosteroid treatment and severe extensive or fulminant disease needs hospital admission and intravenous corticosteroid administration. The aminosalicylate **sulfasalazine** is useful in the treatment of symptomatic disease. It also has value in the maintenance of remission in ulcerative colitis for which corticosteroid treatment is unsuitable because of adverse effects. The most common adverse effects of sulfasalazine are nausea and vomiting, abdominal discomfort, headache, fever, loss of appetite, and rashes. In resistant cases azathioprine 2 mg/kg daily (section 8.1) given under close supervision may be helpful. Laxatives are required to facilitate bowel movement when proctitis is present but a high-fibre diet and bulk-forming drugs are more useful in adjusting faecal consistency. General nutritional care and appropriate supplements are essential.

CROHN DISEASE. Treatment of Crohn disease of the colon is similar to that of ulcerative colitis. In small bowel disease **sulfasalazine** may have marginal benefit. Symptoms and inflammation associated with disease exacerbation are suppressed by oral corticosteroids such as prednisolone. **Metronidazole** may be beneficial possibly through its antibacterial activity. Other antibacterials should be given if specifically indicated and for managing bacterial overgrowth in the small bowel. General nutritional care and appropriate supplements are essential.

Hydrocortisone

Hydrocortisone retention enema is a representative rectal corticosteroid preparation (other than suppository). Various formulations can serve as alternatives

Suppositories, hydrocortisone acetate 25 mg

Retention enema (Rectal solution), hydrocortisone 100 mg, 60-ml bottle

Uses: ulcerative colitis, proctitis, proctosigmoiditis; anaphylaxis (section 3.1); skin (section 13.3); adrenocortical insufficiency (section 18.1)

Contraindications: bowel obstruction, bowel perforation, or extensive fistulas; untreated infections

Precautions: proctological examination required before treatment; systemic absorption may occur (see section 18.1); prolonged use should be avoided; pregnancy (Appendix 2); breastfeeding (Appendix 3); **interactions:** Appendix 1

Dosage:

Ulcerative colitis, proctitis, *by rectum* (suppositories), ADULT 25 mg twice daily for 2 weeks; may be increased to 25 mg 3 times daily *or* 50 mg twice daily in severe cases; in factitial proctitis treatment may be required for 6–8 weeks

Ulcerative colitis, ulcerative proctitis, ulcerative proctosigmoiditis, *by rectum* (retention enema), ADULT 100 mg at night for 21 days or until clinical and proctological remission; if no clinical and proctological improvement after 21 days, discontinue; treatment for 2–3 months may be required for proctological remission; when used for more than 21 days, discontinue gradually using 100 mg every other night for 2–3 weeks

Adverse effects: local pain or burning sensation; rectal bleeding (reported with use of enema); exacerbation of untreated infections; suppositories may stain fabrics; systemic adverse effects (section 18.1)

Sulfasalazine

Sulfasalazine is a representative aminosalicylate. Various drugs can serve as alternatives

Tablets, sulfasalazine 500 mg

Suppositories, sulfasalazine 500 mg

Retention enema (Rectal solution), sulfasalazine 3 g, 100-ml bottle

Uses: ulcerative colitis; Crohn disease; severe rheumatoid arthritis (section 2.4)

Contraindications: hypersensitivity to salicylates or sulfonamides; child under 2 years; porphyria; intestinal or urinary obstruction; severe renal impairment

Precautions: renal impairment (Appendix 4); hepatic impairment; G6PD deficiency; slow acetylator status; monitor blood counts and liver function initially and at monthly intervals for first 3 months; monitor kidney function initially and at intervals during treatment; history of allergy; pregnancy and breastfeeding (Appendices 2 and 3); **interactions:** Appendix 1

BLOOD DISORDERS. Patients should be advised to report any unexplained bleeding, bruising, purpura, sore throat, fever or malaise occurring during treatment; blood count should be performed and sulfasalazine stopped immediately if there is suspicion or evidence of blood disorder

Dosage:

Ulcerative colitis, *by mouth*, ADULT 1–2 g 4 times daily in acute attack until remission, reducing to maintenance dose of 500 mg 4 times daily; CHILD over 2 years, 40–60 mg/kg daily in acute attack, reducing to maintenance dose of 20–30 mg/kg daily

Active Crohn disease, *by mouth*, ADULT 1–2 g 4 times daily in acute attack until remission occurs; CHILD over 2 years, 40–60 mg/kg daily in acute attack

Ulcerative colitis, Crohn colitis, *by rectum* (suppositories, used alone or in conjunction with oral therapy), ADULT 0.5–1 g morning and evening after a bowel movement; *by rectum* (retention enema), ADULT 3 g at night retained for at least an hour; CHILD not a suitable formulation

Adverse effects: nausea, exacerbation of colitis; diarrhoea, loss of appetite, fever, blood disorders (including Heinz body anaemia, megaloblastic anaemia, leukopenia, neutropenia, thrombocytopenia); hypersensitivity reactions (including rash, urticaria, Stevens-Johnson syndrome (erythema multiforme), exfoliative dermatitis, epidermal necrolysis, pruritus, photosensitization, anaphylaxis, serum sickness, interstitial nephritis, lupus erythematosus-like syndrome); lung complications (including eosinophilia, fibrosing alveolitis); ocular complications (including periorbital oedema); stomatitis, parotitis; ataxia, aseptic meningitis, vertigo, tinnitus, alopecia, peripheral neuropathy, insomnia, depression, headache, hallucinations; kidney reactions (including proteinuria, crystalluria, haematuria); oligospermia; rarely acute pancreatitis, hepatitis; urine may be coloured orange; some soft contact lenses may be stained

17.5 Antispasmodic drugs

The smooth muscle relaxant properties of anticholinergic (more correctly, antimuscarinic) and other antispasmodic drugs may be useful as adjunctive treatment in non-ulcer dyspepsia, in irritable bowel syndrome, and in diverticular disease. The gastric antisecretory effects of conventional anticholinergic drugs are of little practical significance since dosage is limited by atropine-like adverse effects. Moreover they have been superseded by more powerful and specific antisecretory drugs, including the histamine H_2-receptor antagonists and the selective anticholinergic drugs.

Anticholinergics that are used for gastrointestinal smooth muscle spasm include **atropine** and hyoscine butylbromide.

Atropine sulfate

Atropine sulfate is a representative antispasmodic drug. Various drugs can
serve as alternatives

Tablets, atropine sulfate 600 micrograms

Uses: dyspepsia, irritable bowel syndrome, diverticular disease;
premedication (section 1.3); mydriasis and cycloplegia
(section 21.5); poisoning (section 4.2.3)

Contraindications: angle-closure glaucoma; myasthenia
gravis; paralytic ileus; pyloric stenosis; prostatic enlargement

Precautions: children, elderly and Down syndrome (increased
risk of adverse effects); gastro-oesophageal reflux; diarrhoea;
ulcerative colitis; acute myocardial infarction; hypertension;
hyperthyroidism; cardiac insufficiency, cardiac surgery—
conditions characterized by tachycardia; pyrexia; pregnancy
(Appendix 2); breastfeeding (Appendix 3); **interactions:**
Appendix 1

Dosage:

Dyspepsia, irritable bowel syndrome, diverticular disease, *by
mouth*, ADULT 0.6–1.2 mg at night

Adverse effects: constipation; transient bradycardia (followed
by tachycardia, palpitations and arrhythmias); reduced
bronchial secretions, urinary urgency and retention; dilatation
of pupils with loss of accommodation, photophobia, dry
mouth, flushing and dryness of skin; occasionally confusion
(particularly in the elderly), nausea, vomiting and giddiness

17.6 Laxatives

A balanced diet, including adequate fluid intake and fibre is of
value in preventing constipation.

Before prescribing laxatives, it is important to be sure that the
patient is constipated and that the constipation is not secondary
to an underlying undiagnosed complaint. It is also important
that the patient understands that bowel habit can vary
considerably in frequency without doing harm. For example
some people consider themselves constipated if they do not
have a bowel movement each day. A useful definition of
constipation is the passage of hard stools less frequently than the
patient's own normal pattern and this should be explained to the
patient since misconceptions about bowel habits have led to
excessive laxative use which in turn has led to hypokalaemia
and an atonic non-functioning colon.

Laxatives should generally be avoided except where straining
will exacerbate a condition such as angina or increase the risk of
rectal bleeding as in haemorrhoids. Laxatives are of value in
drug-induced constipation, for the expulsion of parasites after
anthelminthic treatment and to clear the alimentary tract before
surgery and radiological procedures. Prolonged treatment of
constipation is rarely necessary except occasionally in the
elderly.

There are many different laxatives. These include **bulk-forming laxatives** which relieve constipation by increasing faecal mass and stimulating peristalsis, **stimulant laxatives** which increase intestinal motility and often cause abdominal cramp, **faecal softeners** which lubricate and soften impacted faeces and **osmotic laxatives** which act by retaining fluid in the bowel by osmosis. **Bowel cleansing solutions** are used before colonic surgery, colonoscopy or radiological examination to ensure that the bowel is free of solid contents; they are **not** a treatment for constipation.

Senna

Senna is a representative stimulant laxative. Various drugs can serve as alternatives

Tablets, total sennosides (calculated as sennoside B) 7.5 mg

Uses: constipation; acts in 8–12 hours

Contraindications: intestinal obstruction; undiagnosed abdominal symptoms

Precautions: avoid prolonged use unless indication for prevention of faecal impaction; breastfeeding (Appendix 3)

Dosage:

Constipation, *by mouth*, ADULT 2–4 tablets, usually at night; initial dose should be low, then gradually increased; CHILD over 6 years, half the adult dose in the morning (on doctor's advice)

Adverse effects: abdominal discomfort; atonic non-functioning colon and hypokalaemia (with prolonged use or overdosage)

17.7 Drugs used in diarrhoea

Acute diarrhoeal diseases are a leading cause of childhood morbidity and mortality. In adults acute diarrhoea is the most frequent health problem of travellers to developing countries and is increasingly common among HIV-infected persons. Assessment and correction of dehydration and electrolyte disturbance is the priority in all cases of acute diarrhoea. Symptomatic relief in adults may be warranted in some cases but antidiarrhoeals should never be used in children since they do not reduce fluid and electrolyte loss and may cause adverse effects.

Diarrhoea persisting for longer than a month is known as chronic diarrhoea. A mild malabsorption syndrome, tropical enteropathy, is apparent in most healthy indigenous populations of tropical countries. However the majority of cases of chronic diarrhoea have non-infectious causes including gluten-sensitivity, inherited metabolic disorders or inflammatory bowel disease.

Bloody diarrhoea is usually a sign of invasive enteric infection and should be treated with an appropriate anti-infective agent.

17.7.1 Oral rehydration

Acute diarrhoea in children should always be treated with oral
rehydration solution according to plan A, B or C as shown.
Severely dehydrated patients must be treated initially with
intravenous fluids until they are able take fluids by mouth. For
oral rehydration it is important to administer the solution in
small amounts at regular intervals as indicated below.

Treatment of dehydration: WHO recommendations

According to the degree of dehydration, health professionals are
advised to follow one of 3 management plans.

Plan A: no dehydration. Nutritional advice and increased
fluid intake are sufficient (soup, rice, water and yoghurt, or even
water). For infants aged under 6 months who have not yet
started taking solids, oral rehydration solution must be
presented before offering milk. Mother's milk or dried cow's
milk must be given without any particular restrictions. In the
case of mixed breast-milk/formula feeding, the contribution of
breastfeeding must be increased.

Plan B: moderate dehydration. Whatever the child's age, a
4-hour treatment plan is applied to avoid short-term problems.
Feeding should not therefore be envisaged initially. It is
recommended that parents are shown how to give approximately 75 ml/kg of oral rehydration solution with a spoon over a
4-hour period, and it is suggested that parents should be
watched to see how they cope at the beginning of the treatment.
A larger amount of solution can be given if the child continues
to have frequent stools. In case of vomiting, rehydration must be
discontinued for 10 minutes and then resumed at a slower rate
(about one teaspoonful every 2 minutes). The child's status
must be re-assessed after 4 hours to decide on the most
appropriate subsequent treatment. Oral rehydration solution
should continue to be offered once dehydration has been
controlled, for as long as the child continues to have diarrhoea.

Plan C: severe dehydration. Hospitalization is necessary, but
the most urgent priority is to start rehydration. In hospital (or
elsewhere), if the child can drink, oral rehydration solution must
be given pending, and even during, intravenous infusion (20 ml/
kg every hour by mouth before infusion, then 5 ml/kg every
hour by mouth during intravenous rehydration). For intravenous
supplementation, it is recommended that compound solution of
sodium lactate (see section 26.2) is administered at a rate
adapted to the child's age (infant under 12 months: 30 ml/kg
over 1 hour then 70 ml/kg over 5 hours; child over 12 months:
the same amounts over 30 minutes and 2.5 hours respectively).
If the intravenous route is unavailable, a nasogastric tube is also
suitable for administering oral rehydration solution, at a rate of
20 ml/kg every hour. If the child vomits, the rate of
administration of the oral solution should be reduced.

Oral rehydration salts

Glucose salt solution

sodium chloride	3.5 g/litre of clean water
trisodium citrate	2.9 g/litre of clean water
potassium chloride	1.5 g/litre of clean water
glucose (anhydrous)	20.00 g/litre of clean water

When glucose and trisodium citrate are not available, they may be replaced by

sucrose (common sugar)	40.00 g/litre of clean water
sodium bicarbonate	2.5 g/litre of clean water

NOTE. The solution may be prepared either from prepackaged sugar/salt mixtures or from bulk substances and water. Solutions must be freshly prepared, preferably with recently boiled and cooled water. Accurate weighing and thorough mixing and dissolution of ingredients in the correct volume of clean water is important. Administration of more concentrated solutions can result in hypernatraemia

Uses: dehydration from acute diarrhoea

Precautions: renal impairment

Dosage:

Fluid and electrolyte loss in acute diarrhoea, *by mouth*, ADULT 200–400 ml solution after every loose motion; INFANT and CHILD according to Plan A, B or C (see notes above)

Adverse effects: vomiting—may indicate too rapid administration; hypernatraemia and hyperkalaemia may result from overdose in renal impairment or administration of too concentrated a solution

17.7.2 Antimotility drugs

Opioids such as codeine are used in the symptomatic relief of acute diarrhoea in adults. They act on opioid receptors in the gut wall and decrease bowel motility.

Codeine phosphate

Drug subject to international control under the Single Convention on Narcotic Drugs (1961)

Codeine phosphate is a representative antimotility drug. Various drugs can serve as alternatives

Tablets, codeine phosphate 30 mg

Uses: short-term symptomatic relief of acute diarrhoea in adults; pain (section 2.2)

Contraindications: children; conditions where inhibition of peristalsis should be avoided; abdominal distension; acute diarrhoeal conditions such as ulcerative colitis or antibiotic-associated colitis; acute respiratory depression

Precautions: tolerance or dependence may occur with prolonged use; elderly and debilitated patients; hepatic impairment (Appendix 5); renal impairment (Appendix 4); pregnancy (Appendix 2); breastfeeding (Appendix 3); **overdosage:** see section 4.2.2; **interactions:** Appendix 1

Dosage:

Symptomatic relief of acute diarrhoea, *by mouth*, ADULT 30 mg 3–4 times daily

Adverse effects: nausea, vomiting, drowsiness; respiratory depression and hypotension (large doses); difficulty with micturition; ureteric or biliary spasm; dry mouth, sweating, headache, facial flushing, vertigo, bradycardia, tachycardia, palpitations, hypothermia, hallucinations, dysphoria, mood changes, miosis, decreased libido or potency, rash, urticaria, pruritus; convulsions (large doses)

Section 18: Hormones and other endocrine drugs and contraceptives

18.1 Adrenal hormones and synthetic substances

Corticosteroids are hormones secreted by the adrenal cortex or are synthetic analogues of these hormones. The adrenal cortex normally secretes **hydrocortisone** which has glucocorticoid activity and weak mineralocorticoid activity. It also secretes the mineralocorticoid aldosterone. Synthetic glucocorticoids include beclomethasone, **dexamethasone** and **prednisolone**. **Fludrocortisone** also has glucocorticoid properties but has potent mineralocorticoid properties and is used for its mineralocorticoid effects.

Pharmacology of the corticosteroids is complex and their actions are wide-ranging. In physiologic (low) doses, they are administered to replace deficient endogenous hormones. In pharmacological (high) doses, glucocorticoids decrease inflammation, suppress the immune response, stimulate erythroid cells of the bone marrow, promote protein catabolism, reduce intestinal absorption, increase blood glucose, and elevate blood pressure, increase renal excretion of calcium and promote redistribution of fat and development of cushingoid features.

In therapeutic doses glucocorticoids suppress release of corticotrophin (ACTH) from the pituitary thus the adrenal cortex ceases secretion of endogenous corticosteroids. If suppressive doses are given for prolonged periods, the adrenal cortex may atrophy and this leads to a deficiency on sudden withdrawal or dosage reduction or situations such as stress or trauma where corticosteroid requirements are increased. After high dosage or prolonged therapy, withdrawal should be gradual, the rate depending on various factors including patient response, corticosteroid dose, duration of treatment and disease state. The suppressive action of a corticosteroid on cortisol secretion is least when given in the morning. Corticosteroids should normally be given in a single morning dose to attempt to minimize pituitary-adrenal suppression. Because the therapeutic effects of corticosteroids are of longer duration than the metabolic effects, intermittent therapy may allow the body's normal metabolic rhythm and the therapeutic effects to be maintained. Alternate day dosing is, however, suitable only in certain disease states and with corticosteroids with small mineralocorticoid effects and a relatively short duration of action.

Hydrocortisone is used in adrenal replacement therapy and on a short-term basis by intravenous injection for the emergency management of some conditions. Its mineralocorticoid activity is too high for it to be used on a long-term basis for disease suppression. The mineralocorticoid activity of **fludrocortisone** is also high and its anti-inflammatory activity is of no clinical relevance. It is used together with glucocorticoids in adrenal insufficiency. **Prednisolone** has predominantly glucocorticoid activity and is the corticosteroid most commonly administered for long-term disease suppression. It is the active metabolite of prednisone, conversion of which is variable and prednisone should not be used interchangeably with prednisolone. **Dexamethasone** has very high glucocorticoid activity in conjunction with insignificant mineralocorticoid activity making it particularly suitable for high-dose therapy in conditions where water retention would be a disadvantage such as cerebral oedema. It also has a long duration of action and this, together with its lack of mineralocorticoid activity makes it particularly suitable for conditions requiring suppression of corticotrophin secretion such as congenital adrenal hyperplasia.

DISADVANTAGES OF CORTICOSTEROIDS. Overdosage or prolonged use may exaggerate some of the normal physiological actions of corticosteroids leading to mineralocorticoid and glucocorticoid adverse effects.

Mineralocorticoid adverse effects include hypertension, sodium and water retention and potassium loss. These effects are most marked with fludrocortisone but are significant with hydrocortisone, occur slightly with prednisolone and are negligible with dexamethasone.

Glucocorticoid adverse effects include diabetes mellitus and osteoporosis which is of particular importance in the elderly since it may result in osteoporotic fractures of the hip or vertebrae. High doses may also be associated with avascular necrosis of the femoral neck. Muscle wasting may also occur and there is a weak link with peptic ulceration. Mental disturbances can occur, including serious paranoid state or depression with risk of suicide, particularly in patients with a history of mental disorders; euphoria is also common. High doses may cause Cushing syndrome (typical moon face, striae and acne), which is usually reversible on withdrawal of treatment, but this should always be tapered gradually to avoid symptoms of acute adrenal insufficiency (see also Withdrawal). In children, corticosteroids may result in suppression of growth and corticosteroids administered during pregnancy can affect adrenal development in the fetus. Any adrenal suppression in the neonate following prenatal exposure usually resolves spontaneously after birth and is rarely clinically important. Healing of wounds may be impaired and infections and thinning of the skin may occur; spread of infections may result from modification of tissue reactions.

Adrenal atrophy can persist for years after stopping prolonged therapy; therefore any illness or surgical emergency may require temporary reintroduction of corticosteroid therapy in order to compensate for lack of sufficient adrenocortical response. It is important for anaesthetists to know whether a patient is taking or has been taking corticosteroids in order to avoid a precipitous fall in blood pressure during anaesthesia or in the immediate postoperative period.

DOSAGE AND ADMINISTRATION. Adverse effects of systemic glucocorticoids, including suppression of the HPA (hypothalamo-pituitary-adrenal) axis, are dose and duration dependent; thus patients should be given treatment for the shortest length of time at the lowest dose that is clinically necessary. Patient response is variable and doses should therefore be individualized. In life-threatening diseases, high doses may need to be given because the complications of therapy are likely to be less serious than the disease. In long-term therapy in relatively benign chronic conditions such as rheumatoid arthritis, adverse effects often outweigh the advantages. In order to minimize the adverse effects, the maintenance dose should be kept as low as possible and if possible, single morning doses or alternate day therapy should be used. Glucocorticoids can improve the prognosis of serious conditions such as systemic lupus erythematosus, temporal arteritis and polyarteritis nodosa; in such disorders the effects of the disease process may be suppressed and symptoms relieved but the underlying condition is not cured.

Glucocorticoids are used both topically and systemically. In emergency situations, hydrocortisone may be given intravenously; in the treatment of asthma, inhalation therapy with beclometasone may be used (section 25.1). Whenever possible, local treatment with creams, intra-articular injections, inhalations, eye-drops or enemas should be used in preference to systemic therapy.

WITHDRAWAL OF SYSTEMIC CORTICOSTEROIDS. The rate of withdrawal of systemic glucocorticoids is dependent upon several factors including size of dose, duration of treatment, individual patient's response and the likelihood of relapse of the underlying disease. If there is uncertainty about suppression of the HPA axis, withdrawal should be gradual to enable the adrenal gland to recover. Patients should be advised not to stop taking glucocorticoids abruptly unless permitted by their doctor.

Gradual withdrawal should be considered in those whose disease is unlikely to relapse and who have:
- recently received repeated courses (particularly if taken for longer than 3 weeks)
- taken a short course within 1 year of stopping long-term therapy
- other possible causes of adrenal suppression
- received more than 40 mg daily prednisolone (or equivalent)
- been given repeat doses in the evening
- received more than 3 weeks' treatment

Abrupt withdrawal may be considered in those whose disease is unlikely to relapse *and* who have received treatment for 3 weeks or less *and* are not included in the patient groups described above.

During corticosteroid withdrawal the dose may be reduced rapidly down to the physiological dosage (equivalent to 7.5 mg prednisolone daily) and then reduced more slowly. Assessment of the disease may be needed during withdrawal to ensure that relapse does not occur.

CORTICOSTEROID COVER DURING STRESS. The response of the HPA axis to stress is reduced during long-term therapy and for an extended period after withdrawal of the corticosteroid. If stress (infection, trauma, surgery) occurs during adrenal suppression, corticosteroid cover should be given. Cover should also be given to patients who suffer stress within 1 week of finishing a course of systemic corticosteroids lasting less than three weeks. Patients who are unable to take the dose by mouth should receive parenteral corticosteroid cover.

For patients requiring surgery, parenteral hydrocortisone should be administered as follows:

- 200 mg hydrocortisone *intramuscularly* with premedication
- 100 mg hydrocortisone by *intravenous infusion* in 500 ml 0.9% sodium chloride during surgery
- 100 mg hydrocortisone *intramuscularly* every 6 hours for 72 hours after surgery

For patients requiring minor surgical procedures:

- 100 mg hydrocortisone *intramuscularly* shortly before and after intervention

---

Dexamethasone

Dexamethasone is a representative corticosteroid. Various drugs can serve as alternatives

Tablets, dexamethasone 500 micrograms, 4 mg

Injection (Solution for injection), dexamethasone phosphate (as dexamethasone sodium phosphate) 4 mg/ml, 1-ml ampoule

Uses: suppression of inflammatory and allergic disorders (see also allergy and allergic disorders, section 3.1); diagnosis of Cushing syndrome; congenital adrenal hyperplasia; cerebral oedema

Contraindications: see notes above; systemic infection (unless life-threatening or specific antimicrobial therapy given); avoid live virus vaccines in those receiving immunosuppressive doses (serum antibody response diminished)

Precautions: adrenal suppression during prolonged treatment which persists for years after stopping treatment (see notes above); ensure patients understand importance of compliance with dosage and have guidance on precautions to reduce risks; monitor weight, blood pressure, fluid and electrolyte balance and blood glucose levels throughout prolonged treatment; infections (greater susceptibility, symptoms may be masked until advanced stage; clinical presentation may be atypical; risks of chickenpox and measles increased—passive immunization recommended for non-immune patients in contact with either infection; specialist care required); quiescent tuberculosis—chemoprophylactic therapy during prolonged corticosteroid treatment; elderly; children and adolescents (growth retardation possibly irreversible); hypertension, recent myocardial infarction (rupture reported), congestive heart failure, liver failure, renal impairment, diabetes mellitus including family history, osteoporosis (may be manifested as back pain, postmenopausal women at special risk), glaucoma including family history, severe affective disorder (particularly if history of steroid-induced psychosis), epilepsy, psoriasis, peptic ulcer, hypothyroidism, history of steroid myopathy; pregnancy (Appendix 2); breastfeeding (Appendix 3); **interactions:** Appendix 1

Dosage:

Suppression of inflammatory and allergic disorders, *by mouth*, ADULT usual range 0.5–10 mg daily; *by intramuscular injection or slow intravenous injection or intravenous infusion* (as dexamethasone phosphate), ADULT initially 0.5–20 mg daily; CHILD 200–500 micrograms/kg daily

Cerebral oedema, *by intravenous injection* (as dexamethasone phosphate), ADULT 10 mg initially, then 4 mg *by intramuscular injection* (as dexamethasone phosphate) every 6 hours, as required for 2–10 days

Diagnosis of Cushing syndrome, see manufacturer's literature
NOTE. Dexamethasone 1 mg ≡ dexamethasone phosphate 1.2 mg ≡ dexamethasone sodium phosphate 1.3 mg

Adverse effects: gastrointestinal effects including dyspepsia, peptic ulceration (with perforation), abdominal distension, acute pancreatitis, oesophageal ulceration and candidosis; musculoskeletal effects including proximal myopathy, osteoporosis, vertebral and long bone fractures, avascular osteonecrosis, tendon rupture; endocrine effects including adrenal suppression, menstrual irregularities and amenorrhoea, Cushing syndrome (with high doses, usually reversible on withdrawal), hirsutism, weight gain, negative nitrogen and calcium balance, increased appetite, increased susceptibility to and severity of infection; neuropsychiatric effects including euphoria, psychological dependence, depression, insomnia, increased intracranial pressure with papilloedema in children (usually after withdrawal), psychosis and aggravation of schizophrenia, aggravation of epilepsy; ophthalmic effects including glaucoma, papilloedema, posterior subcapsular cataracts, corneal or scleral thinning and exacerbation of ophthalmic viral or fungal disease; also impaired healing, skin atrophy, bruising, striae, telangiectasia, acne, myocardial rupture following recent myocardial infarction, fluid and electrolyte disturbances, leukocytosis, hypersensitivity reactions (including anaphylaxis), thromboembolism, nausea, malaise and hiccups; perineal irritation may follow intravenous administration of phosphate ester

---

Hydrocortisone
Tablets, hydrocortisone 10 mg
Injection (Powder for solution for injection), hydrocortisone (as sodium succinate) 100-mg vial

Uses: adrenocortical insufficiency; hypersensitivity reactions including anaphylactic shock (section 3.1); inflammatory bowel disease (section 17.4); skin (section 13.3)

Contraindications: see notes above; systemic infection (unless life-threatening or specific antimicrobial therapy given); avoid live virus vaccines in those receiving immunosuppressive doses (serum antibody response diminished)

Precautions: adrenal suppression during prolonged treatment which persists for years after stopping treatment (see notes above); ensure patients understand importance of compliance with dosage and have guidance on precautions to reduce risks; monitor weight, blood pressure, fluid and electrolyte balance and blood glucose levels throughout prolonged treatment; infections (greater susceptibility, symptoms may be masked until advanced stage; clinical presentation may be atypical; risks of chickenpox and measles increased—passive immunization recommended for non-immune patients in contact with either infection; specialist care required); quiescent tuberculosis—chemoprophylactic therapy during prolonged corticosteroid treatment; elderly; children and adolescents (growth retardation possibly irreversible); hypertension, recent myocardial infarction (rupture reported), congestive heart failure, liver failure, renal impairment, diabetes mellitus including family history, osteoporosis (may be manifested as back pain, postmenopausal women at special risk), glaucoma including family history, severe affective disorder (particularly if history of steroid-induced psychosis), epilepsy, psoriasis, peptic ulcer, hypothyroidism, history of steroid myopathy; pregnancy (Appendix 2); breastfeeding (Appendix 3); **interactions:** Appendix 1

Dosage:

Replacement therapy in adrenocortical insufficiency, *by mouth*, ADULT 20–30 mg daily in divided doses (usually 20 mg in the morning and 10 mg in early evening); CHILD 10–30 mg

Acute adrenocortical insufficiency, *by slow intravenous injection or by intravenous infusion*, ADULT 100–500 mg, 3–4 times in 24 hours or as required; *by slow intravenous injection*, CHILD up to 1 year 25 mg, 1–5 years 50 mg, 6–12 years 100 mg

RECONSTITUTION AND ADMINISTRATION. According to manufacturer's directions

Adverse effects: gastrointestinal effects including dyspepsia, peptic ulceration (with perforation), abdominal distension, acute pancreatitis, oesophageal ulceration and candidosis; musculoskeletal effects including proximal myopathy, osteoporosis, vertebral and long bone fractures, avascular osteonecrosis, tendon rupture; endocrine effects including adrenal suppression, menstrual irregularities and amenorrhoea, Cushing syndrome (with high doses, usually reversible on withdrawal), hirsutism, weight gain, negative nitrogen and calcium balance, increased appetite, increased susceptibility to and severity of infection; neuropsychiatric effects including euphoria, psychological dependence, depression, insomnia, increased intracranial pressure with papilloedema in children (usually after withdrawal), psychosis and aggravation of schizophrenia, aggravation of epilepsy; ophthalmic effects including glaucoma, papilloedema, posterior subcapsular cataracts, corneal or scleral thinning and exacerbation of ophthalmic viral or fungal disease; also impaired healing, skin atrophy, bruising, striae, telangiectasia, acne, myocardial rupture following recent myocardial infarction, fluid and electrolyte disturbances, leukocytosis, hypersensitivity reactions (including anaphylaxis), thromboembolism, nausea, malaise and hiccups

Prednisolone

Prednisolone is a representative corticosteroid. Various drugs can serve as alternatives

Tablets, prednisolone 1 mg, 5 mg

Uses: suppression of inflammatory and allergic reactions (see also section 3.1); with antineoplastic drugs for acute leukaemias and lymphomas (section 8.3); eye (section 21.2)

Contraindications: see notes above; systemic infection (unless life-threatening or specific antimicrobial therapy given); avoid live virus vaccines in those receiving immunosuppressive doses (serum antibody response diminished)

Precautions: adrenal suppression during prolonged treatment which persists for years after stopping treatment (see notes above); ensure patients understand importance of compliance with dosage and have guidance on precautions to reduce risks; monitor weight, blood pressure, fluid and electrolyte balance and blood glucose levels throughout prolonged treatment; infections (greater susceptibility, symptoms may be masked until advanced stage; clinical presentation may be atypical; risks of chickenpox and measles increased—passive immunization recommended for non-immune patients in contact with either infection; specialist care required); quiescent tuberculosis—chemoprophylactic therapy during prolonged corticosteroid treatment; elderly; children and adolescents (growth retardation possibly irreversible); hypertension, recent myocardial infarction (rupture reported), congestive heart failure, renal impairment, hepatic impairment (Appendix 5); diabetes mellitus including family history, osteoporosis (may be manifested as back pain, postmenopausal women at special risk), glaucoma including family history, severe affective disorder (particularly if history of steroid-induced psychosis), epilepsy, psoriasis, peptic ulcer, hypothyroidism, history of steroid myopathy; pregnancy (Appendix 2); breastfeeding (Appendix 3); **interactions:** Appendix 1

Dosage:

Suppression of inflammatory and allergic disorders, *by mouth*, ADULT initially up to 10–20 mg daily (severe disease, up to 60 mg daily), preferably taken in the morning after breakfast; dose can often be reduced within a few days, but may need to be continued for several weeks or months; maintenance, 2.5–15 mg daily or higher; cushingoid features are increasingly

likely with doses above 7.5 mg daily; CHILD fractions of adult
dose may be used (for example, at 1 year 25% of adult dose, at
7 years 50%, and at 12 years 75%) but clinical factors must be
given due weight

Adverse effects: gastrointestinal effects including dyspepsia,
peptic ulceration (with perforation), abdominal distension,
acute pancreatitis, oesophageal ulceration and candidosis;
musculoskeletal effects including proximal myopathy, osteoporosis, vertebral and long bone fractures, avascular osteonecrosis, tendon rupture; endocrine effects including adrenal
suppression, menstrual irregularities and amenorrhoea, Cushing syndrome (with high doses, usually reversible on
withdrawal), hirsutism, weight gain, negative nitrogen and
calcium balance, increased appetite, increased susceptibility
to and severity of infection; neuropsychiatric effects including
euphoria, psychological dependence, depression, insomnia,
increased intracranial pressure with papilloedema in children
(usually after withdrawal), psychosis and aggravation of
schizophrenia, aggravation of epilepsy; ophthalmic effects
including glaucoma, papilloedema, posterior subcapsular
cataracts, corneal or scleral thinning and exacerbation of
ophthalmic viral or fungal disease; also impaired healing, skin
atrophy, bruising, striae, telangiectasia, acne, myocardial
rupture following recent myocardial infarction, fluid and
electrolyte disturbances, leukocytosis, hypersensitivity reactions (including anaphylaxis), thromboembolism, nausea,
malaise and hiccups

Fludrocortisone acetate
Fludrocortisone acetate is a complementary drug
Tablets, fludrocortisone acetate 100 micrograms

Uses: mineralocorticoid replacement in adrenocortical insufficiency

Contraindications: see under Prednisolone

Precautions: see under Prednisolone; **interactions:** Appendix 1

Dosage:
Adrenocortical insufficiency, *by mouth*, ADULT 50–300 micrograms daily; CHILD 5 micrograms/kg daily

Adverse effects: *glucocorticoid effects:* see notes above and
under Prednisolone; *mineralocorticoid effects:* oedema,
hypertension, sodium and water retention and potassium loss;
cardiac failure (may be induced in susceptible patients)

18.2 Androgens

Androgens are secreted by the testes and weaker androgens by
the adrenal cortex and ovaries. In the male, they are responsible
for the development and maintenance of the sex organs and the
secondary sexual characteristics, normal reproductive function,
and sexual performance ability in addition to stimulating the
growth and development of the skeleton and skeletal muscle
during puberty. At high doses in the normal male androgens

inhibit pituitary gonadotrophin secretion and depress spermatogenesis. **Testosterone** is used as replacement therapy in those
who are hypogonadal due to either pituitary (secondary
hypogonadism) or testicular disease (primary hypogonadism).
Androgens are useless as a treatment of impotence and impaired
spermatogenesis unless there is associated hypogonadism; they
should not be given until the hypogonadism has been properly
investigated and treatment should always be under expert
supervision. When given to patients with hypopituitarism they
can lead to normal sexual development and potency but not
fertility. If fertility is desired, the usual treatment is with
gonadotrophins or pulsatile gonadotrophin-releasing hormone
which will stimulate spermatogenesis as well as androgen
production. Androgens cannot induce fertility in men with
primary hypogonadism. Caution should be used in treating boys
with delayed puberty with excessive doses of testosterone since
the fusion of epiphyses is hastened and may result in short
stature. Androgens, including testosterone have also been used
in postmenopausal women for the palliative treatment of
androgen-responsive, advanced, metastatic breast cancer; care
is required to prevent masculinizing effects.

Testosterone enantate

Oily injection (Solution for injection), testosterone enantate 200 mg/ml,
250 mg/ml; 1-ml ampoules

Uses: hypogonadism; palliative treatment of advanced breast
cancer in women

Contraindications: breast cancer in men, prostate cancer,
hypercalcaemia, pregnancy (Appendix 2), breastfeeding
(Appendix 3), nephrosis, history of primary liver tumours

Precautions: cardiac, renal or hepatic impairment
(Appendix 5), elderly, ischaemic heart disease, hypertension,
epilepsy, skeletal metastases (risk of hypercalcaemia); regular
examination of prostate during treatment; prepubertal boys;
interactions: Appendix 1

Dosage:

Hypogonadism, *by slow intramuscular injection*; ADULT (males),
initially 200–250 mg every 2–3 weeks; maintenance 200–
250 mg every 3–6 weeks

Breast cancer, *by slow intramuscular injection*, ADULT (females)
250 mg every 2–3 weeks

Adverse effects: prostate abnormalities and prostate cancer,
headache, depression, gastrointestinal bleeding, nausea,
cholestatic jaundice, changes in libido, gynaecomastia,
anxiety, asthenia, generalized paraesthesia, electrolyte disturbances including sodium retention with oedema and
hypercalcaemia; increased bone growth; androgenic effects
such as hirsutism, male pattern baldness, seborrhoea, acne,
priapism, precocious sexual development and premature
closure of epiphyses in pre-pubertal males, virilism in
females, and suppression of spermatogenesis in men

18.3 Contraceptives

18.3.1 Hormonal contraceptives

Hormonal contraception is one of the most effective methods of reversible fertility control, but has unwanted major and minor adverse effects, especially for certain groups of women. Estrogen plus progestogen combinations are the most widely used. They produce a contraceptive effect mainly by suppressing the hypothalamic-pituitary system resulting in prevention of ovulation. In addition, changes in the endometrium make it unreceptive to implantation and changes in the cervical mucus may prevent sperm penetration.

Endometrial proliferation is usually followed by thinning or regression of the endometrium resulting in reduced menstrual flow. Ovulation usually resumes within three menstrual cycles after oral contraception has been discontinued in women who have previously had a baby; but anovulation and amenorrhoea may persist for six months or longer in some women including those who are nulliparous.

Potential non-contraceptive benefits of combined oral contraceptives include improved regularity of the menstrual cycle, decreased blood loss, less iron-deficiency anaemia and significant decrease in dysmenorrhoea. Long-term use is associated with reduced risk of endometrial and ovarian cancer and of some pelvic infections.

An association between the amount of estrogen and progestogen in oral contraceptives and an increased risk of adverse cardiovascular effects has been observed.

The risk of hypertension increases with increasing duration of oral contraceptive use and they should be discontinued if the woman becomes hypertensive during use. Combined oral contraceptives are associated with an increased risk of thromboembolic and thrombotic disorders and an increase in risk of cerebrovascular disorders including stroke and subarachnoid haemorrhage. The use of oral contraceptive combinations containing the progestogens, desogestrel or gestodene are associated with a slightly increased risk of venous thromboembolism compared with oral contraceptives containing the progestogens, levonorgestrel or norethisterone.

RISK FACTORS FOR VENOUS THROMBOEMBOLISM OR ARTERIAL DISEASE. Risk factors for *venous thromboembolism* include family history of venous thromboembolism in first-degree relative aged under 45 years, obesity, long-term immobilization and varicose veins.

Risk factors for *arterial disease* include family history of arterial disease in first-degree relative aged under 45 years, diabetes mellitus, hypertension, smoking, age over 35 years (avoid if over 50 years), obesity and migraine.

If any one of the factors is present, combined oral contraceptives should be used with caution; if 2 or more factors for either venous thromboembolism or arterial disease are present, combined oral contraceptives should be avoided. Combined oral contraceptives are contraindicated if there is severe or focal migraine.

Estrogen-containing oral contraceptives should be discontinued four weeks prior to major elective surgery and all surgery to the legs. When discontinuation is not possible, consideration should be given to the prophylactic use of subcutaneous heparin.

REASONS TO STOP COMBINED ORAL CONTRACEPTIVES IMMEDIATELY. Combined estrogen-containing oral contraceptives should be stopped immediately if any of the following symptoms occur:

- Sudden severe chest pain (even if not radiating to left arm);
- Sudden breathlessness (or cough with blood-stained sputum);
- Severe pain in calf of one leg;
- Severe stomach pain;
- Serious neurological effects including unusual, severe, prolonged headache especially if first time or getting progressively worse or sudden partial or complete loss of vision or sudden disturbance of hearing or other perceptual disorders or dysphagia or bad fainting attack or collapse or first unexplained epileptic seizure or weakness, motor disturbances, very marked numbness suddenly affecting one side or one part of body;
- Hepatitis, jaundice, liver enlargement;
- Severe depression;
- Blood pressure above systolic 160 mmHg and diastolic100 mmHg;
- Detection of a risk factor, see Precautions and Contraindications under Combined Oral Contraceptives

PROGESTOGEN-ONLY CONTRACEPTIVES. Progestogen-only contraceptives, such as oral **levonorgestrel** may offer a suitable alternative when estrogens are contraindicated but the oral progestogen-only preparations do not prevent ovulation in all cycles and have a higher failure rate than combined estrogen-containing preparations. Progestogen-only contraceptives carry less risk of thromboembolic and cardiovascular disease than combined oral contraceptives and are preferable for women over 35 years, for heavy smokers, and for those with hypertension, valvular heart disease, diabetes mellitus, and migraine. They can be used as an alternative to estrogen-containing combined preparations prior to major surgery. Menstrual irregularities (oligomenorrhoea, menorrhagia, amenorrhoea) are common. Injectable preparations of **medroxy-progesterone acetate** or **norethisterone enantate** may be given intramuscularly. They have prolonged action and should only be given with full counselling and manufacturer's information leaflet.

EMERGENCY CONTRACEPTION. Emergency contraception can be obtained using **levonorgestrel**. One tablet of 750 micrograms should be taken as soon as possible after unprotected intercourse followed 12 hours later by another tablet. Under those circumstances it prevents about 86% of pregnancies that would have occurred if no treatment had been given. Adverse effects include nausea, vomiting, headache, dizziness, breast discomfort, and menstrual irregularities. If vomiting occurs within 2–3 hours of taking the tablets, replacement tablets can be given orally with an antiemetic.

It should be explained to the woman that her next period may be early or late; that she needs to use a barrier contraceptive method until her next period, and that she should return promptly if she has any lower abdominal pain or if the subsequent menstrual bleed is abnormally light, heavy, brief or absent. There is no evidence of harmful effects to the fetus if pregnancy should occur.

Combined oral contraceptives

Ethinylestradiol with levonorgestrel and ethinylestradiol with norethisterone are representative combined oral contraceptive preparations. Various combinations can serve as alternatives

Tablets, ethinylestradiol 30 micrograms, levonorgestrel 150 micrograms
Tablets, ethinylestradiol 50 micrograms, levonorgestrel 250 micrograms
Tablets, ethinylestradiol 35 micrograms, norethisterone 1 mg

Uses: contraception; menstrual symptoms; endometriosis (see also progestogens, section 18.5)

Contraindications: pregnancy; twenty-one days post partum; breastfeeding until weaning or for first 6 months post partum (Appendix 3); personal history of venous or arterial thrombosis; heart disease associated with pulmonary hypertension or risk of embolism; migraine (see below); history of sub-acute bacterial endocarditis; ischaemic cerebrovascular disease; liver disease, including disorders of hepatic secretion such as Dubin-Johnson or Rotor syndromes, infectious hepatitis (until liver function normal); porphyria; systemic lupus erythematosus; liver adenoma; history of cholestasis; gallstones; estrogen-dependent neoplasms; neoplasms of breast or genital tract; undiagnosed vaginal bleeding; history during pregnancy of pruritus, chorea, herpes, deteriorating otosclerosis, cholestatic jaundice; pemphigoid gestationis; diabetes mellitus (if either retinopathy, neuropathy or if more than 20 years duration); after evacuation of hydatidiform mole (until return to normal of urine and plasma gonadotrophin values)

Precautions: risk factors for venous thromboembolism and arterial disease (see notes above); migraine (see below); hyperprolactinaemia (seek specialist advice); some types of hyperlipidaemia; gallbladder disease; depression; long-term immobilization; sickle-cell disease; inflammatory bowel disease including Crohn disease; **interactions:** Appendix 1

MIGRAINE. Patients should report any increase in headache frequency or onset of focal symptoms (discontinue immediately and refer urgently to neurology expert if focal neurological symptoms not typical of aura persist for more than one hour); **contraindications:** migraine with typical focal aura; severe migraine of more than 72 hours duration despite treatment; migraine treated with ergot derivatives; **precautions:** migraine without focal aura or controlled with $5HT_1$ agonist

Dosage:

Contraception (21-day combined (monophasic) preparations), *by mouth*, ADULT (female), 1 tablet ('pill') daily for 21 days; subsequent courses repeated after 7-day pill-free interval (during which withdrawal bleeding occurs)

ADMINISTRATION. Each tablet ('pill') should be taken at approximately the same time each day; if delayed by longer than 24 hours contraceptive protection may be lost. It is important to bear in mind that the critical time for loss of protection is when a pill is omitted at the beginning or end of a cycle (which lengthens the pill-free interval).

The following advice is recommended:

If you forget a pill, take it as soon as you remember, and the next one at the normal time. If you are 12 or more hours late, the pill may not work; as soon as you remember, continue normal pill-taking, but for 7 days an additional method of contraception such as the sheath will be required. If the 7 days run beyond the end of your packet, start the next packet when you have finished the present one—do not have a gap between packets.

Adverse effects: nausea, vomiting, headache, breast tenderness, increase in body weight, thrombosis, changes in libido, depression, chorea, skin reactions, chloasma, hypertension, impairment of liver function, 'spotting' in early cycles, absence of withdrawal bleeding, irritation of contact lenses; rarely, photosensitivity and hepatic tumours; breast cancer (small increase in risk of breast cancer during use which reduces during the 10 years after stopping; risk factor seems related to age at which contraceptive is stopped rather than total duration of use; small increase in risk of breast cancer should be weighed against the protective effect against cancers of the ovary and endometrium)

Levonorgestrel

Levonorgestrel 30 micrograms is a complementary drug
Tablets, levonorgestrel 30 micrograms
Tablets, levonorgestrel 750 micrograms, 2-tablet pack

Uses: contraception (particularly when estrogens are contraindicated); emergency hormonal contraception

Contraindications: *progestogen-only oral contraceptives:* pregnancy (Appendix 2); undiagnosed vaginal bleeding; severe arterial disease; liver tumours; breast cancer; thromboembolic disorders; sickle-cell anaemia; porphyria; after evacuation of hydatidiform mole (until return to normal of urine and plasma gonadotrophin values); *progestogen-only emergency hormonal contraceptives:* pregnancy (see Administration, below); severe liver disease; porphyria

Precautions: cardiac disease; sex-steroid dependent cancer; past ectopic pregnancy; malabsorption syndrome; ovarian cysts; active liver disease, recurrent cholestatic jaundice, history of jaundice in pregnancy (Appendix 5); increase in frequency of headache (discontinue pending investigation); breastfeeding (Appendix 3); **interactions:** Appendix 1

Dosage:

Contraception, *by mouth*, ADULT (female), 1 tablet ('pill') (30 micrograms) daily, starting on the first day of the cycle and then continuously

ADMINISTRATION. Each tablet ('pill') should be taken at approximately the same time each day. If delayed for longer than 3 hours contraceptive protection may be lost.

The following advice is recommended:

If you forget a pill, take it as soon as you remember, and the next one at the normal time. If you are more than 3 hours late, the pill may not work; as soon as you remember, continue normal pill-taking, but for 2 days an additional method of contraception such as the sheath will be required.

Emergency (post-coital) contraception, *by mouth*, ADULT (female), 1 tablet (750 micrograms) followed by a second tablet 12 hours later

ADMINISTRATION. Effective if first dose is taken within 72 hours (3 days) of unprotected intercourse; taking the first dose as soon as possible increases efficacy; should not be administered if menstrual bleeding overdue

Adverse effects: menstrual irregularities but tend to resolve on long-term treatment (including oligomenorrhoea and menorrhagia); nausea, vomiting, headache, dizziness, breast discomfort, depression, skin disorders, disturbances of appetite, weight increase, change in libido

---

Medroxyprogesterone acetate

Medroxyprogesterone acetate is a complementary drug

Injection (Suspension for injection), medroxyprogesterone acetate 150 mg/ml, 1-ml vial

Uses: parenteral progestogen-only contraception (short-term or long-term)

Contraindications: pregnancy (Appendix 2); hormone-dependent breast or genital neoplasms; undiagnosed vaginal bleeding; hepatic impairment or active liver disease (Appendix 5); severe arterial disease; porphyria

Precautions: migraine; liver disease; thromboembolic or coronary vascular disease; diabetes mellitus; trophoblastic disease; hypertension; renal disease; breastfeeding (Appendix 3); **interactions:** Appendix 1

Dosage:

Contraception (short-term), *by deep intramuscular injection*, ADULT (female) 150 mg within first 5 days of cycle or within first 5 days after parturition (delay until 6 weeks after parturition if breastfeeding)

Contraception (long-term), *by deep intramuscular injection*, ADULT (female) as for short-term, repeated every 12 weeks

ADMINISTRATION. If interval between injections is greater than 12 weeks and 5 days, exclude pregnancy before next injection and advise patient to use additional contraceptive measures (for example barrier) for 14 days after the injection

PATIENT ADVICE. Women must receive full counselling (backed by manufacturer's approved leaflet) before treatment, concerning menstrual irregularities and because of prolonged activity and the potential for a delay in return to full fertility

---

Adverse effects: menstrual irregularities; delayed return to fertility; reduction in bone mineral density; weight gain; depression; rarely, anaphylaxis

---

Norethisterone enantate

Norethisterone enantate is a complementary drug

Oily injection (Solution for injection), norethisterone enantate 200 mg/ml, 1-ml ampoule

Uses: parenteral progestogen-only contraception (short-term)

Contraindications: pregnancy (Appendix 2); breast or endometrial cancer; severe liver disease (Dubin-Johnson or Rotor syndromes) (Appendix 5); history during pregnancy of jaundice, pruritus, herpes or of deteriorating otosclerosis; severe diabetes mellitus with vascular changes; hypertension; 12 weeks before planned surgery and during immobilization; thromboembolic disease; disturbances of lipid metabolism; undiagnosed vaginal bleeding; porphyria

Precautions: migraine; liver dysfunction; depression; diabetes mellitus; previous ectopic pregnancy; breastfeeding (Appendix 3); cardiac and renal disease; **interactions:** Appendix 1

Dosage:

Short-term contraception, *by deep intramuscular injection* into gluteal muscle, ADULT (female) 200 mg within first five days of cycle or immediately after parturition; may be repeated once after 8 weeks

PATIENT ADVICE. Women must receive full counselling (backed by manufacturer's approved leaflet) before treatment, concerning possible menstrual irregularities and because of prolonged activity

Adverse effects: bloating, breast discomfort, headache, dizziness, depression, nausea; rarely, weight gain; menstrual irregularities

18.3.2 Intrauterine contraceptive devices

Intrauterine devices consist of a plastic carrier wound with copper wire or fitted with copper bands; some also have a central core of silver to prevent fragmentation of copper. Smaller devices have been introduced to minimize adverse effects and the replacement time for these devices is 5 years.

The intrauterine device is suitable for older parous women; they should be used with caution in young nulliparous women because of the increased risk of pelvic inflammatory disease. Insertion of a copper intrauterine contraceptive device is also an effective method of emergency contraception.

The timing and technique of fitting an intrauterine device play a critical part in its subsequent performance and call for proper training and experience. Patients should receive full counselling backed by the manufacturer's approved leaflet. For routine contraception the optimal time for insertion is the three to four day period after the end of menstruation; for emergency contraception the device can be inserted at any time in the menstrual cycle. There is an increased risk of infection for 20 days after insertion and this may be related to existing lower genital tract infection. Pre-screening (at least for chlamydia) should if possible be performed. If sustained pelvic or lower abdominal pain occur during the following 20 days after insertion of the device, the woman should be treated as having acute pelvic inflammatory disease. An intrauterine device should not be removed in mid-cycle unless an additional contraceptive was used for the previous 7 days. If removal is essential (for example to treat severe pelvic infection) post-coital contraception should be considered. If the woman becomes pregnant, the device should be removed in the first trimester.

Copper-containing IUD

Uses: contraception; emergency contraception

Contraindications: pregnancy; severe anaemia; 48 hours–4 weeks post partum; puerperal sepsis; postseptic abortion; cervical or endometrial cancer; pelvic inflammatory disease; recent sexually transmitted disease (if not fully investigated and treated); pelvic tuberculosis; unexplained uterine bleeding; malignant gestational trophoblastic disease; distorted or small uterine cavity; copper allergy; Wilson disease; medical diathermy

Precautions: anaemia; heavy menstrual bleeding, endometriosis, severe primary dysmenorrhoea, history of pelvic inflammatory disease, history of ectopic pregnancy or tubal surgery, diabetes mellitus, fertility problems, nulliparity and young age, severely scarred uterus or severe cervical stenosis, valvular heart disease (requires antibiotic cover)—avoid if prosthetic valve or history of endocarditis; HIV infection or immunosuppressive therapy; joint and other prostheses; epilepsy; increased risk of expulsion if inserted before uterine involution; gynaecological examination before insertion, 6–8 weeks after then annually, but counsel women to see doctor if significant symptoms such as pain; anticoagulant therapy; remove if pregnancy occurs (if pregnancy, increased likelihood of ectopic pregnancy)

Administration: Contraception, the device is best fitted after the end of menstrual bleeding and before the calculated timed of implantation; it should not be fitted during the heavy days of the period

Emergency contraception, the device may be inserted up to 120 hours (5 days) after unprotected intercourse, at any time in the menstrual cycle; if intercourse has occurred more than 5 days previously, the device can still be inserted up to 5 days after the earliest likely calculated ovulation. The device can be removed at the beginning of menstruation if the woman does not wish to continue using it

Adverse effects: uterine or cervical perforation, displacement, expulsion; pelvic infection may be exacerbated; heavy menstrual bleeding; dysmenorrhoea; pain and bleeding and occasionally epileptic seizure, or vasovagal attack on insertion

18.3.3 Barrier and spermicidal methods

NOTE. Barrier methods are not as effective in preventing conception as hormonal contraception and copper intrauterine devices. Spermicidal methods when used alone are generally considered relatively ineffective and such use is not recommended

Barriers, male latex condoms, male non-latex condoms or female non-latex condoms

Spermicidals: film, vaginal tablets, foam, gel or cream containing nonoxinol (various concentrations)

Barriers and spermicidals, diaphragm or cervical caps for use in conjunction with spermicide

Uses: contraception; to decrease risk of transmission of AIDS and other sexually transmitted diseases

Precautions: oil-based products including baby oil, massage oil, lipstick, petroleum jelly, sun-tan oil can damage latex condoms and render them less effective as barrier method of contraception and as a protection from sexually transmitted diseases (including AIDS); if a lubricant required, use one that is water-based; male condom must be put on before the penis touches the vaginal area and the penis must not touch the vaginal area after the condom has been taken off

Adverse effects: vaginal irritation and allergic vaginitis, toxic shock syndrome, increased risk of urinary-tract infection (due to nonoxinol)

18.4 Estrogens

Estrogens are necessary for the development of female secondary sexual characteristics; they also stimulate myometrial hypertrophy with endometrial hyperplasia. They affect bone by increasing calcium deposition and have a favourable effect on blood cholesterol and phospholipid concentrations. They are secreted at varying rates during the menstrual cycle throughout the period of activity of the ovaries. During pregnancy, the placenta becomes the main source of estrogens. At the menopause, ovarian secretion declines at varying rates.

Estrogen therapy is given cyclically or continuously for a number of gynaecological conditions principally contraception and the alleviation of menopausal symptoms. If long-term therapy is required for menopausal hormone therapy a progestogen should be added to prevent cystic hyperplasia of the endometrium and possible transformation to cancer. The addition of a progestogen is not necessary if the patient has had a hysterectomy.

The palliative care of advanced inoperable, metastatic carcinoma of the breast in both men and postmenopausal women is another indication for estrogen therapy.

HORMONE REPLACEMENT THERAPY (HRT). Estrogens are used for replacement therapy in perimenopausal and menopausal women for the treatment of vasomotor instability, vulvar and vaginal atrophy associated with the menopause and for the prevention of osteoporosis and may reduce mortality from ischaemic heart disease. Hormone replacement therapy is indicated for menopausal women whose lives are inconvenienced by vaginal atrophy or vasomotor instability. Vaginal atrophy may respond to a short course of a vaginal estrogen preparation. Systemic treatment is needed for vasomotor symptoms and should be given for at least a year; in women with a uterus, a progestogen should be added to reduce the risk of endometrial cancer.

HRT for 5–10 years is indicated for women with early natural or surgical menopause (before age of 45) since they have a high risk of osteoporosis. Long-term HRT is favourable in risk:benefit terms for women without a uterus, because additional progestogen is not required, but the possible increased risk of breast cancer needs to be taken into account. In women with a uterus, the need for additional progestogen (for example norethisterone 1 mg on days 15–26 of each 28-day estrogen HRT cycle) may blunt the protective effect of low dose estrogen against myocardial infarction and stroke. In these cases, the risk factors for osteoporosis (recent corticosteroid therapy, family history, thinness, lack of exercise, alcoholism or smoking, fractures to the hip or forearm before age 65 years) should be taken into account in deciding risk:benefit before HRT use; women of Afro-Caribbean origin appear to be less susceptible than those who are white or of Asian origin.

Most of the severe adverse effects rarely associated with estrogen/progestogen contraception are not associated with hormonal replacement therapy. There is an increased risk of deep-vein thrombosis and of pulmonary embolism in women taking HRT but the overall balance of benefits outweighs the risk in most women. In women who have predisposing factors such as a personal or family history of deep venous thrombosis or pulmonary embolism, severe varicose veins, obesity, surgery, trauma or prolonged bed-rest, the overall risk may outweigh the benefit.

HRT does not provide contraception. If a potentially fertile woman needs to use HRT, non-hormonal contraceptive measures are necessary.

Ethinylestradiol
Ethinylestradiol is a representative estrogen. Various drugs can serve as alternatives

Tablets, ethinylestradiol 10 micrograms, 50 micrograms

Uses: hormone replacement for menopausal symptoms; osteoporosis prophylaxis; palliation in breast cancer in men and postmenopausal women; contraception in combination with a progestogen (section 18.3.1)

Contraindications: pregnancy; estrogen-dependent cancer; active thrombophlebitis or thromboembolic disorders; undiagnosed vaginal bleeding; breastfeeding (Appendix 3); liver disease (where liver function tests have failed to return to normal), Dubin-Johnson and Rotor syndromes (or monitor closely)

Precautions: progestogen may need to be added to regimen to reduce risk of endometrial cancer due to unopposed estrogen (see notes above); migraine; history of breast nodules of fibrocystic disease; pre-existing uterine fibroids may increase in size; symptoms of endometriosis may be exacerbated; increased risk of gallbladder disease; porphyria; **interactions:** Appendix 1

Dosage:

Hormone replacement, *by mouth*, ADULT (female) 10–20 micrograms daily

Palliation in breast cancer in postmenopausal women, *by mouth*, ADULT 0.1–1 mg 3 times daily

Adverse effects: nausea and vomiting, abdominal cramps and bloating, weight increase; breast enlargement and tenderness; premenstrual-like syndrome; sodium and fluid retention; changes in liver function; cholestatic jaundice; rashes and chloasma; changes in libido; depression, headache, migraine, dizziness, leg cramps (rule out venous thrombosis); contact lenses may irritate

18.5   Progestogens

Progesterone is a hormone secreted by the corpus luteum whose actions include induction of secretory changes in the endometrium, relaxation of uterine smooth muscle and production of changes in the vaginal epithelium. Progesterone is relatively inactive following oral administration and produces local reactions at site of injection. This has led to the development of synthetic progestogens including **levonorgestrel**, **norethisterone** and **medroxyprogesterone**. Where endometriosis requires drug treatment, it may respond to synthetic progestogens on a continuous basis. They may also be used for the treatment of severe dysmenorrhoea. In postmenopausal women receiving long-term estrogen therapy for hormone replacement therapy, a progestogen needs to be added for women with an intact uterus to prevent hyperplasia of the endometrium (section 18.4).

Progestogens are also used in combined oral contraceptives and progestogen-only oral contraceptives (section 18.3.1.).

Norethisterone

Tablets, norethisterone 5 mg

Uses: endometriosis; menorrhagia; severe dysmenorrhoea; contraception (section 18.3.1); HRT (section 18.4)

Contraindications: pregnancy (Appendix 2); undiagnosed vaginal bleeding; hepatic impairment or active liver disease (Appendix 5); severe arterial disease; breast or genital tract cancer; porphyria; history in pregnancy of idiopathic jaundice, severe pruritus or pemphigoid gestationis

Precautions: epilepsy; migraine; diabetes mellitus; hypertension; cardiac or renal disease; breastfeeding (Appendix 3); **interactions:** Appendix 1

Dosage:

Endometriosis, *by mouth*, ADULT (female) 10 mg daily starting on fifth day of cycle (increased if spotting occurs to 20–25 mg daily, reduced once bleeding has stopped)

Menorrhagia, *by mouth*, ADULT (female) 5 mg three times daily for 10 days to stop bleeding; to prevent bleeding 5 mg twice daily from day 19 to 26 of cycle

Dysmenorrhoea, *by mouth*, ADULT (female) 5 mg 2–3 times daily from day 5 to 24 for 3 to 4 cycles

Adverse effects: acne, urticaria, fluid retention, weight increase, gastrointestinal disturbances, changes in libido, breast discomfort, premenstrual symptoms, irregular menstrual cycles, depression, insomnia, somnolence, alopecia, hirsutism, anaphylactoid-like reactions; exacerbation of epilepsy and migraine; rarely jaundice

18.6 Ovulation inducers

The anti-estrogen, **clomifene** is used in the treatment of female infertility due to disturbances in ovulation. It induces gonadotrophin release by occupying estrogen receptors in the hypothalamus, thereby interfering with feedback mechanisms. Patients should be carefully counselled and should be fully aware of the potential adverse effects, including a risk of multiple pregnancy (rarely more than twins), of this treatment. Most patients who are going to respond will do so to the first course; 3 courses should be adequate; long-term cyclical therapy (more than 6 cycles) is not recommended as it may increase risk of ovarian cancer.

Clomifene citrate

Tablets, clomifene citrate 50 mg

Uses: anovulatory infertility

Contraindications: hepatic disease; ovarian cysts; hormone dependent tumours or uterine bleeding of undetermined cause; pregnancy (exclude before treatment, Appendix 2)

Precautions: visual disturbances (discontinue and initiate eye examination) and ovarian hyperstimulation syndrome (discontinue treatment immediately); polycystic ovary syndrome (cysts may enlarge during treatment); uterine fibroids, ectopic pregnancy, incidence of multiple births increased (consider ultrasound monitoring); breastfeeding (Appendix 3)

Dosage:

Anovulatory infertility, *by mouth*, ADULT (female) 50 mg daily for 5 days, starting within 5 days of onset of menstruation, preferably on the second day, or at any time if cycles have ceased; a second course of 100 mg daily for 5 days may be given in the absence of ovulation

Adverse effects: visual disturbances, ovarian hyperstimulation, hot flushes, abdominal discomfort, occasional nausea and vomiting, depression, insomnia, breast tenderness, headache, intermenstrual spotting, menorrhagia, endometriosis, convulsions, weight gain, rashes, dizziness and hair loss

18.7 Insulins and other antidiabetic drugs

Diabetes mellitus is characterized by hyperglycaemia and disturbances of carbohydrate, fat and protein metabolism. There are 2 principal types of diabetes.

Type 1 diabetes or insulin-dependent diabetes mellitus is due to a defiency of insulin caused by autoimmune destruction of pancreatic beta cells. Patients require administration of insulin.

Type 2 diabetes or non-insulin dependent diabetes mellitus is due to reduced secretion of insulin or to peripheral resistance to the action of insulin. Patients may be controlled by diet alone, but often require administration of oral antidiabetic drugs or insulin. The energy and carbohydrate intake must be adequate but obesity should be avoided. In type 2 diabetes, obesity is one of the factors associated with insulin resistance. Diets high in complex carbohydrate and fibre and low in fat are beneficial. Emphasis should be placed on exercise and increased activity.

The aim of treatment is to achieve the best possible control of plasma glucose concentration and prevent or minimize complications including microvascular complications (retinopathy, albuminuria, neuropathy). Diabetes mellitus is a strong risk factor for cardiovascular disease. Other risk factors such as smoking, hypertension, obesity and hyperlipidaemia should also be addressed.

Insulin

For those who require administration of insulin, appropriate combinations of insulin therapy will have to be worked out for the individual patient. Insulin requirements may be affected by variations in lifestyle (diet and exercise) and use of drugs such as corticosteroids, infections, stress, accidental or surgical trauma, puberty and pregnancy (second and third trimesters) may increase insulin requirements; renal or hepatic impairment and some endocrine disorders (for example Addison disease, hypopituitarism) or coelic disease may reduce requirements. In pregnancy insulin requirements should be monitored frequently.

Most patients can and should monitor their own blood glucose concentrations using blood glucose strips. Since blood glucose levels vary throughout the day, it is best to recommend that patients should maintain blood glucose concentrations of between 4 and 10 mmol/litre for most of the day while accepting that on occasions levels will be higher; strenuous efforts should be made to prevent blood glucose concentrations falling below 4 mmol/litre. Patients should be advised to look for troughs and peaks of blood glucose and to adjust their insulin dosage only once or twice a week. Insulin doses are determined on an individual basis, by gradually increasing the dose but avoiding hypoglycaemic reactions.

In the absence of blood glucose monitoring strips, urine glucose can be tested to ensure glucose levels are not too high. It is the method of personal choice for many patients with Type 2 diabetes mellitus. It is less reliable than blood glucose but is easier and costs much less. All patients should monitor either blood or urine glucose levels daily.

Hypoglycaemia is a potential complication in all patients with diabetes mellitus whether they are treated with insulin or oral hypoglycaemic agents. The serious consequences of hypoglycaemia relate to its effects on the brain, including loss of cognitive function, seizures, coma and cerebral infarction.

The risk of hypoglycaemia is particularly high when meticulous glycaemic control is sought in patients receiving insulin. Very tight control lowers the blood glucose concentration needed to trigger hypoglycaemic symptoms; increase in the frequency of hypoglycaemic episodes reduces the warning symptoms experienced by patients. Some patients report loss of hypoglycaemic warning after transfer to human insulin. To restore warning signs, episodes of hypoglycaemia must be reduced to a minimum; this involves an appropriate adjustment of insulin type, dose and frequency and suitable timing and quantity of meals and snacks. Car drivers need to be particularly careful to avoid hypoglycaemia. They should check their blood glucose concentrations before driving and, on long journeys, at intervals of approximately two hours; they should ensure that a supply of sugar is always readily available. If hypoglycaemia occurs the driver should switch off the ignition until recovery is complete (may be 15 minutes or longer). Driving is not permitted when hypoglycaemic awareness has been lost. For sporadic physical activity departing from the patient's usual daily routine extra carbohydrate may need to be taken to avert hypoglycaemia. Blood glucose should be monitored before, during and after exercise. Hypoglycaemia can develop in patients taking oral antidiabetics, notably the sulfonylureas, although this is uncommon and usually indicates excessive dosage. Sulphonylurea-induced hypoglycaemia may persist for several hours and must be treated in hospital.

Diabetic ketoacidosis is a potentially lethal condition caused by an absolute or relative lack of insulin and commonly occurs after failure to adjust insulin dosage in the presence of factors which increase insulin requirements such a severe infection or major intercurrent illness. Diabetes ketoacidosis occurs mostly in patients with Type 1 diabetes mellitus. It also occurs in diabetics who are not insulin-dependent but in whom the need for insulin may be temporarily created. It is characterized by hyperglycaemia, hyperketonaemia and acidaemia with dehydration and electrolyte disturbances. It is essential that insulin (and intravenous fluids) should be readily available for its treatment.

Infections are more likely to develop in patients with poorly controlled diabetes mellitus. These should be treated promptly and effectively to avoid diabetic ketoacidosis.

Surgery. Particular attention should be given to the insulin requirements when an insulin-dependent diabetic patient undergoes surgery that is likely to need an intravenous infusion of insulin for longer than 12 hours. Soluble insulin should be given together with glucose and potassium chloride (provided the patient is not hyperkalaemic) intravenously and adjusted to provide a blood glucose concentration of between 7 and 12 mmol/litre. The duration of action of intravenous insulin is only a few minutes therefore the infusion must not be stopped unless the patient becomes frankly hypoglycaemic. For non-insulin dependent diabetics, insulin treatment is almost always required during surgery (oral antidiabetic drugs having been omitted).

Insulin must be given by injection as it is inactivated by gastrointestinal enzymes. Following subcutaneous or intramuscular injection, it is absorbed directly into the blood. Subcutaneous injection into the upper arms, thighs, buttocks, or abdomen is the route most commonly used. There may be increased absorption from a limb site, if the limb is used in strenuous exercise following the injection. It is essential to use only syringes calibrated for the particular concentration of insulin administered.

There are three main types of insulin preparations, classified according to duration of action after subcutaneous injection:

- those of short duration which have a relatively rapid onset of action, namely soluble or regular insulin;
- those with an intermediate action for example isophane insulin and insulin zinc suspension;
- those with a relatively slow onset and long duration of action for example crystalline insulin zinc suspension.

Soluble insulin is a short-acting form of insulin. When injected subcutaneously, it has a rapid onset of action (after 30–60 minutes), a peak action between 2 and 4 hours, and a duration of action up to 8 hours. When injected intravenously, soluble insulin has a very short half-life of only about 5 minutes.

When administered subcutaneously, **intermediate-acting insulins** have an onset of action of approximately 1–2 hours, a maximal effect at 4–12 hours and a duration of action of 16–24 hours. They can be given twice daily together with short-acting insulin or once daily, particularly in elderly patients. They can be mixed with soluble insulin in the syringe, essentially retaining properties of each component.

The duration of action of different insulin preparations varies considerably from one patient to another and this needs to be assessed for every individual. The type of insulin used and its dose and frequency of administration depend on the needs of each patient. For patients with acute onset diabetes mellitus, treatment should be started with soluble insulin given 3 times daily with medium acting insulin at bedtime. For those less seriously ill, treatment is usually started with a mixture of pre-mixed short and medium acting insulins given twice daily. The proportions of soluble insulin can be increased in patients with excessive post-prandial hyperglycaemia. Patients should remain on the same insulin throughout treatment.

Regimens should be developed by each country.

Soluble insulin

Injection (Solution for injection), soluble insulin 40 units/ml, 10-ml vial; 100 units/ml, 10-ml vial

Uses: diabetes mellitus; diabetic emergencies and at surgery; diabetic ketoacidosis or coma

Precautions: see notes above; reduce dose in renal impairment (Appendix 4); occasionally insulin resistance necessitating large doses; pregnancy and breastfeeding (Appendices 2 and 3); **interactions:** Appendix 1

Dosage:

Diabetes mellitus, *by subcutaneous injection, by intramuscular injection, by intravenous injection or by intravenous infusion*, ADULT and CHILD according to individual requirements

Adverse effects: hypoglycaemia in overdose; localized and rarely, generalized, allergic reactions; lipoatrophy at injection site; insulin resistance

Isophane insulin

Injection (Suspension for injection), isophane insulin 40 units/ml, 10-ml vial; 100 units/ml, 10-ml vial

Uses: diabetes mellitus

Contraindications: intravenous administration

Precautions: see notes above; reduce dose in renal impairment (Appendix 4); occasionally insulin resistance necessitating large doses; pregnancy and breastfeeding (Appendices 2 and 3); **interactions:** Appendix 1

Dosage:

Diabetes mellitus, *by subcutaneous injection*, ADULT and CHILD according to individual requirements

IMPORTANT. Intravenous injection contraindicated

Adverse effects: hypoglycaemia in overdose; localized and rarely generalized, allergic reactions; lipoatrophy at injection site; insulin resistance

Oral antidiabetic drugs

Oral antidiabetic drugs are used for non-insulin-dependent diabetes mellitus in patients who do not respond to dietary adjustment and an increase in physical exercise. They are used to supplement the effect of diet and exercise. There are various types of oral antidiabetic agents. The most commonly used are the **sulfonylureas** and the **biguanide**, metformin.

Sulfonylureas act mainly by augmenting insulin secretion and are therefore only effective if there is some residual pancreatic beta-cell activity. They may occasionally lead to hypoglycaemia 4 hours or more after food. This may be dose-related and usually indicates excessive dose and it occurs more frequently with long-acting sulfonylureas such as **glibenclamide** and occurs particularly in the elderly. The sulfonylureas have the disadvantage that they may encourage weight gain. They should not be used during breastfeeding and caution is required in the elderly and those with renal or hepatic insufficiency because of the risk of hypoglycaemia. Insulin therapy is generally required during intercurrent illness, during surgery and also during pregnancy.

Metformin exerts its effect by decreasing gluconeogenesis and by increasing peripheral utilization of glucose. Metformin can only act in the presence of endogenous insulin therefore is effective only in diabetics with some residual functioning pancreatic islet cells. It is used as a first-line treatment in overweight non-insulin-dependent diabetic patients and in others when strict dieting and sulfonylureas have failed to control the disease. Gastrointestinal adverse effects are common on initial treatment and may persist, particularly when very high doses are given. Metformin should be avoided in situations which might predispose to lactic acidosis including renal and hepatic impairment and severe dehydration. One major advantage of metformin is that it does not usually cause hypoglycaemia. It may be used together with insulin (but weight gain and hypoglycaemia can be problems) or sulfonylureas (but may be increased hazard with such combinations). During medical and surgical emergencies insulin treatment is almost always required; insulin should be substituted for metformin before elective surgery.

Glibenclamide

Glibenclamide is a representative long-acting sulfonylurea. Various drugs can act as alternatives

Tablets, glibenclamide 2.5 mg, 5 mg

Uses: diabetes mellitus

Contraindications: ketoacidosis; porphyria; pregnancy (Appendix 2); breastfeeding (Appendix 3)

Precautions: renal impairment (Appendix 4); hepatic impairment (Appendix 5); elderly; substitute insulin during severe infection, trauma, surgery (see notes above); **interactions:** Appendix 1

Dosage:

Diabetes mellitus, *by mouth*, ADULT initially 5 mg once daily with breakfast (ELDERLY 2.5 mg, but avoid—see notes above), adjusted according to response (maximum 15 mg daily)

Adverse effects: mild and infrequent, including gastrointestinal disturbances and headache; hypersensitivity reactions; hypoglycaemia, particularly in the elderly

Metformin hydrochloride

Tablets, metformin hydrochloride 500 mg, 850 mg

Uses: diabetes mellitus (see notes above)

Contraindications: renal impairment (withdraw if renal impairment suspected; Appendix 4); hepatic impairment (Appendix 5); predisposition to lactic acidosis (see notes above); heart failure; severe infections or trauma; dehydration; alcohol dependence; pregnancy (Appendix 2)

Precautions: substitute insulin during severe infection, trauma, surgery (see notes above); breastfeeding (Appendix 3); **interactions:** Appendix 1

Dosage:

Diabetes mellitus, *by mouth,* ADULT 500 mg every 8 hours *or* 850 mg every 12 hours with or after food (maximum 2 g daily in divided doses)

Adverse effects: anorexia, nausea and vomiting, diarrhoea (usually transient); lactic acidosis most likely in patients with renal failure (discontinue); decreased vitamin B_{12} absorption

18.8 Thyroid hormones and antithyroid drugs

Thyroid agents are natural or synthetic agents containing **levothyroxine** (thyroxine) or **liothyronine** (tri-iodothyronine). The principal effect is to increase the metabolic rate. They also exert a cardiostimulatory effect which may be the result of a direct action on the heart.

Thyroid hormones are used in hypothyroidism (myxoedema) and also in diffuse non-toxic goitre, Hashimoto thyroiditis (lymphadenoid goitre) and thyroid carcinoma. Neonatal hypothyroidism requires prompt treatment for normal development.

Levothyroxine sodium (thyroxine sodium) is the treatment of choice for maintenance therapy. It is almost completely absorbed from the gastrointestinal tract but the full effects are not seen for up to 1 to 3 weeks after beginning therapy; there is a slow response to dose change and effects may persist for several weeks after withdrawal. Dosage of levothyroxine in infants and children for congenital hypothyroidism and juvenile myxoedema should be titrated according to clinical response, growth assessment and measurement of plasma thyroxine and thyroid-stimulating hormone.

Antithyroid drugs such as **propylthiouracil** and carbimazole are used in the management of thyrotoxicosis. They are also used to prepare the patient for thyroidectomy. They are usually well-tolerated, with mild leukopenia or rashes developing in a few percent of cases, usually during the first 6–8 weeks of therapy. During this time the blood count should be checked every 2 weeks or if a sore throat or other signs of infection develop. The drugs are generally given in a high dose in the first instance until the patient becomes euthyroid, the dose may then be gradually reduced to a maintenance dose which is continued for 12–18 months, followed by monitoring to identify relapse.

There is a lag time of some 2 weeks between the achievement of biochemical euthyroidism and clinical euthyroidism. Beta-adrenoceptor antagonists (beta-blockers) (usually propranolol) may be used as a short-term adjunct to antithyroid drugs to control symptoms but their use in heart failure associated with thyrotoxicosis is controversial.

Treatment can be given, if necessary, in pregnancy but antithyroid drugs cross the placenta and in high doses may cause fetal goitre and hypothyroidism. The lowest dose that will control the hyperthyroid state should be used (requirements in Graves disease tend to fall during pregnancy). Propylthiouracil appears in breast milk but does not preclude breastfeeding as long as neonatal development is closely monitored and the lowest effective dose is used.

If surgery (partial thyroidectomy) is contemplated, it may be necessary to give **iodine** for 10 to 14 days in addition to antithyroid drugs to assist control and reduce vascularity of the thyroid. Iodine should not be used for long-term treatment since its antithyroid action tends to diminish. In patients in whom drug therapy fails to achieve long-term remissions definitive treatment with surgery or (increasingly) radioactive iodine is preferable.

Levothyroxine sodium

Tablets, levothyroxine sodium 25 micrograms, 50 micrograms, 100 micrograms

Uses: hypothyroidism

Contraindications: thyrotoxicosis

Precautions: cardiovascular disorders (myocardial insufficiency or ECG evidence of myocardial infarction); hypopituitarism or predisposition to adrenal insufficiency (must be corrected by corticosteroid prior to initial levothyroxine); elderly; long-standing hypothyroidism, diabetes insipidus, diabetes mellitus (may need to increase dose of insulin or oral antidiabetic drug); pregnancy (Appendix 2), breastfeeding (Appendix 3); **interactions:** Appendix 1

Dosage:

Hypothyroidism, *by mouth*, ADULT initially 50–100 micrograms daily (25–50 micrograms for those over 50 years) before breakfast, increased by 25–50 micrograms every 3–4 weeks until normal metabolism maintained (usual maintenance dose, 100–200 micrograms daily); where there is cardiac disease, initially 25 micrograms daily *or* 50 micrograms on alternate days, adjusted in steps of 25 micrograms every 4 weeks

Congenital hypothyroidism and juvenile myxoedema (see notes above), *by mouth*, CHILD up to 1 month, initially 5–10 micrograms/kg daily, CHILD over 1 month, initally 5 micrograms/kg daily, adjusted in steps of 25 micrograms every 2–4 weeks, until mild toxic symptoms appear, then reduce dose slightly

Adverse effects: (usually with excessive dose) anginal pain, arrhythmias, palpitations, tachycardia, skeletal muscle cramps, diarrhoea, vomiting, tremors, restlessness, excitability, insomnia, headache, flushing, sweating, excessive loss of weight and muscular weakness

---

Propylthiouracil

Propylthiouracil is a representative antithyroid drug. Various drugs can serve as alternatives

Tablets, propylthiouracil 50 mg

Uses: hyperthyroidism

Precautions: large goitre; pregnancy and breastfeeding (see also notes; Appendices 2 and 3); hepatic impairment (Appendix 5)—withdraw treatment if hepatic function deteriorates (fatal reactions reported); renal impairment—reduce dosage (Appendix 4)

Dosage:

Hyperthyroidism, *by mouth*, ADULT 300–600 mg daily until patient becomes euthyroid; dose may then be gradually reduced to a maintenance dose of 50–150 mg daily

PATIENT ADVICE. Warn patient to tell doctor immediately if sore throat, mouth ulcers, bruising, fever, malaise, or non-specific illness occurs

Adverse effects: nausea, rashes, pruritus, arthralgia, headache; rarely, alopecia, cutaneous vasculitis, thrombocytopenia, aplastic anaemia, lupus erythematosus-like syndrome, jaundice, hepatitis

---

Potassium iodide

Tablets, potassium iodide 60 mg

Uses: thyrotoxicosis (pre-operative treatment); sporotrichosis, subcutaneous phycomycosis (section 6.3)

Contraindications: breastfeeding (Appendix 3); long-term treatment

Precautions: pregnancy (Appendix 2), children

Dosage:

Pre-operative management of thyrotoxicosis, *by mouth*, ADULT 60–180 mg daily

Adverse effects: hypersensitivity reactions including coryza-like symptoms, headache, lacrimation, conjunctivitis, pain in salivary glands, laryngitis, bronchitis, rashes; on prolonged treatment, depression, insomnia, impotence, goitre in infants of mothers taking iodides

Section 19: Immunologicals

Active immunity

Active immunity may be induced by the administration of micro-organisms or their products which act as antigens to induce antibodies to confer a protective immune response in the host. Vaccination may consist of (a) a **live attenuated** form of a virus or bacteria, (b) **inactivated** preparations of the virus or bacteria, or (c) **extracts of** or **detoxified exotoxins**. Live attenuated vaccines usually confer immunity with a single dose which is of long duration. Inactivated vaccines may require a series of injections in the first instance to produce an adequate antibody response and in most cases, require reinforcing (booster) doses. The duration of immunity varies from months to many years. Extracts of or detoxified exotoxins require a primary series of injections followed by reinforcing doses.

Passive immunity

Passive immunity is conferred by injecting preparations made from the plasma of immune individuals with adequate levels of antibody to the disease for which protection is sought. Treatment has to be given soon after exposure to be effective. This immunity lasts only a few weeks but passive immunization can be repeated where necessary.

19.1 Diagnostic agents

The **tuberculin test** has limited diagnostic value. A positive tuberculin test indicates previous exposure to mycobacterial antigens through infection with one of the tubercle bacilli, or BCG vaccination. The tuberculin test does not distinguish between tuberculosis and other mycobacterial infection, between active and quiescent disease, or between acquired infection and seroconversion induced by BCG vaccination.

Tuberculin purified protein derivative (tuberculin PPD)

All tuberculins should comply with the requirements for tuberculins (revised 1985). who technical report series, no.745, 1987, annex 1.

Injection, tuberculin purified protein derivative 100 units/ml, 10 units/ml

Uses: test for hypersensitivity to tuberculoprotein

Contraindications: should not be used within 3 weeks of receiving a live viral vaccine

Precautions: elderly; malnutrition; viral or bacterial infections (including HIV and severe tuberculosis), malignant disease, corticosteroid or immunosuppressant therapy—diminished sensitivity to tuberculin; avoid contact with open cuts, abraded or diseased skin, eyes or mouth

Dosage:

NOTE. National recommendations may vary

Test for hypersensitivity to tuberculoprotein, *by intradermal injection*, ADULT and CHILD 5 or 10 units (1 unit may be used in hypersensitive patients or if tuberculosis is suspected)

ADMINISTRATION. According to manufacturer's directions

Adverse effects: occasionally nausea, headache, malaise, rash; immediate local reactions (more common in atopic patients); rarely, vesicular or ulcerating local reactions, regional adenopathy and fever

19.2 Sera and immunoglobulins

Antibodies of human origin are usually termed **immunoglobulins**. Material prepared from animals is called **antiserum**. Because of serum sickness and other allergic-type reactions that may follow injections of antisera, this therapy has been replaced wherever possible by the use of immunoglobulins.

All immunoglobulins and antisera should comply with WHO requirements for blood and plasma products.

CONTRAINDICATIONS AND PRECAUTIONS. Anaphylaxis, although rare, can occur and epinephrine must always be immediately available during immunization.

The IgA content of normal immunoglobulins can result in the development of IgE and IgG anti-IgA antibodies in immunodeficient patients with IgA deficiency. Normal immunoglobulin should not be used in patients with known class specific antibody to immunoglobulin A (IgA).

Immunoglobulins may interfere with the immune response to live virus vaccines which should normally be given *either at least 3 weeks before or at least 3 months after* the administration of the immunoglobulin.

ADVERSE REACTIONS. *Intramuscular injection.* Local reactions including pain and tenderness may occur at the injection site. Hypersensitivity reactions may occur including, rarely, anaphylaxis.

Intravenous injection. Systemic reactions including fever, chills, facial flushing, headache and nausea may occur, particularly following high rates of infusion. Hypersensitivity reactions may occur including, rarely, anaphylaxis.

19.2.1 Anti-D immunoglobulin (human)

Anti-D immunoglobulin is prepared from plasma with a high titre of anti-D antibody. It is available to prevent a rhesus-negative mother from forming antibodies to fetal rhesus-positive cells which may pass into the maternal circulation. The aim is to protect any subsequent child from the hazard of haemolytic disease of the newborn. It should be administered following any sensitizing episode (for example abortion, miscarriage, still-birth) immediately or within 72 hours of the episode but even if a longer period has elapsed it may still give protection and should be used. The dose of anti-D immunoglobulin given depends on the level of exposure to rhesus-positive blood. The injection of anti-D immunoglobulin is not effective once the mother has formed anti-D antibodies. It is also given following Rh_O (D) incompatible blood.

Anti-D immunoglobulin (human)

Plasma fractions should comply with the Requirements for the Collection, Processing and Quality Control of Blood, Blood Components and Plasma Derivatives (Revised 1992). WHO Technical Report Series No 840, 1994, Annexe 2

Injection, anti-D immunoglobulin 250-microgram vial

Uses: prevention of formation of antibodies to rhesus-positive blood cells in rhesus-negative patients (see notes above)

Contraindications: see introductory notes; known hypersensitivity

Precautions: see introductory notes; caution in rhesus-positive patients for treatment of blood disorders; caution in rhesus-negative patients with anti-D antibodies in their serum; **interactions:** Appendix 1

RUBELLA VACCINE. Rubella vaccine may be administered in the postpartum period at the same time as anti-D immunoglobulin injection, but only using separate syringes and separate contralateral sites

MMR VACCINE. MMR vaccine should only be given either at least 3 weeks before or at least 3 months after an injection of anti-D immunoglobulin

Dosage:

NOTE. National recommendations may vary

Following birth of a rhesus-positive infant in rhesus-negative mother, *by intramuscular injection,* ADULT 250 micrograms immediately or within 72 hours (see also notes above)

Following any potentially sensitizing episode (for example amniocentesis, still-birth), *by intramuscular injection,* ADULT up to 20 weeks' gestation, 250 micrograms per episode (after 20 weeks, 500 micrograms) immediately or within 72 hours (see notes above)

Following Rh$_O$(D) incompatible blood transfusion, *by intramuscular injection,* ADULT 10–20 micrograms per ml transfused rhesus-positive blood

Adverse effects: see introductory notes

19.2.2 Antitetanus immunoglobulin (human)

Antitetanus immunoglobulin of human origin is a preparation containing immunoglobulins derived from the plasma of adults immunized with tetanus toxoid. It is used for the management of tetanus-prone wounds in addition to wound toilet and if appropriate antibacterial prophylaxis and adsorbed tetanus vaccine (see section 19.3.1.2)

Antitetanus immunoglobulin (human)

Plasma fractions should comply with the Requirements for the Collection, Processing and Quality Control of Blood, Blood Components and Plasma Derivatives (Revised 1992). WHO Technical Report Series No 840, 1994, Annexe 2

Injection, antitetanus immunoglobulin 500 units/vial

Uses: passive immunization against tetanus as part of the management of tetanus-prone wounds

Contraindications: see introductory notes

Precautions: see introductory notes

TETANUS VACCINE. If schedule requires tetanus vaccine and antitetanus immunoglobulin to be administered at the same time, they should be administered using separate syringes and separate sites

Dosage:

NOTE. National recommendations may vary

Management of tetanus-prone wounds, *by intramuscular injection*, ADULT and CHILD 250 units, increased to 500 units if wound older than 12 hours or there is risk of heavy contamination or if patient weighs more than 90 kg; second dose of 250 units given after 3–4 weeks if patient immuno-suppressed or if active immunization with tetanus vaccine contraindicated (see also section 19.3.1.2)

Adverse effects: see introductory notes

19.2.3 Diphtheria antitoxin

Diphtheria antitoxin is prepared from the plasma or serum of healthy horses immunized against diphtheria toxin or diphtheria toxoid. It is used for passive immunization in suspected cases of diphtheria without waiting for bacterial confirmation of the infection. A test dose should be given initially to exclude hypersensitivity. Diphtheria antitoxin is not used for prophy-laxis of diphtheria because of the risk of hypersensitivity.

Diphtheria antitoxin

Injection, diphtheria antitoxin 10 000 units, 20 000 units/ vial

Uses: passive immunization in suspected cases of diphtheria

Precautions: initial test dose to exclude hypersensitivity; observation required after full dose (epinephrine and resuscitation facilities should be available)

Dosage:

NOTE. National recommendations may vary

Passive immunization in suspected diphtheria, *by intramuscular injection*, ADULT and CHILD 10 000–30 000 units in mild to moderate cases; 40 000–100 000 units in severe cases (for doses of more than 40 000 units, a portion should be given *by intramuscular injection* followed by the bulk of the dose *intravenously* after an interval of 0.5–2 hours)

Adverse effects: anaphylaxis with urticaria, hypotension, dyspnoea and shock; serum sickness up to 12 days after injection

19.2.4 Normal immunoglobulin (human)

Normal immunoglobulin is prepared from pools of at least 1000 donations of human plasma; it contains antibodies to measles, mumps, varicella, hepatitis A and other viruses currently prevalent in the general population. Normal immuno-globulin is available as two distinct preparations, one to be given intramuscularly and the other intravenously.

Normal immunoglobulin containing approximately 16% of protein, **administered intramuscularly**, is used for passive immunization for the protection of susceptible contacts against hepatitis A virus, measles and to a lesser extent, rubella.

HEPATITIS A. Control of hepatitis A depends on good hygiene, but normal immunoglobulin has been shown to be of value in the prevention and control of the disease; however, because of changes in the raw materials some brands of normal immuno-globulin may not be suitable for hepatitis A prophylaxis. Normal immunoglobulin is recommended for controlling infections in closed institutions, and under certain conditions, in school and home contacts; it is also used for occasional or short-term travellers to areas where the disease is highly endemic.

MEASLES. Normal immunoglobulin may be given for measles prophylaxis in children with compromised immunity (and adults with compromised immunity who have no measles antibodies). It should be given as soon as possible after contact with measles. It should also be given to children under 12 months with recent severe illness for whom measles should be avoided.

RUBELLA. Normal immunoglobulin does not prevent infection in non-immune contacts after exposure to rubella. It is not recommended for protection of pregnant women exposed to rubella. It may however reduce the likelihood of a clinical attack which may possibly reduce the risk to the fetus. It should only be used when termination of pregnancy is unacceptable, when it should be given as soon as possible after exposure.

Normal immunoglobulin containing 3–6% protein (may contain up to 12%) is **administered intravenously** for primary antibody deficiencies and idiopathic thrombocytopenic purpura, Kawasaki syndrome and for the prophylaxis of infection in bone-marrow transplantation.

Normal immunoglobulin (human) (for intramuscular use)

Plasma fractions should comply with the Requirements for the Collection, Processing and Quality Control of Blood, Blood Components and Plasma Derivatives (Revised 1992). WHO Technical Report Series No 840, 1994, Annexe 2

Injection, normal immunoglobulin for intramuscular use, 250-mg vial, 750-mg vial

Uses: passive immunization of susceptible contacts against hepatitis A, measles or rubella

Contraindications: see introductory notes; intravenous administration

Precautions: see introductory notes; **interactions:** Appendix 1

Dosage:

NOTE. National recommendations may vary

Hepatitis A prophylaxis for travellers (2 months or less abroad), *by deep intramuscular injection*, ADULT 250 mg; CHILD under 10 years, 125 mg

Hepatitis A, control of outbreak, *by deep intramuscular injection*, ADULT 500 mg; CHILD under 10 years, 250 mg

Measles prophylaxis, *by deep intramuscular injection*, ADULT and CHILD over 3 years, 750 mg; CHILD under 1 year 250 mg, 1–2 years, 500 mg

Rubella in pregnancy, prevention of clinical attack, *by deep intramuscular injection*, ADULT 750 mg

Adverse effects: see introductory notes

Normal immunoglobulin (human) (for intravenous use)

Plasma fractions should comply with the Requirements for the Collection, Processing and Quality Control of Blood, Blood Components and Plasma Derivatives (Revised 1992). WHO Technical Report Series No 840, 1994, Annexe 2

Injection, normal immunoglobulin for intravenous use

Uses: replacement therapy in congenital agammaglobulinaemia and hypogammaglobulinaemia; treatment of idiopathic thrombocytopenic purpura and Kawasaki syndrome; prophylaxis of infection following bone-marrow transplant

Contraindications: see introductory notes; intramuscular administration

Precautions: see introductory notes; avoid exceeding recommended rate of infusion; monitor vital signs; **interactions:** Appendix 1

Dosage:

NOTE. National recommendations may vary

According to manufacturer's directions; consult specific product literature

NOTE. Formulations from different manufacturers vary and should not be regarded as equivalent

Adverse effects: see introductory notes

19.2.5 Rabies immunoglobulin (human)

Rabies immunoglobulin is a preparation containing immunoglobulins derived from the plasma of adults immunized with rabies vaccine. It is used as part of the management of potential rabies following exposure of an unimmunized individual to an animal in or from a high-risk country. It should be administered as soon as possible after exposure without waiting for confirmation that the animal is rabid. The rabies immunoglobulin should be infiltrated round the site of the bite and also given intramuscularly. In addition rabies vaccine (see section 19.3.2.3) should be administered at a different site.

Rabies immunoglobulin (human)

Plasma fractions should comply with the Requirements for the Collection, Processing and Quality Control of Blood, Blood Components and Plasma Derivatives (Revised 1992). WHO Technical Report Series No 840, 1994, Annexe 2

Injection, rabies immunoglobulin 300-units vial, 1500-unit vial

Uses: passive immunization either post-exposure or in suspected exposure to rabies in high-risk countries in unimmunized individuals (in conjunction with rabies vaccine)

Contraindications: see introductory notes; avoid repeat doses after vaccine treatment initiated; intravenous administration

---

Precautions: see introductory notes

RABIES VACCINE. If schedule requires rabies vaccine and rabies immuno-globulin to be administered at the same time, they should be administered using seperate syringes and seperate sites

Dosage:

NOTE. National recommendations may vary

Immunization against rabies: post-exposure (or suspected exposure) treatment, *by intramuscular injection* and *wound infiltration*, ADULT and CHILD 20 units/kg (half by intramuscular injection and half by wound infiltration)

Adverse effects: see introductory notes

19.2.6 Antivenom sera

Acute envenoming from snakes or spiders is common in many parts of the world. The bite may cause local and systemic effects.

Local effects include pain, swelling, bruising and tender enlargement of regional lymph nodes. Wounds should be cleaned and pain may be relieved by analgesics.

If significant amounts of toxin are absorbed after a snake bite, this may result in early anaphylactoid symptoms such as transient hypotension, angioedema, abdominal colic, diarrhoea and vomiting, followed by persistent or recurrent hypotension and ECG abnormalities. Spontaneous systemic bleeding, coagulopathy, adult respiratory distress syndrome and acute renal failure may occur. Early anaphylactoid symptoms may be treated with epinephrine. **Snake antivenom sera** are the only specific treatment available but they can produce severe adverse reactions. They are generally only used if there is a clear indication of systemic involvement or severe local involvement or if supplies are not limited in patients at high risk of systemic or severe local involvement.

Spider bites may cause either necrotic or neurotoxic syndromes depending on the species involved. Supportive and symptomatic treatment is required and in the case of necrotic syndrome, surgical repair may be necessary. **Spider antivenom sera**, suitable for the species involved, may prevent symptoms if administered as soon as possible after envenomation.

Antivenom sera

Injection, snake antivenom serum and spider antivenom serum

NOTE. There are many antivenom sera each containing specific venom-neutralizing globulins. It is important that the specific antivenom serum suitable for the species causing the envenomation is administered

Uses: treatment of snake bites and spider bites

Precautions: resuscitation facilities should be immediately available

Dosage:

Depends on the specific antivenom used; consult manufacturer's literature

Adverse effects: serum sickness; anaphylaxis with hypotension, dyspnoea, urticaria and shock

---

19.3 Vaccines

All vaccines should comply with the WHO requirements for biological substances.

CONTRAINDICATIONS AND PRECAUTIONS. Recipients of any vaccine should be observed for an adverse reaction. Anaphylaxis though rare, can occur and epinephrine must always be immediately available whenever immunization is given. If a serious adverse event (including anaphylaxis, collapse, shock, encephalitis, encephalopathy, or non-febrile convulsion) occurs following a dose of any vaccine, a subsequent dose should not be given. In the case of a severe reaction to Diphtheria, Pertussis, and Tetanus vaccine, the pertussis component should be omitted and the vaccination completed with Diphtheria and Tetanus vaccine.

Immunization should be postponed in acute illness which may limit the response to immunization, but minor infections without fever or systemic upset are not contraindications. A definite reaction to a preceding dose is a definite contra-indication.

If alcohol or other disinfecting agent is used to wipe the injection site it must be allowed to evaporate, otherwise inactivation of a live vaccine may occur.

The intramuscular route must not be used in patients with bleeding disorders such as haemophilia or thrombocytopenia.

Some viral vaccines contain small quantities of antibacterials such as polymyxin B or neomycin; such vaccines may need to be withheld from individuals who are sensitive to the antibacterial. Some vaccines are prepared using hens' eggs and a history of anaphylaxis to egg ingestion is a contraindication to the use of such vaccines; caution is required if such vaccines are used in persons with less severe hypersensitivity to egg.

When two live virus vaccines are required (and are not available as a combined preparation) they should be given *either* simultaneously at different sites using separate syringes *or* with an interval of at least 3 weeks. Live virus vaccines should normally be given *either at least 3 weeks before or at least 3 months after* the administration of immunoglobulin.

Live vaccines should not be routinely administered to pregnant women because of the possible harm to the fetus but where there is significant risk of exposure, the need for immunization may outweigh any possible risk to the fetus.

Live vaccines should not be given to anyone with malignant disease such as leukaemia or lymphomas or other tumours of the reticulo-endothelial system. Live vaccines should not be given to individuals with an impaired immune response caused by disease, radiotherapy or drug treatment (for example, high doses of corticosteroids).

However, the WHO recommends that immunocompromised individuals who are HIV-positive should, under certain circumstances, be given some live vaccines. *Asymptomatic* and *symptomatic* HIV-positive children and women of child-bearing age should receive diphtheria, pertussis, tetanus, hepatitis B and oral poliomyelitis vaccines (included in the Expanded Programme on Immunization (EPI)). Because of the risk of early and severe measles infection, infants should receive an extra dose of measles vaccine at 6 months of age with the EPI dose as soon after 9 months of age as possible. Individuals with *symptomatic* HIV infection must **not** be given either BCG or yellow fever vaccines. Individuals with *asymptomatic* HIV infection should only be given BCG or yellow fever vaccines where the prevalence of tuberculosis or yellow fever, respectively, is high. National policies on immunization of HIV-positive individuals may vary.

ADVERSE REACTIONS. Local reactions including inflammation and lymphangitis may occur. Sterile abscess may develop at the injection site; fever, headache, malaise starting a few hours after injection and lasting for 1–2 days may occur. Hypersensitivity reactions can occur including rarely, anaphylaxis.

19.3.1 Vaccines for universal immunization
The WHO Expanded Programme on Immunization (EPI) currently recommends that all countries immunize against diphtheria, hepatitis B, measles, poliomyelitis, pertussis, tetanus and that countries with a high incidence of tuberculosis infections should immunize against tuberculosis. Immunization against yellow fever is recommended in endemic countries. Routine vaccination against *Haemophilus influenzae* type b infection is also recommended in some countries. In geographical regions where the burden of disease is unclear, efforts should be made to evaluate the magnitude of the problem.

IMMUNIZATION SCHEDULE RECOMMENDED BY WHO.

Scheme A

Recommended in countries where perinatal transmission of hepatitis B virus is frequent (for example, South East Asia)

Age	Vaccines
Birth	BCG; Poliomyelitis, oral (1st); Hepatitis B (1st)
6 weeks	Diphtheria, pertussis, tetanus (1st); Poliomyelitis, oral (2nd); Hepatitis B (2nd)
10 weeks	Diphtheria, pertussis, tetanus (2nd); Poliomyelitis, oral (3rd)
14 weeks	Diphtheria, pertussis, tetanus (3rd); Poliomyelitis, oral (4th); Hepatitis B (3rd)
9 months	Yellow fever (in countries where yellow fever poses a risk); Measles

Scheme B

Recommended in countries where perinatal transmission of hepatitis B virus is less frequent (for example, sub-Saharan Africa)

Schedule as Scheme A, but hepatitis B (1st) given at 6 weeks and hepatitis B (2nd) given at 10 weeks

19.3.1.1 BCG vaccine (dried)

Where tuberculosis remains highly prevalent, routine immunization of infants within the first year of life with BCG vaccine, derived from bacillus Calmette-Guérin (an attenuated strain of *Mycobacterium bovis*), is highly cost-effective. This has been estimated, in several settings, to reduce the incidence of meningeal and miliary tuberculosis in early childhood by 50 to 90%. However, estimates of its effectiveness in older children have differed greatly from region to region and because efficacy against pulmonary tuberculosis is doubtful, the mainstay of the tuberculosis control programme is case-finding and treatment.

BCG vaccine

Requirements should comply with the recommendations published in the report of the WHO Expert Committee on Biological Standardization, WHO Technical Report Series, No. 745, 1987 and Amendment 1987, WHO Technical Report Series No. 771, 1988

Injection (Powder for solution for injection), live bacteria of a strain derived from the bacillus of Calmette and Guérin

Uses: active immunization against tuberculosis; see also section 6.2.4

Contraindications: see introductory notes; generalized oedema; antimycobacterial treatment

Precautions: pregnancy (Appendix 2); eczema, scabies— vaccine site must be lesion-free; **interactions:** Appendix 1

Dosage:

NOTE. National immunization schedules may vary

Immunization against tuberculosis, *by intradermal injection*, INFANTS up to 3 months, 0.05 ml; ADULT and CHILD over 3 months 0.1 ml

RECONSTITUTION AND ADMINISTRATION. According to manufacturer's directions

Adverse effects: see introductory notes; lymphadenitis and keloid formation; osteitis and localized necrotic ulceration; rarely, disseminated BCG infection in immunodeficient patients

19.3.1.2 Diphtheria, pertussis and tetanus vaccines

DIPHTHERIA. Diphtheria is a bacterial infection caused by *Corynebacterium diphtheriae*, transmitted person to person through close physical and respiratory contact. Diphtheria vaccine is a formaldehyde-inactivated preparation of diphtheria toxin, adsorbed onto a mineral carrier to increase its antigenicity and reduce adverse reactions. Immunized individuals can be infected by toxin-producing strains of diphtheria but systemic manifestations of the disease do not occur.

When administered for primary immunization in infants, diphtheria vaccine is almost always given together with pertussis and tetanus vaccines as part of a *three-component* preparation (DPT).

A *two-component* diphtheria vaccine with tetanus but without pertussis exists in two forms, DT and Td. Diphtheria-tetanus vaccine for children (DT) is used for primary immunization in infants who have contraindications to pertussis vaccine; it is also used in children under the age of 10 years for reinforcing immunization against diphtheria and tetanus in those countries which recommend it. Tetanus-diphtheria vaccine for adults, adolescents and children over 10 years of age (Td), which has a reduced amount of diphtheria toxoid to reduce the risk of hypersensitivity reactions, is used for primary immunization in persons over the age of 10 years; it is also used for reinforcing immunization in persons over the age of 10 years in those countries that recommend it.

PERTUSSIS. Pertussis (whooping cough) is a bacterial respiratory infection caused by *Bordetella pertussis*. Many of the symptoms are thought to be caused by toxins released by *B. pertussis*. Whole cell vaccine composed of whole pertussis bacteria killed by chemicals or heat is effective in preventing serious illness. It causes frequent local reactions and fever and rarely it may cause neurological reactions. Neurological complications after pertussis infection are considerably more common than after the vaccine. It is combined with diphtheria-tetanus vaccine for primary immunization unless immunization against pertussis is contra-indicated. Single component pertussis vaccines are available in some countries for use when the pertussis component has been omitted from all or part of the primary immunization schedule. An acellular form of the vaccine is also available.

In some countries it is recommended that children with a personal or family history of febrile convulsions or a family history of idiopathic epilepsy should be immunized. It is also recommended that children with well-controlled epilepsy are immunized. Advice on prevention of fever should be given at the time of immunization. In children with evolving neurological problems, immunization with pertussis should be deferred until the condition is stable; in such children diphtheria and tetanus vaccine should be offered for primary immunization, and there may be an opportunity at a later date to complete immunization with a single-component pertussis vaccine. Where there is doubt advice should be sought from a paediatrician.

TETANUS. Tetanus is caused by the action of a neurotoxin of *Clostridium tetani* in necrosed tissues such as occur in dirty wounds. Tetanus vaccine is available as a single component vaccine for primary immunization in adults who have not received childhood immunization against tetanus and for reinforcing immunization. The vaccine is also used in the prevention of neonatal tetanus and in the management of clean wounds and tetanus-prone wounds. Some countries recommend a maximum of 5 doses of tetanus vaccine in a life-time; for the fully immunized patient reinforcing doses at the time of a tetanus-prone injury should only be required if more than 10 years have elapsed since the last dose.

Neonatal tetanus due to infection of the baby's umbilical stump during unclean delivery is the cause of many deaths of newborn infants. Control of neonatal tetanus may be achieved by ensuring adequate hygiene during delivery and by ensuring protective immunity of mothers in late pregnancy. Tetanus vaccine is highly effective and the efficacy of two doses during pregnancy in preventing neonatal tetanus ranges from 80–100%. Women of child-bearing age may be immunized by a course of 5 doses (3 primary and 2 reinforcing) of tetanus vaccine.

Wounds are considered to be tetanus-prone if they are sustained *either* more than 6 hours before surgical treatment of the wound *or* at any interval after injury and show one or more of the following: a puncture-type wound, a significant degree of devitalized tissue, clinical evidence of sepsis, contamination with soil/manure likely to contain tetanus organisms. All wounds should receive thorough surgical toilet. Antibacterial prophylaxis may also be required for tetanus-prone wounds.

Diphtheria, pertussis, and tetanus vaccine (DPT)

Requirements should comply with the recommendations published in the report of the who expert committee on biological standardization, who technical report series, no. 800, 1990

Injection, diphtheria and tetanus toxoids and pertussis vaccine adsorbed onto a mineral carrier

Uses: active immunization against diphtheria, tetanus and pertussis

Contraindications: see introductory notes and notes above

Precautions: see introductory notes and notes above; in cases of severe reaction, the pertussis component should be omitted and the primary course of immunization completed with diphtheria and tetanus vaccine

Dosage:
NOTE. National immunization schedules may vary

Primary immunization of children against diphtheria, pertussis and tetanus, *by intramuscular or deep subcutaneous injection*, INFANT 0.5 ml at 6, 10 and 14 weeks (see WHO schedule, section 19.3.1)

Adverse effects: see introductory notes; tetanus component rarely associated with peripheral neuropathy; pertussis component rarely associated with convulsions and encephalopathy

---

Diphtheria and tetanus vaccine (DT) (For children under 10 years)

Requirements should comply with the recommendations published in the report of the WHO Expert Committee on Biological Standardization, WHO Technical Report Series, No. 800, 1990

Injection, diphtheria and tetanus toxoids adsorbed onto a mineral carrier

Uses: active immunization of children under 10 years against diphtheria and tetanus (see notes above)

Contraindications: see introductory notes; adults and children over 10 years of age (see notes above)

Precautions: see introductory notes

Dosage:

NOTE. National immunization schedules may vary

Primary immunization of children against diphtheria and tetanus when pertussis immunization is contraindicated, *by intramuscular or deep subcutaneous injection*, CHILD under 10 years 3 doses each of 0.5 ml with an interval of not less than 4 weeks between each dose (see also WHO schedule, section 19.3.1)

Reinforcing immunization of children against diphtheria and tetanus, *by intramuscular or deep subcutaneous injection*, CHILD under 10 years of age, 0.5 ml at least 3 years after completion of primary course of DPT or DT immunization

Adverse effects: see introductory notes; tetanus component rarely associated with peripheral neuropathy

Tetanus and diphtheria vaccine (Td) (for adults, adolescents and children over 10 years)

Requirements should comply with the recommendations published in the report of the WHO Expert Committee on Biological Standardization, WHO Technical Report Series, No. 800, 1990

Injection, diphtheria (low dose) and tetanus toxoid adsorbed onto a mineral carrier

Uses: active immunization of adults and children over 10 years of age against tetanus and diphtheria (see notes above)

Contraindications: see introductory notes; children under 10 years (see notes above)

Precautions: see introductory notes

Dosage:

NOTE. National immunization schedules may vary

Primary immunization of unimmunized adults and children over 10 years of age against tetanus and diphtheria, *by intramuscular or deep subcutaneous injection*, ADULT and CHILD over 10 years of age, 3 doses each of 0.5 ml with an interval of not less than 4 weeks between each dose

Reinforcing immunization of adults and children over 10 years of age against tetanus and diphtheria, *by intramuscular or deep subcutaneous injection*, ADULT and CHILD over 10 years of age, 0.5 ml 10 years after completing primary course

Adverse effects: see introductory notes; tetanus component rarely associated with peripheral neuropathy

Tetanus vaccine

Requirements should comply with the recommendations published in the report of the WHO Expert Committee on Biological Standardization, WHO Technical Report Series, No. 800, 1990

Injection, tetanus toxoid adsorbed onto a mineral carrier

Uses: active immunization against tetanus and neonatal tetanus; wound management (tetanus-prone wounds and clean wounds)

Contraindications: see introductory notes and notes above

Precautions: see introductory notes and notes above

ANTITETANUS IMMUNOGLOBULIN. If schedule requires tetanus vaccine and antitetanus immunoglobulin to be administered at the same time, they should be administered using separate syringes and separate sites

Dosage:

NOTE. National immunization schedules may vary; some countries recommend a **maximum** of 5 doses of tetanus vaccine in a life-time

Primary immunization of unimmunized adults against tetanus, *by intramuscular or deep subcutaneous injection,* ADULT 3 doses each of 0.5 ml with an interval of 4 weeks between each dose

Reinforcing immunization of adults against tetanus, *by intramuscular or deep subcutaneous injection,* ADULT 2 doses each of 0.5 ml, the first 10 years after completion of primary course, and the second dose 10 years later

Immunization of women of child-bearing age against tetanus, *by intramuscular or deep subcutaneous injection,* WOMAN OF CHILD-BEARING AGE, 3 primary doses each of 0.5 ml with an interval of not less than 4 weeks between the first and second doses and 6 months between the second and third doses; 2 reinforcing doses each of 0.5 ml, the first 1 year after completion of the primary course and the second dose 1 year later; UNIMMUNIZED PREGNANT WOMAN 2 doses of 0.5 ml with an interval of 4 weeks between each dose, with the second dose at least 2 weeks before delivery

Management of tetanus-prone wounds and clean wounds, *by intramuscular or deep subcutaneous injection,* ADULT 0.5 ml, the dose schedule being dependent upon the immune status of the patient and the level of contamination of the wound (see also notes above and under Antitetanus Immunoglobulin, section 19.2.2)

Adverse effects: see introductory notes; tetanus component rarely associated with peripheral neuropathy

19.3.1.3 Hepatitis B vaccine

Hepatitis B is caused by hepatitis B virus. It is transmitted in blood and blood products, by sexual contact and by contact with infectious body fluids. Persons at increased risk of infection because of their life-style, occupation or other factors include parenteral drug abusers, individuals who change sexual partners frequently, health care workers who are at risk of injury from blood-stained sharp instruments and haemophiliacs. Also at risk are babies born to mothers who are HbsAg (hepatitis B virus surface antigen)-positive and individuals who might acquire the infection as the result of medical or dental procedures in countries of high prevalence. The main public health consequences are chronic liver disease and liver cancer rather than acute infection. Routine immunization is recommended and has been implemented in some countries. Plasma-derived hepatitis B vaccine is highly efficacious. Over 90% of susceptible children develop a protective antibody response. A recombinant DNA vaccine is also available.

Hepatitis B vaccine

Requirements should comply with the recommendations published in the report of the WHO Expert Committee on Biological Standardization, WHO Technical Report Series, No. 858, 1995

Injection, inactivated hepatitis B surface antigen adsorbed onto a mineral carrier

Uses: active immunization against hepatitis B

Contraindications: see introductory notes

Precautions: see introductory notes

Dosage:

NOTE. National immunization schedules may vary

Immunization of children against hepatitis B, *by intramuscular injection*, INFANT 0.5 ml *either Scheme A* at birth and at 6 and 14 weeks of age, *or Scheme B* at 6, 10 and 14 weeks of age (see WHO schedule, section 19.3.1)

Immunization of unimmunized high risk persons against hepatitis B, *by intramuscular injection*, ADULT and CHILD over 15 years of age 3 doses of 1 ml, with an interval of 1 month between the first and second dose and 5 months between the second and third doses; CHILD under 15 years, 0.5 ml

NOTE. Different products may contain different concentrations of antigen per ml. Consult manufacturer's literature

ADMINISTRATION. The vaccine should be given in the deltoid region in adults; anterolateral thigh is the preferred site in infants and children; it should not be injected into the buttock (vaccine efficacy reduced); subcutaneous route used for patients with haemophilia

Adverse effects: see introductory notes; abdominal pain and gastrointestinal disturbances; muscle and joint pain, dizziness and sleep disturbance; occasionally cardiovascular effects

19.3.1.4 Measles vaccines

Measles is an acute viral infection transmitted by close respiratory contact. In some countries routine immunization of children against measles is given as one dose of a single component vaccine; in other areas, a two-dose schedule has been found to be more applicable. In developing countries, clinical efficacy is usually greater than 85%. Convulsions and encephalitis are rare complications. Measles vaccine is administered in some countries as part of a combined preparation with mumps vaccine and rubella vaccine (MMR vaccine); a single-dose primary immunization is followed by a reinforcing dose 2–5 years later.

Single-component vaccines or MMR may be used in the control of outbreaks of measles and should be offered to susceptible children within 3 days of exposure. It is important to note that MMR vaccine is **not** suitable for prophylaxis following exposure to mumps or rubella since the antibody response to the mumps and rubella components is too slow for effective prophylaxis.

Measles vaccine

Requirements should comply with the recommendations published in the reports of the WHO Expert Committee on Biological Standardization, WHO Technical Report Series, No. 840, 1994, and Note, WHO Technical Report Series, No. 848, 1994

Injection (Powder for solution for injection), live, attenuated measles virus

Uses: active immunization against measles

Contraindications: see introductory notes; hypersensitivity to any antibiotic present in vaccine—consult manufacturer's literature; hypersensitivity to egg

Precautions: see introductory notes; pregnancy (Appendix 2); **interactions:** Appendix 1

Dosage:

NOTE. National immunization schedules may vary

Immunization of children against measles, *by intramuscular or deep subcutaneous injection*, INFANT at 9 months of age, 0.5 ml (see WHO schedule, section 19.3.1)

Prophylaxis in susceptible children after exposure to measles, *by intramuscular or deep subcutaneous injection* within 72 hours of contact, CHILD over 9 months of age 0.5 ml

RECONSTITUTION AND ADMINISTRATION. According to manufacturer's directions

Adverse effects: see introductory notes; rashes sometimes accompanied by convulsions; rarely, encephalitis and thrombocytopenia

---

Measles, mumps and rubella vaccine (MMR vaccine)

Requirements should comply with the recommendations published in the reports of the WHO Expert Committee on Biological Standardization, WHO Technical Report Series, No. 840, 1994 and Note, WHO Technical Report Series, No. 848, 1994

Injection, live, attenuated measles virus, mumps virus and rubella virus

Uses: active immunization against measles, mumps and rubella

Contraindications: see introductory notes; pregnancy (Appendix 2); hypersensitivity to any antibiotic present in vaccine—consult manufacturer's literature; hypersensitivity to egg

Precautions: see introductory notes; history of convulsions—advice on controlling fever (see below); **interactions:** Appendix 1

POST-IMMUNIZATION FEVER. Malaise, fever or rash may occur following the first dose of MMR vaccine, most commonly about 1 week after immunization and lasting 2–3 days. Carers should be advised that the child can be given paracetamol to reduce the fever followed if necessary by a second dose 4–6 hours later. If fever persists after the second dose of paracetamol, medical advice should be sought.

After a second dose of MMR vaccine, adverse reactions are considerably less common than after the first dose

Dosage:

NOTE. National immunization schedules may vary

Primary immunization of children against measles, mumps and rubella, *by intramuscular or deep subcutaneous injection*, CHILD 12–15 months, 0.5 ml

Reinforcing immunization of children against measles, mumps and rubella, *by intramuscular or deep subcutaneous injection*, CHILD 0.5 ml 2–5 years after primary dose

Prophylaxis in susceptible children after exposure to measles (see notes above), *by intramuscular or deep subcutaneous injection* within 72 hours of contact, CHILD 12 months of age and older, 0.5 ml

Adverse effects: see introductory notes; malaise, fever, rash most common after first dose (see above); occasionally parotid swelling; rarely meningoencephalitis

19.3.1.5 Poliomyelitis vaccines

Poliomyelitis is an acute viral infection spread by the faecal-oral route which can cause paralysis of varying degree. There are two types of vaccine against poliomyelitis: oral and injectable. Oral poliomyelitis vaccine (OPV) is composed of three types of live attenuated poliomyelitis viruses. The efficacy of OPV in preventing paralytic polio in developing countries ranges from 72% to 98% and is the vaccine of choice in eradication of the disease. Oral poliomyelitis vaccine should not be given to patients with diarrhoea or vomiting and those with immuno-deficiency disorders (or household contacts of patients with immunodeficiency disorders). The need for strict personal hygiene must be stressed as the vaccine virus is excreted in the faeces. The contacts of a recently vaccinated baby should be advised particularly of the need to wash their hands after changing the baby's nappies. After primary immunization reinforcing doses may be given. Inactivated polio vaccine (IPV) is injectable and composed of inactivated strains of three types of poliomyelitis virus. It should be used for individuals who are immunosuppressed or for their household contacts.

Poliomyelitis vaccine (OPV) (live attenuated)

Requirements should comply with the recommendations published in the report of the WHO Expert Committee on Biological Standardization, WHO Technical Report Series, No. 800, 1990

Oral suspension, live, attenuated poliomyelitis virus, types 1, 2, and 3

Uses: active immunization against poliomyelitis

Contraindications: see introductory notes; avoid in patients with diarrhoea or vomiting (vaccine virus excreted in faeces—strict personal hygiene required; see notes above); not to be taken with food which contains a preservative; hypersensitivity to any antibiotic present in vaccine—consult manufacturer's literature

Precautions: see introductory notes; pregnancy (Appendix 2); **interactions:** Appendix 1

Dosage:

NOTE. National immunization schedules may vary

Primary immunization of children against poliomyelitis, *by mouth*, CHILD 3 drops at birth and at 6, 10 and at 14 weeks of age (see WHO schedule, section 19.3.1)

Reinforcing immunization of children against poliomyelitis, *by mouth*, CHILD 3 drops at least 3 years after completion of primary course and a further 3 drops at 15–19 years of age

Primary immunization of unimmunized adult against poliomyelitis, *by mouth*, ADULT 3 doses each of 3 drops with an interval of at least 4 weeks between each dose

Reinforcing immunization of adults against poliomyelitis, *by mouth*, ADULT 3 drops 10 years after completion of primary course

NOTE. Some countries consider reinforcing immunization unnecessary in adults unless travelling to endemic areas

Adverse effects: rarely, vaccine-associated poliomyelitis in recipients of vaccine and contacts of recipients

---

Poliomyelitis vaccine (IPV) (inactivated)

Requirements should comply with the recommendations published in the reports of the WHO Expert Committee on Biological Standardization, WHO Technical Report Series, No. 673, 1982 and Addendum 1985, WHO Technical Report Series, No. 745, 1987

Injection, inactivated poliomyelitis virus, types 1, 2, and 3

Uses: active immunization against poliomyelitis in patients for whom live vaccine is contraindicated (see notes above) or in persons in countries not wishing to use live vaccine

Contraindications: see introductory notes

Precautions: see introductory notes

Dosage:

NOTE. National immunization schedules may vary

Primary immunization of children against poliomyelitis, *by subcutaneous injection*, CHILD 0.5 ml at birth and at 6, 10 and 14 weeks of age (see WHO schedule, section 19.3.1)

Reinforcing immunization of children against poliomyelitis, *by subcutaneous injection*, CHILD 0.5 ml at least 3 years after completion of the primary course and a further 0.5 ml at 15–19 years of age

Primary immunization of unimmunized adults against poliomyelitis, *by subcutaneous injection*, ADULT 3 doses each of 0.5 ml with intervals of at least 4 weeks between each dose

Reinforcing immunization of adults against poliomyelitis, *by subcutaneous injection*, ADULT 0.5 ml 10 years after completion of primary course

NOTE. Some countries consider reinforcing immunization unnecessary in adults unless travelling to endemic areas

Adverse effects: see introductory notes

19.3.2 Vaccines for specific groups of individuals

There are several other vaccines available which are used in different countries but are not yet recommended for routine use throughout the world.

Allergic patients require specific immunotherapy.

19.3.2.1 Influenza vaccine

While most viruses are antigenically stable, the influenza viruses A and B (especially A) are constantly changing their antigenic structure as indicated by changes in the haemagglutinins (H) and neuraminidases (N) on the surface of the viruses. It is essential that **influenza vaccines** in use contain the H and N components of the prevalent strain or strains. The changes are monitored and recommendations are made each year regarding the strains to be included in influenza vaccines for the following season. The recommended vaccine strains are grown on chick embryos and the vaccine is therefore contraindicated in individuals hypersensitive to egg. There are three forms of influenza vaccine; whole virion vaccine (not recommended for use in children because of the increased risk of severe febrile reactions), split-virion vaccine and surface-antigen vaccine.

The vaccines will not control epidemics and they are recommended only for those at high risk. Annual immunization is recommended in the elderly and those of any age with diabetes mellitus, chronic heart disease, chronic renal failure, chronic respiratory disease including asthma, or immunosuppression due to disease or drug treatment.

Influenza vaccine

Requirements should comply with the recommendations published in the report of the WHO Expert Committee on Biological Standardization, WHO Technical Report Series, No. 814, 1991

Injection, inactivated influenza virus, types A and B

Uses: active immunization against influenza in individuals at risk

Contraindications: see introductory notes; whole virion vaccine not recommended in children; hypersensitivity to any antibiotic present in vaccine—consult manufacturer's literature; hypersensitivity to egg

Precautions: see introductory notes; **interactions:** Appendix 1

Dosage:

NOTE. National immunization schedules may vary

Immunization against influenza (annually for high-risk persons), *by intramuscular or deep subcutaneous injection*, ADULT and CHILD over 13 years 0.5 ml as a single dose; CHILD 6–35 months, 0.25–0.5 ml repeated after at least 4 weeks if child not previously infected or vaccinated; CHILD 4–12 years of age, 0.5 ml, with a second dose after at least 4 weeks if child not previously infected or vaccinated

Adverse effects: see introductory notes; occasionally, severe febrile reactions—particularly after whole virion vaccine in children

19.3.2.2 Meningococcal polysaccharide vaccine

Meningococcal polysaccharide vaccine is effective against serogroups A and C of *Neisseria meningitidis* but infants respond less well than adults. Immunity to some meningococcal vaccines may be insufficient to confer adequate protection against infection in infants under about 2 years of age and the minimum age recommended by manufacturers varies from 2 months to 2 years. It is indicated for persons at risk of serogroups A and C meningococcal disease in epidemics (where it must be administered early in the course of the epidemic) or endemic areas and as an adjunct to chemoprophylaxis in close contacts of persons with the disease. It is indicated for visits of longer than 1 month to areas of the world where risk of infection is high.

Meningococcal polysaccharide vaccine

Requirements should comply with the recommendations published in the reports of the WHO Expert Committee on Biological Standardization, WHO Technical Report Series, No. 594, 1976 and Addendum 1980 incorporating Addendum 1976 and 1977, WHO Technical Report Series, No. 658, 1981

Injection (Powder for solution for injection), inactivated polysaccharide antigens of *Neisseria meningitidis* (meningococcus) groups A and C

Uses: active immunization against meningitis and septicaemia caused by *N. meningitidis* group A and C serotypes

Contraindications: see introductory notes

Precautions: see introductory notes

Dosage:

NOTE. National immunization schedules may vary

Immunization against infection by *N. meningitidis* groups A and C, *by deep subcutaneous or by intramuscular injection*, ADULT and CHILD (see notes above and manufacturer's literature), 0.5 ml as a single dose

RECONSTITUTION AND ADMINISTRATION. According to manufacturer's directions

Adverse effects: see introductory notes

19.3.2.3 Rabies vaccine (inactivated)

Rabies vaccine is used as part of the *post-exposure treatment* to prevent rabies in patients who have been bitten by rabid animals or animals suspected of being rabid. Treatment is dependent upon the individual's immune status and upon the level of risk of rabies in the country concerned (consult national immunization schedule); in certain circumstances *passive immunization* with rabies immunoglobulin may be indicated (see Rabies Immunoglobulin, section 19.2.5). Treatment should also include thorough wound cleansing.

The vaccine is also used for *pre-exposure prophylaxis* against rabies in those at high risk such as laboratory workers, veterinary surgeons, animal handlers and health workers who are likely to come into close contact with patients with rabies.

Pre-exposure prophylaxis is also recommended for those living or travelling in enzootic areas who may be exposed to unusual risk.

Rabies vaccine (inactivated) (prepared in cell culture)

Requirements should comply with the recommendations on Rabies Vaccine (inactivated) for Human Use Produced in Continuous Cell Lines, published in the reports of the WHO Expert Committee on Biological Standardization, WHO Technical Report Series, No. 760, 1987 and Amendment 1992, WHO Technical Report Series, No. 840, 1994

Injection, inactivated rabies virus prepared in cell culture

Uses: active immunization against rabies; pre-exposure prophylaxis, post-exposure treatment (see notes above)

Contraindications: see introductory notes

Precautions: see introductory notes; **interactions:** Appendix 1
RABIES IMMUNOGLOBULIN. If schedule requires rabies vaccine and rabies immunoglobulin to be administered at the same time, they should be administered using separate syringes and separate sites

Dosage:
NOTE. National immunization schedules may vary

Immunization against rabies: pre-exposure prophylaxis, *by deep subcutaneous or by intramuscular injection*, ADULT and CHILD 1 ml on days 0, 7 and 28, with reinforcing doses every 2–3 years for those at continued risk

Immunization against rabies: post-exposure treatment, *by deep subcutaneous or by intramuscular injection*, ADULT and CHILD 2–5 doses of 1 ml (see notes above)

Adverse effects: see introductory notes; pain, erythema and induration at injection site; nausea, myalgia; hypersensitivity—less likely with vaccines from human sources

19.3.2.4 Rubella vaccine

Rubella vaccine should be given to women of child-bearing age if they are seronegative to protect them from the risks of rubella in pregnancy. It should not be given in pregnancy and patients should be advised not to become pregnant within one month of vaccination. However, congenital rubella syndrome has not been reported following inadvertent immunization shortly before or during pregnancy. There is no evidence that the vaccine is teratogenic and routine termination of pregnancy following inadvertent immunization should **not** be recommended. There is no risk to a pregnant woman from contact with recently vaccinated persons as the vaccine virus is not transmitted.

The vaccine may contain traces of antibiotics and if so should not be used in individuals with hypersensitivity to them.

In some countries the policy of protecting women of childbearing age has been replaced by a policy of eliminating rubella in children. Rubella vaccine is a component of the MMR vaccine (see section 19.3.1.4).

Rubella vaccine

Requirements should comply with the recommendations published in the report of the WHO Expert Committee on Biological Standardization, WHO Technical Report Series, No. 840, 1994 and Note, WHO Technical Report Series, No. 848, 1994

Injection (Powder for solution for injection), live attenuated rubella virus

Uses: active immunization against rubella in women of child-bearing age

Contraindications: see introductory notes; pregnancy (see notes above); hypersensitivity to any antibiotic present in vaccine—consult manufacturer's literature; hypersensitivity to egg

Precautions: see introductory notes; **interactions:** Appendix 1

Dosage:

NOTE. National immunization schedules may vary

Immunization of women of child-bearing age against rubella, *by deep subcutaneous or by intramuscular injection*, WOMAN OF CHILD-BEARING AGE, 0.5 ml as a single dose

RECONSTITUTION AND ADMINISTRATION. According to the manufacturer's directions

Adverse effects: see introductory notes; rash, lymphadeno-pathy; arthralgia and arthritis; rarely, thrombocytopenia, neurological symptoms

19.3.2.5 Typhoid vaccine

Typhoid vaccine is used for active immunization against typhoid fever and immunization is advised for those travelling to endemic areas. The efficacy of the vaccine is not complete and the importance of maintaining scrupulous attention to food and water hygiene as well as personal hygiene must also be emphasized.

Typhoid vaccine is available as a capsular polysaccharide injection.

In children under 2 years the injection may show sub-optimal response. Immunization is also recommended for laboratory workers handling specimens from suspected cases.

Typhoid vaccine

Requirements should comply with the recommendations published in the report of the WHO Expert Committee on Biological Standardization, WHO Technical Report Series, No. 840, 1994

Injection, Vi capsular polysaccharide typhoid 25 microgram/0.5 ml

Uses: active immunization against typhoid

Contraindications: see introductory notes

Precautions: see introductory notes and notes above

Dosage:

NOTE. National immunization schedules may vary

Immunization against typhoid fever, *by deep subcutaneous or by intramuscular injection*, ADULT and CHILD (see notes above) 0.5 ml, with reinforcing doses every 3 years for those at continued risk

ADMINISTRATION. According to the manufacturer's directions

Adverse effects: see introductory notes

19.3.2.6 Yellow fever vaccine

Yellow fever is a viral haemorrhagic fever endemic in some countries of South America and Africa. The disease is transmitted by *Haemagogus* and *Aedes* mosquito bites. The vaccine is highly immunogenic and offers about 10 years protection. Over 92% of children develop protective antibodies. It is recommended that all countries in which yellow fever is endemic should incorporate this vaccine into their immunization schedule. It is also used for travellers to endemic areas.

Yellow fever vaccine

Requirements should comply with the recommendations published in the reports of the WHO Expert Committee on Biological Standardization, WHO Technical Report Series, No. 872, 1998

Injection (Powder for solution for injection), live, attenuated yellow fever virus

Uses: active immunization against yellow fever

Contraindications: see introductory notes; not recommended for infants under 4 months of age; hypersensitivity to any antibiotic present in vaccine—consult manufacturer's literature; hypersensitivity to egg

Precautions: see introductory notes; pregnancy (Appendix 2); **interactions:** Appendix 1

Dosage:

NOTE. National immunization schedules may vary

Immunization of children against yellow fever, *by subcutaneous injection*, INFANT at 9 months of age, 0.5 ml (see WHO schedule, section 19.3.1)

Immunization of travellers and others at risk against yellow fever, *by subcutaneous injection*, ADULT and CHILD over 9 months of age 0.5 ml; INFANT 4–9 months of age 0.5 ml, only if risk of yellow fever is unavoidable (see Adverse Effects)

RECONSTITUTION AND ADMINISTRATION. According to manufacturer's directions

Adverse effects: see introductory notes; rarely encephalitis, generally in infants under 9 months

Section 20: Muscle relaxants (peripherally acting) and cholinesterase inhibitors

Muscle relaxants used in surgery include **suxamethonium,** **alcuronium,** and **vecuronium**; for further details see section 1.4.

20.1 Cholinesterase inhibitors

MYASTHENIA GRAVIS. Cholinesterase inhibitors, such as **neostigmine** and **pyridostigmine**, are used to treat myasthenia gravis. They act by inhibiting anticholinesterase, thereby prolonging the action of acetylcholine, and thus enhancing neuromuscular transmission; this produces at least a partial improvement in most myasthenic patients but complete restoration of muscle strength is rare. Unless the patient has difficulty in swallowing, cholinesterase inhibitors are given by mouth. Pyridostigmine has a slower onset (usually within 30–60 minutes), but a longer duration of effect than neostigmine; it also tends to cause fewer muscarinic effects such as diarrhoea, abdominal cramps, and excess salivation, so is usually preferred. Doses should be carefully adjusted to avoid precipitating a *cholinergic crisis* due to overdosage; this must be differentiated from a *myasthenic crisis* due to disease progression, and consequent underdosage; the principal effect in both cases is increased muscle weakness.

In myasthenic crisis, if the patient has difficulty in breathing and in swallowing, the cholinesterase inhibitor must be given parenterally; neostigmine is usually used, as intravenous injection of pyridostigmine is hazardous; to reduce muscarinic effects, atropine (section 1.3) should also be given.

For the use of neostigmine in surgery, see section 1.4.

Neostigmine

Neostigmine is a representative cholinesterase inhibitor. Various drugs can serve as alternatives

Tablets, neostigmine bromide 15 mg

Injection, neostigmine metilsulfate 500 micrograms/ml, 1-ml ampoule; 2.5 mg/ml, 1-ml ampoule

Uses: myasthenia gravis; reversal of non-depolarizing block, postoperative urinary retention (section 1.4)

Contraindications: recent intestinal or bladder surgery; mechanical intestinal or urinary tract obstruction; after suxamethonium; pneumonia; peritonitis

Precautions: asthma; urinary tract infections; cardiovascular disease including arrhythmias (especially bradycardia or atrioventricular block); hypotension; peptic ulcer; epilepsy; parkinsonism; renal impairment (Appendix 4); pregnancy and breastfeeding (Appendices 2 and 3); **interactions:** Appendix 1

Dosage:

Myasthenia gravis, *by mouth* as neostigmine bromide, ADULT initially 15 mg 3 times daily, gradually increased until desired response obtained; total daily dose within range 75–300 mg, taken at appropriate intervals when maximum strength required, but doses above 180 mg daily not usually tolerated;

CHILD up to 6 years, initially 7.5 mg, 6–12 years, initially 15 mg; total daily dose usually 15–90 mg in divided doses at appropriate intervals

By subcutaneous or intramuscular injection as neostigmine metilsulfate, ADULT 0.5–2.5 mg as required, total daily dose 5–20 mg; NEONATE 50–250 micrograms before feeds (not usually required beyond 8 weeks of age); CHILD 200–500 micrograms as required

NOTE. To reduce muscarinic effects, atropine sulfate *by intravenous injection* (ADULT 0.6–1.2 mg, CHILD 20 micrograms/kg) with or before neostigmine injection

Adverse effects: increased salivation and bronchial secretions, sweating, nausea and vomiting, abdominal cramps, diarrhoea, miosis, muscle spasm, bradycardia, bronchospasm, allergic reactions; hypotension; cholinergic crisis on overdosage; thrombophlebitis reported; rash associated with bromide salt

---

Pyridostigmine bromide

Tablets, pyridostigmine bromide 60 mg
Injection, pyridostigmine 1 mg/ml, 1-ml ampoule

Uses: myasthenia gravis

Contraindications: recent intestinal or bladder surgery; mechanical intestinal or urinary tract obstruction; after suxamethonium; pneumonia; peritonitis

Precautions: asthma; urinary tract infection; cardiovascular disease including arrhythmias (especially bradycardia or atrioventricular block); hypotension; peptic ulcer; epilepsy; parkinsonism; avoid intravenous injection; renal impairment (Appendix 4); pregnancy and breastfeeding (Appendices 2 and 3); **interactions:** Appendix 1

Dosage:

Myasthenia gravis, *by mouth,* ADULT initially 30–60 mg 3 times daily, gradually increased until desired response obtained; total daily dose within range 0.3–1.2 g, taken at appropriate intervals when maximum strength required, but doses above 720 mg daily not usually advisable; CHILD up to 6 years initially 30 mg, 6–12 years initially 60 mg; total daily dose usually 30–360 mg in divided doses at appropriate intervals

By subcutaneous or intramuscular injection, ADULT 2 mg every 2–3 hours; NEONATE 200–400 micrograms before feeds (but neostigmine usually preferred); CHILD, total daily dose 1–12 mg given in divided doses at appropriate intervals

NOTE. To reduce muscarinic effects, atropine sulfate *by intravenous injection* (ADULT 0.6–1.2 mg, CHILD 20 micrograms/kg) with or before pyridostigmine injection

Adverse effects: muscarinic effects generally weaker than with neostigmine: increased salivation and bronchial secretions, sweating, nausea and vomiting, abdominal cramps, diarrhoea, miosis, muscle spasm; bradycardia, bronchospasm, allergic reactions; hypotension; cholinergic crisis on overdosage; thrombophlebitis; rash associated with bromide salt

---

Section 21:
Ophthalmological preparations

Administration of eye preparations

Preparations for the eye should be sterile when issued. Use of single-application containers is preferable; multiple-application preparations include antimicrobial preservatives and when used particular care should be taken to prevent contamination of the contents, including the avoidance of contact between the applicator and the eye or other surfaces.

Eye drops are generally instilled into the lower conjunctivital sac which is accessed by gently pulling down the lower eyelid to form a pocket into which one drop is instilled. The eye should be kept closed for as long as possible after application, preferably 1–2 minutes. A small amount of eye ointment is applied similarly; the ointment melts rapidly and blinking helps to spread it.

When two different eye drops are required at the same time, dilution and overflow may occur when one immediately follows the other; an interval of 5 minutes should be allowed between the two applications.

Systemic absorption, which may occur after topical application of eye drops, can be minimized by using the finger to compress the lacrimal sac at the medial canthus for at least one minute after instillation of the drops. This helps block the passage of the drops through the naso-lacrimal duct.

PERFORMANCE OF SKILLED TASKS. Application of eye preparations may cause blurring of vision which is generally transient; patients should be advised not to carry out skilled tasks such as operating machinery or driving until their vision has cleared.

21.1 Anti-infective drugs

Blepharitis, conjunctivitis, keratitis and endophthalmitis are common acute infections of the eye and can be treated topically. However, in some cases, for example, in gonococcal conjunctivitis, both topical and systemic anti-infective treatment may be necessary. Blepharitis and conjunctivitis are often caused by staphylococcus, while keratitis and endophthalmitis may be bacterial, viral or fungal. Bacterial blepharitis is treated with an antibacterial eye ointment or drops. Although most cases of acute bacterial conjunctivitis may resolve spontaneously, anti-infective treatment shortens the infectious process and prevents complications. Acute infective conjunctivitis is treated with antibacterial eye drops by day and eye ointment applied at night. A poor response may indicate viral or allergic conjunctivitis. Keratitis requires immediate specialist treatment.

Gentamicin is a broad spectrum bactericidal antibiotic with particular activity against *Pseudomonas aeruginosa*, *Neisseria gonorrhoea* and other bacteria that may be implicated in blepharitis or conjunctivitis. Topical application may lead to systemic absorption and possible adverse effects.

Idoxuridine is used in the treatment of keratitis due to herpes simplex virus. Idoxuridine is effective against epithelial infections of recent origin. These may respond to treatment within a week and resolve completely in 1–2 weeks. Eye drops must be applied frequently to keep the concentration high and achieve a successful therapeutic outcome; however, if there is no relief within 7 days, treatment should be discontinued and alternative treatment is indicated. For systemic treatment, see section 6.5.1.

Silver nitrate is a topical anti-infective. Its antibacterial activity is attributed to precipitation of bacterial proteins by silver ions. It is available in 1% ophthalmic solutions and is used for prophylaxis of gonococcal ophthalmia neonatorum.

Tetracycline is a broad spectrum antibiotic with activity against many Gram-positive and Gram-negative bacteria including *N. gonorrhoea*, and most chlamydia, rickettsia, mycoplasma and spirochetes. Ophthalmic tetracycline is used in blepharitis, conjunctivitis, and keratitis produced by susceptible bacteria. Tetracycline is also used in the treatment of trachoma caused by *Chlamydia trachomatis* and in the prophylaxis of neonatal conjunctivitis (ophthalmia neonatorum) caused by *N. gonorrhoea* and *C. trachomatis*.

Gentamicin

An example of an antibacterial. Various drugs can serve as alternatives
Eye drops, solution, gentamicin (as sulfate) 0.3%

Uses: blepharitis; bacterial conjunctivitis; systemic infections (section 6.2.2.5)

Contraindications: hypersensitivity to aminoglycoside group of antibiotics

Precautions: prolonged use may lead to skin sensitization and emergence of resistant organisms including fungi; discontinue if purulent discharge, inflammation or exacerbation of pain

Administration: Mild to moderate infection, *by instillation into the eye,* ADULT and CHILD 1 drop every 2 hours, reducing frequency as infection is controlled, then continue for 48 hours after healing is complete

Severe infection, *by instillation into the eye,* ADULT and CHILD 1 drop every hour, reducing frequency as infection is controlled, then continue for 48 hours after healing is complete

Adverse effects: burning, stinging, itching, dermatitis

Idoxuridine

An example of an antiviral. Various drugs can serve as alternatives
Eye drops, solution, idoxuridine 0.1%
Eye ointment, idoxuridine 0.2%

Uses: keratitis or keratoconjunctivitis caused by herpes simplex

Contraindications: pregnancy; concurrent use of an eye preparation containing boric acid

---

Precautions: existing deep ulceration of cornea; prolonged or excessive use may damage the cornea; do not exceed frequency or duration of treatment, discontinue if no relief within 7 days; concurrent use of a corticosteroid

Administration: Herpes simplex keratitis, *by instillation into the eye,* ADULT and CHILD 1 drop every hour during daytime and every 2 hours at night-time, reducing frequency as infection is controlled to 1 drop every 2 hours during daytime and every 4 hours at night-time, then continue for 3–5 days after healing is complete; maximum length of treatment 21 days; alternatively, *by application to the eye,* ADULT and CHILD 1 application of ointment every 4 hours during daytime and once at night-time (5 applications), then continue for 3–5 days after healing is complete; maximum length of treatment 21 days

Adverse effects: occasionally burning, itching, irritation, pain, conjunctivitis, oedema, inflammation, photophobia, pruritus; rarely allergic reactions

---

Silver nitrate
Eye drops, solution, silver nitrate 1%

Uses: prophylaxis of neonatal conjunctivitis (ophthalmia neonatorum) due to *Neisseria gonorrhoea,* if tetracycline not available

Precautions: avoid use of old, concentrated drops; wipe excess drops from skin near the eye to prevent staining

Administration: Prophylaxis of neonatal conjunctivitis, *by instillation into the eye,* NEWBORN at birth after cleansing eyes with sterile gauze, 2 drops into each eye

Adverse effects: skin and mucous membrane irritation; mild conjunctivitis; repeated use may cause skin discoloration, corneal cauterization and blindness

---

Tetracycline hydrochloride
An example of an antibacterial. Various drugs can serve as alternatives
Eye ointment, tetracycline hydrochloride 1%

Uses: superficial bacterial infection of the eye; mass treatment of trachoma in endemic areas; prophylaxis of neonatal conjunctivitis (ophthalmia neonatorum) due to *Neisseria gonorrhoea* or *Chlamydia trachomatis*

Contraindications: hypersensitivity to tetracycline group of antibiotics

Precautions: prolonged use may lead to overgrowth of non-susceptible organisms

Administration: Superficial bacterial infection, *by application to the eye,* ADULT and CHILD aged over 8 years 1 application of ointment 3–4 times daily

Prophylaxis of neonatal conjunctivitis, *by application to the eye,* NEWBORN at birth after cleansing eyes with sterile gauze, 1 application of ointment into each eye; close eyelids and massage gently to aid spread of ointment

Trachoma, intermittent treatment, *by application to the eye,* ADULT and CHILD 1 application of ointment into each eye *either* twice daily for 5 days *or* once daily for 10 days, every month for 6 consecutive months each year, repeated as necessary

Trachoma, continuous intensive treatment, *by application to the eye,* ADULT and CHILD 1 application of ointment into each eye twice daily for at least 6 weeks

Adverse effects: rash; rarely stinging, burning

21.2 Anti-inflammatory drugs

Ophthalmic corticosteroids should only be used under supervision of an ophthalmologist as inappropriate use is potentially blinding. Dangers include the development of open-angle glaucoma (chronic simple glaucoma) and cataracts, and the aggravation of a simple herpes simplex epithelial lesion into an extensive amoeboid ulcer and subsequent permanent corneal scarring.

Corticosteroids such as **prednisolone** are useful in the treatment of inflammatory conditions including uveitis and scleritis. They are also used for reducing postoperative ocular inflammation. Before administration of an ophthalmic corticosteroid, the possibility of bacterial, viral or fungal infection should be excluded. Treatment should be the lowest effective dose for the shortest possible time; if long-term therapy (more than 6 weeks) is unavoidable, withdrawal of an ophthalmic corticosteroid should be gradual to avoid relapse.

Prednisolone sodium phosphate

An example of a corticosteroid. Various drugs can serve as alternatives
Eye drops, solution, prednisolone sodium phosphate 0.5%

Uses: short-term local treatment of inflammation of the eye; malignant disease (section 8.3); inflammatory and allergic reactions (section 18.1, also section 3.1)

Contraindications: undiagnosed 'red eye' caused by herpetic keratitis; glaucoma

Precautions: cataract; corneal thinning, corneal or conjunctival infection; discontinue treatment if no improvement within 7 days; risk of adrenal suppression after prolonged use in infants

Administration: Use only under the supervision of an ophthalmologist

Inflammation of the eye, *by instillation into the eye,* ADULT and CHILD 1 drop every 1–2 hours, reducing frequency as inflammation is controlled

Adverse effects: secondary ocular infection; impaired corneal healing (due to corneal thinning), optic nerve damage, cataract; glaucoma, mydriasis, ptosis, epithelial punctate keratitis, delayed hypersensitivity reactions including burning, stinging

21.3 Local anaesthetics

Topical local anaesthetics are employed for simple ophthalmo-
logical procedures and for short operative procedures involving
the cornea and conjunctiva. **Tetracaine**, available in 0.5%
ophthalmic solution, provides a rapid local anaesthesia which
lasts for 15 minutes or more. Prolonged or unsupervized use of
tetracaine is not recommended.

Tetracaine hydrochloride

Amethocaine

An example of a local anaesthetic. Various drugs can serve as alternatives

Eye drops, solution, tetracaine hydrochloride 0.5%

Uses: short-acting local anaesthesia of cornea and conjunctiva

Contraindications: hypersensitivity to ester-type local anaesthetics; eye inflammation or infection

Precautions: avoid prolonged use (cause of severe keratitis,
permanent corneal opacification, scarring, delayed corneal
healing); protect eye from dust and bacterial contamination
until sensation fully restored

Administration: Local anaesthesia, *by instillation into the eye*,
ADULT and CHILD 1 drop

Adverse effects: burning, stinging, redness; rarely, allergic
reactions may occur

21.4 Antiglaucoma drugs

Glaucoma is normally associated with raised intra-ocular
pressure and eventual damage to the optic nerve which may
result in blindness. The rise in pressure is almost always due to
reduced outflow of aqueous humour, the inflow remaining
constant. The most common condition is chronic open-angle
glaucoma (chronic simple glaucoma) in which the intra-ocular
pressure increases gradually and the condition is usually
asymptomatic until well advanced. In contrast, angle-closure
glaucoma (closed-angle glaucoma) usually occurs as an acute
emergency resulting from a rapid rise in intra-ocular pressure; if
treatment is delayed, chronic angle-closure glaucoma may
develop. Ocular hypertension is a condition in which intra-
ocular pressure is raised without signs of optic nerve damage.

Drugs used in the treatment of glaucoma lower the intra-ocular
pressure by a variety of mechanisms including reduction in
secretion of aqueous humour by the ciliary body, or increasing
the outflow of the aqueous humour by opening of the trabecular
network. Antiglaucoma drugs used include topical application
of a beta-blocker (beta-adrenoceptor antagonist), a miotic, or a
sympathomimetic such as epinephrine; systemic administration
of a carbonic anhydrase inhibitor may be used as an adjunct.

Timolol is a non-selective beta-blocker which acts by reducing
the secretion of aqueous humour. A beta-blocker is usually the
drug of choice for initial and maintenance treatment of chronic
open-angle glaucoma. If further reduction in intra-ocular

pressure is required a miotic, epinephrine or a systemic carbonic anhydrase inhibitor may be used with timolol. If it is used to reduce elevated intra-ocular pressure in angle-closure glaucoma, timolol should be used with a miotic and not alone. Since systemic absorption can occur, an ophthalmic beta-blocker should be used with caution in certain individuals.

A miotic such as **pilocarpine**, through its parasympathomimetic action, contracts the iris sphincter muscle and the ciliary muscle, and opens the trabecular network. It is used in chronic open-angle glaucoma either alone or, if required, as an adjunct with a beta-blocker, epinephrine or a systemic carbonic anhydrase inhibitor. Pilocarpine is used with systemic acetazolamide in an acute attack of angle-closure glaucoma prior to surgery; however, it is not advisable to use pilocarpine after surgery because of a risk of posterior synechiae forming. Systemic absorption of topically applied pilocarpine can occur producing muscarinic-like adverse effects.

The sympathomimetic drug **epinephrine** probably acts by reducing the rate of production of aqueous humour and increasing the outflow through the trabecular network. Epinephrine is usually used in combination with a miotic, a beta-blocker or a systemic carbonic anhydrase inhibitor in the treatment of chronic open-angle glaucoma; however, because epinephrine is also a mydriatic, it is contraindicated for angle-closure glaucoma unless an iridectomy has been carried out.

Acetazolamide, by reducing carbonic anhydrase in the eye, reduces the production of aqueous humour and so reduces intra-ocular pressure. It is used systemically as an adjunct in chronic open-angle glaucoma unresponsive to treatment with topically applied antiglaucoma drugs. Prolonged therapy with acetazolamide is not normally recommended, but if treatment is unavoidable blood count and plasma electrolyte concentration should be monitored. Acetazolamide is also used as part of emergency treatment for an acute attack of angle-closure glaucoma; however it should not be used in chronic angle-closure glaucoma as it may mask deterioration of the condition.

21.4.1 Miotics

Pilocarpine
An example of a miotic. Various drugs can serve as alternatives
Eye drops, solution, pilocarpine hydrochloride 2%, 4%; pilocarpine nitrate 2%, 4%

Uses: chronic open-angle glaucoma, ocular hypertension; emergency treatment of acute angle-closure glaucoma; to antagonize effects of mydriasis and cycloplegia following surgery or ophthalmoscopic examination

Contraindications: acute iritis, acute uveitis, anterior uveitis, some forms of secondary glaucoma; acute inflammation of anterior segment; not advisable after angle-closure surgery (risk of posterior synechiae)

Precautions: retinal disease, conjunctival or corneal damage; monitor intra-ocular pressure in chronic open-angle glaucoma and in long-term treatment; cardiac disease, hypertension, asthma, peptic ulceration, urinary-tract obstruction, Parkinson disease; stop treatment if symptoms of systemic toxicity develop

SKILLED TASKS. Causes difficulty with dark adaptation; may cause accommodation spasm. Do not carry out skilled tasks, for example operating machinery or driving until vision is clear

Administration: Chronic open-angle glaucoma, *by instillation into the eye*, ADULT 1 drop (2% or 4%) up to 4 times daily

Acute angle-closure glaucoma before surgery, *by instillation into the eye*, ADULT 1 drop (2%) every 10 minutes for 30–60 minutes, then 1 drop every 1–3 hours until intra-ocular pressure subsides

Adverse effects: eye pain, blurred vision, ciliary spasm, lacrimation, myopia, browache; conjunctival vascular congestion, superficial keratitis, vitreous haemorrhage and increased pupillary block have been reported; lens opacities have occurred following prolonged use; rarely systemic effects including hypertension, tachycardia, bronchial spasm, pulmonary oedema, salivation, sweating, nausea, vomiting, diarrhoea

21.4.2 Beta-blockers

Timolol

An example of a beta-blocker. Various drugs can serve as alternatives

Eye drops, solution, timolol (as maleate) 0.25%, 0.5%

Uses: ocular hypertension; chronic open-angle glaucoma, aphakic glaucoma, some secondary glaucomas

Contraindications: uncontrolled heart failure, bradycardia, heart block; asthma, obstructive airways disease

Precautions: older people (risk of keratitis); if used in angle-closure glaucoma, use with a miotic, and not alone; **interactions:** see Appendix 1

Administration: Ocular hypertension, chronic open-angle glaucoma, aphakic glaucoma, some secondary glaucomas, *by instillation into the eye*, ADULT 1 drop (0.25% or 0.5%) twice daily

Adverse effects: stinging, burning, pain, itching, erythema, transient dryness, allergic blepharitis, transient conjunctivitis, keratitis, decreased corneal sensitivity, diplopia, ptosis; systemic effects, particularly on the pulmonary, cardiovascular and central nervous systems, may follow absorption

21.4.3 Sympathomimetics

Epinephrine (Adrenaline)

A complementary drug.

Eye drops, solution, epinephrine (as hydrochloride) 0.5%, 1%

Uses: chronic open-angle glaucoma, ocular hypertension; anaphylaxis (section 3.1); cardiac arrest (section 12.2)

Contraindications: angle-closure glaucoma, unless an iridectomy has been carried out

Precautions: hypertension, heart disease, aneurysm, arrhythmia, tachycardia, hyperthyroidism, cerebral arteriosclerosis, diabetes mellitus

Administration: Chronic open-angle glaucoma, *by instillation into the eye*, ADULT 1–2 drops (0.5% or 1%) 1–2 times daily

Adverse effects: stinging, blurred vision, photophobia, eye pain, conjunctival hyperaemia, headache or browache; occasionally, conjunctival sensitization and local skin reactions; after prolonged use conjunctival pigmentation and macular oedema in aphakia; systemic adverse reactions are rare following topical use at normal dosage but tachycardia, hypertension, arrhythmia, dizziness, sweating may occur

21.4.4 Carbonic anhydrase inhibitors

Acetazolamide
Tablets, acetazolamide 250 mg

Uses: as an adjunct in the treatment of chronic open-angle glaucoma; secondary glaucoma; as part of pre-operative treatment of acute angle-closure glaucoma

Contraindications: hypersensitivity to sulfonamides; chronic angle-closure glaucoma (may mask deterioration); hypokalaemia, hyponatraemia, hyperchloraemic acidosis; renal impairment (Appendix 4); severe hepatic impairment

Precautions: elderly; pregnancy (Appendix 2); breastfeeding (Appendix 3); diabetes; pulmonary obstruction; monitor blood count and electrolytes if used for long periods; **interactions:** see Appendix 1

SKILLED TASKS. May impair ability to perform skilled tasks, for example operating machinery, driving

Dosage:

Chronic open-angle glaucoma, secondary glaucoma, *by mouth*, ADULT 0.25–1 g daily in divided doses

Adverse effects: nausea, vomiting, diarrhoea, taste disturbance; loss of appetite, paraesthesia, flushing, headache, dizziness, fatigue, irritability, depression; thirst, polyuria; reduced libido; metabolic acidosis and electrolyte disturbances on long-term therapy; occasionally drowsiness, confusion, hearing disturbances, urticaria, melaena, glycosuria, haematuria, abnormal liver function, renal calculi, blood disorders including agranulocytosis and thrombocytopenia, rashes including Stevens-Johnson syndrome and toxic epidermal necrolysis; transient myopia reported

21.5 Mydriatics and cycloplegics

Antimuscarinics, by blocking the cholinergic effects of acetylcholine, paralyse the pupillary constrictor muscles causing dilation of the pupil (mydriasis) and paralyse the ciliary muscles resulting in paralysis of accommodation (cycloplegia). Mydriasis may precipitate acute angle-closure glaucoma particularly in elderly or long-sighted patients. In patients with dark iridic pigmentation, higher concentrations of mydriatic drugs are usually required and care should be taken to avoid overdosing.

Atropine is a long-acting antimuscarinic used for cycloplegic refraction procedures, particularly in children. It is also used to immobilize the ciliary muscle and iris and to prevent formation of posterior synechiae in the treatment of inflammatory eye disorders such as iritis and uveitis.

Atropine sulfate

Eye drops, solution, atropine sulfate 0.1%, 0.5%, 1%

Uses: iritis, uveitis; cycloplegic refraction procedures; premedication (section 1.3); organophosphate poisoning (section 4.2.3); antispasmodic (section 17.5)

Contraindications: angle-closure glaucoma

Precautions: may precipitate acute attack of angle-closure glaucoma, particularly in the elderly or long-sighted; risk of systemic effects with eye drops in infants under 3 months—eye ointment preferred

SKILLED TASKS. May cause sensitivity to light and blurred vision. Do not carry out skilled tasks, for example operating machinery or driving, until vision is clear

Administration: Cycloplegic refraction, *by instillation into the eye,* ADULT 1 drop (1%) twice daily for 1–2 days before procedure *or* a single application of 1 drop (1%) 1 hour before procedure; CHILD over 5 years (0.5–1%), 1–5 years (0.1–0.5%), under 1 year (0.1%), 1 drop twice daily for 1–3 days before procedure with a further dose given 1 hour before procedure (child under 3 months, see Precautions)

Iritis, uveitis, *by instillation into the eye,* ADULT 1–2 drops (0.5% or 1%) up to 4 times daily; CHILD 1–2 drops (0.5%) or 1 drop (1%) up to 3 times daily

Adverse effects: transient stinging and raised intra-ocular pressure; on prolonged administration, local irritation, hyperaemia, oedema and conjunctivitis may occur; contact dermatitis; systemic toxicity may occur in the very young and the elderly

Section 22: Drugs used in Obstetrics

22.1 Drugs used in obstetrics

Drugs may be used to modify uterine contractions. These include oxytocic drugs used to stimulate uterine contractions both in induction of labour and to control postpartum haemorrhage and beta$_2$-adrenoceptor agonists used to relax the uterus and prevent premature labour.

POSTPARTUM HAEMORRHAGE. **Ergometrine** and **oxytocin** differ in their actions on the uterus. In moderate doses oxytocin produces slow generalized contractions with full relaxation in between; ergometrine produces faster contractions superimposed on a tonic contraction. High doses of both substances produce sustained tonic contractions. Oxytocin is now recommended for routine use in postpartum and post-abortion haemorrhage since it is more stable than ergometrine. However, ergometrine may be used if oxytocin is not available or in emergency situations.

PREMATURE LABOUR. **Salbutamol** is a beta$_2$-adrenoceptor agonist which relaxes the uterus and can be used to prevent premature labour in uncomplicated cases between 24 and 33 weeks of gestation. Its main purpose is to permit a delay in delivery of at least 48 hours. The greatest benefit is obtained by using this delay to administer corticosteroid therapy or to implement other measures known to improve perinatal health. Prolonged therapy should be avoided since the risks to the mother increase after 48 hours and the response of the myometrium is reduced.

ECLAMPSIA. **Magnesium sulfate** has been shown to have a major role in eclampsia for the prevention of recurrent seizures. Monitoring of blood pressure, respiratory rate and urinary output is carried out, as is monitoring for clinical signs of overdosage (loss of patellar reflexes, weakness, nausea, sensation of warmth, flushing, double vision and slurred speech—calcium gluconate injection (section 27.2) is used for the management of magnesium toxicity).

Ergometrine maleate

Ergometrine is subject to international control under the United Nations Convention against Illicit Traffic in Narcotic Drugs and Psychotropic Substances (1988)

Ergometrine is a representative oxytocic drug. Various drugs can serve as alternatives

Tablets, ergometrine maleate 200 micrograms

Injection (Solution for injection), ergometrine maleate 200 micrograms/ml, 1-ml ampoule

NOTE. Injection requires transport by 'cold chain' and refrigerated storage

Uses: prevention and treatment of postpartum and post-abortion haemorrhage in emergency situations and where oxytocin not available

Contraindications: induction of labour, first and second stages of labour; vascular disease, severe cardiac disease especially angina pectoris; severe hypertension; impaired respiratory function; severe renal and hepatic impairment; sepsis; eclampsia

Precautions: cardiac disease, hypertension, hepatic impairment (Appendix 5) and renal failure (Appendix 4), multiple pregnancy, porphyria

Dosage:

Prevention and treatment of postpartum haemorrhage, when oxytocin is not available, *by intramuscular injection,* ADULT 200 micrograms

Prevention of postpartum haemorrhage in high risk cases, *by intravenous injection,* ADULT 250–500 micrograms

Secondary postpartum haemorrhage, *by mouth,* ADULT 400 micrograms 3 times daily for 3 days

Adverse effects: nausea, vomiting, headache, dizziness, tinnitus, abdominal pain, chest pain, palpitations, dyspnoea, bradycardia, transient hypertension, vasoconstriction; stroke, myocardial infarction and pulmonary oedema also reported

---

Magnesium sulfate

Injection (Solution for injection), magnesium sulfate 500 mg/ml, 2-ml ampoule, 10-ml ampoule

Uses: prevention of recurrent seizures in eclampsia

Precautions: hepatic impairment (Appendix 5); renal failure (Appendix 4); in severe hypomagnesaemia administer initially via a controlled infusion device; **interactions:** Appendix 1

Dosage:

Prevention of recurrent seizures in eclampsia, *by intravenous injection,* ADULT initially 4 g over 5–10 minutes followed *by intravenous infusion* at a rate of 1 g every hour for at least 24 hours after the last seizure; recurrence of seizures may require additional *intravenous bolus* of 2 g

DILUTION AND ADMINISTRATION. According to manufacturer's directions

Adverse effects: generally associated with hypermagnesaemia, nausea, vomiting, thirst, flushing of skin, hypotension, arrhythmias, coma, respiratory depression, drowsiness, confusion, loss of tendon reflexes, muscle weakness; see also Appendix 2

Oxytocin

Injection (Solution for injection), oxytocin 10 units/ml, 1-ml ampoule

Uses: routine prevention and treatment of postpartum and post-abortion haemorrhage; induction of labour

Contraindications: hypertonic uterine contractions, mechanical obstruction to delivery, fetal distress; any condition where spontaneous labour or vaginal delivery inadvisable; avoid prolonged administration in oxytocin-resistant uterine inertia, in severe pre-eclamptic toxaemia or in severe cardiovascular disease

Precautions: induction or enhancement of labour in presence of borderline cephalopelvic disproportion (avoid if significant); mild to moderate pregnancy-associated hypertension or cardiac disease; age over 35 years; history of low-uterine segment caesarean section; avoid tumultuous labour if fetal death or meconium-stained amniotic fluid (risk of amniotic fluid embolism); water intoxication and hyponatraemia (avoid large volume infusions and restrict fluid intake); caudal block anaesthesia (risk of severe hypertension due to enhanced vasopressor effect of sympathomimetics); **interactions:** Appendix 1

Dosage:

Induction of labour, *by intravenous infusion,* ADULT, initially 0.0005–0.001 unit/minute increased in 0.001–0.002 unit/minute increments at intervals of 30–60 minutes until labour pattern similar to normal established; no more than 5 units should be administered in 24 hours

Prevention of postpartum haemorrhage, *by slow intravenous injection,* ADULT 5–10 units after placenta is delivered

Postpartum haemorrhage; *by intravenous infusion,* ADULT a total of 40 units should be infused at a rate of 0.02–0.04 units/minute; this should be started after the placenta is delivered

DILUTION AND ADMINISTRATION. According to manufacturer's directions

Adverse effects: uterine spasm, uterine hyperstimulation; water intoxication and hyponatraemia associated with high doses and large-volume infusions; nausea, vomiting, arrhythmias, rashes and anaphylactoid reactions also reported

---

Salbutamol

Salbutamol is a representative myometrial relaxant. Various drugs can serve as alternatives

Tablets, salbutamol (as sulfate) 4 mg

Injection (Solution for injection), salbutamol (as sulfate) 50 micrograms/ml, 5-ml ampoule

Uses: uncomplicated premature labour between 24–33 weeks gestation; asthma (section 25.1)

Contraindications: first and second trimester of pregnancy; cardiac disease, eclampsia and pre-eclampsia, intra-uterine infection, intra-uterine fetal death, antepartum haemorrhage, placenta praevia, cord compression, ruptured membranes

Precautions: monitor pulse and blood pressure and avoid over-hydration; suspected cardiac disease, hypertension, hyperthyroidism, hypokalaemia, diabetes mellitus; if pulmonary oedema suspected, discontinue immediately and institute diuretic therapy; **interactions:** Appendix 1

Dosage:

Premature labour, *by intravenous infusion*, ADULT initially 10 micrograms/minute, gradually increased according to response at 10-minute intervals until contractions diminish then increase rate (maximum of 45 micrograms/minute) until contractions have ceased, maintain rate for 1 hour then gradually reduce; *or by intravenous or intramuscular injection*, ADULT 100–250 micrograms repeated according to response, then *by mouth*, 4 mg every 6–8 hours (use for more than 48 hours not recommended)

Adverse effects: nausea, vomiting, flushing, sweating, tremor; hypokalaemia, tachycardia, palpitations, and hypotension, increased tendency to uterine bleeding; pulmonary oedema; chest pain or tightness and arrhythmias; hypersensitivity reactions including bronchospasm, urticaria and angioedema reported

Section 23: Peritoneal dialysis solution

23.1 Peritoneal dialysis solution

Solutions for peritoneal dialysis are preparations for intraperitoneal use which contain electrolytes in a similar concentration to that in plasma, and also contain glucose or another suitable osmotic agent. Peritoneal dialysis solutions always contain sodium, chloride, and hydrogen carbonate or a precursor; they may also contain calcium, magnesium, and potassium.

In renal failure haemodialysis is the preferred method to correct the accumulation of toxins, electrolytes and fluid. Peritoneal dialysis is less efficient than haemodialysis, but it is preferred in children, diabetic patients, and patients with unstable cardiovascular disease; it is also used in patients who can manage their condition, or those who live far from a dialysis centre. It is unsuitable for patients who have had significant abdominal surgery.

In peritoneal dialysis, the solution is infused into the peritoneal cavity, where exchange of electrolytes takes place by diffusion and convection, and excess fluid is removed by osmosis, using the peritoneal membrane as an osmotic membrane. There are two forms of peritoneal dialysis:

- *continuous ambulatory peritoneal dialysis* (CAPD), in which dialysis is performed manually by the patient several times each day
- *automated peritoneal dialysis* (APD), in which dialysis is performed by machine overnight.

The main complication of peritoneal dialysis is peritonitis, which often results from poor exchange technique; infections of the catheter exit site may also occur, again because of poor technique.

Peritoneal dialysis solution

Dialysis solution (Solution for peritoneal dialysis), intraperitoneal dialysis solution of appropriate composition

Uses: to correct electrolyte imbalance and fluid overload, and to remove metabolites, in renal failure

Contraindications: abdominal sepsis; previous abdominal surgery; severe inflammatory bowel disease

Precautions: care required with technique to reduce risk of infection; warm dialysis solution to body temperature before use; some drugs may be removed by dialysis

Dosage:
Individualized according to clinical condition, and based on blood results

Adverse effects: infection, including peritonitis; hernia; haemoperitoneum; hyperglycaemia, protein malnutrition; blocked catheter

---

Section 24:
Psychotherapeutic drugs

24.1 Drugs used in psychotic disorders

Treatment of psychotic disorders is both pharmacological and psychosocial. Individual and community programmes for relearning old skills and developing new ones and for learning to cope with the illness should be initiated. Classes of antipsychotic drugs include phenothiazines (for example chlorpromazine), butyrophenones (for example haloperidol), thioxanthenes (for example flupentixol) and newer 'atypical' neuroleptics including clozapine and risperidone. The various antipsychotic drugs do not, in general, differ in their antipsychotic activity, but differ in range and quality of adverse effects (see below).

ACUTE PHASE TREATMENT. The administration of **chlorpromazine** or **haloperidol** will relieve symptoms such as thought disorder, hallucinations and delusions and prevent relapse. They are usually less effective in apathetic, withdrawn patients. However, haloperidol may restore an acutely ill schizophrenic, who was previously withdrawn, or even mute and akinetic, to normal activity and social behaviour. In the acute phase chlorpromazine may be administered by intramuscular injection in a dose of 25–50 mg which can be repeated every 6–8 hours while observing the patient for possible hypotension. In most cases, however, the intramuscular injection is not needed and patients can be treated with an oral dose. Haloperidol may be administered in the acute phase.

MAINTENANCE THERAPY. Long-term treatment in patients with a definite diagnosis of schizophrenia may be necessary after the first episode to prevent the manifest illness from becoming chronic.

The lowest possible dose of antipsychotic drug that will prevent major exacerbations of florid symptoms is used for long-term management. Too rapid a dose reduction should be avoided. Intramuscular depot preparations such as **fluphenazine decanoate** may be used as an alternative to oral maintenance therapy especially when compliance with oral treatment is unreliable. Exacerbations of illness in patients on maintenance drug therapy can be precipitated by stress.

Withdrawal of maintenance drug treatment requires careful surveillance since it is not possible to predict the course of the disease and the patient may suffer a relapse if treatment is withdrawn inappropriately. Further, the need for continuation of treatment may not be evident on withdrawal of treatment because relapse may be delayed for several weeks.

ADVERSE EFFECTS. They are very common with long-term administration of antipsychotic medicines. Hypotension and interference with temperature regulation, neuroleptic malignant syndrome and bone-marrow depression are the most life-threatening. Hypotension and interference with temperature regulation are dose-related. They can result in dangerous falls and hypothermia in the elderly and this must be considered before prescribing these drugs for patients over 70 years of age.

Neuroleptic malignant syndrome (hypothermia, fluctuating levels of consciousness, muscular rigidity and autonomic dysfunction with pallor, tachycardia, labile blood pressure, sweating and urinary incontinence) is a rare adverse effect of drugs including haloperidol, chlorpromazine and flupentixol decanoate. It is managed by discontinuation of the antipsychotic medication, attention to fluid and electrolyte balance, and administration of bromocriptine and sometimes dantrolene.

Extrapyramidal symptoms are the most troublesome and are caused most frequently by the piperazine phenothiazines such as fluphenazine, the butyrophenones such as haloperidol and the depot preparations. Although easily recognized, they are not so easy to predict because they depend in part on the dose and patient susceptibility as well as the type of drug. However, there is a general tendency for low-potency drugs to have less extrapyramidal adverse effects, while high-potency drugs such as haloperidol have more extrapyramidal effects but less sedation and anticholinergic (more correctly antimuscarinic) effects. Sedation and anticholinergic effects usually diminish with continued use. Extrapyramidal symptoms consist of parkinsonian-type symptoms including tremor which may occur gradually, dystonia (abnormal face and body movements) which may appear after only a few doses, akathisia (restlessness) and tardive dyskinesia (an orofacial dyskinesia) which usually takes longer to develop. Parkinsonian symptoms are usually reversible on withdrawal of the drug and may be suppressed by anticholinergic (antimuscarinic) drugs but tardive dyskinesia may be irreversible. Tardive dyskinesia is usually associated with long-term treatment and high dosage of neuroleptics, particularly in elderly patients. There is no established treatment for tardive dyskinesias and treatment of all patients on neuroleptic medication must be carefully and regularly reviewed.

Chlorpromazine hydrochloride

Chlorpromazine is a representative antipsychotic. Various drugs can serve as alternatives

WARNING. Owing to the risk of contact sensitization, pharmacists, nurses, and other health workers should avoid direct contact with chlorpromazine; tablets should not be crushed and solutions should be handled with care

Tablets, chlorpromazine hydrochloride 100 mg

Syrup, chlorpromazine hydrochloride 25 mg/5 ml

Injection (Solution for injection), chlorpromazine hydrochloride 25 mg/ml, 2-ml ampoule

Uses: schizophrenia and other psychotic disorders, mania, psychomotor agitation and violent behaviour; adjunct in severe anxiety

Contraindications: impaired consciousness due to CNS depression; bone-marrow depression; phaeochromocytoma

Precautions: cardiovascular and cerebrovascular disorders, respiratory disease, parkinsonism, epilepsy, acute infections, pregnancy (Appendix 2), breastfeeding (Appendix 3), renal and hepatic impairment (avoid if severe; Appendices 4 and 5), history of jaundice, leukopenia (blood counts if unexplained fever or infection); hypothyroidism, myasthenia gravis, prostatic hypertrophy, angle-closure glaucoma; elderly (particularly in very hot or very cold weather); avoid abrupt withdrawal; patients should remain supine and the blood pressure monitored for 30 minutes after intramuscular injection; **interactions:** Appendix 1

SKILLED TASKS. May impair ability to perform skilled tasks, for example operating machinery, driving

Dosage:

Schizophrenia and other psychoses, mania, psychomotor agitation, violent behaviour, and severe anxiety (adjunct), *by mouth*, ADULT initially 25 mg 3 times daily (*or* 75 mg at night) adjusted according to response to usual maintenance dose of 100–300 mg daily (but up to 1.2 g daily may be required in psychoses); ELDERLY (or debilitated) third to half adult dose; CHILD (childhood schizophrenia and autism) 1–5 years 500 micrograms/kg every 4–6 hours (maximum 40 mg daily); 6–12 years, third to half adult dose (maximum 75 mg daily)

For relief of acute symptoms, *by deep intramuscular injection*, ADULT 25–50 mg every 6–8 hours; CHILD 500 micrograms/kg every 6–8 hours (1–5 years, maximum 40 mg daily; 6–12 years, maximum 75 mg daily) (see also Precautions and Adverse effects)

Adverse effects: extrapyramidal symptoms and on prolonged administration, occasionally potentially irreversible tardive dyskinesias (see notes above); hypothermia (occasionally pyrexia), drowsiness, apathy, pallor, nightmares, depression; more rarely, agitation, EEG changes, convulsions, nasal congestion; anticholinergic symptoms including dry mouth, constipation, blurred vision, difficulty in micturition; hypotension, tachycardia and arrhythmias; ECG changes; respiratory depression; menstrual disturbances, galactorrhoea, gynaecomastia, impotence, weight gain; sensitivity reactions such as agranulocytosis, leukopenia, leukocytosis, haemolytic anaemia, photosensitization, contact sensitization and rashes, jaundice and alterations in liver function; neuroleptic malignant syndrome; lupus erythematosus-like syndrome; with prolonged high dosage, corneal and lens opacities, and purplish pigmentation of the skin, cornea and retina; intramuscular injection may be painful and cause hypotension and tachycardia (see Precautions) and nodule formation

---

Haloperidol

Haloperidol is a representative antipsychotic. Various drugs can serve as alternatives

Tablets, haloperidol 2 mg, 5 mg

Injection (Solution for injection), haloperidol 5 mg/ml, 1-ml ampoule

Uses: schizophrenia and other psychotic disorders, mania, psychomotor agitation and violent behaviour; adjunct in severe anxiety

Contraindications: impaired consciousness due to CNS depression; bone-marrow depression; phaeochromocytoma; porphyria; basal ganglia disease

Precautions: cardiovascular and cerebrovascular disorders, respiratory disease, parkinsonism, epilepsy, acute infections, pregnancy (Appendix 2), breastfeeding (Appendix 3), renal and hepatic impairment (avoid if severe; Appendices 4 and 5), history of jaundice, leukopenia (blood counts if unexplained fever or infection); hypothyroidism, myasthenia gravis, prostatic hypertrophy, angle-closure glaucoma; elderly (particularly in very hot or very cold weather); children and adolescents; avoid abrupt withdrawal; patients should remain supine and the blood pressure monitored for 30 minutes after intramuscular injection; **interactions:** Appendix 1

SKILLED TASKS. May impair ability to perform skilled tasks, for example operating machinery, driving

Dosage:

Schizophrenia and other psychoses, mania, psychomotor agitation, violent behaviour, and severe anxiety (adjunct), *by mouth*, ADULT initially 1.5–3 mg 2–3 times daily *or* 3–5 mg 2–3 times daily in severely affected or resistant patients (up to 30 mg daily in resistant schizophrenia); ELDERLY (or debilitated) initially half adult dose; CHILD initially 25–50 micrograms/kg daily in 2 divided doses (maximum 10 mg daily)

Acute psychotic conditions, *by deep intramuscular injection*, ADULT 2–10 mg, subsequent doses every 4–8 hours according to response (up to every hour if necessary) to total maximum of 18 mg; severely disturbed patients may require initial dose of up to 18 mg; CHILD not recommended

Adverse effects: as for Chlorpromazine Hydrochloride (see above), but less sedating and fewer hypotensive and anticholinergic symptoms; pigmentation and photosensitivity reactions rare; extrapyramidal symptoms are common, particularly acute dystonia and akathisia (especially in thyrotoxic patients); rarely weight loss

---

Fluphenazine

Fluphenazine is a representative depot antipsychotic, used if compliance unlikely to be reliable. Various drugs can serve as alternatives

Oily injection (Solution for injection), fluphenazine decanoate 25 mg/ml, 1-ml ampoule

Oily injection (Solution for injection), fluphenazine enantate 25 mg/ml, 1-ml ampoule

Uses: maintenance treatment of schizophrenia and other psychoses

Contraindications: children; confusional states; impaired consciousness due to CNS depression; parkinsonism; intolerance to antipsychotics; depression; bone-marrow depression; phaeochromocytoma

Precautions: treatment requires careful monitoring for optimum effect; extrapyramidal symptoms occur frequently; when transferring from oral to depot therapy, dosage by mouth should be gradually phased out; cardiovascular and cerebrovascular disorders, respiratory disease, epilepsy, acute infections, pregnancy (Appendix 2), breastfeeding (Appendix 3), renal and hepatic impairment (avoid if severe; Appendices 4 and 5), history of jaundice, leukopenia (blood counts if unexplained fever or infection); hypothyroidism, myasthenia gravis, prostatic hypertrophy, angle-closure glaucoma; elderly (particularly in very hot or very cold weather); **interactions:** Appendix 1

SKILLED TASKS. May impair ability to perform skilled tasks, for example operating machinery, driving

Dosage:

Maintenance in schizophrenia and other psychoses, *by deep intramuscular injection* into gluteal muscle, ADULT test dose of 12.5 mg (6.25 mg in elderly), then after 4–7 days 12.5–100 mg repeated at intervals of 2–5 weeks, adjusted according to response; CHILD not recommended

ADMINISTRATION. According to manufacturer's directions

Adverse effects: as for Chlorpromazine Hydrochloride (see above), but less sedating and fewer hypotensive and anticholinergic symptoms; higher incidence of extrapyramidal symptoms (most likely to occur a few hours after injection and continue for about 2 days but may be delayed); pain at injection site, occasionally erythema, swelling, nodules

24.2 Drugs used in mood disorders

Mood disorders can be classified as depression (unipolar disorder) and mania; alternating episodes of mania and depression (manic depression) are termed bipolar disorder.

Electroconvulsive therapy (ECT) has been shown to be rapidly effective in the urgent treatment of severe depression. Counselling and psychotherapy have an important role in treating some forms of depression.

24.2.1 Drugs used in depressive disorders

Tricyclic and related antidepressants and the more recently introduced selective serotonin reuptake inhibitors (SSRIs) are the most widely used drugs in the treatment of depressive disorders. The response to antidepressant therapy is usually delayed with a lag-period of up to two weeks and at least six weeks before maximum improvement occurs. It is important to use doses that are sufficiently high for effective treatment, but not so high as to cause toxic effects. Low doses should be used for initial treatment in the elderly. The use of more than one antidepressant at a time is not recommended since this does not enhance effectiveness and it may result in enhanced adverse effects or interactions. The response of the patient should be monitored carefully especially during the first few weeks after diagnosis to detect any suicidal tendencies. Minimal quantities of antidepressants should be prescribed at any one time since they may be dangerous in overdosage. The natural history of depressive illness suggests that remission usually occurs after three months to one year. Treatment at full therapeutic dose should be continued for at least 6 months after resolution of symptoms. Treatment should not be withdrawn prematurely otherwise symptoms are likely to recur. Reduction in dose should be gradually carried out over a period of about four weeks.

Tricyclic and related antidepressants can be divided into those with more or less sedative effect. Those with sedative properties include **amitriptyline** and those with less sedative effects include **imipramine**. These drugs are most effective in the treatment of depression associated with psychomotor and physiological disturbances. Adverse effects include anticholinergic (more correctly amtimuscarinic) symptoms of dry mouth, blurred vision, constipation and urinary retention. Arrhythmias and heart block can occur.

The SSRIs characteristically cause gastrointestinal disturbances and sleep disturbances but they are less sedating and have fewer anticholinergic (antimuscarinic) and cardiotoxic effects than tricyclic antidepressants. The SSRIs are less toxic in overdose than the older tricyclic compounds. They may be preferred in patients in whom the risk of suicide is strong, although there is some concern that SSRIs, especially fluoxetine, may increase suicidal ideation.

Amitriptyline hydrochloride

Amitriptyline hydrochloride is a representative tricyclic antidepressant. Various drugs can serve as alternatives

Tablets, amitriptyline hydrochloride 25 mg

Uses: moderate to severe depression

Contraindications: recent myocardial infarction, arrhythmias (especially heart block); manic phase in bipolar disorders; severe liver disease; children; porphyria

Precautions: cardiac disease (see Contraindications above), history of epilepsy; pregnancy (Appendix 2); breastfeeding (Appendix 3); elderly; hepatic impairment (Appendix 5); thyroid disease; phaeochromocytoma; history of mania, psychoses (may aggravate psychotic symptoms); angle-closure glaucoma, history of urinary retention; concurrent electroconvulsive therapy; avoid abrupt withdrawal; anaesthesia (increased risk of arrhythmias and hypotension); **interactions:** Appendix 1

SKILLED TASKS. May impair ability to perform skilled tasks, for example operating machinery, driving

Dosage:

Depression, *by mouth*, ADULT initially 75 mg (elderly and adolescents 30–75 mg) daily in divided doses *or* as a single dose at bedtime increased gradually as necessary to 150 mg daily; CHILD under 16 years not recommended for depression

Adverse effects: sedation, dry mouth, blurred vision (disturbance of accommodation, increased intra-ocular pressure), constipation, nausea, difficulty in micturition; cardiovascular adverse effects particularly with high dosage including ECG changes, arrhythmias, postural hypotension, tachycardia, syncope; sweating, tremor, rash and hypersensitivity reactions (urticaria, photosensitivity); behavioural disturbances; hypomania or mania, confusion (particularly in elderly), interference with sexual function, blood sugar changes; increased appetite and weight gain (occasional weight loss); endocrine adverse effects such as testicular enlargement, gynaecomastia and galactorrhoea; convulsions, movement disorders and dyskinesias, fever, agranulocytosis, leukopenia, eosinophilia, purpura, thrombocytopenia, hyponatraemia (may be due to inappropriate antidiuretic hormone secretion); abnormal liver function test

In overdose, excitement, restlessness, marked anticholinergic effects; severe symptoms including unconsciousness, convulsions, myoclonus, hyperreflexia, hypotension, acidosis, respiratory and cardiac depression with arrhythmias

24.2.2 Drugs used in bipolar disorders

Treatment of bipolar disorders has to take account of three stages: treatment of the acute episode, continuation phase and prophylaxis to prevent further episodes. **Lithium** is effective in acute mania but symptomatic control of the florid symptoms with an antipsychotic or benzodiazepine is often necessary whilst waiting for the antimania drug to exert its effect. Benzodiazepines may be given during the initial stages until lithium becomes effective but they should not be used for long periods because of the risk of dependence. Lithium may be given concurrently with antipsychotics and treatment with the antipsychotic should be tailed off as lithium becomes effective. Alternatively, lithium therapy may be delayed until the patient's mood is stabilized with the antipsychotic. However, there is a risk of interactions including neurotoxicity and increased extrapyramidal disorders when lithium and antipsychotics are used concurrently. Lithium is the mainstay of treatment but its narrow therapeutic range is a disadvantage. **Sodium valproate** is effective and **carbamazepine** may also be used and it is a valuable drug in areas where there are few effective treatments.

Treatment of depressive episodes in bipolar disorders will mostly involve combination treatment using either lithium or sodium valproate together with a tricyclic antidepressant. Increased adverse effects are a problem which may compromise treatment.

Lithium prophylaxis should usually only be undertaken with specialist advice and consideration of the likelihood of recurrence in the individual patient and with the benefits carefully weighed against the risks. Long-term lithium therapy has been associated with thyroid disorders and mild cognitive and memory impairment. Patients should continue the treatment for longer than three to five years only if, on assessment, benefit persists.

Withdrawal appears to produce high levels of relapse. If lithium is to be discontinued, the dose should be reduced gradually over a period of a few weeks and patients should be warned of possible relapses if discontinued abruptly.

Lithium salts have a narrow therapeutic/toxic ratio and should only be prescribed if there are facilities for monitoring serum lithium concentrations. Doses are adjusted to achieve serum-lithium concentrations of 0.4–1 mmol/litre (lower end of range for maintenance therapy and the elderly) on samples taken 12 hours after the preceding dose. The optimum range for each patient should be determined.

Overdosage with lithium carbonate (plasma concentrations of over 1.5 mmol lithium/litre) may be fatal. Toxic effects include coarse tremor, ataxia, dysarthria, nystagmus, renal impairment and convulsions. If any of these toxic effects occur, treatment should be stopped, plasma lithium levels determined and in mild overdosage large amounts of sodium and fluid should be given to reverse the toxicity; in severe toxicity, haemodialysis may be required.

For patients who are unresponsive to or intolerant of lithium, carbamazepine may be used in the prophylaxis of bipolar illness in patients with rapid cycling affective disorders (more than four affective episodes per year).

Lithium carbonate
Tablets, capsules, lithium carbonate 300 mg

Uses: treatment and prophylaxis of mania, prophylaxis of bipolar disorder and recurrent depression

Contraindications: renal impairment (Appendix 4); cardiac insufficiency; conditions with sodium imbalance such as Addison disease

Precautions: measure serum-lithium concentration about 4 days after starting treatment, then weekly until stabilized, then at least every 3 months; monitor thyroid function and renal function; maintain adequate fluid and sodium intake; reduction of dose or discontinuation may be necessary in diarrhoea, vomiting and intercurrent infection (especially if associated with profuse sweating); pregnancy (Appendix 2); breastfeeding (Appendix 3); elderly (reduce dose); diuretic treatment; myasthenia gravis; surgery; if possible, avoid abrupt withdrawal (see notes above); **interactions:** Appendix 1

PATIENT ADVICE. Patients should maintain adequate fluid intake and should avoid dietary changes which may reduce or increase sodium intake

NOTE. Different preparations vary widely in bioavailability; a change in the preparation used requires the same precautions as initiation of treatment

Dosage:

Treatment of mania (general guidelines only, see also note below) *by mouth,* ADULT initially 0.6–1.8 g daily (elderly 300–900 mg daily)

Prophylaxis of mania, bipolar disorder and recurrent depression (general guidelines only, see also note below), *by mouth*, ADULT initially 0.6–1.2 g daily (elderly 300–900 mg daily)

NOTE. Dosage of lithium depends on the preparation chosen since different preparations vary widely in bioavailability. Dosage should be adjusted to achieve a serum-lithium concentration of 0.4–1 mmol/litre (lower end of range for maintenance therapy and in elderly) on samples taken 12 hours after a dose and 4–7 days after starting treatment

For dose information for a specific preparation, consult manufacturer's literature

Adverse effects: gastrointestinal disturbances, fine tremor, polyuria, polydipsia, weight gain and oedema (may respond to dose reduction); signs of intoxication include blurred vision, muscle weakness, increasing gastrointestinal disturbances (anorexia, vomiting, diarrhoea), increased CNS disturbances (mild drowsiness and sluggishness, increasing to giddiness with ataxia, coarse tremor, lack of co-ordination, dysarthria) and require withdrawal of treatment; with severe overdosage (serum concentrations above 2 mmol/litre) hyperreflexia and hyperextension of the limbs, convulsions, toxic psychoses, syncope, oliguria, circulatory failure, coma, occasionally death; goitre, raised antidiuretic hormone concentration, hypothyroidism, hypokalaemia, ECG changes, exacerbation of psoriasis and kidney changes may occur

---

Carbamazepine

Tablets, carbamazepine 100 mg, 200 mg

Uses: prophylaxis of bipolar disorder unresponsive to or intolerant of lithium; epilepsy, trigeminal neuralgia (section 5.1)

Contraindications: atrioventricular conduction abnormalities; history of bone-marrow depression; porphyria

Precautions: hepatic impairment (Appendix 5); renal impairment (Appendix 4); cardiac disease (see also Contraindications); skin reactions (see Adverse effects); history of blood disorders (blood counts before and during treatment); glaucoma; pregnancy (Appendix 2); breastfeeding (Appendix 3); avoid sudden withdrawal; **interactions:** Appendix 1

BLOOD, HEPATIC OR SKIN DISORDERS. Patients or their carers should be told how to recognize signs of blood, liver or skin disorders, and advised to seek immediate medical attention if symptoms such as fever, sore throat, rash, mouth ulcers, bruising or bleeding develop. Leukopenia which is severe, progressive and associated with clinical symptoms requires withdrawal (if necessary under cover of suitable alternative)

SKILLED TASKS. May impair ability to perform skilled tasks, for example operating machinery, driving

Dosage:

Prophylaxis of bipolar disorder, *by mouth*, ADULT initially 400 mg daily in divided doses increased until symptoms are controlled to a maximum of 1.6 g daily; usual maintenance range 400–600 mg daily

Adverse effects: dizziness, drowsiness, headache, ataxia, blurred vision, diplopia (may be associated with high plasma concentrations); gastrointestinal intolerance including nausea and vomiting, anorexia, abdominal pain, dry mouth, diarrhoea or constipation; commonly, mild transient generalized erythematous rash (withdraw if worsens or is accompanied by other symptoms); leukopenia and other blood disorders (including thrombocytopenia, agranulocytosis and aplastic anaemia); cholestatic jaundice, hepatitis, acute renal failure, Stevens-Johnson syndrome (erythema multiforme), toxic epidermal necrolysis, alopecia, thromboembolism, arthralgia, fever, proteinuria, lymph node enlargement, arrhythmias, heart block and heart failure, dyskinesias, paraesthesia, depression, impotence, male infertility, gynaecomastia, galactorrhoea, aggression, activation of psychosis, photosensitivity, pulmonary hypersensitivity, hyponatraemia, oedema, disturbances of bone metabolism with osteomalacia also reported; confusion and agitation in elderly

Sodium valproate

Enteric-coated tablets (Gastro-resistant tablets), sodium valproate 200 mg, 500 mg

Uses: acute mania; epilepsy (section 5.1)

Contraindications: active liver disease, family history of severe hepatic dysfunction; pancreatitis; porphyria

Precautions: monitor liver function before and during therapy (Appendix 5), especially in patients at most risk (those with metabolic disorders, degenerative disorders, organic brain disease or severe seizure disorders associated with mental retardation); ensure no undue potential for bleeding before starting and before major surgery or anticoagulant therapy; renal impairment (Appendix 4); pregnancy (Appendix 2 (neural tube screening)); breastfeeding (Appendix 3); systemic lupus erythematosus; false-positive urine tests for ketones; avoid sudden withdrawal; **interactions:** Appendix 1
BLOOD OR HEPATIC DISORDERS. Patients or their carers should be told how to recognize signs of blood or liver disorders, and advised to seek immediate medical attention if symptoms including malaise, weakness, anorexia, lethargy, oedema, vomiting, abdominal pain, drowsiness, jaundice, or spontaneous bruising or bleeding develop

Dosage:

Acute mania, *by mouth*, ADULT initially 750 mg daily in divided doses, increased as quickly as possible to achieve the optimal response (maximum 60 mg/kg daily)

Adverse effects: gastrointestinal irritation, nausea, increased appetite and weight gain, hyperammonaemia; ataxia, tremor; transient hair loss (regrowth may be curly); oedema, thrombocytopenia, inhibition of platelet aggregation; impaired hepatic function and rarely fatal hepatic failure (see Precautions—withdraw treatment immediately if malaise, weakness, lethargy, oedema, abdominal pain, vomiting, anorexia, jaundice, drowsiness); sedation reported and also increased alertness; behavioural disturbances; rarely pancreatitis (measure plasma amylase if acute abdominal pain), leukopenia, pancytopenia, red cell hypoplasia, fibrinogen reduction; irregular periods, amenorrhoea, gynaecomastia, hearing loss, Fanconi syndrome, dementia, toxic epidermal necrolysis, Stevens-Johnson syndrome (erythema multiforme) and vasculitis reported

24.3 Drugs used in anxiety and sleep disorders

The most widely used anxiolytics and hypnotics are the benzodiazepines. Treatment of anxiety should be limited to the lowest effective dose for the shortest possible time. The cause of insomnia should be established and appropriate treatment for underlying factors instituted before hypnotics are considered. Hypnotics may be of value for a few days but rarely longer than a week.

Tolerance and dependence (both physical and psychological) and subsequent difficulty in withdrawing the drug may occur after regular use for more than a few weeks. Patients with chronic anxiety, alcohol or drug dependence or those with personality disorders are more likely to become dependent. Anxiolytics and hypnotics should be prescribed in carefully individualized dosage and use should be limited to control of acute conditions such as panic attacks and acute anxiety and severe, incapacitating insomnia. There is usually no justification for prolonging treatment with anxiolytics and hypnotics for more than one to two weeks.

If used for longer periods, withdrawal should be gradual by reduction of the dose over a period of weeks or months, as abrupt discontinuation may produce confusion, toxic psychosis, convulsions or a condition resembling delirium tremens. The benzodiazepine withdrawal syndrome may not develop until up to three weeks after stopping a long-acting benzodiazepine but may occur within a few hours in the case of a short-acting one. The syndrome is characterized by insomnia, anxiety, loss of appetite and body-weight, tremor, perspiration, tinnitus and perceptual disturbances. These symptoms may be similar to the original complaint and encourage further prescribing.

Patients should be warned that their ability to drive or operate machinery may be impaired and that the effects of alcohol may be enhanced.

Diazepam

Drug subject to international control under the Convention on Psychotropic Substances (1971)

Diazepam is a representative benzodiazepine anxiolytic and hypnotic. Various drugs can serve as alternatives

Tablets, diazepam 2 mg, 5 mg

Uses: short-term treatment of anxiety and insomnia; status epilepticus, recurrent seizures; febrile convulsions, adjunct in acute alcohol withdrawal (section 5.1); premedication (section 1.3)

Contraindications: respiratory depression; acute pulmonary insufficiency; sleep apnoea; severe hepatic impairment; myasthenia gravis

Precautions: respiratory disease, muscle weakness, history of alcohol or drug abuse, marked personality disorder; pregnancy (Appendix 2); breastfeeding (Appendix 3); reduce dose in elderly or debilitated and in hepatic impairment (avoid if severe, Appendix 5), renal impairment (Appendix 4); avoid prolonged use and abrupt withdrawal; porphyria; **interactions:** Appendix 1

SKILLED TASKS. May impair ability to perform skilled tasks, for example operating machinery, driving

Dosage:

Anxiety, *by mouth*, ADULT 2 mg 3 times daily increased if necessary to 15–30 mg daily in divided doses; ELDERLY (or debilitated) half adult dose

Insomnia, *by mouth*, ADULT 5–15 mg at bedtime

Adverse effects: drowsiness and lightheadedness the next day; confusion and ataxia (especially in the elderly); amnesia; dependence; paradoxical increase in aggression; muscle weakness; occasionally headache, vertigo, salivation changes, gastrointestinal disturbances, visual disturbances, dysarthria, tremor, changes in libido, incontinence, urinary retention; blood disorders and jaundice; skin reactions; raised liver enzymes

24.4 Obsessive-compulsive disorders and panic attacks

Obsessive-compulsive disorders can be treated with a combination of pharmacological, behavioural and psychological treatments. Antidepressants such as **clomipramine** which inhibit reuptake of serotonin have been found to be effective. Panic attacks may be treated with behavioural or cognitive therapy. If this management fails, drug therapy may be tried. Some tricyclic antidepressants including clomipramine, or SSRIs can reduce frequency of attacks or prevent them completely. Benzodiazepines may be used in panic attacks resistant to antidepressants.

Clomipramine hydrochloride
Capsules, clomipramine hydrochloride 10 mg, 25 mg

Uses: phobic and obsessional states; panic attacks

Contraindications: recent myocardial infarction, arrhythmias (especially heart block); manic phase in bipolar disorders; severe liver disease; children; porphyria

Precautions: cardiac disease (see Contraindications above), history of epilepsy; pregnancy (Appendix 2); breastfeeding (Appendix 3); elderly; hepatic impairment (Appendix 5); thyroid disease; phaeochromocytoma; history of mania, psychoses (may aggravate psychotic symptoms); angle-closure glaucoma, history of urinary retention; concurrent electroconvulsive therapy; avoid abrupt withdrawal; anaesthesia (increased risk of arrhythmias and hypotension); **interactions:** Appendix 1

SKILLED TASKS. May impair ability to perform skilled tasks, for example operating machinery, driving

Dosage:

Phobic and obsessional states, *by mouth*, ADULT initially 25 mg daily, usually at bedtime (ELDERLY 10 mg daily) increased over 2 weeks to 100–150 mg daily; CHILD not recommended

Adverse effects: sedation, dry mouth, blurred vision (disturbance of accommodation, increased intra-ocular pressure), constipation, nausea, difficulty in micturition; cardiovascular adverse effects particularly with high dosage including ECG changes, arrhythmias, postural hypotension, tachycardia, syncope; sweating, tremor, rash and hypersensitivity reactions (urticaria, photosensitivity); behavioural disturbances; hypomania or mania, confusion (particularly in elderly), interference with sexual function, blood sugar changes; increased appetite and weight gain (occasional weight loss); endocrine adverse effects such as testicular enlargement, gynaecomastia and galactorrhoea; convulsions, movement disorders and dyskinesias, fever, agranulocytosis, leukopenia, eosinophilia, purpura, thrombocytopenia, hyponatraemia (may be due to inappropriate antidiuretic hormone secretion); abnormal liver function test

Section 25: Drugs acting on the respiratory tract

25.1 Antiasthmatic drugs

Asthma

Asthma is a chronic inflammatory disease characterized by episodes of reversible airways obstruction due to bronchial hyperresponsiveness; inflammation may lead to irreversible obstruction in a few patients. A classification based on severity before the start of treatment and disease progression is of importance when decisions have to be made about management. It can be divided by severity into intermittent, mild persistent, moderate persistent and severe persistent. These are useful in the management of the disease since therapy has a stepwise approach which must be discussed with the patient before commencing therapy. The level of therapy is increased as the severity of the asthma increases with stepping-down if control is sustained (see tables on treatment below).

INHALATION. Medications for asthma can be administered in several different ways, including inhaled, oral and parenteral (subcutaneous, intramuscular, or intravenous). The main advantage of delivering drugs directly into the airways via inhalation is that high concentrations can be delivered more effectively and rapidly to the airways, and systemic adverse effects avoided or minimized.

It is important that patients receive careful instruction in the use of pressurized (aerosol) inhalation (using a metered-dose inhaler) to obtain optimum results. Before use, the inhaler should be shaken well. After exhaling as completely as possible, the mouthpiece of the inhaler should be placed well into the mouth and the lips firmly closed around it. The patient should inhale deeply through the mouth while actuating the inhaler. After holding the breath for 10 seconds or as long as is comfortable, the mouthpiece should be removed and the patient should exhale slowly.

It is important to check that patients continue to use their inhalers correctly as inadequate technique may be mistaken for drug failure. Spacing devices provide a space between the inhaler and the mouth. They may be of benefit for patients such as the elderly, small children and the asthmatic who find inhalers difficult to use or for those who have difficulty synchronizing their breathing with administration of the aerosol. A large volume spacing device is also recommended for inhalation of high doses of corticosteroids to reduce oropharyngeal deposition which can cause candidosis. The use of metered-dose inhalers with spacers is less expensive and may be as effective as use of nebulizers, although drug delivery may be affected by choice of spacing device.

PREGNANCY. Poorly controlled asthma in pregnant women can have an adverse effect on the fetus, resulting in perinatal mortality, increased prematurity and low birth-weight. For this reason using medications to obtain optimal control of asthma is justified. Administration of drugs by inhalation during pregnancy has the advantage that plasma drug concentrations are not likely to be high enough to have an effect on the fetus. Acute exacerbations should be treated aggressively in order to avoid fetal hypoxia.

Acute exacerbation of asthma

Severe asthma can be fatal and **must** be treated promptly and energetically. Acute severe asthma attacks require hospital admission where resuscitation facilities are immediately available.

Severe asthma is characterized by persistent dyspnoea poorly relieved by bronchodilators, exhaustion, a high pulse rate (usually more than 110/minute) and a very low peak expiratory flow.

As asthma becomes more severe, wheezing may be absent. Patients should be given oxygen 40–60% (if available) (see also section 1.1.3) and **corticosteroids;** for adults, prednisolone 30–60 mg by mouth *or* hydrocortisone 200 mg (preferably as sodium succinate) intravenously; for children, prednisolone 1–2 mg/kg by mouth (1–4 years, maximum 20 mg, 5–15 years, maximum 40 mg) *or* hydrocortisone 100 mg (preferably as sodium succinate) intravenously; if the patient experiences vomiting the parenteral route may be preferred for the first dose.

Patients should also be given **salbutamol** or terbutaline via a nebulizer. In emergency situations where delivery via a nebulizer is not available, salbutamol 100 micrograms by aerosol inhalation can be repeated 10–20 times preferably using a large volume spacing device.

If there is little response, the following additional treatment should be considered: **ipratropium** by nebulizer, **aminophylline** by slow intravenous injection if the patient has **not** been receiving theophylline, or administer the beta$_2$-selective adrenoceptor agonist by the intravenous route.

The use of **epinephrine (adrenaline)** (see section 3.1) in asthma has generally been superseded by beta$_2$-selective adrenoceptor agonists.

Treatment should **never** be delayed for investigations, patients should **never** be sedated and the possibility of pneumothorax should also be considered. Patients who deteriorate further despite treatment may need intermittent positive pressure ventilation.

Asthma tables.

TREATMENT OF CHRONIC ASTHMA:
INFANTS AND YOUNG CHILDREN UNDER 5 YEARS OLD
Preferred treatments are in bold print

	Long-term Preventive	**Quick Relief**
STEP 4 **Severe** **Persistent**	Daily medications •**Inhaled corticosteroid**, beclometasone dipropionate MDI with spacer and face mask > 1 mg daily *or* nebulized beclometasone > 1 mg twice daily Consider short course of soluble prednisolone tablets, regular inhaled long-acting beta$_2$-agonist *or* modified-release theophylline *Also*, nebulized beta$_2$-agonist	• Inhaled short-acting bronchodilator: **inhaled beta$_2$-agonist** *or* ipratropium bromide as needed for symptoms, not to exceed 3–4 times daily
STEP 3 **Moderate** **Persistent**	Daily medications •**Inhaled corticosteroid**, beclometasone dipropionate MDI with spacer and face mask 400–800 micrograms daily *or* nebulized beclometasone ≤ 1 mg twice daily Consider short course of soluble prednisolone tablets, regular inhaled long-acting beta$_2$-agonist *or* modified-release theophylline	• Inhaled short-acting bronchodilator: **inhaled beta$_2$-agonist** *or* ipratropium bromide as needed for symptoms, not to exceed 3–4 times daily
STEP 2 **Mild** **Persistent**	Daily medications • *Either* **inhaled corticosteroid**, beclometasone dipropionate, 400–800 micrograms, *or* cromoglicate (use MDI with a spacer and face mask *or* use a nebulizer)	• Inhaled short-acting bronchodilator: **inhaled beta$_2$-agonist** *or* ipratropium bromide as needed for symptoms, not to exceed 3–4 times daily
STEP 1 **Intermittent**	• None needed	• Inhaled short-acting bronchodilator: **inhaled beta$_2$-agonist** *or* ipratropium bromide as needed for symptoms, but not more than once daily • Intensity of treatment will depend on severity of attack

Step down
Review treatment every 3 to 6 months. If control is sustained for at least 3 months, a gradual stepwise reduction in treatment may be possible.

Step up
If control is not achieved, consider step up. But first: review patient medication technique, compliance and environmental control.

TREATMENT OF CHRONIC ASTHMA:
ADULTS AND CHILDREN OVER 5 YEARS OLD
Preferred treatments are in bold print

	Long-term Preventive	**Quick Relief**
STEP 4 **Severe** **Persistent**	Daily medications • **Inhaled corticosteroid**, beclometasone dipropionate 0.8–2 mg + • Long-acting bronchodilator: *either* **long-acting inhaled beta₂-agonist**, *and/or* modified-release theophylline, *and/or* long-acting beta₂-agonist tablets or syrup + • Corticosteroid tablets or syrup long term	• Short-acting bronchodilator: **inhaled beta₂-agonist** as needed for symptoms
STEP 3 **Moderate** **Persistent**	Daily medications • **Inhaled corticosteroid**, beclometasone diproprionate 0.8–2 mg daily in divided doses + if needed • Long-acting bronchodilator: *either* **long-acting inhaled beta₂-agonist**, modified-release theophylline, *or* long-acting beta₂-agonist tablets or syrup	• Short-acting bronchodilator: **inhaled beta₂-agonist** as needed for symptoms, not to exceed 3–4 times daily
STEP 2 **Mild** **Persistent**	Daily medications • *Either* **inhaled corticosteroid**, beclometasone dipropionate 100–400 micrograms twice daily, sodium cromoglicate *or* modified-release theophylline	• Short-acting bronchodilator: **inhaled beta₂-agonist** as needed for symptoms, not to exceed 3–4 times daily
STEP 1 **Intermittent**	• None needed	• Short-acting bronchodilator: **inhaled beta₂-agonist** as needed for symptoms (up to once daily) • Intensity of treatment will depend on severity of attack • Inhaled beta₂-agonist or sodium cromoglicate before exercise or exposure to allergen
Step down Review treatment every 3 to 6 months. If control is sustained for at least 3 months, a gradual stepwise reduction in treatment may be possible.		Step up If control is not achieved, consider step up. But first: review patient medication technique, compliance and environmental control.

Chronic obstructive pulmonary disease

Chronic obstructive pulmonary disease (chronic bronchitis and emphysema) may be helped by an inhaled short-acting **beta₂-adrenoceptor agonist** used as required *or* when the airways obstruction is more severe, by an inhaled **anticholinergic (antimuscarinic) bronchodilator** or both if necessary. Although many patients are treated with an inhaled corticosteroid its role in chronic obstructive pulmonary disease is not clear at present. A limited trial of high-dose inhaled corticosteroid *or* an oral corticosteroid is recommended for patients with moderate airflow obstruction to determine the extent of the airway reversibility and to ensure that asthma has not been overlooked.

Beta₂-adrenoceptor agonists (beta₂-adrenoceptor stimulants)

The adrenoreceptors in bronchi are mainly $beta_2$ type and their stimulation causes bronchial muscles to relax. The $beta_2$-adrenoceptor agonists include **salbutamol**, salmeterol, terbutaline, fenoterol, pirbuterol, reproterol and rimiterol.

When salbutamol is given by inhalation (100–200 micrograms) the effect can last as long as four hours thus making it suitable for both the treatment (see Tables) and prevention of asthma. It can also be taken orally, 2–4 mg up to four times a day but is less effective and causes more adverse effects. It can also be given by injection for severe bronchospasm.

ADVERSE EFFECTS. Cardiovascular adverse effects (arrhythmias, palpitations and tachycardia) may occur with salbutamol, but are infrequent with inhaled preparations. Hypokalaemia may result from $beta_2$-adrenoceptor agonist therapy. Particular caution is required in severe asthma because this effect may be potentiated by concomitant treatment with xanthines (for example theophylline), corticosteroids, diuretics and hypoxia. Plasma potassium concentrations should be monitored in severe asthma.

Xanthines

Xanthines include **theophylline** and **aminophylline**. They relax bronchial smooth muscle. Absorption of theophylline from the gastrointestinal tract is usually rapid and complete. It is metabolized by the liver but its half-life can vary considerably in certain diseases including hepatic impairment and cardiac failure and with some coadministered drugs (see Appendix 1). The half-life variations are important because theophylline has a narrow margin between therapeutic and toxic effects. At therapeutic doses some patients experience nausea and diarrhoea and when plasma concentrations exceed the recommended range of 10–20 mg/litre (55–110 micromol/litre) arrhythmias and convulsions which may be fatal can occur. Monitoring of plasma concentrations is therefore recommended. Theophylline is used to treat chronic asthma, usually in the form of modified-release preparations which produce adequate plasma concentrations for up to 12 hours. It is used as an adjunct to $beta_2$-agonist or corticosteroid therapy when additional bronchodilation is required but there is an increased risk of adverse effects with beta$_2$-agonists (see above). When given as a single dose at night, modified-release preparations may be useful in controlling nocturnal asthma and early morning wheezing.

The absorption characteristics of modified-release theophylline peparations vary considerably and therefore it is important to keep the patient on the same brand-name formulation.

Theophylline is given by injection as aminophylline (a mixture of theophylline with ethylenediamine) which is 20 times more soluble in water than theophylline alone. It is administered by slow intravenous injection in severe asthma attacks.

Corticosteroids

INHALED CORTICOSTEROIDS. Inhaled corticosteroids are antiinflammatory agents. They include **beclometasone**, budesonide and fluticasone, all of which appear equally effective. They are currently the most effective anti-inflammatory medications for the treatment of asthma. Several studies have now demonstrated that treatment with inhaled corticosteroids for one month or more significantly reduces the pathological signs of airway inflammation in asthma. They are recommended for the prophylaxis of asthma in patients using a beta$_2$-adrenoceptor agonist more than once a day. They must be used regularly to obtain maximum benefit. Symptom control is usually effective after 3 to 7 days treatment. Long-term high-dose regimens of inhaled corticosteroids are useful for the treatment of severe persistent asthma because they both reduce the need for the long-term use of oral corticosteroids and have fewer systemic adverse effects.

Local adverse effects from inhaled corticosteroids include oropharyngeal candidosis, dysphonia and occasional coughing from upper airway irritation. The use of spacing devices reduces oropharyngeal deposition and thus reduces the incidence of candidosis. The risk for systemic effects of inhaled corticosteroids is small and is dependent upon the dose and potency of the corticosteroid as well as its bioavailability and the plasma halflife of its systemically absorbed fraction. Systemic effects are very rare and include skin thinning and easy bruising, a small increased risk of glaucoma and cataracts, adrenal suppression, decrease of bone metabolism and growth retardation in children.

SYSTEMIC CORTICOSTEROIDS. Oral **corticosteroids** may be used as 'maximum therapy' to achieve control of a patient's asthma. This may be useful either when initiating long-term therapy for a patient with uncontrolled asthma or as a short 'rescue' course at any stage for acute exacerbation.

Long-term oral corticosteroid therapy may be required to control severe persistent asthma, but its use is limited by the risk of significant adverse effects. In these cases high-dose inhaled corticosteroids should be continued so that oral requirements are reduced to a minimum. Oral doses should be given as a single dose in the morning to reduce the disturbance to the circadian cortisol secretion. Dosage should always be adjusted to the lowest dose which controls symptoms.

Sodium cromoglicate

Sodium cromoglicate prevents the asthmatic response to certain allergic and nonallergic stimuli. It may be used as long-term therapy early in the course of asthma. It reduces symptoms and the frequency of exacerbations and allows dosage reduction of bronchodilators and oral corticosteroids. Prophylaxis with sodium cromoglicate is generally less effective in adults than prophylaxis with inhaled corticosteroids, but long-tem use of inhaled corticosteroids may be associated with more adverse effects. Children may respond better than adults to sodium cromoglicate. Sodium cromoglicate is of value in the prevention of exercise-induced asthma, a single dose being inhaled 30 minutes beforehand. Sodium cromoglicate is of **no** value for the treatment of acute attacks of asthma. In general, sodium cromoglicate produces only minimal adverse effects such as occasional coughing upon inhalation of the powder formulation.

Anticholinergic (antimuscarinic) bronchodilators

Ipratropium bromide may be given by inhalation in the management of chronic asthma in those who cannot be managed with beta$_2$-agonists and inhaled corticosteroids. Ipratropium bromide is also used as a bronchodilator in chronic obstructive pulmonary disease.

Salbutamol

Salbutamol is a representative beta$_2$-adrenoceptor agonist. Various drugs can serve as alternatives

Tablets, salbutamol (as sulfate) 2 mg, 4 mg

Syrup, salbutamol (as sulfate) 2 mg/5 ml

Injection (Solution for injection), salbutamol (as sulfate) 50 micrograms/ml, 5-ml ampoule

Pressurized inhalation solution (Aerosol), salbutamol (as sulfate) 100 micrograms/metered inhalation

Nebulizer solution, salbutamol (as sulfate) 5 mg/ml, 20-ml ampoules

Uses: prophylaxis and treatment of asthma; premature labour (section 22.1)

Precautions: hyperthyroidism, myocardial insufficiency, arrhythmias, susceptibility to QT-interval prolongation, hypertension, pregnancy (but appropriate to use; see also notes above); breastfeeding (Appendix 3); diabetes mellitus—especially intravenous administration (monitor blood glucose; ketoacidosis reported); **interactions:** Appendix 1

Dosage:

Chronic asthma (when inhalation is ineffective), *by mouth*, ADULT 2–4 mg 3 or 4 times daily; in some patients up to maximum of 8 mg 3 or 4 times daily; CHILD under 2 years, 100 micrograms/kg 4 times daily, 2–6 years, 1–2 mg 3–4 times daily, 6–12 years, 2 mg 3–4 times daily

Severe acute bronchospasm, *by slow intravenous injection*, ADULT 250 micrograms, repeated if necessary

Relief of acute bronchospasm, *by aerosol inhalation*, ADULT 100–200 micrograms (1–2 puffs); CHILD 100 micrograms (1 puff) increased to 200 micrograms (2 puffs) if necessary; *by intramuscular or subcutaneous injection*, ADULT 500 micrograms repeated every 4 hours if necessary

Prophylaxis of exercise-induced bronchospasm, *by aerosol inhalation*, ADULT 200 micrograms (2 puffs); CHILD 100 micrograms (1 puff) increased to 200 micrograms (2 puffs) if required

Chronic asthma (as adjunct in stepped treatment), *by aerosol inhalation*, ADULT 100–200 micrograms (1–2 puffs) up to 3–4 times daily; CHILD 100 micrograms (1 puff) 3–4 times daily, increased to 200 micrograms (2 puffs) 3–4 times daily if necessarySevere acute asthma or chronic bronchospasm unresponsive to conventional treatment, *by inhalation of nebulized solution*, ADULT and CHILD over 18 months, 2.5 mg repeated up to 4 times daily; may be increased to 5 mg if necessary—medical assessment should be considered since alternative therapy may be indicated; CHILD under 18 months, clinical efficacy uncertain (transient hypoxaemia may occur—consider oxygen supplementation)

Adverse effects: hypokalaemia after high doses (see notes above); arrhythmias, tachycardia, palpitations, peripheral vasodilation, fine tremor (usually hands), muscle cramps, headache, insomnia, behavioural disturbances in children; hypersensitivity reactions including paradoxical bronchospasm, urticaria and angioedema; slight pain on intramuscular injection

---

Beclometasone dipropionate

Beclometasone dipropionate is a representative corticosteroid. Various drugs can serve as alternatives

Pressurized inhalation solution (Aerosol), beclometasone dipropionate 50 micrograms/metered inhalation (standard dose inhaler), 250 micrograms/metered inhalation (high dose inhaler)

Uses: chronic asthma not controlled by short-acting beta$_2$-adrenoceptor agonists

Precautions: see notes above; active or quiescent tuberculosis; systemic therapy may be required during periods of stress or when airway obstruction or mucus prevent drug access to smaller airways; not for relief of acute symptoms; monitor height of children receiving prolonged treatment—if growth slowed, review therapy

---

Dosage:

Chronic asthma, *by aerosol inhalation* (standard dose inhaler), ADULT 200 micrograms twice daily *or* 100 micrograms 3–4 times daily (in more severe cases, initially 600–800 micrograms daily); CHILD 50–100 micrograms 2–4 times daily *or* 100–200 micrograms twice daily;

Chronic asthma, *by aerosol inhalation* (high dose inhaler), ADULT 500 micrograms twice daily *or* 250 micrograms 4 times daily; if necessary may be increased to 500 micrograms 4 times daily; CHILD not recommended

Adverse effects: oropharyngeal candidosis, cough and dysphonia (usually only with high doses); adrenal suppression, growth retardation in children and adolescents, impaired bone metabolism, glaucoma and cataract (with high doses, but less frequent than with systemic corticosteroids); paradoxical bronchospasm—requires discontinuation and alternative therapy (if mild, may be prevented by inhalation of beta$_2$-adrenoceptor agonist *or* by transfer from aerosol to powder inhalation); rarely, urticaria, rash, angioedema

CANDIDOSIS. Candidosis can be reduced by use of a spacing device (see notes above); rinsing the mouth with water after inhalation may help to prevent candidosis

---

Theophylline and Aminophylline

Aminophylline is a representative xanthine bronchodilator. Various drugs including theophylline can serve as alternatives

Tablets, theophylline 100 mg
Modified-release tablets, theophylline 200 mg, 300 mg
Injection (Solution for injection), aminophylline 25 mg/ml, 10-ml ampoule

Uses: chronic asthma including nocturnal asthma; acute severe asthma

Contraindications: porphyria; known hypersensitivity to ethylenediamine (for aminophylline)

Precautions: cardiac disease, hypertension, hyperthyroidism, peptic ulcer, epilepsy, hepatic impairment (Appendix 5), pregnancy (Appendix 2), breastfeeding (Appendix 3), elderly, fever; smokers may require larger or more frequent doses; **interactions:** Appendix 1

Dosage:

Chronic asthma, *by mouth* (as tablets), ADULT and CHILD over 12 years, 100–200 mg 3–4 times daily after food; *by mouth* (as modified-release tablets) ADULT 300–450 mg every 12 hours

Nocturnal asthma, *by mouth* (as modified-release tablets), ADULT total daily requirement as single evening dose

NOTE. Plasma theophylline concentration for optimum response 10–20 mg/litre (55–110 micromol/litre); narrow margin between therapeutic and toxic dose; see notes above; a range of 5–15 mg/litre (27.5–82.5 micromol/litre) may be effective and associated with fewer adverse effects

Acute severe asthma (**not** previously treated with theophylline), *by slow intravenous injection* (over at least 20 minutes), ADULT and CHILD 5 mg/kg; maintenance, *by intravenous infusion*, ADULT 500 micrograms/kg/hour; CHILD 6

months–9 years, 1 mg/kg/hour, 10–16 years, 800 micrograms/
kg/hour, adjusted according to plasma-theophylline concentration

NOTE. Patients taking oral theophylline (or aminophylline) should not
normally receive intravenous aminophylline unless plasma-theophylline
concentration is available to guide dosage

Adverse effects: gastrointestinal irritation, restlessness,
anxiety, tremor, palpitations, headache, insomnia, dizziness;
convulsions, arrhythmias and hypotension—especially if
given by rapid injection; urticaria, erythema and exfoliative
dermatitis—resulting from hypersensitivity to ethylenediamine component of aminophylline

---

Sodium cromoglicate

Sodium cromoglicate is a representative antiasthma drug. Various drugs can
serve as alternatives

Sodium cromoglicate is a complementary drug

Pressurized inhalation suspension (Aerosol), sodium cromoglicate 5 mg/
metered inhalation

Uses: prophylaxis of asthma; prevention of exercise-induced
asthma

Precautions: pregnancy (appropriate to use; see notes above
and Appendix 2); breastfeeding (Appendix 3)

Dosage:

Prophylaxis of asthma and exercise-induced asthma, *by aerosol
inhalation,* ADULT and CHILD 10 mg 4 times daily, increased in
severe cases or during periods of risk to 6–8 times daily;
additional doses may be taken before exercise; when
stabilized, may be possible to reduce to maintenance of
5 mg 4 times daily

Adverse effects: coughing, transient bronchospasm

Ipratropium bromide

Pressurized inhalation solution (Aerosol), ipratropium bromide 20 mic-
rograms/metered dose

Uses: chronic asthma; chronic obstructive pulmonary disease

Precautions: prostatic hypertrophy; pregnancy; glaucoma
(standard doses unlikely to be harmful; reported with
nebulized drug, particularly in association with nebulized
salbutamol)

Dosage:

Chronic asthma or chronic obstructive pulmonary disease, *by
aerosol inhalation,* ADULT 20–40 micrograms, in early treatment up to 80 micrograms at a time, 3–4 times daily; CHILD up
to 6 years, 20 micrograms 3 times daily, 6–12 years, 20–
40 micrograms 3 times daily

Adverse effects: occasionally, dry mouth; rarely, urinary
retention, constipation

25.2 Antitussives

Cough is an important physiological protective mechanism, but may also occur as a symptom of an underlying disorder. Treatment of the disease should be the first step in therapy to stop the cough. Upper respiratory tract infections often produce a self-limiting non-productive cough which serves no useful purpose and cough suppressants such as **dextromethorphan** may provide the patient with relief, although they control the cough rather than eliminate it. Cough suppressants must not be used to treat productive cough.

Cough suppressants should not be combined with expectorants in the treatment of cough since the combination is illogical and there is little evidence for their efficacy, but patients may be exposed to unnecessary adverse effects. Inhibition of cough reflex will lead to retention of phlegm.

Dextromethorphan hydrobromide

Drug subject to international control under Single Convention on Narcotic Drugs (1961)

Dextromethorphan hydrobromide is a representative antitussive. Various drugs can serve as alternatives
Oral solution, dextromethorphan hydrobromide 13.5 mg/5 ml

Uses: dry unproductive cough

Precautions: avoid in patients with or at risk of respiratory failure; history of asthma (avoid in asthma attack); history of drug abuse; pregnancy (Appendix 2); renal and hepatic impairment (Appendices 4 and 5)

Dosage:

Dry unproductive cough, *by mouth*, ADULT 10–20 mg every 4 hours *or* 30 mg every 6–8 hours (usual maximum 120 mg in 24 hours); CHILD 2–6 years, 2.5–5 mg every 4 hours *or* 7.5 mg every 6–8 hours (maximum 30 mg in 24 hours), 6–12 years, 5–10 mg every 4 hours *or* 15 mg every 6–8 hours (maximum 60 mg in 24 hours)

Adverse effects: dizziness, gastrointestinal disturbances; in overdose, excitation, confusion, respiratory depression

Section 26: Solutions correcting water, electrolyte and acid-base disturbances

26.1 Oral solutions

26.1.1 Oral rehydration

Replacement of fluid and electrolytes orally can be achieved by giving oral rehydration salts—solutions containing sodium, potassium and glucose. Acute diarrhoea in children should always be treated with oral rehydration solution according to plans A, B, or C as shown.

Treatment of dehydration: WHO recommendations

According to the degree of dehydration, health professionals are advised to follow one of 3 management plans.

Plan A: no dehydration. Nutritional advice and increased fluid intake are sufficient (soup, rice, water and yoghurt, or even water). For infants aged under 6 months who have not yet started taking solids, oral rehydration solution must be presented before offering milk. Mother's milk or dried cow's milk must be given without any particular restrictions. In the case of mixed breast-milk/formula feeding, the contribution of breastfeeding must be increased.

Plan B: moderate dehydration. Whatever the child's age, a 4-hour treatment plan is applied to avoid short-term problems. Feeding should not therefore be envisaged initially. It is recommended that parents are shown how to give approximately 75 ml/kg of oral rehydration solution with a spoon over a 4-hour period, and it is suggested that parents should be watched to see how they cope at the beginning of the treatment. A larger amount of solution can be given if the child continues to have frequent stools. In case of vomiting, rehydration must be discontinued for 10 minutes and then resumed at a slower rate (about one teaspoonful every 2 minutes). The child's status must be re-assessed after 4 hours to decide on the most appropriate subsequent treatment. Oral rehydration solution should continue to be offered once dehydration has been controlled, for as long as the child continues to have diarrhoea.

Plan C: severe dehydration. Hospitalization is necessary, but most urgent priority is to start rehydration. In hospital (or elsewhere), if the child can drink, oral rehydration solution must be given pending, and even during, intravenous infusion (20 ml/kg every hour by mouth before infusion, then 5 ml/kg every hour by mouth during intravenous rehydration. For intravenous supplementation, it is recommended that compound solution of sodium lactate (see section 26.2) is administered at a rate adapted to the child's age (infant under 12 months: 30 ml/kg over 1 hour then 70 ml/kg over 5 hours; child over 12 months: the same amounts over 30 minutes and 2.5 hours respectively). If the intravenous route is unavailable, a nasogastric tube is also suitable for administering oral rehydration solution, at a rate of 20 ml/kg every hour. If the child vomits, the rate of administration of the oral solution should be reduced.

Oral rehydration salts
Glucose salt solution

sodium chloride	3.5 g/litre of clean water
trisodium citrate	2.9 g/litre of clean water
potassium chloride	1.5 g/litre of clean water
glucose (anhydrous)	20.00 g/litre of clean water

When glucose and trisodium citrate are not available, they may be replaced by

sucrose (common sugar)	40.00 g/litre of clean water
sodium bicarbonate	2.5 g/litre of clean water

NOTE. The solution may be prepared either from prepackaged sugar/salt mixtures or from bulk substances and water. Solutions must be freshly prepared, preferably with recently boiled and cooled water. Accurate weighing and thorough mixing and dissolution of ingredients in the correct volume of clean water is important. Administration of more concentrated solutions can result in hypernatraemia

Uses: dehydration from acute diarrhoea

Precautions: renal impairment

Dosage:

Fluid and electrolyte loss in acute diarrhoea, *by mouth*, ADULT 200–400 ml solution after every loose motion; INFANT and CHILD according to Plans A, B or C (see above)

Adverse effects: vomiting—may indicate too rapid administration; hypernatraemia and hyperkalaemia may result from overdose in renal impairment or administration of too concentrated a solution

26.1.2 Oral potassium

Compensation for potassium loss is necessary in patients taking digoxin or antiarrhythmic drugs where potassium depletion may induce arrhythmias. It is also necessary in patients with secondary hyperaldosteronism (renal artery stenosis, liver cirrhosis, the nephrotic syndrome, severe heart failure) and those with excessive loss of potassium in the faeces (chronic diarrhoea associated with intestinal malabsorption or laxative abuse).

Measures to compensate for potassium loss may also be required in the elderly since they often take inadequate amounts in the diet (but see warning on use in renal insufficiency, below). Measures may also be required during long-term administration of drugs known to induce potassium loss (for example, corticosteroids). Potassium supplements are seldom required with the small doses of diuretics given to treat hypertension. Potassium-sparing diuretics (rather than potassium supplements) are recommended for prevention of hypokalaemia due to diuretics such as furosemide or the thiazides when these are given to eliminate oedema (see section 16.3).

For the prevention of hypokalaemia doses of potassium chloride 1.5 g (approximately 20 mmol) daily by mouth are suitable in patients taking a normal diet. Smaller doses must be used if there is renal insufficiency (common in the elderly) otherwise there is a danger of hyperkalaemia.

Larger doses may be required in established potassium depletion, the quantity depending on the severity of any continuing potassium loss (monitoring of plasma potassium and specialist advice required).

Potassium depletion is frequently associated with metabolic alkalosis and chloride depletion and these disorders require correction.

Potassium chloride

Powder for oral solution, potassium chloride 1.5 g (potassium 20 mmol, chloride 20 mmol)

Uses: prevention and treatment of hypokalaemia (see notes above)

Contraindications: severe renal impairment; plasma potassium concentration above 5 mmol/litre

Precautions: elderly , mild to moderate renal impairment (close monitoring required, Appendix 4), history of peptic ulcer; **important:** special hazard if given with drugs liable to raise plasma potassium concentrations such as potassium-sparing diuretics, ACE inhibitors or ciclosporin, for other **interactions:** Appendix 1

Dosage:

Prevention of hypokalaemia (see notes above), *by mouth*, ADULT 20–50 mmol daily after meals

Potassium depletion (see notes above), *by mouth*, ADULT 40–100 mmol daily in divided doses after meals: adjust dose according to severity of deficiency and any continuing loss of potassium

RECONSTITUTION AND ADMINISTRATION. According to manufacturer's directions

Adverse effects: nausea and vomiting, gastrointestinal irritation

---

26.2 Parenteral solutions

Solutions of electrolytes are given intravenously, to meet normal fluid and electrolyte requirements or to replenish substantial deficits or continuing losses, when the patient is nauseated or vomiting and is unable to take adequate amounts by mouth.

In an individual patient the nature and severity of the electrolyte imbalance must be assessed from the history and clinical and biochemical examination. Sodium, potassium, chloride, magnesium, phosphate, and water depletion can occur singly and in combination with or without disturbances of acid-base balance.

Isotonic solutions may be infused safely into a peripheral vein. More concentrated solutions, for example 20% glucose, are best given through an indwelling catheter positioned in a large vein.

Sodium chloride in isotonic solution provides the most important extracellular ions in near physiological concentrations and is indicated in *sodium depletion* which may arise from conditions such as gastroenteritis, diabetic ketoacidosis, ileus and ascites. In a severe deficit of from 4 to 8 litres, 2 to 3 litres of isotonic sodium chloride may be given over 2 to 3 hours; thereafter infusion can usually be at a slower rate.

Excessive administration should be avoided; the jugular venous pressure should be assessed; the bases of the lungs should be examined for crepitations, and in elderly or seriously ill patients it is often helpful to monitor the right atrial (central) venous pressure.

The more physiologically appropriate **compound solution of sodium lactate** can be used instead of isotonic sodium chloride solution during surgery or in the initial management of the injured or wounded.

Sodium chloride and glucose solutions are indicated when there is *combined water and sodium depletion*. A 1:1 mixture of isotonic sodium chloride and 5% glucose allows some of the water (free of sodium) to enter body cells which suffer most from dehydration while the sodium salt with a volume of water determined by the normal plasma Na^+ remains extracellular. Combined sodium, potassium, chloride, and water depletion may occur, for example, with severe diarrhoea or persistent vomiting; replacement is carried out with sodium chloride intravenous infusion 0.9% and glucose intravenous infusion 5% with potassium as appropriate.

Glucose solutions (5%) are mainly used to replace *water deficits* and should be given alone when there is no significant loss of electrolytes. Average water requirement in a healthy adult are 1.5 to 2.5 litres daily and this is needed to balance unavoidable losses of water through the skin and lungs and to provide sufficient for urinary excretion. Water depletion (dehydration) tends to occur when these losses are not matched by a comparable intake, as for example may occur in coma or dysphagia or in the aged or apathetic who may not drink water in sufficient amount on their own initiative.

Excessive loss of water without loss of electrolytes is uncommon, occurring in fevers, hyperthyroidism, and in uncommon water-losing renal states such as diabetes insipidus or hypercalcaemia. The volume of glucose solution needed to replace deficits varies with the severity of the disorder, but usually lies within the range of 2 to 6 litres.

Glucose solutions are also given in regimens with calcium, bicarbonate, and insulin for the emergency treatment of *hyperkalaemia*. They are also given, after correction of hyperglycaemia, during treatment of diabetic ketoacidosis, when they must be accompanied by continuing insulin infusion. A concentrated solution of glucose (50%) is used to treat *hypoglycaemia*.

Sodium hydrogen carbonate (sodium bicarbonate) is used to control severe *metabolic acidosis* (as in renal failure). Since this condition is usually attended by sodium depletion, it is reasonable to correct this first by the administration of isotonic sodium chloride intravenous infusion, provided the kidneys are not primarily affected and the degree of acidosis is not so severe as to impair renal function. In these circumstances, isotonic sodium chloride alone is usually effective as it restores the ability of the kidneys to generate bicarbonate. In renal acidosis or in severe metabolic acidosis of any origin, for example blood pH < 7.1, sodium hydrogen carbonate (1.4%) may be infused with isotonic sodium chloride when the acidosis remains unresponsive to correction of anoxia or fluid depletion; a total volume of up to 6 litres (4 litres of sodium chloride and 2 litres of sodium hydrogen carbonate) may be necessary in the adult. In severe shock due for example to cardiac arrest, metabolic acidosis may develop without sodium depletion; in these circumstances sodium hydrogen carbonate is best given in a small volume of hypertonic solution (for example 50 ml of 8.4% solution intravenously); plasma pH should be monitored. Sodium hydrogen carbonate is also used in the emergency management of *hyperkalaemia*.

Intravenous **potassium chloride** and sodium chloride infusion is used to correct *severe hypokalaemia* and depletion when sufficient potassium cannot be taken by mouth. Potassium chloride may be added to sodium chloride 0.9% infusion and given slowly over 2 to 3 hours with specialist advice and ECG monitoring in difficult cases. Repeated measurements of plasma potassium are necessary to determine whether further infusions are required and to avoid the development of hyperkalaemia which is especially likely to occur in renal impairment.

Initial potassium replacement therapy should **not** involve glucose infusions because glucose may cause a further decrease in the plasma-potassium concentration.

Glucose

Infusion (Solution for infusion), glucose 5% (isotonic), 10% (hypertonic), 50% (hypertonic)

Uses: fluid replacement without significant electrolyte deficit (see notes above); treatment of hypoglycaemia

Precautions: diabetes mellitus (may require additional insulin)

Dosage:

Fluid replacement, *by intravenous infusion*, ADULT and CHILD determined on the basis of clinical and, whenever possible, electrolyte monitoring (see notes above)

Treatment of hypoglycaemia, *by intravenous infusion* of 50% glucose solution into a large vein, ADULT, 25 ml

Adverse effects: glucose injections, especially if hypertonic, may have a low pH and cause venous irritation and thrombophlebitis; fluid and electrolyte disturbances; oedema or water intoxication (on prolonged administration or rapid infusion of large volumes of isotonic solutions); hyperglyc-aemia (on prolonged administration of hypertonic solutions)

Glucose with sodium chloride

Infusion (Solution for infusion), glucose 4%, sodium chloride 0.18% (1.8 g, 30 mmol each of Na$^+$ and Cl$^-$/litre)

Uses: fluid and electrolyte replacement

Precautions: restrict intake in impaired renal function, cardiac failure, hypertension, pulmonary oedema, toxaemia of pregnancy

Dosage:

Fluid replacement, *by intravenous infusion*, ADULT and CHILD determined on the basis of clinical and, whenever possible, electrolyte monitoring (see notes above)

Adverse effects: administration of large doses may give rise to oedema

Sodium chloride

Infusion (Solution for infusion), sodium chloride 0.9% (9 g, 154 mmol each of Na$^+$ and Cl$^-$/litre)

Uses: electrolyte and fluid replacement

Precautions: restrict intake in impaired renal function (Appendix 4), cardiac failure, hypertension, pulmonary oedema, toxaemia of pregnancy

Dosage:

Fluid and electrolyte replacement, *by intravenous infusion*, ADULT and CHILD determined on the basis of clinical and, whenever possible, electrolyte monitoring (see notes above)

Adverse effects: administration of large doses may give rise to sodium accumulation and oedema

Sodium lactate, compound solution of

Compound solution of sodium lactate is a representative intravenous electrolyte solution. Various solutions can serve as alternatives

Infusion (Solution for infusion), sodium chloride 0.6%, sodium lactate 0.25%, potassium chloride 0.04%, calcium chloride 0.027% (containing Na$^+$ 131 mmol, K$^+$ 5 mmol, Ca^{2+} 2 mmol, HCO$_3^-$ (as lactate) 29 mmol, Cl$^-$ 111 mmol/litre)

Uses: pre- and perioperative fluid and electrolyte replacement; hypovolaemic shock

Contraindications: metabolic or respiratory alkalosis; hypocalcaemia or hypochlorhydria

Precautions: restrict intake in impaired renal function, cardiac failure, hypertension, pulmonary oedema, toxaemia of pregnancy; **interactions:** Appendix 1

Dosage:

Fluid and electrolyte replacement or hypovolaemic shock, *by intravenous infusion*, ADULT and CHILD determined on the basis of clinical and, whenever possible, electrolyte monitoring (see notes above)

Adverse effects: excessive administration may cause metabolic alkalosis; administration of large doses may give rise to oedema

Sodium hydrogen carbonate

Infusion (Solution for infusion), sodium hydrogen carbonate 1.4% (14 g, 166.7 mmol each of Na^+ and HCO_3^-/litre)

Injection (Solution for injection), sodium hydrogen carbonate 8.4% (840 mg, 10 mmol each of Na^+ and HCO_3^-/10 ml)

Uses: metabolic acidosis

Contraindications: metabolic or respiratory alkalosis, hypocalcaemia, hypochlorhydria

Precautions: restrict intake in impaired renal function (Appendix 4), cardiac failure, hypertension, pulmonary oedema, toxaemia of pregnancy; monitor electrolytes and acid-base status; **interactions:** Appendix 1

Dosage:

Metabolic acidosis, *by slow intravenous injection*, ADULT and CHILD a strong solution (up to 8.4%) **or** *by continuous intravenous infusion*, ADULT and CHILD a weaker solution (usually 1.4%), an amount appropriate to the body base deficit (see notes above)

Adverse effects: excessive administration may cause hypokalaemia and metabolic alkalosis, especially in renal impairment; large doses may give rise to sodium accumulation and oedema

---

Potassium chloride

Concentrate for infusion (Concentrate for solution for infusion), potassium chloride 11.2% (112 mg, approximately 1.5 mmol each of K^+ and Cl^-/ml), 20-ml ampoule

Uses: electrolyte imbalance

Precautions: for intravenous infusion the concentration of solution should not usually exceed 3.2 g (43 mmol)/litre; specialist advice and ECG monitoring (see notes above); renal impairment (Appendix 4); **interactions:** Appendix 1

Dosage:

Electrolyte imbalance, *by slow intravenous infusion*, ADULT and CHILD depending on the deficit or the daily maintenance requirements (see also notes above)

DILUTION AND ADMINISTRATION. **Must** be diluted before use and administered according to manufacturer's directions

Adverse effects: rapid infusion is toxic to the heart

26.3 Water

Water for injections

Injection, sterile distilled water free from pyrogens, 2-ml, 5-ml, 10-ml ampoules

Uses: in preparations intended for parenteral administration and in other sterile preparations

Section 27: Vitamins and minerals

27.1 Vitamins

Vitamins are used for the prevention and treatment of specific deficiency states or when the diet is known to be inadequate. It has often been suggested but never convincingly proved, that subclinical vitamin deficiencies cause much chronic ill-health and liability to infections. This has led to enormous consumption of vitamin preparations, which have no more than placebo value. Most vitamins are comparatively non-toxic but prolonged administration of high doses of retinol (vitamin A), ergocalciferol (vitamin D_2) and pyridoxine (vitamin B_6) may have severe adverse effects.

Retinol (vitamin A) is a fat-soluble substance stored in body organs, principally the liver. Periodic high-dose supplementation is intended to protect against vitamin A deficiency which is associated with ocular defects particularly xerophthalmia (including night blindness which may progress to severe eye lesions and blindness), and an increased susceptibility to infections, particularly measles and diarrhoea. Universal vitamin A distribution involves the periodic administration of supplemental doses to all preschool-age children with priority given to age groups, 6 months to 3 years, or regions at greatest risk. All mothers in high-risk regions should also receive a high dose of vitamin A within 8 weeks of delivery. Since vitamin A is associated with a teratogenic effect it should be given in smaller doses (no more than 10 000 IU/day) to women of child-bearing age. It is also used in the treatment of active xerophthalmia. Doses of vitamin A should be administered orally immediately upon diagnosis of xerophthalmia and thereafter patients with acute corneal lesions should be referred to a hospital on an emergency basis. In women of child-bearing age there is a need to balance the possible teratogenic effects of vitamin A should they be pregnant with the serious consequences of xerophthalmia. Where there are severe signs of xerophthalmia high dose treatment as for patients over 1 year should be given. When less severe symptoms are present (for example night blindness) a much lower dose is recommended. Vitamin A therapy should also be given during epidemics of measles to reduce complications.

Vitamin B is composed of widely differing substances which are, for convenience, classed as 'vitamin B complex'. **Thiamine (vitamin B_1)** is used orally for deficiency due to to inadequate dietary intake. Severe deficiency may result in 'beri-beri'. Chronic dry 'beri-beri' is characterized by peripheral neuropathy, muscle wasting and weakness, and paralysis; wet 'beri-beri' is characterized by cardiac failure and oedema. Wernicke-Korsakoff syndrome (demyelination of the CNS) may develop in severe deficiency. Thiamine is given by intravenous injection in doses of up to 300 mg daily (parenteral preparations may contain several B group vitamins) as initial treatment in severe deficiency states. Potentially severe allergic reactions may occur after parenteral administration. Facilities for resuscitation should be immediately available. **Riboflavin (vitamin B$_2$)** deficiency may result from reduced dietary intake or reduced absorption due to liver disease, alcoholism, chronic infection or probenecid therapy. It may also occur in association with other deficiency states such as pellagra. **Pyridoxine (vitamin B$_6$)** deficiency is rare as the vitamin is widely distributed in foods, but deficiency may occur during isoniazid therapy and is characterized by peripheral neuritis. High doses are given in some metabolic disorders, such as hyperoxaluria. **Nicotinic acid** inhibits the synthesis of cholesterol and triglyceride and is used in some hyperlipidaemias. Nicotinic acid and **nicotinamide** are used to prevent and treat nicotinic acid deficiency (pellagra). Nicotinamide is generally preferred as it does not cause vasodilation. **Hydroxocobalamin** is the form of **vitamin B$_{12}$** used to treat vitamin B$_{12}$ deficiency due to dietary deficiency or malabsorption (see section 10.1).

Folic acid is essential for the synthesis of DNA and certain proteins. Deficiency of folic acid or vitamin B$_{12}$ is associated with megaloblastic anaemia. Folic acid should not be used in undiagnosed megaloblastic anaemia unless vitamin B$_{12}$ is administered concurrently, otherwise neuropathy may be precipitated (see section 10.1). Supplementation with folic acid 400 micrograms daily is recommended for women of child-bearing potential in order to reduce the risk of serious neural tube defects in their offspring (see section 10.1).

Ascorbic acid (vitamin C) is used for the prevention and treatment of scurvy. Claims that ascorbic acid is of value in the treatment of common colds are unsubstantiated.

The term **vitamin D** covers a range of compounds including **ergocalciferol (vitamin D$_2$)** and **colecalciferol (vitamin D$_3$)**. These two compounds are equipotent and either can be used to prevent and treat rickets.

Simple deficiency of vitamin D occurs in those who have an inadequate dietary intake or who fail to produce enough colecalciferol (vitamin D$_3$) in their skin from the precursor 7-dehydrocholesterol in response to ultraviolet light.

Children with dark skin must continue vitamin D prophylaxis for up to 24 months because of their inability to produce enough vitamin D$_3$ in their skin. Dark skin with a high melanin content must be exposed to daylight longer than light skin in order to obtain the same synthesis of vitamin D$_3$. Vitamin D is also used in deficiency states caused by intestinal malabsorption or chronic liver disease and for the hypocalcaemia of hypoparathyroidism.

Vitamin K is necessary for the production of blood clotting factors (see section 10.2).

Ascorbic acid

Vitamin C

Tablets, ascorbic acid 50 mg

Uses: prevention and treatment of scurvy

Dosage:

Prophylaxis of scurvy, *by mouth*, ADULT and CHILD 25–75 mg daily

Treatment of scurvy, *by mouth*, ADULT and CHILD not less than 250 mg daily in divided doses

Adverse effects: gastrointestinal disturbances reported with large doses

---

Ergocalciferol

Vitamin D$_2$

Ergocalciferol is a representative vitamin D compound. Various vitamin D compounds can serve as alternatives

Tablets, ergocalciferol 1.25 mg (50 000 units)

Capsules, ergocalciferol 1.25 mg (50 000 units)

Oral solution, ergocalciferol 250 micrograms/ml (10 000 units/ml)

NOTE. There is no plain vitamin D tablet available for the treatment of simple deficiency. Alternatives include calcium and ergocalciferol tablets, although the calcium is unnecessary

Tablets, ergocalciferol 10 micrograms (400 units), calcium lactate 300 mg, calcium phosphate 150 mg

Uses: prevention of vitamin D deficiency; vitamin D deficiency caused by malabsorption or chronic liver disease; hypocalcaemia of hypoparathyroidism

Contraindications: hypercalcaemia; metastatic calcification

Precautions: take care to ensure correct dose in infants; monitor plasma calcium at weekly intervals in patients receiving high doses or those with renal impairment; nausea and vomiting— may indicate overdose and hypercalcaemia; pregnancy and breastfeeding (Appendices 2 and 3); **interactions:** Appendix 1

Dosage:

Prevention of vitamin D deficiency, *by mouth*, ADULT and CHILD 10 micrograms (400 units) daily

Treatment of vitamin D deficiency, *by mouth*, ADULT 1.25 mg (50 000 units) daily for a limited period; CHILD 75–125 micrograms (3000–5000 units) daily

Hypocalcaemia associated with hypoparathyroidism, *by mouth*, ADULT 2.5 mg (100 000 units) daily; CHILD up to 1.5 mg (60 000 units) daily

Adverse effects: symptoms of overdosage include anorexia, lassitude, nausea and vomiting, diarrhoea, weight loss, polyuria, sweating, headache, thirst, vertigo, and raised concentrations of calcium and phosphate in plasma and urine; calcification of tissues may occur if dose of 1.25 mg continued for several months

---

Nicotinamide

Nicotinamide is a representative vitamin B substance. Various compounds can serve as alternatives

Tablets, nicotinamide 50 mg

Uses: treatment of pellagra

Dosage:

Treatment of pellagra, *by mouth*, ADULT up to 500 mg daily in divided doses

Pyridoxine hydrochloride

Vitamin B$_6$

Tablets, pyridoxine hydrochloride 25 mg

Uses: treatment of pyridoxine deficiency due to metabolic disorders; isoniazid neuropathy; sideroblastic anaemia

Precautions: interactions: Appendix 1

Dosage:

Deficiency states, *by mouth*, ADULT 25–50 mg up to 3 times daily

Isoniazid neuropathy, prophylaxis, *by mouth*, ADULT 10 mg daily

Isoniazid neuropathy, treatment, *by mouth*, ADULT 50 mg 3 times daily

Sideroblastic anaemia, *by mouth*, ADULT 100–400 mg daily in divided doses

Adverse effects: generally well tolerated, but chronic administration of high doses may cause peripheral neuropathies

Retinol

Vitamin A

Retinol is a representative vitamin A compound. Various compounds can serve as alternatives

Sugar-coated tablets (Coated tablets), retinol (as palmitate) 10 000 units

Capsules, retinol (as palmitate) 200 000 units

Oral solution (oily), retinol (as palmitate) 100 000 units/ml

Water-miscible injection (Solution for injection), retinol (as palmitate) 50 000 units/ml, 2-ml ampoule

Uses: prevention and treatment of vitamin A deficiency; prevention of complications of measles

Precautions: pregnancy (teratogenic; see notes above and Appendix 2); breastfeeding (Appendix 3)

Dosage:

Prevention of vitamin A deficiency (universal or targeted distribution programmes), *by mouth*, INFANTS less than 6 months, 50 000 units before 6 weeks of age, followed by 2 further doses of 50 000 units at intervals of 1 month (total dose 150 000 units), 6–12 months, 100 000 units, preferably at measles vaccination; CHILD over 1 year (preschool), 200 000 units every 4–6 months; ADULTS women of child-bearing age or pregnant, maximum of 10 000 units daily *or* maximum 25 000 units weekly; ADULTS in high-risk regions, mothers at or soon after delivery 200 000 units, then further dose within 6 weeks

Treatment of xerophthalmia, *by mouth*, INFANTS less than 6 months, 50 000 units on diagnosis, repeated the next day and then after 2 weeks; 6–12 months, 100 000 units immediately on diagnosis, repeated the next day and then after 2 weeks; CHILD over one year and ADULT (except women of child-bearing age) 200 000 units on diagnosis, repeated the next day and then after 2 weeks; ADULT (women of child-bearing age, see notes above), severe signs of xerophthalmia, as for other adults; less severe cases (for example, night blindness), 5000–10 000 units daily for at least 4 weeks *or* up to 25 000 units weekly

NOTE. Oral vitamin A preparations are preferred for the prevention and treatment of vitamin A deficiency. However, in situations where patients have severe anorexia or vomiting or are suffering from malabsorption, a water-miscible injection preparation may be administered intramuscularly

Adverse effects: no serious or irreversible adverse effects in recommended doses; high levels may cause birth defects; transient increased intracranial pressure in adults or a tense and bulging fontanelle in infants (with high dosage); massive overdose can cause rough skin, dry hair, an enlarged liver, a raised erythrocyte sedimentation rate, raised serum calcium and raised serum alkaline phosphatase concentrations

---

Riboflavin

Vitamin B_2

Tablets, riboflavin 5 mg

Uses: vitamin B_2 deficiency

Dosage:

Treatment of vitamin B_2 deficiency, *by mouth*, ADULT and CHILD up to 30 mg daily in single or divided doses

Prophylaxis of vitamin B_2 deficiency, *by mouth*, ADULT and CHILD 1–2 mg daily

---

Thiamine hydrochloride

Vitamin B_1

Tablets, thiamine hydrochloride 50 mg

Uses: prevention and treatment of vitamin B_1 deficiency

Precautions: parenteral administration (see notes above); breastfeeding (Appendix 3)

Dosage:

Mild chronic thiamine deficiency, *by mouth*, ADULT 10–25 mg daily

27.2 Minerals

Calcium gluconate. Calcium supplements are usually only required where dietary calcium intake is deficient. This dietary requirement varies with age and is relatively greater in childhood, pregnancy and lactation due to an increased demand, and in old age, due to impaired absorption. In osteoporosis, a calcium intake which is double the recommended daily amount reduces the rate of bone loss. In hypocalcaemic tetany calcium gluconate must be given parenterally but plasma calcium must be monitored. Calcium gluconate is also used in cardiac resuscitation.

Iodine is among the body's essential trace elements. The recommended intake of iodine is 150 micrograms daily (200 micrograms daily in pregnant and breastfeeding women); in children the recommended intake of iodine is 50 micrograms daily for infants under 1 year, 90 micrograms daily for children aged 2–6 years, and 120 micrograms daily for children aged 7–12 years. Deficiency causes endemic goitre and results in endemic cretinism (characterized by deaf-mutism, intellectual deficit, spasticity and sometimes hypothyroidism), impaired mental function in children and adults and an increased incidence of still-births and perinatal and infant mortality. Iodine and iodides may suppress neonatal thyroid function and in general iodine compounds should be avoided in pregnancy. Where it is essential to prevent neonatal goitre and cretinism, iodine should not be witheld from pregnant women. Control of iodine deficiency largely depends upon salt iodization with potassium iodide or potassium iodate and through dietary diversification. In areas where iodine deficiency disorders are moderate to severe, **iodized oil** given either before or at any stage of pregnancy is found to be beneficial.

Sodium fluoride. Availability of adequate fluoride confers significant resistance to dental caries. It is now considered that the topical action of fluoride on enamel and plaque is more important than the systemic effect. Where the natural fluoride content of the drinking water is significantly less than 1 mg per litre, artificial fluoridation is the most economical method of supplementing fluoride intake. Daily administration of fluoride tablets or drops is a suitable alternative, but systemic fluoride supplements should not be prescribed without reference to the fluoride content of the local water supply; they are not advisable when the water contains more than 700 micrograms per litre. In addition, infants need not receive fluoride supplements until the age of 6 months. Use of dentifrices which incorporate sodium fluoride is a convenient source of fluoride. Individuals who are either particularly caries prone or medically compromised may be given additional protection by the use of fluoride rinses or by application of fluoride gels. Rinses may be used daily or weekly; daily use of a less concentrated rinse is more effective than weekly use of a more concentrated one. High-strength gels must be applied on a regular basis under professional supervision; extreme caution is necessary to prevent the child from swallowing any excess.

For the use of **iron** preparations in the treatment of anaemia see section 10.1.

Calcium gluconate

Calcium gluconate is a complementary drug

Injection (Solution for injection), calcium gluconate (monohydrate) 100 mg (Ca^{2+} 220 micromol)/ml, 10-ml ampoule

Uses: hypocalcaemic tetany

Contraindications: conditions associated with hypercalcaemia and hypercalciuria (for example some forms of malignant disease)

Precautions: monitor plasma calcium concentration; **interactions:** Appendix 1

Dosage:

Hypocalcaemic tetany, *by slow intravenous injection*, ADULT 1 g (2.2 mmol) followed *by continuous intravenous infusion* of about 4 g (8.8 mmol) daily

DILUTION AND ADMINISTRATION. According to manufacturer's directions

Adverse effects: mild gastrointestinal disturbances; bradycardia, arrhythmia; irritation at injection site

---

Iodine

Oily injection (Solution for injection), iodine (as iodized oil) 240 mg/ml, 480 mg/ml

NOTE. Iodized oil may also be given by mouth

Uses: prevention and treatment of iodine deficiency

Contraindications: breastfeeding (Appendix 3)

Precautions: over 45 years old or with nodular goitre (especially susceptible to hyperthyroidism when given iodine supplements—iodized oil may not be appropriate); may interfere with thyroid-function tests; pregnancy (see notes above and Appendix 2)

Dosage:

Endemic moderate to severe iodine deficiency, *by intramuscular injection*, ADULT women of child-bearing age, including any stage of pregnancy, 480 mg once each year; *by mouth*, ADULT during pregnancy and one year postpartum, 300–480 mg once a year *or* 100–300 mg every 6 months; women of child-bearing age, 400–960 mg once a year *or* 200–480 mg every 6 months

Iodine deficiency, *by intramuscular injection*, INFANT up to 1 year, 190 mg; CHILD and ADULT 380 mg (aged over 45 years or with nodular goitre, 76 mg but see also Precautions) (provides up to 3 years protection)

Iodine deficiency, *by mouth*, ADULT (except during pregnancy) and CHILD above 6 years, 400 mg once a year; ADULT during pregnancy, single dose of 200 mg; INFANT under 1 year, single dose of 100 mg; CHILD 1–5 years, 200 mg once a year

Adverse effects: hypersensitivity reactions; goitre and hypothyroidism; hyperthyroidism

---

Sodium fluoride

Sodium fluoride is a representative fluoride. Various fluorides can serve as alternatives

Mouth wash, sodium fluoride 0.05%, 0.2%

Uses: prevention of dental caries

Contraindications: not for areas where drinking water is fluoridated or where fluorine content is naturally high

---

Dosage:

Prevention of dental caries, *as oral rinse*, CHILD over 6 years, 10 ml 0.05% solution daily *or* 10 ml 0.2% solution weekly

NOTE. Fluoridated toothpastes are also a convenient source of fluoride for prophylaxis of dental caries

Adverse effects: in recommended doses toxicity unlikely; occasional white flecks on teeth at recommended doses; rarely yellowish-brown discoloration if recommended doses are exceeded

Appendix 1: Interactions

Two or more drugs given at the same time may exert their effects independently or may interact. The interaction may be potentiation or antagonism of one drug by another, or occasionally some other effect. Drug interactions may be pharmacodynamic or pharmacokinetic.

Pharmacodynamic interactions occur between drugs which have similar or antagonistic pharmacological effects or adverse effects. They are usually predictable from a knowledge of the pharmacology of the interacting drugs and an interaction occurring with one drug is likely to occur with a related drug. Pharmacodynamic interactions may be due to

- competition at receptor sites
- drugs acting on the same physiological system

Pharmacodynamic interactions usually occur in most patients who receive the interacting drugs.

Pharmacokinetic interactions occur when one drug increases or reduces the amount of another drug available to produce its pharmacological action. They are not easily predicted and an interaction occurring with one drug cannot be assumed to occur with a related drug unless their pharmacokinetic properties are known to be similar. Pharmacokinetic interactions may be due to

- interference with absorption
- changes in protein binding
- modification of drug metabolism
- interference with renal excretion

Many pharmacokinetic interactions affect only a small proportion of patients taking the combination of drugs.

Many drug interactions do not have serious consequences and many which are potentially harmful occur only in a small proportion of patients. A known interaction will not necessarily occur to the same extent in all patients. Drugs with a small therapeutic ratio (such as phenytoin) and drugs which require careful dose control (such as anticoagulants, antihypertensives or antidiabetics) are most often involved.

Patients at increased risk from drug interactions include the elderly and those with impaired renal or liver function.

In the following table the symbol * indicates a **potentially hazardous interaction** and the combined administration of the drugs involved should be **avoided**, or only taken with caution and appropriate monitoring. Interactions with no symbol do not usually have serious consequences.

Acetazolamide

 Acetylsalicylic acid: Reduced excretion of acetazolamide (risk of toxicity)

 Alcohol: Enhanced hypotensive effect

 Amitriptyline: Increased risk of postural hypotension

 Atenolol: Enhanced hypotensive effect

 * Captopril: Enhanced hypotensive effect (can be extreme)

 * Carbamazepine: Increased risk of hyponatraemia; acetazolamide
    increases plasma-carbamazepine concentration

 Chloral hydrate: Enhanced hypotensive effect

 Chlorpromazine: Enhanced hypotensive effect

 Cisplatin: Increased risk of nephrotoxicity and ototoxicity

 Clomipramine: Increased risk of postural hypotension

 Clonazepam: Enhanced hypotensive effect

 Contraceptives, Oral: Antagonism of diuretic effect

 Dexamethasone: Increased risk of hypokalaemia; antagonism of diuretic
    effect

 Diazepam: Enhanced hypotensive effect

 * Digoxin: Cardiac toxicity of digoxin increased if hypokalaemia occurs

 Ether, Anaesthetic: Enhanced hypotensive effect

 Fludrocortisone: Increased risk of hypokalaemia; antagonism of diuretic
    effect

 Fluphenazine: Enhanced hypotensive effect

 Furosemide: Increased risk of hypokalaemia

 Glyceryl trinitrate: Enhanced hypotensive effect

 Halothane: Enhanced hypotensive effect

 Hydralazine: Enhanced hypotensive effect

 Hydrochlorothiazide: Increased risk of hypokalaemia

 Hydrocortisone: Increased risk of hypokalaemia; antagonism of diuretic
    effect

 Ibuprofen: Risk of nephrotoxicity of ibuprofen increased; antagonism of
    diuretic effect

 Isosorbide dinitrate: Enhanced hypotensive effect

 Ketamine: Enhanced hypotensive effect

 Levodopa: Enhanced hypotensive effect

 * Lidocaine: Action of lidocaine antagonised by hypokalaemia

 * Lithium: Excretion of lithium increased

 Methyldopa: Enhanced hypotensive effect

 Nifedipine: Enhanced hypotensive effect

 Nitrous oxide: Enhanced hypotensive effect

 Phenytoin: Increased risk of osteomalacia

 * Prazosin: Enhanced hypotensive effect; increased risk of first-dose
    hypotensive effect of prazosin

 Prednisolone: Increased risk of hypokalaemia; antagonism of diuretic
    effect

 Propranolol: Enhanced hypotensive effect

 * Quinidine: Cardiac toxicity of quinidine increased if hypokalaemia
    occurs; acetazolamide reduces excretion of quinidine (occasionally
    increased plasma concentration)

 Reserpine: Enhanced hypotensive effect

 Salbutamol: Increased risk of hypokalaemia with high doses of salbu-
    tamol

 Sodium nitroprusside: Enhanced hypotensive effect

 Theophylline: Increased risk of hypokalaemia

 Thiopental: Enhanced hypotensive effect

 Timolol: Enhanced hypotensive effect

 Verapamil: Enhanced hypotensive effect

Acetylsalicylic acid

 Acetazolamide: Reduced excretion of acetazolamide (risk of toxicity)

 Antacids (Aluminium hydroxide; Magnesium hydroxide): Excretion of
    acetylsalicylic acid increased in alkaline urine

 * Captopril: Antagonism of hypotensive effect; increased risk of renal
    impairment

 Dexamethasone: Increased risk of gastrointestinal bleeding and ulcera-
    tion; dexamethasone reduces plasma-salicylate concentration

Acetylsalicylic acid (Continued)

Fludrocortisone: Increased risk of gastrointestinal bleeding and ulceration; fludrocortisone reduces plasma-salicylate concentration

* Heparin: Enhanced anticoagulant effect

Hydrocortisone: Increased risk of gastrointestinal bleeding and ulceration; hydrocortisone reduces plasma-salicylate concentration

* Ibuprofen: Avoid concurrent administration (increased adverse effects, including gastrointestinal damage)

* Methotrexate: Reduced excretion of methotrexate (increased toxicity)

Metoclopramide: Enhanced effect of acetylsalicylic acid (increased rate of absorption)

Phenytoin: Enhancement of effect of phenytoin

Prednisolone: Increased risk of gastrointestinal bleeding and ulceration; prednisolone reduces plasma-salicylate concentration

Spironolactone: Antagonism of diuretic effect

Valproic acid: Enhancement of effect of valproic acid

* Warfarin: Increased risk of bleeding due to antiplatelet effect

Alcohol

Acetazolamide: Enhanced hypotensive effect

Amiloride: Enhanced hypotensive effect

* Amitriptyline: Enhanced sedative effect

Atenolol: Enhanced hypotensive effect

Captopril: Enhanced hypotensive effect

Carbamazepine: Possibly enhanced CNS adverse effects of carbamazepine

Chloral hydrate: Enhanced sedative effect

Chlorphenamine: Enhanced sedative effect

Chlorpromazine: Enhanced sedative effect

* Clomipramine: Enhanced sedative effect

Clonazepam: Enhanced sedative effect

Codeine: Enhanced sedative and hypotensive effect

Diazepam: Enhanced sedative effect

Fluphenazine: Enhanced sedative effect

Furosemide: Enhanced hypotensive effect

Glibenclamide: Enhanced hypoglycaemic effect

Glyceryl trinitrate: Enhanced hypotensive effect

Haloperidol: Enhanced sedative effect

Hydralazine: Enhanced hypotensive effect

Hydrochlorothiazide: Enhanced hypotensive effect

Insulins: Enhanced hypoglycaemic effect

Isosorbide dinitrate: Enhanced hypotensive effect

Metformin: Enhanced hypoglycaemic effect; increased risk of lactic acidosis

Methyldopa: Enhanced hypotensive effect

Metronidazole: Disulfiram-like reaction

Morphine: Enhanced sedative and hypotensive effect

Nifedipine: Enhanced hypotensive effect

Paracetamol: Increased risk of liver damage with regular large amounts of alcohol

Pethidine: Enhanced sedative and hypotensive effect

Phenobarbital: Enhanced sedative effect

Phenytoin: Plasma-phenytoin concentration reduced with regular large amounts of alcohol

Prazosin: Enhanced hypotensive effect

Procarbazine: Disulfiram-like reaction

Promethazine: Enhanced sedative effect

Propranolol: Enhanced hypotensive effect

Reserpine: Enhanced hypotensive effect

Sodium nitroprusside: Enhanced hypotensive effect

Spironolactone: Enhanced hypotensive effect

Timolol: Enhanced hypotensive effect

Verapamil: Enhanced hypotensive effect; plasma concentration of alcohol possibly increased by verapamil

Alcohol (Continued)
> * Warfarin: Enhanced anticoagulant effect with large amounts of alcohol; major changes in alcohol consumption may affect anticoagulant control

Alcuronium
> Carbamazepine: Antagonism of muscle relaxant effect (recovery from neuromuscular blockade accelerated)
> Clindamycin: Enhanced muscle relaxant effect
> * Gentamicin: Enhanced muscle relaxant effect
> Lithium: Enhanced muscle relaxant effect
> Magnesium (parenteral): Enhanced muscle relaxant effect
> Neostigmine: Antagonism of muscle relaxant effect
> Nifedipine: Enhanced muscle relaxant effect
> Phenytoin: Antagonism of muscle relaxant effect (accelerated recovery from neuromuscular blockade)
> * Procainamide: Enhanced muscle relaxant effect
> Propranolol: Enhanced muscle relaxant effect
> Pyridostigmine: Antagonism of muscle relaxant effect
> * Quinidine: Enhanced muscle relaxant effect
> * Streptomycin: Enhanced muscle relaxant effect
> Verapamil: Enhanced muscle relaxant effect

Allopurinol
> Amoxicillin: Increased risk of rash
> Ampicillin: Increased risk of rash
> * Azathioprine: Effects of azathioprine enhanced with increased toxicity, reduce dose when given with allopurinol
> Captopril: Increased risk of toxicity especially in renal impairment
> Ciclosporin: Plasma-ciclosporin concentration possibly increased (risk of nephrotoxicity)
> * Mercaptopurine: Effects of mercaptopurine enhanced with increased toxicity, reduce dose when given with allopurinol
> Theophylline: Plasma-theophylline concentration possibly increased
> Warfarin: Anticoagulant effect possibly enhanced

Aluminium hydroxide *see* Antacids

Amiloride
> Alcohol: Enhanced hypotensive effect
> Amitriptyline: Increased risk of postural hypotension
> * Artemether+Lumefantrine: Increased risk of ventricular arrhythmias if electrolyte disturbance occurs
> Atenolol: Enhanced hypotensive effect
> * Captopril: Enhanced hypotensive effect (can be extreme); risk of severe hyperkalaemia
> Carbamazepine: Increased risk of hyponatraemia
> Chloral hydrate: Enhanced hypotensive effect
> Chlorpromazine: Enhanced hypotensive effect
> * Ciclosporin: Increased risk of hyperkalaemia
> Cisplatin: Increased risk of nephrotoxicity and ototoxicity
> Clomipramine: Increased risk of postural hypotension
> Clonazepam: Enhanced hypotensive effect
> Contraceptives, Oral: Antagonism of diuretic effect
> Dexamethasone: Antagonism of diuretic effect
> Diazepam: Enhanced hypotensive effect
> Ether, Anaesthetic: Enhanced hypotensive effect
> Fludrocortisone: Antagonism of diuretic effect
> Fluphenazine: Enhanced hypotensive effect
> Glyceryl trinitrate: Enhanced hypotensive effect
> Halothane: Enhanced hypotensive effect
> Hydralazine: Enhanced hypotensive effect
> Hydrocortisone: Antagonism of diuretic effect
> Ibuprofen: Risk of nephrotoxicity of ibuprofen increased; antagonism of diuretic effect; possibly increased risk of hyperkalaemia
> Isosorbide dinitrate: Enhanced hypotensive effect
> Ketamine: Enhanced hypotensive effect
> Levodopa: Enhanced hypotensive effect
> * Lithium: Reduced lithium excretion (increased plasma-lithium concentration and risk of toxicity)

Amiloride (Continued)
> Methyldopa: Enhanced hypotensive effect
> Nifedipine: Enhanced hypotensive effect
> Nitrous oxide: Enhanced hypotensive effect
> * Potassium salts: Risk of hyperkalaemia
> * Prazosin: Enhanced hypotensive effect; increased risk of first-dose hypotensive effect of prazosin
> Prednisolone: Antagonism of diuretic effect
> Propranolol: Enhanced hypotensive effect
> Reserpine: Enhanced hypotensive effect
> Sodium nitroprusside: Enhanced hypotensive effect
> Thiopental: Enhanced hypotensive effect
> Timolol: Enhanced hypotensive effect
> Verapamil: Enhanced hypotensive effect

Aminophylline *see* Theophylline

Amitriptyline
> Acetazolamide: Increased risk of postural hypotension
> * Alcohol: Enhanced sedative effect
> Amiloride: Increased risk of postural hypotension
> * Artemether+Lumefantrine: Increased risk of ventricular arrhythmias
> Atropine: Increased antimuscarinic adverse effects
> Biperiden: Increased antimuscarinic adverse effects
> * Carbamazepine: Antagonism (convulsive threshold lowered); possibly accelerated metabolism of amitriptyline (reduced plasma concentration; reduced antidepressant effect)
> Chloral hydrate: Enhanced sedative effect
> Chlorphenamine: Increased antimuscarinic and sedative effects
> * Chlorpromazine: Increased antimuscarinic adverse effects; increased plasma-amitriptyline concentration; possibly increased risk of ventricular arrhythmias
> Cimetidine: Plasma concentration of amitriptyline increased (inhibition of metabolism)
> Clonazepam: Enhanced sedative effect
> Codeine: Possibly increased sedation
> Contraceptives, Oral: Antagonism of antidepressant effect but adverse effects possibly increased due to increased plasma concentration of amitriptyline
> Diazepam: Enhanced sedative effect
> * Epinephrine: Hypertension and arrhythmias (but local anaesthetics with epinephrine appear to be safe)
> Ether, Anaesthetic: Increased risk of arrhythmias and hypotension
> * Ethosuximide: Antagonism (convulsive threshold lowered)
> * Fluphenazine: Increased antimuscarinic adverse effects; increased plasma-amitriptyline concentration; possibly increased risk of ventricular arrhythmias
> Furosemide: Increased risk of postural hypotension
> Glyceryl trinitrate: Reduced effect of sublingual glyceryl trinitrate (owing to dry mouth)
> * Haloperidol: Increased plasma-amitriptyline concentration; possibly increased risk of ventricular arrhythmias
> Halothane: Increased risk of arrhythmias and hypotension
> Hydralazine: Enhanced hypotensive effect
> Hydrochlorothiazide: Increased risk of postural hypotension
> Isosorbide dinitrate: Reduced effect of sublingual isosorbide dinitrate (owing to dry mouth)
> Ketamine: Increased risk of arrhythmias and hypotension
> Methyldopa: Enhanced hypotensive effect
> Morphine: Possibly increased sedation
> Nitrous oxide: Increased risk of arrhythmias and hypotension
> Pethidine: Possibly increased sedation
> * Phenobarbital: Antagonism of anticonvulsant effect (convulsive threshold lowered); metabolism of amitriptyline possibly accelerated (reduced plasma concentration)
> * Phenytoin: Antagonism (convulsive threshold lowered); possibly reduced plasma-amitriptyline concentration

Amitriptyline (Continued)
* Procainamide: Increased risk of ventricular arrhythmias

  Promethazine: Increased antimuscarinic and sedative effects
* Quinidine: Increased risk of ventricular arrhythmias

  Reserpine: Enhanced hypotensive effect

  Rifampicin: Plasma concentration of amitriptyline possibly reduced (reduced antidepressant effect)
* Ritonavir: Plasma concentration possibly increased by ritonavir

  Sodium nitroprusside: Enhanced hypotensive effect

  Spironolactone: Increased risk of postural hypotension

  Thiopental: Increased risk of arrhythmias and hypotension
* Valproic acid: Antagonism (convulsive threshold lowered)

  Verapamil: Possibly increased plasma concentration of amitriptyline

Amoxicillin
Allopurinol: Increased risk of rash
* Contraceptives, Oral: Possibility of reduced contraceptive effect

  Methotrexate: Reduced excretion of methotrexate (increased risk of toxicity)

  Warfarin: Studies have failed to demonstrate an interaction, but common experience in anticoagulant clinics is that INR can be altered by a course of amoxicillin

Amoxicillin+Clavulanic acid *see* Amoxicillin

Amphotericin *NOTE.* Close monitoring required with concomitant administration of nephrotoxic drugs or cytotoxics
* Ciclosporin: Increased risk of nephrotoxicity
* Dexamethasone: Increased risk of hypokalaemia (avoid concomitant use unless dexamethasone needed to control reactions)
* Digoxin: Increased digoxin toxicity if hypokalaemia occurs

  Fluconazole: Possible antagonism of effect of amphotericin

  Flucytosine: Renal excretion of flucytosine decreased and cellular uptake increased (flucytosine toxicity possibly increased)
* Fludrocortisone: Increased risk of hypokalaemia

  Furosemide: Increased risk of hypokalaemia

  Gentamicin: Increased risk of nephrotoxicity

  Hydrochlorothiazide: Increased risk of hypokalaemia
* Hydrocortisone: Increased risk of hypokalaemia (avoid concomitant use unless hydrocortisone needed to control reactions)
* Prednisolone: Increased risk of hypokalaemia (avoid concomitant use unless prednisolone needed to control reactions)

  Streptomycin: Increased risk of nephrotoxicity

Ampicillin
Allopurinol: Increased risk of rash
* Contraceptives, Oral: Possibility of reduced contraceptive effect

  Methotrexate: Reduced excretion of methotrexate (increased risk of toxicity)

  Warfarin: Studies have failed to demonstrate an interaction, but common experience in anticoagulant clinics is that INR can be altered by a course of ampicillin

Antacids (Aluminium hydroxide; Magnesium hydroxide) *NOTE.* Antacids should preferably not be taken at the same time as other drugs since they may impair absorption
Acetylsalicylic acid: Excretion of acetylsalicylic acid increased in alkaline urine

Captopril: Absorption of captopril reduced

Chloroquine: Reduced absorption

Chlorpromazine: Reduced absorption of chlorpromazine

Ciprofloxacin: Reduced absorption of ciprofloxacin

Digoxin: Possibly reduced absorption of digoxin

Doxycycline: Reduced absorption of doxycycline

Isoniazid: Reduced absorption of isoniazid

Minocycline: Reduced absorption of minocycline

Ofloxacin: Reduced absorption of ofloxacin

Penicillamine: Reduced absorption of penicillamine

Phenytoin: Reduced absorption of phenytoin

Antacids (Aluminium hydroxide; Magnesium hydroxide) (Continued)

> Quinidine: Reduced quinidine excretion in alkaline urine (plasma-quinidine concentration occasionally increased)
>
> Rifampicin: Reduced absorption of rifampicin

Artemether+Lumefantrine

> * Amiloride: Increased risk of ventricular arrhythmias if electrolyte disturbance occurs
> * Amitriptyline: Increased risk of ventricular arrhythmias
> * Chloroquine: Increased risk of ventricular arrhythmias
> * Chlorpromazine: Increased risk of ventricular arrhythmias
> * Clomipramine: Increased risk of ventricular arrhythmias
> * Fluphenazine: Increased risk of ventricular arrhythmias
> * Furosemide: Increased risk of ventricular arrhythmias if electrolyte disturbance occurs
>
> Grapefruit Juice: Metabolism of artemether and lumefantrine may be inhibited
>
> * Hydrochlorothiazide: Increased risk of ventricular arrhythmias if electrolyte disturbance occurs
> * Mefloquine: Increased risk of ventricular arrhythmias
> * Procainamide: Increased risk of ventricular arrhythmias
> * Quinidine: Increased risk of ventricular arrhythmias
> * Quinine: Increased risk of ventricular arrhythmias
> * Spironolactone: Increased risk of ventricular arrhythmias if electrolyte disturbance occurs

Asparaginase

> Vaccine, Live: Avoid use of live vaccines with asparaginase (impairment of immune response)

Atenolol

> Acetazolamide: Enhanced hypotensive effect
> Alcohol: Enhanced hypotensive effect
> Amiloride: Enhanced hypotensive effect
> Captopril: Enhanced hypotensive effect
> Chloral hydrate: Enhanced hypotensive effect
> Chlorpromazine: Enhanced hypotensive effect
> Clonazepam: Enhanced hypotensive effect
> Contraceptives, Oral: Antagonism of hypotensive effect
> Dexamethasone: Antagonism of hypotensive effect
> Diazepam: Enhanced hypotensive effect
> Digoxin: Increased AV block and bradycardia
> * Epinephrine: Severe hypertension
> Ergotamine: Increased peripheral vasoconstriction
> Ether, Anaesthetic: Enhanced hypotensive effect
> Fludrocortisone: Antagonism of hypotensive effect
> Fluphenazine: Enhanced hypotensive effect
> Furosemide: Enhanced hypotensive effect
> Glibenclamide: Masking of warning signs of hypoglycaemia such as tremor
> Glyceryl trinitrate: Enhanced hypotensive effect
> Halothane: Enhanced hypotensive effect
> Hydralazine: Enhanced hypotensive effect
> Hydrochlorothiazide: Enhanced hypotensive effect
> Hydrocortisone: Antagonism of hypotensive effect
> Ibuprofen: Antagonism of hypotensive effect
> Insulins: Enhanced hypoglycaemic effect; masking of warning signs of hypoglycaemia such as tremor
> Isosorbide dinitrate: Enhanced hypotensive effect
> Ketamine: Enhanced hypotensive effect
> Levodopa: Enhanced hypotensive effect
> * Lidocaine: Increased risk of myocardial depression
> Mefloquine: Increased risk of bradycardia
> Metformin: Masking of warning signs of hypoglycaemia such as tremor
> Methyldopa: Enhanced hypotensive effect
> * Nifedipine: Severe hypotension and heart failure occasionally
> Nitrous oxide: Enhanced hypotensive effect

Atenolol (Continued)

* Prazosin: Enhanced hypotensive effect; increased risk of first-dose hypotensive effect of prazosin

    Prednisolone: Antagonism of hypotensive effect

* Procainamide: Increased risk of myocardial depression
* Quinidine: Increased risk of myocardial depression

    Reserpine: Enhanced hypotensive effect

    Sodium nitroprusside: Enhanced hypotensive effect

    Spironolactone: Enhanced hypotensive effect

    Theophylline: Avoid concomitant use on pharmacological grounds (bronchospasm)

    Thiopental: Enhanced hypotensive effect

* Verapamil: Asystole, severe hypotension and heart failure

Atropine

Amitriptyline: Increased antimuscarinic adverse effects

Chlorphenamine: Increased antimuscarinic adverse effects

Chlorpromazine: Increased antimuscarinic adverse effects of chlorpromazine (but reduced plasma concentration)

Clomipramine: Increased antimuscarinic adverse effects

Fluphenazine: Increased antimuscarinic adverse effects of fluphenazine (but reduced plasma concentration)

Glyceryl trinitrate: Possibly reduced effect of sublingual nitrates (failure to dissolve under the tongue owing to dry mouth)

Isosorbide dinitrate: Possibly reduced effect of sublingual nitrates (failure to dissolve under the tongue owing to dry mouth)

Levodopa: Absorption of levodopa possibly reduced

Metoclopramide: Antagonism of effect on gastrointestinal activity

Neostigmine: Antagonism of effect

Promethazine: Increased antimuscarinic adverse effects

Pyridostigmine: Antagonism of effect

Azathioprine

* Allopurinol: Effects of azathioprine enhanced with increased toxicity, reduce dose when given with allopurinol

    Captopril: Increased risk of leukopenia

    Phenytoin: Reduced absorption of phenytoin

* Rifampicin: Manufacturer reports interaction (transplants possibly rejected)
* Sulfamethoxazole+Trimethoprim: Increased risk of haematological toxicity
* Trimethoprim: Increased risk of haematological toxicity
* Vaccine, Live: Avoid use of live vaccines with azathioprine (impairment of immune response)
* Warfarin: Anticoagulant effect possibly reduced

Benzathine benzylpenicillin *see* Benzylpenicillin

Benzylpenicillin

Methotrexate: Reduced excretion of methotrexate (increased risk of toxicity)

BCG vaccine *see* Vaccine, live

Biperiden

Amitriptyline: Increased antimuscarinic adverse effects

Chlorphenamine: Increased antimuscarinic adverse effects

Chlorpromazine: Increased antimuscarinic adverse effects of chlorpromazine (but reduced plasma concentration)

Clomipramine: Increased antimuscarinic adverse effects

Fluphenazine: Increased antimuscarinic adverse effects of fluphenazine (but reduced plasma concentration)

Glyceryl trinitrate: Possibly reduced effect of sublingual nitrates (failure to dissolve under the tongue owing to dry mouth)

Isosorbide dinitrate: Possibly reduced effect of sublingual nitrates (failure to dissolve under the tongue owing to dry mouth)

Levodopa: Absorption of levodopa possibly reduced

Metoclopramide: Antagonism of effect on gastrointestinal activity

Neostigmine: Antagonism of effect

Promethazine: Increased antimuscarinic adverse effects

Pyridostigmine: Antagonism of effect

Bleomycin
* Oxygen: Increased risk of pulmonary toxicity
  Vaccine, Live: Avoid use of live vaccines with bleomycin (impairment of immune response)

Bupivacaine
  Lidocaine: Increased myocardial depression
  Procainamide: Increased myocardial depression
* Propranolol: Increased risk of bupivacaine toxicity
  Quinidine: Increased myocardial depression

Calcium folinate *see* Folic acid and Folinic acid

Calcium gluconate *see* Calcium salts

Calcium salts
  Digoxin: Large intravenous doses of calcium can precipitate arrhythmias
  Hydrochlorothiazide: Increased risk of hypercalcaemia

Captopril
* Acetazolamide: Enhanced hypotensive effect (can be extreme)
* Acetylsalicylic acid: Antagonism of hypotensive effect; increased risk of renal impairment
  Alcohol: Enhanced hypotensive effect
  Allopurinol: Increased risk of toxicity especially in renal impairment
* Amiloride: Enhanced hypotensive effect (can be extreme); risk of severe hyperkalaemia
  Antacids (Aluminium hydroxide; Magnesium hydroxide): Absorption of captopril reduced
  Atenolol: Enhanced hypotensive effect
  Azathioprine: Increased risk of leukopenia
  Chloral hydrate: Enhanced hypotensive effect
  Chlorpromazine: Enhanced hypotensive effect
* Ciclosporin: Increased risk of hyperkalaemia
  Clonazepam: Enhanced hypotensive effect
  Contraceptives, Oral: Antagonism of hypotensive effect
  Dexamethasone: Antagonism of hypotensive effect
  Diazepam: Enhanced hypotensive effect
  Digoxin: Plasma concentration of digoxin possibly increased
  Ether, Anaesthetic: Enhanced hypotensive effect
  Fludrocortisone: Antagonism of hypotensive effect
  Fluphenazine: Enhanced hypotensive effect
* Furosemide: Enhanced hypotensive effect (can be extreme)
  Glibenclamide: Hypoglycaemic effect possibly enhanced
  Glyceryl trinitrate: Enhanced hypotensive effect
  Halothane: Enhanced hypotensive effect
  Heparin: Increased risk of hyperkalaemia
  Hydralazine: Enhanced hypotensive effect
* Hydrochlorothiazide: Enhanced hypotensive effect (can be extreme)
  Hydrocortisone: Antagonism of hypotensive effect
  Ibuprofen: Antagonism of hypotensive effect, increased risk of renal impairment
  Insulins: Hypoglycaemic effect possibly enhanced
  Isosorbide dinitrate: Enhanced hypotensive effect
  Ketamine: Enhanced hypotensive effect
  Levodopa: Enhanced hypotensive effect
* Lithium: Captopril reduces excretion of lithium (increased plasma-lithium concentration)
  Metformin: Hypoglycaemic effect possibly enhanced
  Methyldopa: Enhanced hypotensive effect
  Nifedipine: Enhanced hypotensive effect
  Nitrous oxide: Enhanced hypotensive effect
* Potassium salts: Risk of severe hyperkalaemia
  Prazosin: Enhanced hypotensive effect
  Prednisolone: Antagonism of hypotensive effect
  Procainamide: Increased risk of toxicity, especially in renal impairment
  Propranolol: Enhanced hypotensive effect
  Reserpine: Enhanced hypotensive effect
  Sodium nitroprusside: Enhanced hypotensive effect

Captopril (Continued)
  * Spironolactone: Enhanced hypotensive effect (can be extreme); risk of severe hyperkalaemia
  Thiopental: Enhanced hypotensive effect
  Timolol: Enhanced hypotensive effect
  Verapamil: Enhanced hypotensive effect

Carbamazepine
  * Acetazolamide: Increased risk of hyponatraemia; acetazolamide increases plasma-carbamazepine concentration
  Alcohol: Possibly enhanced CNS adverse effects of carbamazepine
  Alcuronium: Antagonism of muscle relaxant effect (recovery from neuromuscular blockade accelerated)
  Amiloride: Increased risk of hyponatraemia
  * Amitriptyline: Antagonism (convulsive threshold lowered); possibly accelerated metabolism of amitriptyline (reduced plasma concentration; reduced antidepressant effect)
  * Chloroquine: Antagonism of anticonvulsant effect
  * Chlorpromazine: Antagonism of anticonvulsant effect (convulsive threshold lowered)
  * Ciclosporin: Accelerated metabolism (reduced plasma-ciclosporin concentration)
  * Cimetidine: Metabolism of carbamazepine inhibited (increased plasma-carbamazepine concentration)
  * Clomipramine: Antagonism (convulsive threshold lowered); possibly accelerated metabolism of clomipramine (reduced plasma concentration; reduced antidepressant effect)
  * Clonazepam: May be enhanced toxicity without corresponding increase in antiepileptic effect; plasma concentration of clonazepam often lowered
  * Contraceptives, Oral: Accelerated metabolism (reduced contraceptive effect)
  * Dexamethasone: Accelerated metabolism of dexamethasone (reduced effect)
  Doxycycline: Accelerated doxycycline metabolism (reduced effect)
  Ergocalciferol: Ergocalciferol requirements possibly increase
  * Erythromycin: Increased plasma-carbamazepine concentration
  * Ethosuximide: May be enhanced toxicity without corresponding increase in antiepileptic effect; plasma concentration of ethosuximide sometimes lowered
  * Fludrocortisone: Accelerated metabolism of fludrocortisone (reduced effect)
  * Fluphenazine: Antagonism of anticonvulsant effect (convulsive threshold lowered)
  Furosemide: Increased risk of hyponatraemia
  * Haloperidol: Antagonism of anticonvulsant effect (convulsive threshold lowered); metabolism of haloperidol accelerated (reduced plasma concentration)
  Hydrochlorothiazide: Increased risk of hyponatraemia
  * Hydrocortisone: Accelerated metabolism of hydrocortisone (reduced effect)
  Indinavir: Possibly reduced plasma-indinavir concentration
  * Isoniazid: Increased plasma-carbamazepine concentration (also isoniazid hepatotoxicity possibly increased)
  * Levonorgestrel: Accelerated metabolism (reduced contraceptive effect)
  Levothyroxine: Accelerated metabolism of levothyroxine (may increase levothyroxine requirements in hypothyroidism)
  Lithium: Neurotoxicity may occur without increased plasma-lithium concentration
  Lopinavir: Possibly reduced plasma-lopinavir concentration
  * Medroxyprogesterone: Accelerated metabolism (reduced contraceptive effect)
  * Mefloquine: Antagonism of anticonvulsant effect
  Nelfinavir: Possibly reduced plasma-nelfinavir concentration
  Nifedipine: Probably reduced effect of nifedipine
  * Norethisterone: Accelerated metabolism (reduced contraceptive effect)

Carbamazepine (Continued)

* Phenobarbital: May be enhanced toxicity without corresponding increase in antiepileptic effect; plasma concentration of carbamazepine often lowered
* Phenytoin: May be enhanced toxicity without corresponding increase in antiepileptic effect; plasma concentration of phenytoin often lowered but may be raised; plasma concentration of carbamazepine often lowered

    Praziquantel: Plasma-praziquantel concentration reduced
* Prednisolone: Accelerated metabolism of prednisolone (reduced effect)
* Ritonavir: Plasma concentration possibly increased by ritonavir

    Saquinavir: Possibly reduced plasma-saquinavir concentration

    Spironolactone: Increased risk of hyponatraemia

    Theophylline: Accelerated metabolism of theophylline (reduced effect)
* Valproic acid: May be enhanced toxicity without corresponding increase in antiepileptic effect; plasma concentration of valproic acid often lowered; plasma concentration of active metabolite of carbamazepine often raised

    Vecuronium: Antagonism of muscle relaxant effect (recovery from neuromuscular blockade accelerated)
* Verapamil: Enhanced effect of carbamazepine
* Warfarin: Accelerated metabolism of warfarin (reduced anticoagulant effect)

Ceftazidime

    Contraceptives, Oral: Possibility of reduced contraceptive effect

    Furosemide: Nephrotoxicity of ceftazidime possibly increased
* Warfarin: Possibly enhanced anticoagulant effect

Ceftriaxone

    Contraceptives, Oral: Possibility of reduced contraceptive effect

    Furosemide: Nephrotoxicity of ceftriaxone possibly increased
* Warfarin: Possibly enhanced anticoagulant effect

Chloral hydrate

    Acetazolamide: Enhanced hypotensive effect

    Alcohol: Enhanced sedative effect

    Amiloride: Enhanced hypotensive effect

    Amitriptyline: Enhanced sedative effect

    Atenolol: Enhanced hypotensive effect

    Captopril: Enhanced hypotensive effect

    Chlorphenamine: Enhanced sedative effect

    Chlorpromazine: Enhanced sedative effect

    Clomipramine: Enhanced sedative effect

    Codeine: Enhanced sedative effect

    Ether, Anaesthetic: Enhanced sedative effect

    Fluphenazine: Enhanced sedative effect

    Furosemide: Administration of chloral hydrate with parenteral furosemide may displace thyroid hormone from binding sites; enhanced hypotensive effect

    Glyceryl trinitrate: Enhanced hypotensive effect

    Haloperidol: Enhanced sedative effect

    Halothane: Enhanced sedative effect

    Hydralazine: Enhanced hypotensive effect

    Hydrochlorothiazide: Enhanced hypotensive effect

    Isosorbide dinitrate: Enhanced hypotensive effect

    Ketamine: Enhanced sedative effect

    Methyldopa: Enhanced hypotensive effect

    Morphine: Enhanced sedative effect

    Nifedipine: Enhanced hypotensive effect

    Nitrous oxide: Enhanced sedative effect

    Pethidine: Enhanced sedative effect

    Prazosin: Enhanced hypotensive and sedative effects

    Promethazine: Enhanced sedative effect

    Propranolol: Enhanced hypotensive effect

    Reserpine: Enhanced hypotensive effect
* Ritonavir: Plasma concentration possibly increased by ritonavir

    Sodium nitroprusside: Enhanced hypotensive effect

Chloral hydrate (Continued)

Spironolactone: Enhanced hypotensive effect

Thiopental: Enhanced sedative effect

Timolol: Enhanced hypotensive effect

Verapamil: Enhanced hypotensive effect

Warfarin: May transiently enhance anticoagulant effect

Chlorambucil

Vaccine, Live: Avoid use of live vaccines with chlorambucil (impairment of immune response)

Chloramphenicol

* Ciclosporin: Plasma concentration of ciclosporin possibly increased
* Glibenclamide: Enhanced effect of glibenclamide
* Phenobarbital: Metabolism of chloramphenicol accelerated (reduced chloramphenicol concentration)
* Phenytoin: Plasma-phenytoin concentration increased (risk of toxicity)

Rifampicin: Accelerated metabolism of chloramphenicol (reduced plasma-chloramphenicol concentration)

* Warfarin: Enhanced anticoagulant effect

Chlormethine

Vaccine, Live: Avoid use of live vaccines with chlormethine (impairment of immune response)

Chloroquine

Antacids (Aluminium hydroxide; Magnesium hydroxide): Reduced absorption

* Artemether+Lumefantrine: Increased risk of ventricular arrhythmias
* Carbamazepine: Antagonism of anticonvulsant effect
* Ciclosporin: Increased plasma-ciclosporin concentration (increased risk of toxicity)

Cimetidine: Inhibition of chloroquine metabolism (increased plasma concentration)

* Digoxin: Plasma-digoxin concentration possibly increased
* Ethosuximide: Antagonism of anticonvulsant effect
* Mefloquine: Increased risk of convulsions

Neostigmine: Chloroquine has potential to increase symptoms of myasthenia gravis and thus diminish effect of neostigmine

* Phenytoin: Antagonism of anticonvulsant effect

Pyridostigmine: Chloroquine has potential to increase symptoms of myasthenia gravis and thus diminish effect of pyridostigmine

Quinidine: Increased risk of ventricular arrhythmias

Quinine: Increased risk of ventricular arrhythmias

Vaccine, Rabies: Concomitant administration of chloroquine may affect antibody response

* Valproic acid: Antagonism of anticonvulsant effect

Chlorphenamine

Alcohol: Enhanced sedative effect

Amitriptyline: Increased antimuscarinic and sedative effects

Atropine: Increased antimuscarinic adverse effects

Biperiden: Increased antimuscarinic adverse effects

Chloral hydrate: Enhanced sedative effect

Clomipramine: Increased antimuscarinic and sedative effects

Clonazepam: Enhanced sedative effect

Diazepam: Enhanced sedative effect

Chlorpromazine

Acetazolamide: Enhanced hypotensive effect

Alcohol: Enhanced sedative effect

Amiloride: Enhanced hypotensive effect

* Amitriptyline: Increased antimuscarinic adverse effects; increased plasma-amitriptyline concentration; possibly increased risk of ventricular arrhythmias

Antacids (Aluminium hydroxide; Magnesium hydroxide): Reduced absorption of chlorpromazine

* Artemether+Lumefantrine: Increased risk of ventricular arrhythmias

Atenolol: Enhanced hypotensive effect

Atropine: Increased antimuscarinic adverse effects of chlorpromazine (but reduced plasma concentration)

Chlorpromazine (Continued)

Biperiden: Increased antimuscarinic adverse effects of chlorpromazine (but reduced plasma concentration)

Captopril: Enhanced hypotensive effect

* Carbamazepine: Antagonism of anticonvulsant effect (convulsive threshold lowered)

Chloral hydrate: Enhanced sedative effect

Cimetidine: Possibly enhanced effects of chlorpromazine

* Clomipramine: Increased antimuscarinic adverse effects; increased plasma-clomipramine concentration; possibly increased risk of ventricular arrhythmias

Clonazepam: Enhanced sedative effect

Codeine: Enhanced sedative and hypotensive effect

Diazepam: Enhanced sedative effect

Dopamine: Antagonism of pressor action

Ephedrine: Antagonism of pressor action

Epinephrine: Antagonism of pressor action

* Ether, Anaesthetic: Enhanced hypotensive effect

* Ethosuximide: Antagonism (convulsive threshold lowered)

Furosemide: Enhanced hypotensive effect

Glibenclamide: Possible antagonism of hypoglycaemic effect

Glyceryl trinitrate: Enhanced hypotensive effect

* Halothane: Enhanced hypotensive effect

Hydralazine: Enhanced hypotensive effect

Hydrochlorothiazide: Enhanced hypotensive effect

Isoprenaline: Antagonism of pressor action

Isosorbide dinitrate: Enhanced hypotensive effect

* Ketamine: Enhanced hypotensive effect

Levodopa: Antagonism of effects of levodopa

Lithium: Increased risk of extrapyramidal effects and possibility of neurotoxicity

Methyldopa: Enhanced hypotensive effect; increased risk of extrapyramidal effects

Metoclopramide: Increased risk of extrapyramidal effects

Morphine: Enhanced sedative and hypotensive effect

Nifedipine: Enhanced hypotensive effect

* Nitrous oxide: Enhanced hypotensive effect

Pethidine: Enhanced sedative and hypotensive effect

* Phenobarbital: Antagonism of anticonvulsant effect (convulsive threshold lowered)

* Phenytoin: Antagonism of anticonvulsant effect (convulsive threshold lowered)

Prazosin: Enhanced hypotensive effect

* Procainamide: Increased risk of ventricular arrhythmias

* Propranolol: Concomitant administration may increase plasma concentration of both drugs; enhanced hypotensive effect

* Quinidine: Increased risk of ventricular arrhythmias

Reserpine: Enhanced hypotensive effect; increased risk of extrapyramidal effects

* Ritonavir: Plasma concentration possibly increased by ritonavir

Sodium nitroprusside: Enhanced hypotensive effect

Spironolactone: Enhanced hypotensive effect

* Thiopental: Enhanced hypotensive effect

Timolol: Enhanced hypotensive effect

* Valproic acid: Antagonism of anticonvulsant effect (convulsive threshold lowered)

Verapamil: Enhanced hypotensive effect

Ciclosporin

Allopurinol: Plasma-ciclosporin concentration possibly increased (risk of nephrotoxicity)

* Amiloride: Increased risk of hyperkalaemia

* Amphotericin: Increased risk of nephrotoxicity

* Captopril: Increased risk of hyperkalaemia

* Carbamazepine: Accelerated metabolism (reduced plasma-ciclosporin concentration)

Ciclosporin (Continued)
* Chloramphenicol: Plasma concentration of ciclosporin possibly increased
* Chloroquine: Increased plasma-ciclosporin concentration (increased risk of toxicity)
* Cimetidine: Possibly increased plasma-ciclosporin concentration
* Ciprofloxacin: Increased risk of nephrotoxicity
* Colchicine: Possibly increased risk of nephrotoxicity and myotoxicity (increased plasma-ciclosporin concentration)
  Contraceptives, Oral: Possibly increased plasma-ciclosporin concentration
* Doxorubicin: Increased risk of neurotoxicity
* Doxycycline: Possibly increased plasma-ciclosporin concentration
* Erythromycin: Increased plasma-ciclosporin concentration (inhibition of metabolism)
* Fluconazole: Metabolism of ciclosporin possibly inhibited (possibly increased plasma concentration)
* Gentamicin: Increased risk of nephrotoxicity
* Grapefruit Juice: Increased plasma-ciclosporin concentration (risk of toxicity)
  Griseofulvin: Plasma-ciclosporin concentration possibly reduced
* Ibuprofen: Increased risk of nephrotoxicity
* Levonorgestrel: Inhibition of ciclosporin metabolism (increased plasma-ciclosporin concentration)
* Medroxyprogesterone: Inhibition of ciclosporin metabolism (increased plasma-ciclosporin concentration)
* Methotrexate: Increased toxicity
* Nalidixic acid: Increased risk of nephrotoxicity
  Nifedipine: Possibly increased plasma-nifedipine concentration (increased risk of adverse effects such as gingival hyperplasia)
* Norethisterone: Inhibition of ciclosporin metabolism (increased plasma-ciclosporin concentration)
* Ofloxacin: Increased risk of nephrotoxicity
* Phenobarbital: Metabolism of ciclosporin accelerated (reduced effect)
* Phenytoin: Accelerated metabolism (reduced plasma-ciclosporin concentration)
* Potassium salts: Increased risk of hyperkalaemia
  Prednisolone: Increased plasma concentration of prednisolone
* Rifampicin: Accelerated metabolism (reduced plasma-ciclosporin concentration)
* Ritonavir: Plasma concentration possibly increased by ritonavir
* Spironolactone: Increased risk of hyperkalaemia
* Streptomycin: Increased risk of nephrotoxicity
* Sulfadiazine: Plasma-ciclosporin concentration possibly reduced; increased risk of nephrotoxicity
* Sulfadoxine+Pyrimethamine: Increased risk of nephrotoxicity
* Sulfamethoxazole+Trimethoprim: Increased risk of nephrotoxicity; plasma-ciclosporin concentration possibly reduced by intravenous trimethoprim
* Trimethoprim: Increased risk of nephrotoxicity; plasma-ciclosporin concentration possibly reduced by intravenous trimethoprim
* Vaccine, Live: Avoid use of live vaccines with ciclosporin (impairment of immune response)
* Verapamil: Increased plasma-ciclosporin concentration

Cimetidine
  Amitriptyline: Plasma concentration of amitriptyline increased (inhibition of metabolism)
* Carbamazepine: Metabolism of carbamazepine inhibited (increased plasma-carbamazepine concentration)
  Chloroquine: Inhibition of chloroquine metabolism (increased plasma concentration)
  Chlorpromazine: Possibly enhanced effects of chlorpromazine
* Ciclosporin: Possibly increased plasma-ciclosporin concentration
  Clomipramine: Plasma concentration of clomipramine possibly increased

Cimetidine (Continued)

Clonazepam: Inhibition of clonazepam metabolism (increased plasma concentration)

Codeine: Metabolism of codeine inhibited (increased plasma concentration)

Diazepam: Inhibition of diazepam metabolism (increased plasma concentration)

Erythromycin: Increased plasma-erythromycin concentration (increased risk of toxicity, including deafness)

Fluorouracil: Metabolism of fluorouracil inhibited (increased plasma-fluorouracil concentration)

Fluphenazine: Possibly enhanced effects of fluphenazine

Glibenclamide: Enhanced hypoglycaemic effect

Haloperidol: Possibly enhanced effects of haloperidol

* Lidocaine: Increased plasma concentration of lidocaine (increased risk of toxicity)

Mebendazole: Metabolism of mebendazole possibly inhibited (increased plasma concentration)

Metformin: Renal excretion of metformin inhibited; increased plasma-metformin concentration

Metronidazole: Metabolism of metronidazole inhibited (increased plasma-metronidazole concentration)

Morphine: Metabolism of morphine inhibited (increased plasma concentration)

Nifedipine: Metabolism of nifedipine possibly inhibited (increased plasma concentration)

Pethidine: Metabolism of pethidine inhibited (increased plasma concentration)

* Phenytoin: Metabolism of phenytoin inhibited (increased plasma concentration)

* Procainamide: Increased plasma concentration of procainamide

Propranolol: Increased plasma-propranolol concentration

* Quinidine: Increased plasma concentration of quinidine

Quinine: Metabolism of quinine inhibited (increased plasma concentration)

Rifampicin: Accelerated metabolism of cimetidine (reduced plasma-cimetidine concentration)

* Theophylline: Metabolism of theophylline inhibited (plasma-theophylline concentration increased)

* Valproic acid: Metabolism of valproic acid inhibited (increased plasma concentration)

Verapamil: Metabolism of verapamil possibly inhibited (increased plasma concentration)

* Warfarin: Enhanced anticoagulant effect (inhibition of metabolism)

Ciprofloxacin

Antacids (Aluminium hydroxide; Magnesium hydroxide): Reduced absorption of ciprofloxacin

* Ciclosporin: Increased risk of nephrotoxicity

Ferrous salts: Absorption of ciprofloxacin reduced by oral ferrous salts

Glibenclamide: Possibly enhanced effect of glibenclamide

* Ibuprofen: Possibly increased risk of convulsions

Morphine: Manufacturer of ciprofloxacin advises avoid premedication with morphine (reduced plasma-ciprofloxacin concentration)

Pethidine: Manufacturer of ciprofloxacin advises avoid premedication with pethidine (reduced plasma-ciprofloxacin concentration)

Phenytoin: Plasma-phenytoin concentration possibly altered by ciprofloxacin

* Theophylline: Increased plasma-theophylline concentration; possible increased risk of convulsions

* Warfarin: Enhanced anticoagulant effect

Cisplatin

Acetazolamide: Increased risk of nephrotoxicity and ototoxicity

Amiloride: Increased risk of nephrotoxicity and ototoxicity

Furosemide: Increased risk of nephrotoxicity and ototoxicity

* Gentamicin: Increased risk of nephrotoxicity and possibly of ototoxicity

Cisplatin (Continued)

  Hydrochlorothiazide: Increased risk of nephrotoxicity and ototoxicity

  Phenytoin: Reduced absorption of phenytoin

  Spironolactone: Increased risk of nephrotoxicity and ototoxicity

* Streptomycin: Increased risk of nephrotoxicity and possibly of ototoxicity

  Vaccine, Live: Avoid use of live vaccines with cisplatin (impairment of immune response)

  Vancomycin: Increased risk of nephrotoxicity and possibly of ototoxicity

Clindamycin

  Alcuronium: Enhanced muscle relaxant effect

  Neostigmine: Antagonism of effects of neostigmine

  Pyridostigmine: Antagonism of effects of pyridostigmine

  Vecuronium: Enhanced muscle relaxant effect

Clomipramine

  Acetazolamide: Increased risk of postural hypotension

* Alcohol: Enhanced sedative effect

  Amiloride: Increased risk of postural hypotension

* Artemether+Lumefantrine: Increased risk of ventricular arrhythmias

  Atropine: Increased antimuscarinic adverse effects

  Biperiden: Increased antimuscarinic adverse effects

* Carbamazepine: Antagonism (convulsive threshold lowered); possibly accelerated metabolism of clomipramine (reduced plasma concentration; reduced antidepressant effect)

  Chloral hydrate: Enhanced sedative effect

  Chlorphenamine: Increased antimuscarinic and sedative effects

* Chlorpromazine: Increased antimuscarinic adverse effects; increased plasma-clomipramine concentration; possibly increased risk of ventricular arrhythmias

  Cimetidine: Plasma concentration of clomipramine possibly increased

  Clonazepam: Enhanced sedative effect

  Codeine: Possibly increased sedation

  Contraceptives, Oral: Antagonism of antidepressant effect but adverse effects possibly increased due to increased plasma concentration of clomipramine

  Diazepam: Enhanced sedative effect

* Epinephrine: Hypertension and arrhythmias (but local anaesthetics with epinephrine appear to be safe)

  Ether, Anaesthetic: Increased risk of arrhythmias and hypotension

* Ethosuximide: Antagonism (convulsive threshold lowered)

* Fluphenazine: Increased antimuscarinic adverse effects; increased plasma-clomipramine concentration; possibly increased risk of ventricular arrhythmias

  Furosemide: Increased risk of postural hypotension

  Glyceryl trinitrate: Reduced effect of sublingual glyceryl trinitrate (owing to dry mouth)

* Haloperidol: Increased plasma-clomipramine concentration; possibly increased risk of ventricular arrhythmias

  Halothane: Increased risk of arrhythmias and hypotension

  Hydralazine: Enhanced hypotensive effect

  Hydrochlorothiazide: Increased risk of postural hypotension

  Isosorbide dinitrate: Reduced effect of sublingual isosorbide dinitrate (owing to dry mouth)

  Ketamine: Increased risk of arrhythmias and hypotension

  Methyldopa: Enhanced hypotensive effect

  Morphine: Possibly increased sedation

  Nitrous oxide: Increased risk of arrhythmias and hypotension

  Pethidine: Possibly increased sedation

* Phenobarbital: Antagonism of anticonvulsant effect (convulsive threshold lowered); metabolism of clomipramine possibly accelerated (reduced plasma concentration)

* Phenytoin: Antagonism (convulsive threshold lowered); possibly reduced plasma-clomipramine concentration

* Procainamide: Increased risk of ventricular arrhythmias

  Promethazine: Increased antimuscarinic and sedative effects

Clomipramine (Continued)

    * Quinidine: Increased risk of ventricular arrhythmias

    Reserpine: Enhanced hypotensive effect

    Rifampicin: Plasma concentration of clomipramine possibly reduced (reduced antidepressant effect)

    * Ritonavir: Plasma concentration possibly increased by ritonavir

    Sodium nitroprusside: Enhanced hypotensive effect

    Spironolactone: Increased risk of postural hypotension

    Thiopental: Increased risk of arrhythmias and hypotension

    * Valproic acid: Antagonism (convulsive threshold lowered)

    Verapamil: Possibly increased plasma concentration of clomipramine

Clonazepam

    Acetazolamide: Enhanced hypotensive effect

    Alcohol: Enhanced sedative effect

    Amiloride: Enhanced hypotensive effect

    Amitriptyline: Enhanced sedative effect

    Atenolol: Enhanced hypotensive effect

    Captopril: Enhanced hypotensive effect

    * Carbamazepine: May be enhanced toxicity without corresponding increase in antiepileptic effect; plasma concentration of clonazepam often lowered

    Chlorphenamine: Enhanced sedative effect

    Chlorpromazine: Enhanced sedative effect

    Cimetidine: Inhibition of clonazepam metabolism (increased plasma concentration)

    Clomipramine: Enhanced sedative effect

    Codeine: Enhanced sedative effect

    Ether, Anaesthetic: Enhanced sedative effect

    Fluphenazine: Enhanced sedative effect

    Furosemide: Enhanced hypotensive effect

    Glyceryl trinitrate: Enhanced hypotensive effect

    Haloperidol: Enhanced sedative effect

    Halothane: Enhanced sedative effect

    Hydralazine: Enhanced hypotensive effect

    Hydrochlorothiazide: Enhanced hypotensive effect

    Isosorbide dinitrate: Enhanced hypotensive effect

    Ketamine: Enhanced sedative effect

    Levodopa: Possibly occasional antagonism of levodopa effects

    Methyldopa: Enhanced hypotensive effect

    Morphine: Enhanced sedative effect

    Nifedipine: Enhanced hypotensive effect

    Nitrous oxide: Enhanced sedative effect

    Pethidine: Enhanced sedative effect

    * Phenobarbital: May be enhanced toxicity without corresponding increase in antiepileptic effect; plasma concentration of clonazepam often lowered

    * Phenytoin: May be enhanced toxicity without corresponding increase in antiepileptic effect; plasma concentration of clonazepam often lowered

    Prazosin: Enhanced hypotensive and sedative effects

    Promethazine: Enhanced sedative effect

    Propranolol: Enhanced hypotensive effect

    Reserpine: Enhanced hypotensive effect

    Rifampicin: Metabolism of clonazepam possibly accelerated (possibly reduced plasma concentration)

    * Ritonavir: Plasma concentration possibly increased by ritonavir

    Sodium nitroprusside: Enhanced hypotensive effect

    Spironolactone: Enhanced hypotensive effect

    Thiopental: Enhanced sedative effect

    Timolol: Enhanced hypotensive effect

    Verapamil: Enhanced hypotensive effect

Cloxacillin *see* Benzylpenicillin

Codeine

    Alcohol: Enhanced sedative and hypotensive effect

    Amitriptyline: Possibly increased sedation

    Chloral hydrate: Enhanced sedative effect

Codeine (Continued)

> Chlorpromazine: Enhanced sedative and hypotensive effect
> Cimetidine: Metabolism of codeine inhibited (increased plasma concentration)
> Clomipramine: Possibly increased sedation
> Clonazepam: Enhanced sedative effect
> Diazepam: Enhanced sedative effect
> Fluphenazine: Enhanced sedative and hypotensive effect
> Haloperidol: Enhanced sedative and hypotensive effect
> Metoclopramide: Antagonism of effect of metoclopramide on gastro-intestinal activity
> * Ritonavir: Ritonavir possibly increases plasma concentration of codeine

Colchicine

> * Ciclosporin: Possibly increased risk of nephrotoxicity and myotoxicity (increased plasma-ciclosporin concentration)

Contraceptives, Oral *NOTE.* Interactions also apply to ethinylestradiol taken alone. In hormone replacement therapy low dose unlikely to induce interactions

> Acetazolamide: Antagonism of diuretic effect
> Amiloride: Antagonism of diuretic effect
> Amitriptyline: Antagonism of antidepressant effect but adverse effects possibly increased due to increased plasma concentration of amitriptyline
> * Amoxicillin: Possibility of reduced contraceptive effect
> * Ampicillin: Possibility of reduced contraceptive effect
> Atenolol: Antagonism of hypotensive effect
> Captopril: Antagonism of hypotensive effect
> * Carbamazepine: Accelerated metabolism (reduced contraceptive effect)
> Ceftazidime: Possibility of reduced contraceptive effect
> Ceftriaxone: Possibility of reduced contraceptive effect
> Ciclosporin: Possibly increased plasma-ciclosporin concentration
> Clomipramine: Antagonism of antidepressant effect but adverse effects possibly increased due to increased plasma concentration of clomipramine
> Dexamethasone: Oral contraceptives increase plasma concentration of dexamethasone
> * Doxycycline: Possibility of reduced contraceptive effect
> Efavirenz: Efficacy of oral contraceptives possibly reduced
> Fluconazole: Anecdotal reports of contraceptive failure
> Fludrocortisone: Oral contraceptives increase plasma concentration of fludrocortisone
> Furosemide: Antagonism of diuretic effect
> Glibenclamide: Antagonism of hypoglycaemic effect
> Glyceryl trinitrate: Antagonism of hypotensive effect
> * Griseofulvin: Accelerated metabolism (reduced contraceptive effect)
> Hydralazine: Antagonism of hypotensive effect
> Hydrochlorothiazide: Antagonism of diuretic effect
> Hydrocortisone: Oral contraceptives increase plasma concentration of hydrocortisone
> Insulins: Antagonism of hypoglycaemic effect
> Isosorbide dinitrate: Antagonism of hypotensive effect
> Metformin: Antagonism of hypoglycaemic effect
> Methyldopa: Antagonism of hypotensive effect
> * Minocycline: Possibility of reduced contraceptive effect
> * Nelfinavir: Accelerated metabolism (reduced contraceptive effect)
> * Nevirapine: Accelerated metabolism (reduced contraceptive effect)
> Nifedipine: Antagonism of hypotensive effect
> * Phenobarbital: Metabolism accelerated (reduced contraceptive effect)
> * Phenytoin: Accelerated metabolism (reduced contraceptive effect)
> Prazosin: Antagonism of hypotensive effect
> Prednisolone: Oral contraceptives increase plasma concentration of prednisolone
> Propranolol: Antagonism of hypotensive effect
> Reserpine: Antagonism of hypotensive effect

Contraceptives, Oral (Continued)
  * Rifampicin: Accelerated metabolism of oral contraceptives (reduced contraceptive effect)
  * Ritonavir: Accelerated metabolism (reduced contraceptive effect)
    Sodium nitroprusside: Antagonism of hypotensive effect
    Spironolactone: Antagonism of diuretic effect
    Theophylline: Delayed excretion of theophylline (increased plasma concentration)
    Verapamil: Antagonism of hypotensive effect
  * Warfarin: Antagonism of anticoagulant effect

Cyclophosphamide
    Phenytoin: Reduced absorption of phenytoin
    Suxamethonium: Enhanced effect of suxamethonium
    Vaccine, Live: Avoid use of live vaccines with cyclophosphamide (impairment of immune response)

Cytarabine
    Flucytosine: Plasma-flucytosine concentration possibly reduced
    Phenytoin: Reduced absorption of phenytoin
    Vaccine, Live: Avoid use of live vaccines with cytarabine (impairment of immune response)

Dacarbazine
    Vaccine, Live: Avoid use of live vaccines with dacarbazine (impairment of immune response)

Dactinomycin
    Vaccine, Live: Avoid use of live vaccines with dactinomycin (impairment of immune response)

Dapsone
    Rifampicin: Reduced plasma-dapsone concentration

Daunorubicin
    Vaccine, Live: Avoid use of live vaccines with daunorubicin (impairment of immune response)

Dexamethasone
    Acetazolamide: Increased risk of hypokalaemia; antagonism of diuretic effect
    Acetylsalicylic acid: Increased risk of gastrointestinal bleeding and ulceration; dexamethasone reduces plasma-salicylate concentration
    Amiloride: Antagonism of diuretic effect
  * Amphotericin: Increased risk of hypokalaemia (avoid concomitant use unless dexamethasone needed to control reactions)
    Atenolol: Antagonism of hypotensive effect
    Captopril: Antagonism of hypotensive effect
  * Carbamazepine: Accelerated metabolism of dexamethasone (reduced effect)
    Contraceptives, Oral: Oral contraceptives increase plasma concentration of dexamethasone
    Digoxin: Increased risk of hypokalaemia
    Ephedrine: Metabolism of dexamethasone accelerated
    Erythromycin: Erythromycin possibly inhibits metabolism of dexamethasone
    Furosemide: Antagonism of diuretic effect; increased risk of hypokalaemia
    Glibenclamide: Antagonism of hypoglycaemic effect
    Glyceryl trinitrate: Antagonism of hypotensive effect
    Hydralazine: Antagonism of hypotensive effect
    Hydrochlorothiazide: Antagonism of diuretic effect; increased risk of hypokalaemia
    Indinavir: Possibly reduced plasma-indinavir concentration
    Ibuprofen: Increased risk of gastrointestinal bleeding and ulceration
    Insulins: Antagonism of hypoglycaemic effect
    Isosorbide dinitrate: Antagonism of hypotensive effect
    Levonorgestrel: Levonorgestrel increases plasma concentration of dexamethasone
    Lopinavir: Possibly reduced plasma-lopinavir concentration
    Medroxyprogesterone: Medroxyprogesterone increases plasma concentration of dexamethasone

Dexamethasone (Continued)

Metformin: Antagonism of hypoglycaemic effect

Methotrexate: Increased risk of haematological toxicity

Methyldopa: Antagonism of hypotensive effect

Nifedipine: Antagonism of hypotensive effect

Norethisterone: Norethisterone increases plasma concentration of dexamethasone

* Phenobarbital: Metabolism of dexamethasone accelerated (reduced effect)

* Phenytoin: Metabolism of dexamethasone accelerated (reduced effect)

Praziquantel: Plasma-praziquantel concentration reduced

Prazosin: Antagonism of hypotensive effect

Propranolol: Antagonism of hypotensive effect

Reserpine: Antagonism of hypotensive effect

* Rifampicin: Accelerated metabolism of dexamethasone (reduced effect)

Ritonavir: Plasma concentration possibly increased by ritonavir

Salbutamol: Increased risk of hypokalaemia if high doses of dexamethasone given with high doses of salbutamol

Saquinavir: Possibly reduced plasma-saquinavir concentration

Sodium nitroprusside: Antagonism of hypotensive effect

Spironolactone: Antagonism of diuretic effect

Theophylline: Increased risk of hypokalaemia

Vaccine, Live: High doses of dexamethasone impair immune response; avoid use of live vaccines

Verapamil: Antagonism of hypotensive effect

* Warfarin: Anticoagulant effect possibly altered

Diazepam

Acetazolamide: Enhanced hypotensive effect

Alcohol: Enhanced sedative effect

Amiloride: Enhanced hypotensive effect

Amitriptyline: Enhanced sedative effect

Atenolol: Enhanced hypotensive effect

Captopril: Enhanced hypotensive effect

Chlorphenamine: Enhanced sedative effect

Chlorpromazine: Enhanced sedative effect

Cimetidine: Inhibition of diazepam metabolism (increased plasma concentration)

Clomipramine: Enhanced sedative effect

Codeine: Enhanced sedative effect

Ether, Anaesthetic: Enhanced sedative effect

Fluphenazine: Enhanced sedative effect

Furosemide: Enhanced hypotensive effect

Glyceryl trinitrate: Enhanced hypotensive effect

Haloperidol: Enhanced sedative effect

Halothane: Enhanced sedative effect

Hydralazine: Enhanced hypotensive effect

Hydrochlorothiazide: Enhanced hypotensive effect

Isoniazid: Metabolism of diazepam inhibited

Isosorbide dinitrate: Enhanced hypotensive effect

Ketamine: Enhanced sedative effect

Levodopa: Occasional antagonism of levodopa effects

Methyldopa: Enhanced hypotensive effect

Morphine: Enhanced sedative effect

Nifedipine: Enhanced hypotensive effect

Nitrous oxide: Enhanced sedative effect

Pethidine: Enhanced sedative effect

Phenytoin: Plasma-phenytoin concentrations increased or decreased by diazepam

Prazosin: Enhanced hypotensive and sedative effects

Promethazine: Enhanced sedative effect

Propranolol: Enhanced hypotensive effect

Reserpine: Enhanced hypotensive effect

Rifampicin: Metabolism of diazepam accelerated (reduced plasma concentration)

Diazepam (Continued)

   * Ritonavir: Plasma concentration possibly increased by ritonavir (risk of extreme sedation and respiratory depression—avoid concomitant use)

    Sodium nitroprusside: Enhanced hypotensive effect

    Spironolactone: Enhanced hypotensive effect

    Thiopental: Enhanced sedative effect

    Timolol: Enhanced hypotensive effect

    Verapamil: Enhanced hypotensive effect

Didanosine NOTE. Antacids present in tablet formulation may affect absorption of other drugs; *see also* Antacids

Digoxin

   * Acetazolamide: Cardiac toxicity of digoxin increased if hypokalaemia occurs

   * Amphotericin: Increased digoxin toxicity if hypokalaemia occurs

    Antacids (Aluminium hydroxide; Magnesium hydroxide): Possibly reduced absorption of digoxin

    Atenolol: Increased AV block and bradycardia

    Calcium salts: Large intravenous doses of calcium can precipitate arrhythmias

    Captopril: Plasma concentration of digoxin possibly increased

   * Chloroquine: Plasma-digoxin concentration possibly increased

    Dexamethasone: Increased risk of hypokalaemia

    Erythromycin: Enhanced effect of digoxin

    Fludrocortisone: Increased risk of hypokalaemia

   * Furosemide: Cardiac toxicity of digoxin increased if hypokalaemia occurs

   * Hydrochlorothiazide: Cardiac toxicity of digoxin increased if hypokalaemia occurs

    Hydrocortisone: Increased risk of hypokalaemia

    Ibuprofen: Possibly exacerbation of heart failure, reduced GFR, and increased plasma-digoxin concentration

    Mefloquine: Possibly increased risk of bradycardia

   * Nifedipine: Possibly increased plasma concentration of digoxin

    Prednisolone: Increased risk of hypokalaemia

    Propranolol: Increased AV block and bradycardia

   * Quinidine: Plasma concentration of digoxin increased (halve maintenance dose of digoxin)

   * Quinine: Plasma concentration of digoxin increased

   * Spironolactone: Enhanced effect of digoxin

    Sulfamethoxazole+Trimethoprim: Plasma concentration of digoxin possibly increased

    Sulfasalazine: Absorption of digoxin possibly reduced

    Suxamethonium: Risk of arrhythmias

    Timolol: Increased AV block and bradycardia

    Trimethoprim: Plasma concentration of digoxin possibly increased

   * Verapamil: Increased plasma concentration of digoxin; increased AV block and bradycardia

Dopamine

    Chlorpromazine: Antagonism of pressor action

    Fluphenazine: Antagonism of pressor action

    Haloperidol: Antagonism of pressor action

Doxorubicin

   * Ciclosporin: Increased risk of neurotoxicity

    Phenytoin: Reduced absorption of phenytoin

    Stavudine: Doxorubicin may inhibit effect of stavudine

    Vaccine, Live: Avoid use of live vaccines with doxorubicin (impairment of immune response)

Doxycycline

    Antacids (Aluminium hydroxide; Magnesium hydroxide): Reduced absorption of doxycycline

    Carbamazepine: Accelerated doxycycline metabolism (reduced effect)

   * Ciclosporin: Possibly increased plasma-ciclosporin concentration

   * Contraceptives, Oral: Possibility of reduced contraceptive effect

    Ferrous salts: Reduced absorption of oral ferrous salts by doxycycline; reduced absorption of doxycycline by oral ferrous salts

Doxycycline (Continued)

Phenobarbital: Metabolism of doxycycline accelerated (reduced plasma concentration)

Phenytoin: Increased metabolism of doxycycline (reduced plasma concentration)

Rifampicin: Plasma-doxycycline concentration possibly reduced

* Warfarin: Anticoagulant effect possibly enhanced

Efavirenz

Contraceptives, Oral: Efficacy of oral contraceptives possibly reduced

Grapefruit Juice: Plasma concentration of efavirenz may be affected

Indinavir: Efavirenz reduces plasma concentration of indinavir (increase indinavir dose)

Lopinavir: Plasma concentration of lopinavir reduced

Rifampicin: Reduced plasma concentration of efavirenz (increase efavirenz dose)

Ritonavir: Increased risk of toxicity (monitor liver function)

Saquinavir: Efavirenz significantly reduces plasma concentration of saquinavir

Ephedrine

Chlorpromazine: Antagonism of pressor action

Dexamethasone: Metabolism of dexamethasone accelerated

Fluphenazine: Antagonism of pressor action

Haloperidol: Antagonism of pressor action

Oxytocin: Hypertension due to enhanced vasopressor effect of ephedrine

Epinephrine

* Amitriptyline: Hypertension and arrhythmias (but local anaesthetics with epinephrine appear to be safe)

* Atenolol: Severe hypertension

Chlorpromazine: Antagonism of pressor action

* Clomipramine: Hypertension and arrhythmias (but local anaesthetics with epinephrine appear to be safe)

* Ether, Anaesthetic: Risk of arrhythmias

Fluphenazine: Antagonism of pressor action

Haloperidol: Antagonism of pressor action

* Halothane: Risk of arrhythmias

Oxytocin: Hypertension due to enhanced vasopressor effect of epinephrine

* Propranolol: Severe hypertension

* Timolol: Severe hypertension

Ergocalciferol

Carbamazepine: Ergocalciferol requirements possibly increase

Hydrochlorothiazide: Increased risk of hypercalcaemia

Phenobarbital: Ergocalciferol requirements possibly increased

Phenytoin: Ergocalciferol requirements possibly increased

Ergotamine

Atenolol: Increased peripheral vasoconstriction

* Erythromycin: Risk of ergotism (avoid concomitant use)

* Indinavir: Increased risk of ergotism (avoid concomitant use)

* Nelfinavir: Increased risk of ergotism (avoid concomitant use)

Propranolol: Increased peripheral vasoconstriction

* Ritonavir: Increased risk of ergotism (avoid concomitant use)

* Saquinavir: Possible increased risk of ergotism (avoid concomitant use)

Timolol: Increased peripheral vasoconstriction

Erythromycin

* Carbamazepine: Increased plasma-carbamazepine concentration

* Ciclosporin: Increased plasma-ciclosporin concentration (inhibition of metabolism)

Cimetidine: Increased plasma-erythromycin concentration (increased risk of toxicity, including deafness)

Dexamethasone: Erythromycin possibly inhibits metabolism of dexamethasone

Digoxin: Enhanced effect of digoxin

* Ergotamine: Risk of ergotism (avoid concomitant use)

Fludrocortisone: Erythromycin possibly inhibits metabolism of fludrocortisone

Erythromycin (Continued)

Hydrocortisone: Erythromycin possibly inhibits metabolism of hydrocortisone

Prednisolone: Erythromycin possibly inhibits metabolism of prednisolone

Ritonavir: Plasma concentration possibly increased by ritonavir

* Theophylline: Inhibition of theophylline metabolism (increased plasma-theophylline concentration); if erythromycin given by mouth, also decreased plasma-erythromycin concentration

Valproic acid: Metabolism of valproic acid possibly inhibited (increased plasma concentration)

* Warfarin: Enhanced anticoagulant effect

Ether, Anaesthetic

Acetazolamide: Enhanced hypotensive effect

Amiloride: Enhanced hypotensive effect

Amitriptyline: Increased risk of arrhythmias and hypotension

Atenolol: Enhanced hypotensive effect

Captopril: Enhanced hypotensive effect

Chloral hydrate: Enhanced sedative effect

* Chlorpromazine: Enhanced hypotensive effect

Clomipramine: Increased risk of arrhythmias and hypotension

Clonazepam: Enhanced sedative effect

Diazepam: Enhanced sedative effect

* Epinephrine: Risk of arrhythmias

* Fluphenazine: Enhanced hypotensive effect

Furosemide: Enhanced hypotensive effect

Glyceryl trinitrate: Enhanced hypotensive effect

* Haloperidol: Enhanced hypotensive effect

Hydralazine: Enhanced hypotensive effect

Hydrochlorothiazide: Enhanced hypotensive effect

Isoniazid: Possible potentiation of isoniazid hepatotoxicity

* Isoprenaline: Risk of arrhythmias

Isosorbide dinitrate: Enhanced hypotensive effect

* Levodopa: Risk of arrhythmias

Methyldopa: Enhanced hypotensive effect

Nifedipine: Enhanced hypotensive effect

Oxytocin: Oxytocic effect possibly reduced; enhanced hypotensive effect and risk of arrhythmias

* Prazosin: Enhanced hypotensive effect

Propranolol: Enhanced hypotensive effect

Sodium nitroprusside: Enhanced hypotensive effect

Spironolactone: Enhanced hypotensive effect

Timolol: Enhanced hypotensive effect

Vancomycin: Hypersensitivity-like reactions can occur with concomitant intravenous vancomycin

* Verapamil: Enhanced hypotensive effect and AV delay

Ethinylestradiol see Contraceptives, Oral

Ethosuximide

* Amitriptyline: Antagonism (convulsive threshold lowered)

* Carbamazepine: May be enhanced toxicity without corresponding increase in antiepileptic effect; plasma concentration of ethosuximide sometimes lowered

* Chloroquine: Antagonism of anticonvulsant effect

* Chlorpromazine: Antagonism (convulsive threshold lowered)

* Clomipramine: Antagonism (convulsive threshold lowered)

* Fluphenazine: Antagonism (convulsive threshold lowered)

* Haloperidol: Antagonism (convulsive threshold lowered)

* Isoniazid: Metabolism of ethosuximide inhibited (increased plasma-ethosuximide concentration and risk of toxicity)

* Mefloquine: Antagonism of anticonvulsant effect

* Phenobarbital: May be enhanced toxicity without corresponding increase in antiepileptic effect; plasma concentration of ethosuximide sometimes lowered

Ethosuximide (Continued)

  * Phenytoin: May be enhanced toxicity without corresponding increase in antiepileptic effect; plasma concentration of phenytoin sometimes raised; plasma concentration of ethosuximide sometimes lowered
  * Valproic acid: May be enhanced toxicity without corresponding increase in antiepileptic effect; plasma concentration of ethosuximide sometimes raised

Etoposide

  Vaccine, Live: Avoid use of live vaccines with etoposide (impairment of immune response)

Ferrous salt and Folic acid *see* Ferrous salts; Folic acid

Ferrous salts

  Ciprofloxacin: Absorption of ciprofloxacin reduced by oral ferrous salts
  Doxycycline: Reduced absorption of oral ferrous salts by doxycycline; reduced absorption of doxycycline by oral ferrous salts
  Levodopa: Absorption of levodopa may be reduced
  Methyldopa: Reduced hypotensive effect of methyldopa
  Minocycline: Reduced absorption of oral ferrous salts by minocycline; reduced absorption of minocycline by oral ferrous salts
  Ofloxacin: Absorption of ofloxacin reduced by oral ferrous salts
  Penicillamine: Reduced absorption of penicillamine

Fluconazole

  Amphotericin: Possible antagonism of effect of amphotericin
  * Ciclosporin: Metabolism of ciclosporin possibly inhibited (possibly increased plasma concentration)
  Contraceptives, Oral: Anecdotal reports of contraceptive failure
  * Glibenclamide: Plasma concentration of glibenclamide increased
  Hydrochlorothiazide: Plasma concentration of fluconazole increased
  * Phenytoin: Effect of phenytoin enhanced; plasma concentration increased
  * Rifampicin: Accelerated metabolism of fluconazole (reduced plasma concentration)
  * Ritonavir: Plasma concentration possibly increased by ritonavir
  Saquinavir: Plasma concentration of saquinavir possibly increased
  * Theophylline: Plasma-theophylline concentration possibly increased
  * Warfarin: Enhanced anticoagulant effect
  * Zidovudine: Increased plasma concentration of zidovudine (increased risk of toxicity)

Flucytosine

  Amphotericin: Renal excretion of flucytosine decreased and cellular uptake increased (flucytosine toxicity possibly increased)
  Cytarabine: Plasma-flucytosine concentration possibly reduced

Fludrocortisone

  Acetazolamide: Increased risk of hypokalaemia; antagonism of diuretic effect
  Acetylsalicylic acid: Increased risk of gastrointestinal bleeding and ulceration; fludrocortisone reduces plasma-salicylate concentration
  Amiloride: Antagonism of diuretic effect
  * Amphotericin: Increased risk of hypokalaemia
  Atenolol: Antagonism of hypotensive effect
  Captopril: Antagonism of hypotensive effect
  * Carbamazepine: Accelerated metabolism of fludrocortisone (reduced effect)
  Contraceptives, Oral: Oral contraceptives increase plasma concentration of fludrocortisone
  Digoxin: Increased risk of hypokalaemia
  Erythromycin: Erythromycin possibly inhibits metabolism of fludrocortisone
  Furosemide: Antagonism of diuretic effect; increased risk of hypokalaemia
  Glibenclamide: Antagonism of hypoglycaemic effect
  Glyceryl trinitrate: Antagonism of hypotensive effect
  Hydralazine: Antagonism of hypotensive effect
  Hydrochlorothiazide: Antagonism of diuretic effect; increased risk of hypokalaemia
  Ibuprofen: Increased risk of gastrointestinal bleeding and ulceration

Fludrocortisone (Continued)

Insulins: Antagonism of hypoglycaemic effect

Isosorbide dinitrate: Antagonism of hypotensive effect

Levonorgestrel: Levonorgestrel increases plasma concentration of fludrocortisone

Medroxyprogesterone: Medroxyprogesterone increases plasma concentration of fludrocortisone

Metformin: Antagonism of hypoglycaemic effect

Methotrexate: Increased risk of haematological toxicity

Methyldopa: Antagonism of hypotensive effect

Nifedipine: Antagonism of hypotensive effect

Norethisterone: Norethisterone increases plasma concentration of fludrocortisone

* Phenobarbital: Metabolism of fludrocortisone accelerated (reduced effect)

* Phenytoin: Metabolism of fludrocortisone accelerated (reduced effect)

Prazosin: Antagonism of hypotensive effect

Propranolol: Antagonism of hypotensive effect

Reserpine: Antagonism of hypotensive effect

* Rifampicin: Accelerated metabolism of fludrocortisone (reduced effect)

Ritonavir: Plasma concentration possibly increased by ritonavir

Salbutamol: Increased risk of hypokalaemia if high doses of fludrocortisone given with high doses of salbutamol

Sodium nitroprusside: Antagonism of hypotensive effect

Spironolactone: Antagonism of diuretic effect

Theophylline: Increased risk of hypokalaemia

Vaccine, Live: High doses of fludrocortisone impair immune response; avoid use of live vaccines

Verapamil: Antagonism of hypotensive effect

* Warfarin: Anticoagulant effect possibly altered

Fluorouracil

Cimetidine: Metabolism of fluorouracil inhibited (increased plasma-fluorouracil concentration)

Metronidazole: Metabolism of fluorouracil inhibited (increased toxicity)

Phenytoin: Reduced absorption of phenytoin

Vaccine, Live: Avoid use of live vaccines with fluorouracil (impairment of immune response)

Fluphenazine

Acetazolamide: Enhanced hypotensive effect

Alcohol: Enhanced sedative effect

Amiloride: Enhanced hypotensive effect

* Amitriptyline: Increased antimuscarinic adverse effects; increased plasma-amitriptyline concentration; possibly increased risk of ventricular arrhythmias

* Artemether+Lumefantrine: Increased risk of ventricular arrhythmias

Atenolol: Enhanced hypotensive effect

Atropine: Increased antimuscarinic adverse effects of fluphenazine (but reduced plasma concentration)

Biperiden: Increased antimuscarinic adverse effects of fluphenazine (but reduced plasma concentration)

Captopril: Enhanced hypotensive effect

* Carbamazepine: Antagonism of anticonvulsant effect (convulsive threshold lowered)

Chloral hydrate: Enhanced sedative effect

Cimetidine: Possibly enhanced effects of fluphenazine

* Clomipramine: Increased antimuscarinic adverse effects; increased plasma-clomipramine concentration; possibly increased risk of ventricular arrhythmias

Clonazepam: Enhanced sedative effect

Codeine: Enhanced sedative and hypotensive effect

Diazepam: Enhanced sedative effect

Dopamine: Antagonism of pressor action

Ephedrine: Antagonism of pressor action

Epinephrine: Antagonism of pressor action

* Ether, Anaesthetic: Enhanced hypotensive effect

Fluphenazine (Continued)
* Ethosuximide: Antagonism (convulsive threshold lowered)
  Furosemide: Enhanced hypotensive effect
  Glibenclamide: Possible antagonism of hypoglycaemic effect
  Glyceryl trinitrate: Enhanced hypotensive effect
* Halothane: Enhanced hypotensive effect
  Hydralazine: Enhanced hypotensive effect
  Hydrochlorothiazide: Enhanced hypotensive effect
  Isoprenaline: Antagonism of pressor action
  Isosorbide dinitrate: Enhanced hypotensive effect
* Ketamine: Enhanced hypotensive effect
  Levodopa: Antagonism of effects of levodopa
  Lithium: Increased risk of extrapyramidal effects and possibility of neurotoxicity
  Methyldopa: Enhanced hypotensive effect; increased risk of extrapyramidal effects
  Metoclopramide: Increased risk of extrapyramidal effects
  Morphine: Enhanced sedative and hypotensive effect
  Nifedipine: Enhanced hypotensive effect
* Nitrous oxide: Enhanced hypotensive effect
  Pethidine: Enhanced sedative and hypotensive effect
* Phenobarbital: Antagonism of anticonvulsant effect (convulsive threshold lowered)
* Phenytoin: Antagonism of anticonvulsant effect (convulsive threshold lowered)
  Prazosin: Enhanced hypotensive effect
* Procainamide: Increased risk of ventricular arrhythmias
  Propranolol: Enhanced hypotensive effect
* Quinidine: Increased risk of ventricular arrhythmias
  Reserpine: Enhanced hypotensive effect; increased risk of extrapyramidal effects
* Ritonavir: Plasma concentration possibly increased by ritonavir
  Sodium nitroprusside: Enhanced hypotensive effect
  Spironolactone: Enhanced hypotensive effect
* Thiopental: Enhanced hypotensive effect
  Timolol: Enhanced hypotensive effect
* Valproic acid: Antagonism of anticonvulsant effect (convulsive threshold lowered)
  Verapamil: Enhanced hypotensive effect

Folic acid and Folinic acid
  Phenobarbital: Plasma concentration of phenobarbital possibly reduced
  Phenytoin: Plasma-phenytoin concentration possibly reduced

Furosemide
  Acetazolamide: Increased risk of hypokalaemia
  Alcohol: Enhanced hypotensive effect
  Amitriptyline: Increased risk of postural hypotension
  Amphotericin: Increased risk of hypokalaemia
* Artemether+Lumefantrine: Increased risk of ventricular arrhythmias if electrolyte disturbance occurs
  Atenolol: Enhanced hypotensive effect
* Captopril: Enhanced hypotensive effect (can be extreme)
  Carbamazepine: Increased risk of hyponatraemia
  Ceftazidime: Nephrotoxicity of ceftazidime possibly increased
  Ceftriaxone: Nephrotoxicity of ceftriaxone possibly increased
  Chloral hydrate: Administration of chloral hydrate with parenteral furosemide may displace thyroid hormone from binding sites; enhanced hypotensive effect
  Chlorpromazine: Enhanced hypotensive effect
  Cisplatin: Increased risk of nephrotoxicity and ototoxicity
  Clomipramine: Increased risk of postural hypotension
  Clonazepam: Enhanced hypotensive effect
  Contraceptives, Oral: Antagonism of diuretic effect
  Dexamethasone: Antagonism of diuretic effect; increased risk of hypokalaemia
  Diazepam: Enhanced hypotensive effect

Furosemide (Continued)

* Digoxin: Cardiac toxicity of digoxin increased if hypokalaemia occurs

Ether, Anaesthetic: Enhanced hypotensive effect

Fludrocortisone: Antagonism of diuretic effect; increased risk of hypokalaemia

Fluphenazine: Enhanced hypotensive effect

* Gentamicin: Increased risk of ototoxicity

Glibenclamide: Antagonism of hypoglycaemic effect

Glyceryl trinitrate: Enhanced hypotensive effect

Halothane: Enhanced hypotensive effect

Hydralazine: Enhanced hypotensive effect

Hydrochlorothiazide: Increased risk of hypokalaemia

Hydrocortisone: Antagonism of diuretic effect; increased risk of hypokalaemia

Ibuprofen: Risk of nephrotoxicity of ibuprofen increased; antagonism of diuretic effect

Insulins: Antagonism of hypoglycaemic effect

Isosorbide dinitrate: Enhanced hypotensive effect

Ketamine: Enhanced hypotensive effect

Levodopa: Enhanced hypotensive effect

* Lidocaine: Action of lidocaine antagonised by hypokalaemia

* Lithium: Reduced lithium excretion (increased plasma-lithium concentration and risk of toxicity); furosemide safer than hydrochlorothiazide

Metformin: Antagonism of hypoglycaemic effect

Methyldopa: Enhanced hypotensive effect

Nifedipine: Enhanced hypotensive effect

Nitrous oxide: Enhanced hypotensive effect

* Prazosin: Enhanced hypotensive effect; increased risk of first-dose hypotensive effect of prazosin

Prednisolone: Antagonism of diuretic effect; increased risk of hypokalaemia

Propranolol: Enhanced hypotensive effect

* Quinidine: Cardiac toxicity of quinidine increased if hypokalaemia occurs

Reserpine: Enhanced hypotensive effect

Salbutamol: Increased risk of hypokalaemia with high doses of salbutamol

Sodium nitroprusside: Enhanced hypotensive effect

* Streptomycin: Increased risk of ototoxicity

Theophylline: Increased risk of hypokalaemia

Thiopental: Enhanced hypotensive effect

Timolol: Enhanced hypotensive effect

* Vancomycin: Increased risk of ototoxicity

Verapamil: Enhanced hypotensive effect

Gentamicin

* Alcuronium: Enhanced muscle relaxant effect

Amphotericin: Increased risk of nephrotoxicity

* Ciclosporin: Increased risk of nephrotoxicity

* Cisplatin: Increased risk of nephrotoxicity and possibly of ototoxicity

* Furosemide: Increased risk of ototoxicity

* Neostigmine: Antagonism of effect of neostigmine

Polygeline: Increased risk of nephrotoxicity

* Pyridostigmine: Antagonism of effect of pyridostigmine

* Suxamethonium: Enhanced muscle relaxant effect

Vancomycin: Increased risk of nephrotoxicity and ototoxicity

* Vecuronium: Enhanced muscle relaxant effect

Glibenclamide

Alcohol: Enhanced hypoglycaemic effect

Atenolol: Masking of warning signs of hypoglycaemia such as tremor

Captopril: Hypoglycaemic effect possibly enhanced

* Chloramphenicol: Enhanced effect of glibenclamide

Chlorpromazine: Possible antagonism of hypoglycaemic effect

Cimetidine: Enhanced hypoglycaemic effect

Ciprofloxacin: Possibly enhanced effect of glibenclamide

Contraceptives, Oral: Antagonism of hypoglycaemic effect

Glibenclamide (Continued)

Dexamethasone: Antagonism of hypoglycaemic effect
* Fluconazole: Plasma concentration of glibenclamide increased
Fludrocortisone: Antagonism of hypoglycaemic effect
Fluphenazine: Possible antagonism of hypoglycaemic effect
Furosemide: Antagonism of hypoglycaemic effect
Hydrochlorothiazide: Antagonism of hypoglycaemic effect
Hydrocortisone: Antagonism of hypoglycaemic effect
* Ibuprofen: Possibly enhanced effect of glibenclamide
Levonorgestrel: Antagonism of hypoglycaemic effect
Lithium: May occasionally impair glucose tolerance
Medroxyprogesterone: Antagonism of hypoglycaemic effect
Norethisterone: Antagonism of hypoglycaemic effect
Prednisolone: Antagonism of hypoglycaemic effect
Propranolol: Masking of warning signs of hypoglycaemia such as tremor
* Rifampicin: Possibly accelerated metabolism (reduced effect) of glibenclamide
* Sulfadiazine: Enhanced effect of glibenclamide
* Sulfadoxine+Pyrimethamine: Enhanced effect of glibenclamide
* Sulfamethoxazole+Trimethoprim: Enhanced effect of glibenclamide
Testosterone: Hypoglycaemic effect possibly enhanced
Timolol: Masking of warning signs of hypoglycaemia such as tremor
* Warfarin: Possibly enhanced hypoglycaemic effects and changes to anticoagulant effect

Glyceryl trinitrate

Acetazolamide: Enhanced hypotensive effect
Alcohol: Enhanced hypotensive effect
Amiloride: Enhanced hypotensive effect
Amitriptyline: Reduced effect of sublingual glyceryl trinitrate (owing to dry mouth)
Atenolol: Enhanced hypotensive effect
Atropine: Possibly reduced effect of sublingual nitrates (failure to dissolve under the tongue owing to dry mouth)
Biperiden: Possibly reduced effect of sublingual nitrates (failure to dissolve under the tongue owing to dry mouth)
Captopril: Enhanced hypotensive effect
Chloral hydrate: Enhanced hypotensive effect
Chlorpromazine: Enhanced hypotensive effect
Clomipramine: Reduced effect of sublingual glyceryl trinitrate (owing to dry mouth)
Clonazepam: Enhanced hypotensive effect
Contraceptives, Oral: Antagonism of hypotensive effect
Dexamethasone: Antagonism of hypotensive effect
Diazepam: Enhanced hypotensive effect
Ether, Anaesthetic: Enhanced hypotensive effect
Fludrocortisone: Antagonism of hypotensive effect
Fluphenazine: Enhanced hypotensive effect
Furosemide: Enhanced hypotensive effect
Halothane: Enhanced hypotensive effect
Hydralazine: Enhanced hypotensive effect
Hydrochlorothiazide: Enhanced hypotensive effect
Hydrocortisone: Antagonism of hypotensive effect
Ibuprofen: Antagonism of hypotensive effect
Ketamine: Enhanced hypotensive effect
Levodopa: Enhanced hypotensive effect
Methyldopa: Enhanced hypotensive effect
Nifedipine: Enhanced hypotensive effect
Nitrous oxide: Enhanced hypotensive effect
Prazosin: Enhanced hypotensive effect
Prednisolone: Antagonism of hypotensive effect
Propranolol: Enhanced hypotensive effect
Reserpine: Enhanced hypotensive effect
Sodium nitroprusside: Enhanced hypotensive effect
Spironolactone: Enhanced hypotensive effect
Thiopental: Enhanced hypotensive effect

Glyceryl trinitrate (Continued)
  Timolol: Enhanced hypotensive effect
  Verapamil: Enhanced hypotensive effect
Grapefruit Juice
  Artemether+Lumefantrine: Metabolism of artemether and lumefantrine
    may be inhibited
  * Ciclosporin: Increased plasma-ciclosporin concentration (risk of toxicity)
  Efavirenz: Plasma concentration of efavirenz may be affected
  Nifedipine: Increased plasma-nifedipine concentration
  Verapamil: Increased plasma-verapamil concentration
Griseofulvin
  Ciclosporin: Plasma-ciclosporin concentration possibly reduced
  * Contraceptives, Oral: Accelerated metabolism (reduced contraceptive
    effect)
  * Levonorgestrel: Accelerated metabolism (reduced contraceptive effect)
  * Medroxyprogesterone: Accelerated metabolism (reduced contraceptive
    effect)
  * Norethisterone: Accelerated metabolism (reduced contraceptive effect)
  Phenobarbital: Reduction in absorption of griseofulvin (reduced effect)
  * Warfarin: Metabolism of warfarin accelerated (reduced anticoagulant
    effect)
Haloperidol
  Alcohol: Enhanced sedative effect
  * Amitriptyline: Increased plasma-amitriptyline concentration; possibly
    increased risk of ventricular arrhythmias
  * Carbamazepine: Antagonism of anticonvulsant effect (convulsive
    threshold lowered); metabolism of haloperidol accelerated (reduced
    plasma concentration)
  Chloral hydrate: Enhanced sedative effect
  Cimetidine: Possibly enhanced effects of haloperidol
  * Clomipramine: Increased plasma-clomipramine concentration; possibly
    increased risk of ventricular arrhythmias
  Clonazepam: Enhanced sedative effect
  Codeine: Enhanced sedative and hypotensive effect
  Diazepam: Enhanced sedative effect
  Dopamine: Antagonism of pressor action
  Ephedrine: Antagonism of pressor action
  Epinephrine: Antagonism of pressor action
  * Ether, Anaesthetic: Enhanced hypotensive effect
  * Ethosuximide: Antagonism (convulsive threshold lowered)
  * Halothane: Enhanced hypotensive effect
  Isoprenaline: Antagonism of pressor action
  * Ketamine: Enhanced hypotensive effect
  Levodopa: Antagonism of effects of levodopa
  Lithium: Increased risk of extrapyramidal effects and possibility of
    neurotoxicity
  Methyldopa: Enhanced hypotensive effect; increased risk of extrapyr-
    amidal effects
  Metoclopramide: Increased risk of extrapyramidal effects
  Morphine: Enhanced sedative and hypotensive effect
  Nifedipine: Enhanced hypotensive effect
  * Nitrous oxide: Enhanced hypotensive effect
  Pethidine: Enhanced sedative and hypotensive effect
  * Phenobarbital: Antagonism of anticonvulsant effect (convulsive
    threshold lowered); metabolism of haloperidol accelerated (reduced
    plasma concentration)
  * Phenytoin: Antagonism of anticonvulsant effect (convulsive threshold
    lowered)
  Prazosin: Enhanced hypotensive effect
  * Procainamide: Increased risk of ventricular arrhythmias
  * Quinidine: Increased risk of ventricular arrhythmias
  Reserpine: Enhanced hypotensive effect; increased risk of extrapyramidal
    effects
  * Rifampicin: Accelerated metabolism of haloperidol (reduced plasma-
    haloperidol concentration)

Haloperidol (Continued)
  * Ritonavir: Plasma concentration possibly increased by ritonavir
  * Thiopental: Enhanced hypotensive effect
  * Valproic acid: Antagonism of anticonvulsant effect (convulsive threshold lowered)
    Verapamil: Enhanced hypotensive effect
Halothane
    Acetazolamide: Enhanced hypotensive effect
    Amiloride: Enhanced hypotensive effect
    Amitriptyline: Increased risk of arrhythmias and hypotension
    Atenolol: Enhanced hypotensive effect
    Captopril: Enhanced hypotensive effect
    Chloral hydrate: Enhanced sedative effect
  * Chlorpromazine: Enhanced hypotensive effect
    Clomipramine: Increased risk of arrhythmias and hypotension
    Clonazepam: Enhanced sedative effect
    Diazepam: Enhanced sedative effect
  * Epinephrine: Risk of arrhythmias
  * Fluphenazine: Enhanced hypotensive effect
    Furosemide: Enhanced hypotensive effect
    Glyceryl trinitrate: Enhanced hypotensive effect
  * Haloperidol: Enhanced hypotensive effect
    Hydralazine: Enhanced hypotensive effect
    Hydrochlorothiazide: Enhanced hypotensive effect
    Isoniazid: Possible potentiation of isoniazid hepatotoxicity
  * Isoprenaline: Risk of arrhythmias
    Isosorbide dinitrate: Enhanced hypotensive effect
  * Levodopa: Risk of arrhythmias
    Methyldopa: Enhanced hypotensive effect
    Nifedipine: Enhanced hypotensive effect
    Oxytocin: Oxytocic effect possibly reduced; enhanced hypotensive effect and risk of arrhythmias
  * Prazosin: Enhanced hypotensive effect
    Propranolol: Enhanced hypotensive effect
    Reserpine: Enhanced hypotensive effect
    Sodium nitroprusside: Enhanced hypotensive effect
    Spironolactone: Enhanced hypotensive effect
    Theophylline: Increased risk of arrhythmias
    Timolol: Enhanced hypotensive effect
    Vancomycin: Hypersensitivity-like reactions can occur with concomitant intravenous vancomycin
  * Verapamil: Enhanced hypotensive effect and AV delay
Heparin
  * Acetylsalicylic acid: Enhanced anticoagulant effect
    Captopril: Increased risk of hyperkalaemia
    Ibuprofen: Possibly increased risk of bleeding
Hydralazine
    Acetazolamide: Enhanced hypotensive effect
    Alcohol: Enhanced hypotensive effect
    Amiloride: Enhanced hypotensive effect
    Amitriptyline: Enhanced hypotensive effect
    Atenolol: Enhanced hypotensive effect
    Captopril: Enhanced hypotensive effect
    Chloral hydrate: Enhanced hypotensive effect
    Chlorpromazine: Enhanced hypotensive effect
    Clomipramine: Enhanced hypotensive effect
    Clonazepam: Enhanced hypotensive effect
    Contraceptives, Oral: Antagonism of hypotensive effect
    Dexamethasone: Antagonism of hypotensive effect
    Diazepam: Enhanced hypotensive effect
    Ether, Anaesthetic: Enhanced hypotensive effect
    Fludrocortisone: Antagonism of hypotensive effect
    Fluphenazine: Enhanced hypotensive effect
    Furosemide: Enhanced hypotensive effect
    Glyceryl trinitrate: Enhanced hypotensive effect

Hydralazine (Continued)

Halothane: Enhanced hypotensive effect
Hydrochlorothiazide: Enhanced hypotensive effect
Hydrocortisone: Antagonism of hypotensive effect
Ibuprofen: Antagonism of hypotensive effect
Isosorbide dinitrate: Enhanced hypotensive effect
Ketamine: Enhanced hypotensive effect
Levodopa: Enhanced hypotensive effect
Methyldopa: Enhanced hypotensive effect
Nifedipine: Enhanced hypotensive effect
Nitrous oxide: Enhanced hypotensive effect
Prazosin: Enhanced hypotensive effect
Prednisolone: Antagonism of hypotensive effect
Propranolol: Enhanced hypotensive effect
Reserpine: Enhanced hypotensive effect
Sodium nitroprusside: Enhanced hypotensive effect
Spironolactone: Enhanced hypotensive effect
Thiopental: Enhanced hypotensive effect
Timolol: Enhanced hypotensive effect
Verapamil: Enhanced hypotensive effect

Hydrochlorothiazide

Acetazolamide: Increased risk of hypokalaemia
Alcohol: Enhanced hypotensive effect
Amitriptyline: Increased risk of postural hypotension
Amphotericin: Increased risk of hypokalaemia
* Artemether+Lumefantrine: Increased risk of ventricular arrhythmias if electrolyte disturbance occurs
Atenolol: Enhanced hypotensive effect
Calcium salts: Increased risk of hypercalcaemia
* Captopril: Enhanced hypotensive effect (can be extreme)
Carbamazepine: Increased risk of hyponatraemia
Chloral hydrate: Enhanced hypotensive effect
Chlorpromazine: Enhanced hypotensive effect
Cisplatin: Increased risk of nephrotoxicity and ototoxicity
Clomipramine: Increased risk of postural hypotension
Clonazepam: Enhanced hypotensive effect
Contraceptives, Oral: Antagonism of diuretic effect
Dexamethasone: Antagonism of diuretic effect; increased risk of hypokalaemia
Diazepam: Enhanced hypotensive effect
* Digoxin: Cardiac toxicity of digoxin increased if hypokalaemia occurs
Ergocalciferol: Increased risk of hypercalcaemia
Ether, Anaesthetic: Enhanced hypotensive effect
Fluconazole: Plasma concentration of fluconazole increased
Fludrocortisone: Antagonism of diuretic effect; increased risk of hypokalaemia
Fluphenazine: Enhanced hypotensive effect
Furosemide: Increased risk of hypokalaemia
Glibenclamide: Antagonism of hypoglycaemic effect
Glyceryl trinitrate: Enhanced hypotensive effect
Halothane: Enhanced hypotensive effect
Hydralazine: Enhanced hypotensive effect
Hydrocortisone: Antagonism of diuretic effect; increased risk of hypokalaemia
Ibuprofen: Risk of nephrotoxicity of ibuprofen increased; antagonism of diuretic effect
Insulins: Antagonism of hypoglycaemic effect
Isosorbide dinitrate: Enhanced hypotensive effect
Ketamine: Enhanced hypotensive effect
Levodopa: Enhanced hypotensive effect
* Lidocaine: Action of lidocaine antagonised by hypokalaemia
* Lithium: Reduced lithium excretion (increased plasma-lithium concentration and risk of toxicity); furosemide safer than hydrochlorothiazide
Metformin: Antagonism of hypoglycaemic effect
Methyldopa: Enhanced hypotensive effect

Hydrochlorothiazide (Continued)

Nifedipine: Enhanced hypotensive effect

Nitrous oxide: Enhanced hypotensive effect

* Prazosin: Enhanced hypotensive effect; increased risk of first-dose hypotensive effect of prazosin

Prednisolone: Antagonism of diuretic effect; increased risk of hypokalaemia

Propranolol: Enhanced hypotensive effect

* Quinidine: Cardiac toxicity of quinidine increased if hypokalaemia occurs

Reserpine: Enhanced hypotensive effect

Salbutamol: Increased risk of hypokalaemia with high doses of salbutamol

Sodium nitroprusside: Enhanced hypotensive effect

Theophylline: Increased risk of hypokalaemia

Thiopental: Enhanced hypotensive effect

Timolol: Enhanced hypotensive effect

Verapamil: Enhanced hypotensive effect

Hydrocortisone *NOTE*. Interactions do not generally apply to hydrocortisone used for topical application

Acetazolamide: Increased risk of hypokalaemia; antagonism of diuretic effect

Acetylsalicylic acid: Increased risk of gastrointestinal bleeding and ulceration; hydrocortisone reduces plasma-salicylate concentration

Amiloride: Antagonism of diuretic effect

* Amphotericin: Increased risk of hypokalaemia (avoid concomitant use unless hydrocortisone needed to control reactions)

Atenolol: Antagonism of hypotensive effect

Captopril: Antagonism of hypotensive effect

* Carbamazepine: Accelerated metabolism of hydrocortisone (reduced effect)

Contraceptives, Oral: Oral contraceptives increase plasma concentration of hydrocortisone

Digoxin: Increased risk of hypokalaemia

Erythromycin: Erythromycin possibly inhibits metabolism of hydrocortisone

Furosemide: Antagonism of diuretic effect; increased risk of hypokalaemia

Glibenclamide: Antagonism of hypoglycaemic effect

Glyceryl trinitrate: Antagonism of hypotensive effect

Hydralazine: Antagonism of hypotensive effect

Hydrochlorothiazide: Antagonism of diuretic effect; increased risk of hypokalaemia

Ibuprofen: Increased risk of gastrointestinal bleeding and ulceration

Insulins: Antagonism of hypoglycaemic effect

Isosorbide dinitrate: Antagonism of hypotensive effect

Levonorgestrel: Levonorgestrel increases plasma concentration of hydrocortisone

Medroxyprogesterone: Medroxyprogesterone increases plasma concentration of hydrocortisone

Metformin: Antagonism of hypoglycaemic effect

Methotrexate: Increased risk of haematological toxicity

Methyldopa: Antagonism of hypotensive effect

Nifedipine: Antagonism of hypotensive effect

Norethisterone: Norethisterone increases plasma concentration of hydrocortisone

* Phenobarbital: Metabolism of hydrocortisone accelerated (reduced effect)

* Phenytoin: Metabolism of hydrocortisone accelerated (reduced effect)

Prazosin: Antagonism of hypotensive effect

Propranolol: Antagonism of hypotensive effect

Reserpine: Antagonism of hypotensive effect

* Rifampicin: Accelerated metabolism of hydrocortisone (reduced effect)

Ritonavir: Plasma concentration possibly increased by ritonavir

Hydrocortisone (Continued)

Salbutamol: Increased risk of hypokalaemia if high doses of hydrocortisone given with high doses of salbutamol

Sodium nitroprusside: Antagonism of hypotensive effect

Spironolactone: Antagonism of diuretic effect

Theophylline: Increased risk of hypokalaemia

Vaccine, Live: High doses of hydrocortisone impair immune response; avoid use of live vaccines

Verapamil: Antagonism of hypotensive effect

* Warfarin: Anticoagulant effect possibly altered

Ibuprofen

Acetazolamide: Risk of nephrotoxicity of ibuprofen increased; antagonism of diuretic effect

* Acetylsalicylic acid: Avoid concurrent administration (increased adverse effects, including gastrointestinal damage)

Amiloride: Risk of nephrotoxicity of ibuprofen increased; antagonism of diuretic effect; possibly increased risk of hyperkalaemia

Atenolol: Antagonism of hypotensive effect

Captopril: Antagonism of hypotensive effect, increased risk of renal impairment

* Ciclosporin: Increased risk of nephrotoxicity

* Ciprofloxacin: Possibly increased risk of convulsions

Dexamethasone: Increased risk of gastrointestinal bleeding and ulceration

Digoxin: Possibly exacerbation of heart failure, reduced GFR, and increased plasma-digoxin concentration

Fludrocortisone: Increased risk of gastrointestinal bleeding and ulceration

Furosemide: Risk of nephrotoxicity of ibuprofen increased; antagonism of diuretic effect

* Glibenclamide: Possibly enhanced effect of glibenclamide

Glyceryl trinitrate: Antagonism of hypotensive effect

Heparin: Possibly increased risk of bleeding

Hydralazine: Antagonism of hypotensive effect

Hydrochlorothiazide: Risk of nephrotoxicity of ibuprofen increased; antagonism of diuretic effect

Hydrocortisone: Increased risk of gastrointestinal bleeding and ulceration

Isosorbide dinitrate: Antagonism of hypotensive effect

* Lithium: Reduced excretion of lithium (risk of toxicity)

* Methotrexate: Excretion of methotrexate reduced (increased risk of toxicity)

Methyldopa: Antagonism of hypotensive effect

* Nalidixic acid: Possibly increased risk of convulsions

Nifedipine: Antagonism of hypotensive effect

* Ofloxacin: Possible increased risk of convulsions

* Phenytoin: Effect of phenytoin possibly enhanced

Prazosin: Antagonism of hypotensive effect

Prednisolone: Increased risk of gastrointestinal bleeding and ulceration

Propranolol: Antagonism of hypotensive effect

Ritonavir: Plasma concentration possibly increased by ritonavir

Sodium nitroprusside: Antagonism of hypotensive effect

Spironolactone: Risk of nephrotoxicity of ibuprofen increased; antagonism of diuretic effect; possibly increased risk of hyperkalaemia

Verapamil: Antagonism of hypotensive effect

* Warfarin: Anticoagulant effect possibly enhanced

Zidovudine: Increased risk of haematological toxicity

Immunoglobulin, Anti-D

* Vaccine, MMR: Avoid use of MMR vaccine during *3 weeks before* or during *3 months after* injection of anti-D immunoglobulin (impairment of immune response)

Immunoglobulin, Normal

* Vaccine, Live: Avoid use of live vaccine during *3 weeks before* or during *3 months after* injection of normal immunoglobulin (impairment of immune response)

Indinavir

   Carbamazepine: Possibly reduced plasma-indinavir concentration
   Dexamethasone: Possibly reduced plasma-indinavir concentration
   Efavirenz: Efavirenz reduces plasma concentration of indinavir (increase
      indinavir dose)
 * Ergotamine: Increased risk of ergotism (avoid concomitant use)
   Nelfinavir: Combination may lead to increased plasma concentration of
      either drug (or both)
   Nevirapine: Nevirapine reduces plasma concentration of indinavir
 * Phenobarbital: Plasma concentration of indinavir possibly reduced
   Phenytoin: Plasma-indinavir concentration possibly reduced
 * Rifampicin: Metabolism enhanced by rifampicin (plasma-indinavir
      concentration significantly reduced—avoid concomitant use)
   Ritonavir: Ritonavir increases plasma concentration of indinavir
   Saquinavir: Indinavir increases plasma concentration of saquinavir

Insulins

   Alcohol: Enhanced hypoglycaemic effect
   Atenolol: Enhanced hypoglycaemic effect; masking of warning signs of
      hypoglycaemia such as tremor
   Captopril: Hypoglycaemic effect possibly enhanced
   Contraceptives, Oral: Antagonism of hypoglycaemic effect
   Dexamethasone: Antagonism of hypoglycaemic effect
   Fludrocortisone: Antagonism of hypoglycaemic effect
   Furosemide: Antagonism of hypoglycaemic effect
   Hydrochlorothiazide: Antagonism of hypoglycaemic effect
   Hydrocortisone: Antagonism of hypoglycaemic effect
   Levonorgestrel: Antagonism of hypoglycaemic effect
   Lithium: May occasionally impair glucose tolerance
   Medroxyprogesterone: Antagonism of hypoglycaemic effect
   Nifedipine: Occasionally impaired glucose tolerance
   Norethisterone: Antagonism of hypoglycaemic effect
   Prednisolone: Antagonism of hypoglycaemic effect
   Propranolol: Enhanced hypoglycaemic effect; masking of warning signs
      of hypoglycaemia such as tremor
   Testosterone: Hypoglycaemic effect possibly enhanced
   Timolol: Enhanced hypoglycaemic effect; masking of warning signs of
      hypoglycaemia such as tremor

Isoniazid

   Antacids (Aluminium hydroxide; Magnesium hydroxide): Reduced
      absorption of isoniazid
 * Carbamazepine: Increased plasma-carbamazepine concentration (also
      isoniazid hepatotoxicity possibly increased)
   Diazepam: Metabolism of diazepam inhibited
   Ether, Anaesthetic: Possible potentiation of isoniazid hepatotoxicity
 * Ethosuximide: Metabolism of ethosuximide inhibited (increased plasma-
      ethosuximide concentration and risk of toxicity)
   Halothane: Possible potentiation of isoniazid hepatotoxicity
   Ketamine: Possible potentiation of isoniazid hepatotoxicity
   Nitrous oxide: Possible potentiation of isoniazid hepatotoxicity
 * Phenytoin: Metabolism of phenytoin inhibited (enhanced effect)
   Theophylline: Plasma-theophylline concentration possibly increased
   Thiopental: Possible potentiation of isoniazid hepatotoxicity

Isophane insulin *see* Insulins

Isoprenaline

   Chlorpromazine: Antagonism of pressor action
 * Ether, Anaesthetic: Risk of arrhythmias
   Fluphenazine: Antagonism of pressor action
   Haloperidol: Antagonism of pressor action
 * Halothane: Risk of arrhythmias

Isosorbide dinitrate

   Acetazolamide: Enhanced hypotensive effect
   Alcohol: Enhanced hypotensive effect
   Amiloride: Enhanced hypotensive effect
   Amitriptyline: Reduced effect of sublingual isosorbide dinitrate (owing to
      dry mouth)

Isosorbide dinitrate (Continued)

Atenolol: Enhanced hypotensive effect
Atropine: Possibly reduced effect of sublingual nitrates (failure to dissolve under the tongue owing to dry mouth)
Biperiden: Possibly reduced effect of sublingual nitrates (failure to dissolve under the tongue owing to dry mouth)
Captopril: Enhanced hypotensive effect
Chloral hydrate: Enhanced hypotensive effect
Chlorpromazine: Enhanced hypotensive effect
Clomipramine: Reduced effect of sublingual isosorbide dinitrate (owing to dry mouth)
Clonazepam: Enhanced hypotensive effect
Contraceptives, Oral: Antagonism of hypotensive effect
Dexamethasone: Antagonism of hypotensive effect
Diazepam: Enhanced hypotensive effect
Ether, Anaesthetic: Enhanced hypotensive effect
Fludrocortisone: Antagonism of hypotensive effect
Fluphenazine: Enhanced hypotensive effect
Furosemide: Enhanced hypotensive effect
Halothane: Enhanced hypotensive effect
Hydralazine: Enhanced hypotensive effect
Hydrochlorothiazide: Enhanced hypotensive effect
Hydrocortisone: Antagonism of hypotensive effect
Ibuprofen: Antagonism of hypotensive effect
Ketamine: Enhanced hypotensive effect
Levodopa: Enhanced hypotensive effect
Methyldopa: Enhanced hypotensive effect
Nifedipine: Enhanced hypotensive effect
Nitrous oxide: Enhanced hypotensive effect
Prazosin: Enhanced hypotensive effect
Prednisolone: Antagonism of hypotensive effect
Propranolol: Enhanced hypotensive effect
Reserpine: Enhanced hypotensive effect
Sodium nitroprusside: Enhanced hypotensive effect
Spironolactone: Enhanced hypotensive effect
Thiopental: Enhanced hypotensive effect
Timolol: Enhanced hypotensive effect
Verapamil: Enhanced hypotensive effect

Ketamine

Acetazolamide: Enhanced hypotensive effect
Amiloride: Enhanced hypotensive effect
Amitriptyline: Increased risk of arrhythmias and hypotension
Atenolol: Enhanced hypotensive effect
Captopril: Enhanced hypotensive effect
Chloral hydrate: Enhanced sedative effect
* Chlorpromazine: Enhanced hypotensive effect
Clomipramine: Increased risk of arrhythmias and hypotension
Clonazepam: Enhanced sedative effect
Diazepam: Enhanced sedative effect
* Fluphenazine: Enhanced hypotensive effect
Furosemide: Enhanced hypotensive effect
Glyceryl trinitrate: Enhanced hypotensive effect
* Haloperidol: Enhanced hypotensive effect
Hydralazine: Enhanced hypotensive effect
Hydrochlorothiazide: Enhanced hypotensive effect
Isoniazid: Possible potentiation of isoniazid hepatotoxicity
Isosorbide dinitrate: Enhanced hypotensive effect
Methyldopa: Enhanced hypotensive effect
Nifedipine: Enhanced hypotensive effect
* Prazosin: Enhanced hypotensive effect
Propranolol: Enhanced hypotensive effect
Reserpine: Enhanced hypotensive effect
Sodium nitroprusside: Enhanced hypotensive effect
Spironolactone: Enhanced hypotensive effect
Theophylline: Increased risk of convulsions

Ketamine (Continued)
    Timolol: Enhanced hypotensive effect
    Vancomycin: Hypersensitivity-like reactions can occur with concomitant intravenous vancomycin
  * Verapamil: Enhanced hypotensive effect and AV delay
Lamivudine
    Sulfamethoxazole+Trimethoprim: Plasma concentration of lamivudine increased (avoid concomitant use of high-dose sulfamethoxazole+trimethoprim)
    Trimethoprim: Plasma concentration of lamivudine increased (avoid concomitant use of high-dose trimethoprim)
Levodopa
    Acetazolamide: Enhanced hypotensive effect
    Amiloride: Enhanced hypotensive effect
    Atenolol: Enhanced hypotensive effect
    Atropine: Absorption of levodopa possibly reduced
    Biperiden: Absorption of levodopa possibly reduced
    Captopril: Enhanced hypotensive effect
    Chlorpromazine: Antagonism of effects of levodopa
    Clonazepam: Possibly occasional antagonism of levodopa effects
    Diazepam: Occasional antagonism of levodopa effects
  * Ether, Anaesthetic: Risk of arrhythmias
    Ferrous salts: Absorption of levodopa may be reduced
    Fluphenazine: Antagonism of effects of levodopa
    Furosemide: Enhanced hypotensive effect
    Glyceryl trinitrate: Enhanced hypotensive effect
    Haloperidol: Antagonism of effects of levodopa
  * Halothane: Risk of arrhythmias
    Hydralazine: Enhanced hypotensive effect
    Hydrochlorothiazide: Enhanced hypotensive effect
    Isosorbide dinitrate: Enhanced hypotensive effect
    Methyldopa: Enhanced hypotensive effect; antagonism of antiparkinsonian effect
    Nifedipine: Enhanced hypotensive effect
    Prazosin: Enhanced hypotensive effect
    Propranolol: Enhanced hypotensive effect
    Pyridoxine: Antagonism of levodopa unless carbidopa also given
    Reserpine: Enhanced hypotensive effect; antagonism of antiparkinsonian effect
    Sodium nitroprusside: Enhanced hypotensive effect
    Spironolactone: Enhanced hypotensive effect
    Timolol: Enhanced hypotensive effect
    Verapamil: Enhanced hypotensive effect
Levonorgestrel *see also Contraceptives, Oral*
  * Carbamazepine: Accelerated metabolism (reduced contraceptive effect)
  * Ciclosporin: Inhibition of ciclosporin metabolism (increased plasma-ciclosporin concentration)
    Dexamethasone: Levonorgestrel increases plasma concentration of dexamethasone
    Fludrocortisone: Levonorgestrel increases plasma concentration of fludrocortisone
    Glibenclamide: Antagonism of hypoglycaemic effect
  * Griseofulvin: Accelerated metabolism (reduced contraceptive effect)
    Hydrocortisone: Levonorgestrel increases plasma concentration of hydrocortisone
    Insulins: Antagonism of hypoglycaemic effect
    Metformin: Antagonism of hypoglycaemic effect
  * Nevirapine: Accelerated metabolism (reduced contraceptive effect)
  * Phenobarbital: Accelerated metabolism (reduced contraceptive effect)
  * Phenytoin: Accelerated metabolism (reduced contraceptive effect)
    Prednisolone: Levonorgestrel increases plasma concentration of prednisolone
  * Rifampicin: Accelerated metabolism of levonorgestrel (reduced contraceptive effect)
  * Warfarin: Antagonism of anticoagulant effect

Levothyroxine

> Carbamazepine: Accelerated metabolism of levothyroxine (may increase levothyroxine requirements in hypothyroidism)
>
> Phenobarbital: Metabolism of levothyroxine accelerated (may increase levothyroxine requirements in hypothyroidism)
>
> Phenytoin: Accelerated metabolism of levothyroxine (may increase levothyroxine requirements in hypothyroidism)
>
> Propranolol: Metabolism of propranolol accelerated (reduced effect)
>
> Rifampicin: Accelerated metabolism of levothyroxine (may increase levothyroxine requirements in hypothyroidism)
>
> * Warfarin: Enhanced anticoagulant effect

Lidocaine

> * Acetazolamide: Action of lidocaine antagonised by hypokalaemia
> * Atenolol: Increased risk of myocardial depression
>   Bupivacaine: Increased myocardial depression
> * Cimetidine: Increased plasma concentration of lidocaine (increased risk of toxicity)
> * Furosemide: Action of lidocaine antagonised by hypokalaemia
> * Hydrochlorothiazide: Action of lidocaine antagonised by hypokalaemia
> * Procainamide: Increased myocardial depression
> * Propranolol: Increased risk of myocardial depression; increased risk of lidocaine toxicity
> * Quinidine: Increased myocardial depression
>   Suxamethonium: Action of suxamethonium prolonged
> * Timolol: Increased risk of myocardial depression

Lithium

> * Acetazolamide: Excretion of lithium increased
>   Alcuronium: Enhanced muscle relaxant effect
> * Amiloride: Reduced lithium excretion (increased plasma-lithium concentration and risk of toxicity)
> * Captopril: Captopril reduces excretion of lithium (increased plasma-lithium concentration)
>   Carbamazepine: Neurotoxicity may occur without increased plasma-lithium concentration
>   Chlorpromazine: Increased risk of extrapyramidal effects and possibility of neurotoxicity
>   Fluphenazine: Increased risk of extrapyramidal effects and possibility of neurotoxicity
> * Furosemide: Reduced lithium excretion (increased plasma-lithium concentration and risk of toxicity); furosemide safer than hydrochlorothiazide
>   Glibenclamide: May occasionally impair glucose tolerance
>   Haloperidol: Increased risk of extrapyramidal effects and possibility of neurotoxicity
> * Hydrochlorothiazide: Reduced lithium excretion (increased plasma-lithium concentration and risk of toxicity); furosemide safer than hydrochlorothiazide
> * Ibuprofen: Reduced excretion of lithium (risk of toxicity)
>   Insulins: May occasionally impair glucose tolerance
>   Metformin: May occasionally impair glucose tolerance
> * Methyldopa: Neurotoxicity may occur without increased plasma-lithium concentration
>   Metronidazole: Increased lithium toxicity reported
>   Neostigmine: Antagonism of effect of neostigmine
>   Phenytoin: Neurotoxicity may occur without increased plasma-lithium concentration
>   Pyridostigmine: Antagonism of effect of pyridostigmine
>   Sodium hydrogen carbonate: Increased excretion; reduced plasma-lithium concentration
> * Spironolactone: Reduced lithium excretion (increased plasma-lithium concentration and risk of toxicity)
>   Suxamethonium: Enhanced muscle relaxant effect
>   Theophylline: Increased lithium excretion (reduced plasma-lithium concentration)
>   Vecuronium: Enhanced muscle relaxant effect

Lithium (Continued)

    Verapamil: Neurotoxicity may occur without increased plasma-lithium concentration

Lopinavir

    Carbamazepine: Possibly reduced plasma-lopinavir concentration

    Dexamethasone: Possibly reduced plasma-lopinavir concentration

    Efavirenz: Plasma concentration of lopinavir reduced

    Nevirapine: Plasma concentration of lopinavir possibly reduced

    * Phenobarbital: Plasma concentration of lopinavir possibly reduced

    Phenytoin: Plasma-lopinavir concentration possibly reduced

    * Rifampicin: Reduced plasma concentration of lopinavir (avoid concomitant use)

Magnesium hydroxide *see* Antacids

Magnesium (parenteral)

    Alcuronium: Enhanced muscle relaxant effect

    * Nifedipine: Profound hypotension reported with nifedipine and intravenous magnesium sulfate in pre-eclampsia

    Suxamethonium: Enhanced muscle relaxant effect

    Vecuronium: Enhanced muscle relaxant effect

Magnesium sulfate *see* Magnesium (parenteral)

Measles vaccine *see* Vaccine, live

Mebendazole

    Cimetidine: Metabolism of mebendazole possibly inhibited (increased plasma concentration)

Medroxyprogesterone *see also* Contraceptives, Oral

    * Carbamazepine: Accelerated metabolism (reduced contraceptive effect)

    * Ciclosporin: Inhibition of ciclosporin metabolism (increased plasma-ciclosporin concentration)

    Dexamethasone: Medroxyprogesterone increases plasma concentration of dexamethasone

    Fludrocortisone: Medroxyprogesterone increases plasma concentration of fludrocortisone

    Glibenclamide: Antagonism of hypoglycaemic effect

    * Griseofulvin: Accelerated metabolism (reduced contraceptive effect)

    Hydrocortisone: Medroxyprogesterone increases plasma concentration of hydrocortisone

    Insulins: Antagonism of hypoglycaemic effect

    Metformin: Antagonism of hypoglycaemic effect

    * Nevirapine: Accelerated metabolism (reduced contraceptive effect)

    * Phenobarbital: Accelerated metabolism (reduced contraceptive effect)

    * Phenytoin: Accelerated metabolism (reduced contraceptive effect)

    * Prednisolone: Medroxyprogesterone increases plasma concentration of prednisolone

    * Rifampicin: Accelerated metabolism of medroxyprogesterone (reduced contraceptive effect)

    * Warfarin: Antagonism of anticoagulant effect

Mefloquine

    * Artemether+Lumefantrine: Increased risk of ventricular arrhythmias

    Atenolol: Increased risk of bradycardia

    * Carbamazepine: Antagonism of anticonvulsant effect

    * Chloroquine: Increased risk of convulsions

    Digoxin: Possibly increased risk of bradycardia

    * Ethosuximide: Antagonism of anticonvulsant effect

    Nifedipine: Possibly increased risk of bradycardia

    * Phenytoin: Antagonism of anticonvulsant effect

    Propranolol: Increased risk of bradycardia

    * Quinidine: Increased risk of ventricular arrhythmias

    * Quinine: Increased risk of convulsions, but should not prevent the use of intravenous quinine in severe cases

    Timolol: Increased risk of bradycardia

    * Valproic acid: Antagonism of anticonvulsant effect

    Verapamil: Possibly increased risk of bradycardia

Mercaptopurine

    * Allopurinol: Effects of mercaptopurine enhanced with increased toxicity, reduce dose when given with allopurinol

Mercaptopurine (Continued)

Phenytoin: Reduced absorption of phenytoin

* Sulfamethoxazole+Trimethoprim: Increased risk of haematological toxicity

* Trimethoprim: Increased risk of haematological toxicity

Vaccine, Live: Avoid use of live vaccines with mercaptopurine (impairment of immune response)

Metformin

Alcohol: Enhanced hypoglycaemic effect; increased risk of lactic acidosis

Atenolol: Masking of warning signs of hypoglycaemia such as tremor

Captopril: Hypoglycaemic effect possibly enhanced

Cimetidine: Renal excretion of metformin inhibited; increased plasma-metformin concentration

Contraceptives, Oral: Antagonism of hypoglycaemic effect

Dexamethasone: Antagonism of hypoglycaemic effect

Fludrocortisone: Antagonism of hypoglycaemic effect

Furosemide: Antagonism of hypoglycaemic effect

Hydrochlorothiazide: Antagonism of hypoglycaemic effect

Hydrocortisone: Antagonism of hypoglycaemic effect

Levonorgestrel: Antagonism of hypoglycaemic effect

Lithium: May occasionally impair glucose tolerance

Medroxyprogesterone: Antagonism of hypoglycaemic effect

Norethisterone: Antagonism of hypoglycaemic effect

Prednisolone: Antagonism of hypoglycaemic effect

Propranolol: Masking of warning signs of hypoglycaemia such as tremor

Testosterone: Hypoglycaemic effect possibly enhanced

Timolol: Masking of warning signs of hypoglycaemia such as tremor

Methotrexate

* Acetylsalicylic acid: Reduced excretion of methotrexate (increased toxicity)

Amoxicillin: Reduced excretion of methotrexate (increased risk of toxicity)

Ampicillin: Reduced excretion of methotrexate (increased risk of toxicity)

Benzylpenicillin: Reduced excretion of methotrexate (increased risk of toxicity)

* Ciclosporin: Increased toxicity

Dexamethasone: Increased risk of haematological toxicity

Fludrocortisone: Increased risk of haematological toxicity

Hydrocortisone: Increased risk of haematological toxicity

* Ibuprofen: Excretion of methotrexate reduced (increased risk of toxicity)

Phenoxymethylpenicillin: Reduced excretion of methotrexate (increased risk of toxicity)

Phenytoin: Reduced absorption of phenytoin; antifolate effect of methotrexate increased

Prednisolone: Increased risk of haematological toxicity

* Pyrimethamine: Antifolate effect of methotrexate increased

Sulfadiazine: Risk of methotrexate toxicity increased

* Sulfadoxine+Pyrimethamine: Antifolate effect of methotrexate increased; risk of methotrexate toxicity increased

* Sulfamethoxazole+Trimethoprim: Antifolate effect of methotrexate increased; risk of methotrexate toxicity increased

* Trimethoprim: Antifolate effect of methotrexate increased

Vaccine, Live: Avoid use of live vaccines with methotrexate (impairment of immune response)

Methyldopa

Acetazolamide: Enhanced hypotensive effect

Alcohol: Enhanced hypotensive effect

Amiloride: Enhanced hypotensive effect

Amitriptyline: Enhanced hypotensive effect

Atenolol: Enhanced hypotensive effect

Captopril: Enhanced hypotensive effect

Chloral hydrate: Enhanced hypotensive effect

Chlorpromazine: Enhanced hypotensive effect; increased risk of extrapyramidal effects

Clomipramine: Enhanced hypotensive effect

Methyldopa (Continued)

Clonazepam: Enhanced hypotensive effect

Contraceptives, Oral: Antagonism of hypotensive effect

Dexamethasone: Antagonism of hypotensive effect

Diazepam: Enhanced hypotensive effect

Ether, Anaesthetic: Enhanced hypotensive effect

Ferrous salts: Reduced hypotensive effect of methyldopa

Fludrocortisone: Antagonism of hypotensive effect

Fluphenazine: Enhanced hypotensive effect; increased risk of extrapyramidal effects

Furosemide: Enhanced hypotensive effect

Glyceryl trinitrate: Enhanced hypotensive effect

Haloperidol: Enhanced hypotensive effect; increased risk of extrapyramidal effects

Halothane: Enhanced hypotensive effect

Hydralazine: Enhanced hypotensive effect

Hydrochlorothiazide: Enhanced hypotensive effect

Hydrocortisone: Antagonism of hypotensive effect

Ibuprofen: Antagonism of hypotensive effect

Isosorbide dinitrate: Enhanced hypotensive effect

Ketamine: Enhanced hypotensive effect

Levodopa: Enhanced hypotensive effect; antagonism of antiparkinsonian effect

* Lithium: Neurotoxicity may occur without increased plasma-lithium concentration

Nifedipine: Enhanced hypotensive effect

Nitrous oxide: Enhanced hypotensive effect

Prazosin: Enhanced hypotensive effect

Prednisolone: Antagonism of hypotensive effect

Propranolol: Enhanced hypotensive effect

Reserpine: Enhanced hypotensive effect; increased risk of extrapyramidal effects

* Salbutamol: Acute hypotension reported with salbutamol infusion

Sodium nitroprusside: Enhanced hypotensive effect

Spironolactone: Enhanced hypotensive effect

Thiopental: Enhanced hypotensive effect

Timolol: Enhanced hypotensive effect

Verapamil: Enhanced hypotensive effect

Metoclopramide

Acetylsalicylic acid: Enhanced effect of acetylsalicylic acid (increased rate of absorption)

Atropine: Antagonism of effect on gastrointestinal activity

Biperiden: Antagonism of effect on gastrointestinal activity

Chlorpromazine: Increased risk of extrapyramidal effects

Codeine: Antagonism of effect of metoclopramide on gastrointestinal activity

Fluphenazine: Increased risk of extrapyramidal effects

Haloperidol: Increased risk of extrapyramidal effects

Morphine: Antagonism of effect of metoclopramide on gastrointestinal activity

Paracetamol: Increased absorption of paracetamol (enhanced effect)

Pethidine: Antagonism of effect of metoclopramide on gastrointestinal activity

Metronidazole

Alcohol: Disulfiram-like reaction

Cimetidine: Metabolism of metronidazole inhibited (increased plasma-metronidazole concentration)

Fluorouracil: Metabolism of fluorouracil inhibited (increased toxicity)

Lithium: Increased lithium toxicity reported

Phenobarbital: Metabolism of metronidazole accelerated (reduced plasma concentration)

* Phenytoin: Metabolism of phenytoin inhibited (increased plasma-phenytoin concentration)

* Warfarin: Enhanced anticoagulant effect

Minocycline

Antacids (Aluminium hydroxide; Magnesium hydroxide): Reduced absorption of minocycline

* Contraceptives, Oral: Possibility of reduced contraceptive effect

Ferrous salts: Reduced absorption of oral ferrous salts by minocycline; reduced absorption of minocycline by oral ferrous salts

* Warfarin: Anticoagulant effect possibly enhanced

MMR vaccine *see* Vaccine, MMR

Morphine

Alcohol: Enhanced sedative and hypotensive effect

Amitriptyline: Possibly increased sedation

Chloral hydrate: Enhanced sedative effect

Chlorpromazine: Enhanced sedative and hypotensive effect

Cimetidine: Metabolism of morphine inhibited (increased plasma concentration)

Ciprofloxacin: Manufacturer of ciprofloxacin advises avoid premedication with morphine (reduced plasma-ciprofloxacin concentration)

Clomipramine: Possibly increased sedation

Clonazepam: Enhanced sedative effect

Diazepam: Enhanced sedative effect

Fluphenazine: Enhanced sedative and hypotensive effect

Haloperidol: Enhanced sedative and hypotensive effect

Metoclopramide: Antagonism of effect of metoclopramide on gastro-intestinal activity

* Ritonavir: Ritonavir possibly increases plasma concentration of morphine

Nalidixic acid

* Ciclosporin: Increased risk of nephrotoxicity

* Ibuprofen: Possibly increased risk of convulsions

* Theophylline: Possible increased risk of convulsions

* Warfarin: Enhanced anticoagulant effect

Nelfinavir

Carbamazepine: Possibly reduced plasma-nelfinavir concentration

* Contraceptives, Oral: Accelerated metabolism (reduced contraceptive effect)

* Ergotamine: Increased risk of ergotism (avoid concomitant use)

Indinavir: Combination may lead to increased plasma concentration of either drug (or both)

* Phenobarbital: Plasma concentration of nelfinavir possibly reduced

Phenytoin: Possibly reduced plasma-nelfinavir concentration

* Quinidine: Increased risk of ventricular arrhythmias (avoid concomitant use)

* Rifampicin: Plasma concentration of nelfinavir significantly reduced (avoid concomitant use)

Ritonavir: Combination may lead to increased plasma concentration of either drug (or both)

Saquinavir: Combination may lead to increased plasma concentration of either drug (or both)

Neostigmine

Alcuronium: Antagonism of muscle relaxant effect

Atropine: Antagonism of effect

Biperiden: Antagonism of effect

Chloroquine: Chloroquine has potential to increase symptoms of myasthenia gravis and thus diminish effect of neostigmine

Clindamycin: Antagonism of effects of neostigmine

* Gentamicin: Antagonism of effect of neostigmine

Lithium: Antagonism of effect of neostigmine

Procainamide: Antagonism of effect of neostigmine

Propranolol: Antagonism of effect of neostigmine

Quinidine: Antagonism of effect of neostigmine

* Streptomycin: Antagonism of effect of neostigmine

Suxamethonium: Effect of suxamethonium enhanced

Vecuronium: Antagonism of muscle relaxant effect

Nevirapine

 * Contraceptives, Oral: Accelerated metabolism (reduced contraceptive effect)

   Indinavir: Nevirapine reduces plasma concentration of indinavir
 * Levonorgestrel: Accelerated metabolism (reduced contraceptive effect)

   Lopinavir: Plasma concentration of lopinavir possibly reduced
 * Medroxyprogesterone: Accelerated metabolism (reduced contraceptive effect)
 * Norethisterone: Accelerated metabolism (reduced contraceptive effect)

   Rifampicin: Reduced plasma concentration of nevirapine
 * Saquinavir: Plasma concentration of saquinavir reduced (avoid concomitant use)

Nifedipine

   Acetazolamide: Enhanced hypotensive effect

   Alcohol: Enhanced hypotensive effect

   Alcuronium: Enhanced muscle relaxant effect

   Amiloride: Enhanced hypotensive effect
 * Atenolol: Severe hypotension and heart failure occasionally

   Captopril: Enhanced hypotensive effect

   Carbamazepine: Probably reduced effect of nifedipine

   Chloral hydrate: Enhanced hypotensive effect

   Chlorpromazine: Enhanced hypotensive effect

   Ciclosporin: Possibly increased plasma-nifedipine concentration (increased risk of adverse effects such as gingival hyperplasia)

   Cimetidine: Metabolism of nifedipine possibly inhibited (increased plasma concentration)

   Clonazepam: Enhanced hypotensive effect

   Contraceptives, Oral: Antagonism of hypotensive effect

   Dexamethasone: Antagonism of hypotensive effect

   Diazepam: Enhanced hypotensive effect
 * Digoxin: Possibly increased plasma concentration of digoxin

   Ether, Anaesthetic: Enhanced hypotensive effect

   Fludrocortisone: Antagonism of hypotensive effect

   Fluphenazine: Enhanced hypotensive effect

   Furosemide: Enhanced hypotensive effect

   Glyceryl trinitrate: Enhanced hypotensive effect

   Grapefruit juice: Increased plasma-nifedipine concentration

   Haloperidol: Enhanced hypotensive effect

   Halothane: Enhanced hypotensive effect

   Hydralazine: Enhanced hypotensive effect

   Hydrochlorothiazide: Enhanced hypotensive effect

   Hydrocortisone: Antagonism of hypotensive effect

   Ibuprofen: Antagonism of hypotensive effect

   Insulins: Occasionally impaired glucose tolerance

   Isosorbide dinitrate: Enhanced hypotensive effect

   Ketamine: Enhanced hypotensive effect

   Levodopa: Enhanced hypotensive effect
 * Magnesium (parenteral): Profound hypotension reported with nifedipine and intravenous magnesium sulfate in pre-eclampsia

   Mefloquine: Possibly increased risk of bradycardia

   Methyldopa: Enhanced hypotensive effect

   Nitrous oxide: Enhanced hypotensive effect
 * Phenobarbital: Effect of nifedipine probably reduced
 * Phenytoin: Increased plasma-phenytoin concentration; probably reduced effect of nifedipine
 * Prazosin: Enhanced hypotensive effect; increased risk of first-dose hypotensive effect of prazosin

   Prednisolone: Antagonism of hypotensive effect
 * Propranolol: Severe hypotension and heart failure occasionally

   Quinidine: Reduced plasma-quinidine concentration

   Reserpine: Enhanced hypotensive effect
 * Ritonavir: Plasma concentration possibly increased by ritonavir
 * Rifampicin: Accelerated metabolism of nifedipine (plasma concentration significantly reduced)

   Sodium nitroprusside: Enhanced hypotensive effect

Nifedipine (Continued)
Spironolactone: Enhanced hypotensive effect
* Theophylline: Possibly enhanced theophylline effect (possibly increased plasma-theophylline concentration)
Thiopental: Enhanced hypotensive effect
* Timolol: Severe hypotension and heart failure occasionally
Vecuronium: Enhanced muscle relaxant effect

Nitrous oxide
Acetazolamide: Enhanced hypotensive effect
Amiloride: Enhanced hypotensive effect
Amitriptyline: Increased risk of arrhythmias and hypotension
Atenolol: Enhanced hypotensive effect
Captopril: Enhanced hypotensive effect
Chloral hydrate: Enhanced sedative effect
* Chlorpromazine: Enhanced hypotensive effect
Clomipramine: Increased risk of arrhythmias and hypotension
Clonazepam: Enhanced sedative effect
Diazepam: Enhanced sedative effect
* Fluphenazine: Enhanced hypotensive effect
Furosemide: Enhanced hypotensive effect
Glyceryl trinitrate: Enhanced hypotensive effect
* Haloperidol: Enhanced hypotensive effect
Hydralazine: Enhanced hypotensive effect
Hydrochlorothiazide: Enhanced hypotensive effect
Isoniazid: Possible potentiation of isoniazid hepatotoxicity
Isosorbide dinitrate: Enhanced hypotensive effect
Methyldopa: Enhanced hypotensive effect
Nifedipine: Enhanced hypotensive effect
* Prazosin: Enhanced hypotensive effect
Propranolol: Enhanced hypotensive effect
Reserpine: Enhanced hypotensive effect
Sodium nitroprusside: Enhanced hypotensive effect
Spironolactone: Enhanced hypotensive effect
Timolol: Enhanced hypotensive effect
Vancomycin: Hypersensitivity-like reactions can occur with concomitant intravenous vancomycin
* Verapamil: Enhanced hypotensive effect and AV delay

Norethisterone see also Contraceptives, Oral
* Carbamazepine: Accelerated metabolism (reduced contraceptive effect)
* Ciclosporin: Inhibition of ciclosporin metabolism (increased plasma-ciclosporin concentration)
Dexamethasone: Norethisterone increases plasma concentration of dexamethasone
Fludrocortisone: Norethisterone increases plasma concentration of fludrocortisone
Glibenclamide: Antagonism of hypoglycaemic effect
* Griseofulvin: Accelerated metabolism (reduced contraceptive effect)
Hydrocortisone: Norethisterone increases plasma concentration of hydrocortisone
Insulins: Antagonism of hypoglycaemic effect
Metformin: Antagonism of hypoglycaemic effect
* Nevirapine: Accelerated metabolism (reduced contraceptive effect)
* Phenobarbital: Accelerated metabolism (reduced contraceptive effect)
* Phenytoin: Accelerated metabolism (reduced contraceptive effect)
* Prednisolone: Norethisterone increases plasma concentration of prednisolone
* Rifampicin: Accelerated metabolism of norethisterone (reduced contraceptive effect)
* Warfarin: Antagonism of anticoagulant effect

Ofloxacin
Antacids (Aluminium hydroxide; Magnesium hydroxide): Reduced absorption of ofloxacin
* Ciclosporin: Increased risk of nephrotoxicity
Ferrous salts: Absorption of ofloxacin reduced by oral ferrous salts
* Ibuprofen: Possible increased risk of convulsions

Ofloxacin (Continued)
  * Theophylline: Possible increased risk of convulsions
  * Warfarin: Enhanced anticoagulant effect
Oxygen
  * Bleomycin: Increased risk of pulmonary toxicity
Oxytocin
  Ephedrine: Hypertension due to enhanced vasopressor effect of ephedrine
  Epinephrine: Hypertension due to enhanced vasopressor effect of epinephrine
  Ether, Anaesthetic: Oxytocic effect possibly reduced; enhanced hypotensive effect and risk of arrhythmias
  Halothane: Oxytocic effect possibly reduced; enhanced hypotensive effect and risk of arrhythmias
Paracetamol
  Alcohol: Increased risk of liver damage with regular large amounts of alcohol
  Metoclopramide: Increased absorption of paracetamol (enhanced effect)
  Warfarin: Prolonged regular use of paracetamol possibly enhances anticoagulant effect
Penicillamine
  Antacids (Aluminium hydroxide; Magnesium hydroxide): Reduced absorption of penicillamine
  Ferrous salts: Reduced absorption of penicillamine
Pethidine
  Alcohol: Enhanced sedative and hypotensive effect
  Amitriptyline: Possibly increased sedation
  Chloral hydrate: Enhanced sedative effect
  Chlorpromazine: Enhanced sedative and hypotensive effect
  Cimetidine: Metabolism of pethidine inhibited (increased plasma concentration)
  Ciprofloxacin: Manufacturer of ciprofloxacin advises avoid premedication with pethidine (reduced plasma-ciprofloxacin concentration)
  Clomipramine: Possibly increased sedation
  Clonazepam: Enhanced sedative effect
  Diazepam: Enhanced sedative effect
  Fluphenazine: Enhanced sedative and hypotensive effect
  Haloperidol: Enhanced sedative and hypotensive effect
  Metoclopramide: Antagonism of effect of metoclopramide on gastro-intestinal activity
  * Ritonavir: Increased plasma-pethidine concentration (risk of toxicity—avoid concomitant use)
Phenobarbital
  Alcohol: Enhanced sedative effect
  * Amitriptyline: Antagonism of anticonvulsant effect (convulsive threshold lowered); metabolism of amitriptyline possibly accelerated (reduced plasma concentration)
  * Carbamazepine: May be enhanced toxicity without corresponding increase in antiepileptic effect; plasma concentration of carbamazepine often lowered
  * Chloramphenicol: Metabolism of chloramphenicol accelerated (reduced chloramphenicol concentration)
  * Chlorpromazine: Antagonism of anticonvulsant effect (convulsive threshold lowered)
  * Ciclosporin: Metabolism of ciclosporin accelerated (reduced effect)
  * Clomipramine: Antagonism of anticonvulsant effect (convulsive threshold lowered); metabolism of clomipramine possibly accelerated (reduced plasma concentration)
  * Clonazepam: May be enhanced toxicity without corresponding increase in antiepileptic effect; plasma concentration of clonazepam often lowered
  * Contraceptives, Oral: Metabolism accelerated (reduced contraceptive effect)
  * Dexamethasone: Metabolism of dexamethasone accelerated (reduced effect)

Phenobarbital (Continued)

Doxycycline: Metabolism of doxycycline accelerated (reduced plasma concentration)

Ergocalciferol: Ergocalciferol requirements possibly increased

* Ethosuximide: May be enhanced toxicity without corresponding increase in antiepileptic effect; plasma concentration of ethosuximide sometimes lowered

* Fludrocortisone: Metabolism of fludrocortisone accelerated (reduced effect)

* Fluphenazine: Antagonism of anticonvulsant effect (convulsive threshold lowered)

Folic acid and Folinic acid: Plasma concentration of phenobarbital possibly reduced

Griseofulvin: Reduction in absorption of griseofulvin (reduced effect)

* Haloperidol: Antagonism of anticonvulsant effect (convulsive threshold lowered); metabolism of haloperidol accelerated (reduced plasma concentration)

* Hydrocortisone: Metabolism of hydrocortisone accelerated (reduced effect)

* Indinavir: Plasma concentration of indinavir possibly reduced

* Levonorgestrel: Accelerated metabolism (reduced contraceptive effect)

Levothyroxine: Metabolism of levothyroxine accelerated (may increase levothyroxine requirements in hypothyroidism)

* Lopinavir: Plasma concentration of lopinavir possibly reduced

* Medroxyprogesterone: Accelerated metabolism (reduced contraceptive effect)

Metronidazole: Metabolism of metronidazole accelerated (reduced plasma concentration)

* Nelfinavir: Plasma concentration of nelfinavir possibly reduced

* Nifedipine: Effect of nifedipine probably reduced

* Norethisterone: Accelerated metabolism (reduced contraceptive effect)

* Phenytoin: May be enhanced toxicity without corresponding increase in antiepileptic effect; plasma concentration of phenytoin often lowered but may be raised; plasma concentration of phenobarbital often raised

* Prednisolone: Metabolism of prednisolone accelerated (reduced effect)

Quinidine: Metabolism of quinidine accelerated (reduced plasma concentration)

* Saquinavir: Plasma concentration of saquinavir possibly reduced

Theophylline: Metabolism of theophylline accelerated (reduced effect)

* Valproic acid: May be enhanced toxicity without corresponding increase in antiepileptic effect; plasma concentration of valproic acid often lowered; phenobarbital concentration often raised

* Verapamil: Effect of verapamil probably reduced

* Warfarin: Metabolism of warfarin accelerated (reduced anticoagulant effect)

Phenoxymethylpenicillin

Methotrexate: Reduced excretion of methotrexate (increased risk of toxicity)

Phenytoin

Acetazolamide: Increased risk of osteomalacia

Acetylsalicylic acid: Enhancement of effect of phenytoin

Alcohol: Plasma-phenytoin concentration reduced with regular large amounts of alcohol

Alcuronium: Antagonism of muscle relaxant effect (accelerated recovery from neuromuscular blockade)

* Amitriptyline: Antagonism (convulsive threshold lowered); possibly reduced plasma-amitriptyline concentration

Antacids (Aluminium hydroxide; Magnesium hydroxide): Reduced absorption of phenytoin

Azathioprine: Reduced absorption of phenytoin

* Carbamazepine: May be enhanced toxicity without corresponding increase in antiepileptic effect; plasma concentration of phenytoin often lowered but may be raised; plasma concentration of carbamazepine often lowered

Phenytoin (Continued)

* Chloramphenicol: Plasma-phenytoin concentration increased (risk of toxicity)
* Chloroquine: Antagonism of anticonvulsant effect
* Chlorpromazine: Antagonism of anticonvulsant effect (convulsive threshold lowered)
* Ciclosporin: Accelerated metabolism (reduced plasma-ciclosporin concentration)
* Cimetidine: Metabolism of phenytoin inhibited (increased plasma concentration)

  Ciprofloxacin: Plasma-phenytoin concentration possibly altered by ciprofloxacin

  Cisplatin: Reduced absorption of phenytoin
* Clomipramine: Antagonism (convulsive threshold lowered); possibly reduced plasma- clomipramine concentration
* Clonazepam: May be enhanced toxicity without corresponding increase in antiepileptic effect; plasma concentration of clonazepam often lowered
* Contraceptives, Oral: Accelerated metabolism (reduced contraceptive effect)

  Cyclophosphamide: Reduced absorption of phenytoin

  Cytarabine: Reduced absorption of phenytoin
* Dexamethasone: Metabolism of dexamethasone accelerated (reduced effect)

  Diazepam: Plasma-phenytoin concentrations increased or decreased by diazepam

  Doxorubicin: Reduced absorption of phenytoin

  Doxycycline: Increased metabolism of doxycycline (reduced plasma concentration)

  Ergocalciferol: Ergocalciferol requirements possibly increased
* Ethosuximide: May be enhanced toxicity without corresponding increase in antiepileptic effect; plasma concentration of phenytoin sometimes raised; plasma concentration of ethosuximide sometimes lowered
* Fluconazole: Effect of phenytoin enhanced; plasma concentration increased
* Fludrocortisone: Metabolism of fludrocortisone accelerated (reduced effect)

  Fluorouracil: Reduced absorption of phenytoin
* Fluphenazine: Antagonism of anticonvulsant effect (convulsive threshold lowered)

  Folic acid and Folinic acid: Plasma-phenytoin concentration possibly reduced
* Haloperidol: Antagonism of anticonvulsant effect (convulsive threshold lowered)
* Hydrocortisone: Metabolism of hydrocortisone accelerated (reduced effect)
* Ibuprofen: Effect of phenytoin possibly enhanced

  Indinavir: Plasma-indinavir concentration possibly reduced
* Isoniazid: Metabolism of phenytoin inhibited (enhanced effect)
* Levonorgestrel: Accelerated metabolism (reduced contraceptive effect)

  Levothyroxine: Accelerated metabolism of levothyroxine (may increase levothyroxine requirements in hypothyroidism)

  Lithium: Neurotoxicity may occur without increased plasma-lithium concentration

  Lopinavir: Plasma-lopinavir concentration possibly reduced
* Medroxyprogesterone: Accelerated metabolism (reduced contraceptive effect)
* Mefloquine: Antagonism of anticonvulsant effect

  Mercaptopurine: Reduced absorption of phenytoin

  Methotrexate: Reduced absorption of phenytoin; antifolate effect of methotrexate increased
* Metronidazole: Metabolism of phenytoin inhibited (increased plasma-phenytoin concentration)

  Nelfinavir: Possibly reduced plasma-nelfinavir concentration

Phenytoin (Continued)

* Nifedipine: Increased plasma-phenytoin concentration; probably reduced effect of nifedipine
* Norethisterone: Accelerated metabolism (reduced contraceptive effect)
* Phenobarbital: May be enhanced toxicity without corresponding increase in antiepileptic effect; plasma concentration of phenytoin often lowered but may be raised; plasma concentration of phenobarbital often raised

    Praziquantel: Plasma-praziquantel concentration reduced
* Prednisolone: Metabolism of prednisolone accelerated (reduced effect)

    Procarbazine: Reduced absorption of phenytoin
* Pyrimethamine: Antagonism of anticonvulsant effect; increased antifolate effect
* Quinidine: Accelerated metabolism (reduced plasma-quinidine concentration)
* Rifampicin: Accelerated metabolism of phenytoin (reduced plasma concentration)

    Saquinavir: Plasma-saquinavir concentration possibly reduced

    Sulfadiazine: Plasma-phenytoin concentration possibly increased
* Sulfadoxine+Pyrimethamine: Plasma-phenytoin concentration possibly increased; increased antifolate effect
* Sulfamethoxazole+Trimethoprim: Antifolate effect and plasma-phenytoin concentration increased

    Theophylline: Accelerated metabolism of theophylline (reduced plasma concentration)
* Trimethoprim: Antifolate effect and plasma-phenytoin concentration increased

    Vaccine, Influenza: Enhanced effect of phenytoin
* Valproic acid: May be enhanced toxicity without corresponding increase in antiepileptic effect; plasma concentration of valproic acid often lowered; plasma concentration of phenytoin often raised (but may also be lowered)

    Vecuronium: Antagonism of muscle relaxant effect (accelerated recovery from neuromuscular blockade)

    Verapamil: Reduced effect of verapamil

    Vincristine: Reduced absorption of phenytoin
* Warfarin: Accelerated metabolism of warfarin (possibility of reduced anticoagulant effect, but enhancement also reported)

    Zidovudine: Plasma-phenytoin concentration increased or decreased by zidovudine

Phytomenadione

* Warfarin: Antagonism of anticoagulant effect by phytomenadione

Poliomyelitis, oral vaccine *see* Vaccine, live

Polygeline

    Gentamicin: Increased risk of nephrotoxicity

Potassium chloride *see* Potassium salts

Potassium salts

* Amiloride: Risk of hyperkalaemia
* Captopril: Risk of severe hyperkalaemia
* Ciclosporin: Increased risk of hyperkalaemia
* Spironolactone: Risk of hyperkalaemia

Praziquantel

    Carbamazepine: Plasma-praziquantel concentration reduced

    Dexamethasone: Plasma-praziquantel concentration reduced

    Phenytoin: Plasma-praziquantel concentration reduced

Prazosin

* Acetazolamide: Enhanced hypotensive effect; increased risk of first-dose hypotensive effect of prazosin

    Alcohol: Enhanced hypotensive effect
* Amiloride: Enhanced hypotensive effect; increased risk of first-dose hypotensive effect of prazosin
* Atenolol: Enhanced hypotensive effect; increased risk of first-dose hypotensive effect of prazosin

    Captopril: Enhanced hypotensive effect

    Chloral hydrate: Enhanced hypotensive and sedative effects

    Chlorpromazine: Enhanced hypotensive effect

Prazosin (Continued)

Clonazepam: Enhanced hypotensive and sedative effects
Contraceptives, Oral: Antagonism of hypotensive effect
Dexamethasone: Antagonism of hypotensive effect
Diazepam: Enhanced hypotensive and sedative effects
* Ether, Anaesthetic: Enhanced hypotensive effect
Fludrocortisone: Antagonism of hypotensive effect
Fluphenazine: Enhanced hypotensive effect
* Furosemide: Enhanced hypotensive effect; increased risk of first-dose hypotensive effect of prazosin
Glyceryl trinitrate: Enhanced hypotensive effect
Haloperidol: Enhanced hypotensive effect
* Halothane: Enhanced hypotensive effect
Hydralazine: Enhanced hypotensive effect
* Hydrochlorothiazide: Enhanced hypotensive effect; increased risk of first-dose hypotensive effect of prazosin
Hydrocortisone: Antagonism of hypotensive effect
Ibuprofen: Antagonism of hypotensive effect
Isosorbide dinitrate: Enhanced hypotensive effect
* Ketamine: Enhanced hypotensive effect
Levodopa: Enhanced hypotensive effect
Methyldopa: Enhanced hypotensive effect
* Nifedipine: Enhanced hypotensive effect; increased risk of first-dose hypotensive effect of prazosin
* Nitrous oxide: Enhanced hypotensive effect
Prednisolone: Antagonism of hypotensive effect
* Propranolol: Enhanced hypotensive effect; increased risk of first-dose hypotensive effect of prazosin
Reserpine: Enhanced hypotensive effect
Sodium nitroprusside: Enhanced hypotensive effect
* Spironolactone: Enhanced hypotensive effect; increased risk of first-dose hypotensive effect of prazosin
* Thiopental: Enhanced hypotensive effect
* Timolol: Enhanced hypotensive effect; increased risk of first-dose hypotensive effect of prazosin
* Verapamil: Enhanced hypotensive effect; increased risk of first-dose hypotensive effect of prazosin

Prednisolone

Acetazolamide: Increased risk of hypokalaemia; antagonism of diuretic effect
Acetylsalicylic acid: Increased risk of gastrointestinal bleeding and ulceration; prednisolone reduces plasma-salicylate concentration
Amiloride: Antagonism of diuretic effect
* Amphotericin: Increased risk of hypokalaemia (avoid concomitant use unless prednisolone needed to control reactions)
Atenolol: Antagonism of hypotensive effect
Captopril: Antagonism of hypotensive effect
* Carbamazepine: Accelerated metabolism of prednisolone (reduced effect)
Ciclosporin: Increased plasma concentration of prednisolone
Contraceptives, Oral: Oral contraceptives increase plasma concentration of prednisolone
Digoxin: Increased risk of hypokalaemia
Erythromycin: Erythromycin possibly inhibits metabolism of prednisolone
Furosemide: Antagonism of diuretic effect; increased risk of hypokalaemia
Glibenclamide: Antagonism of hypoglycaemic effect
Glyceryl trinitrate: Antagonism of hypotensive effect
Hydralazine: Antagonism of hypotensive effect
Hydrochlorothiazide: Antagonism of diuretic effect; increased risk of hypokalaemia
Ibuprofen: Increased risk of gastrointestinal bleeding and ulceration
Insulins: Antagonism of hypoglycaemic effect
Isosorbide dinitrate: Antagonism of hypotensive effect

Prednisolone (Continued)

Levonorgestrel: Levonorgestrel increases plasma concentration of prednisolone

* Medroxyprogesterone: Medroxyprogesterone increases plasma concentration of prednisolone

Metformin: Antagonism of hypoglycaemic effect

Methotrexate: Increased risk of haematological toxicity

Methyldopa: Antagonism of hypotensive effect

Nifedipine: Antagonism of hypotensive effect

* Norethisterone: Norethisterone increases plasma concentration of prednisolone

* Phenobarbital: Metabolism of prednisolone accelerated (reduced effect)

* Phenytoin: Metabolism of prednisolone accelerated (reduced effect)

Prazosin: Antagonism of hypotensive effect

Propranolol: Antagonism of hypotensive effect

Reserpine: Antagonism of hypotensive effect

* Rifampicin: Accelerated metabolism of prednisolone (reduced effect)

Ritonavir: Plasma concentration possibly increased by ritonavir

Salbutamol: Increased risk of hypokalaemia if high doses of prednisolone given with high doses of salbutamol

Sodium nitroprusside: Antagonism of hypotensive effect

Spironolactone: Antagonism of diuretic effect

Theophylline: Increased risk of hypokalaemia

Vaccine, Live: High doses of prednisolone impair immune response; avoid use of live vaccines

Verapamil: Antagonism of hypotensive effect

* Warfarin: Anticoagulant effect possibly altered

Procainamide

* Alcuronium: Enhanced muscle relaxant effect

* Amitriptyline: Increased risk of ventricular arrhythmias

* Artemether+Lumefantrine: Increased risk of ventricular arrhythmias

* Atenolol: Increased risk of myocardial depression

Bupivacaine: Increased myocardial depression

Captopril: Increased risk of toxicity, especially in renal impairment

* Chlorpromazine: Increased risk of ventricular arrhythmias

* Cimetidine: Increased plasma concentration of procainamide

* Clomipramine: Increased risk of ventricular arrhythmias

* Fluphenazine: Increased risk of ventricular arrhythmias

* Haloperidol: Increased risk of ventricular arrhythmias

* Lidocaine: Increased myocardial depression

Neostigmine: Antagonism of effect of neostigmine

* Propranolol: Increased risk of myocardial depression

Pyridostigmine: Antagonism of effect of pyridostigmine

* Quinidine: Increased myocardial depression

Sulfamethoxazole+Trimethoprim: Increased plasma-procainamide concentration

* Suxamethonium: Enhanced muscle relaxant effect

* Timolol: Increased risk of myocardial depression

Trimethoprim: Increased plasma-procainamide concentration

* Vecuronium: Enhanced muscle relaxant effect

Procaine benzylpenicillin *see* Benzylpenicillin

Procarbazine

Alcohol: Disulfiram-like reaction

Phenytoin: Reduced absorption of phenytoin

Vaccine, Live: Avoid use of live vaccines with procarbazine (impairment of immune response)

Proguanil

* Warfarin: Possibly enhanced anticoagulant effect

Promethazine

Alcohol: Enhanced sedative effect

Amitriptyline: Increased antimuscarinic and sedative effects

Atropine: Increased antimuscarinic adverse effects

Biperiden: Increased antimuscarinic adverse effects

Chloral hydrate: Enhanced sedative effect

Clomipramine: Increased antimuscarinic and sedative effects

Promethazine (Continued)
    Clonazepam: Enhanced sedative effect
    Diazepam: Enhanced sedative effect
Propranolol
    Acetazolamide: Enhanced hypotensive effect
    Alcohol: Enhanced hypotensive effect
    Alcuronium: Enhanced muscle relaxant effect
    Amiloride: Enhanced hypotensive effect
* Bupivacaine: Increased risk of bupivacaine toxicity
    Captopril: Enhanced hypotensive effect
    Chloral hydrate: Enhanced hypotensive effect
* Chlorpromazine: Concomitant administration may increase plasma concentration of both drugs; enhanced hypotensive effect
    Cimetidine: Increased plasma-propranolol concentration
    Clonazepam: Enhanced hypotensive effect
    Contraceptives, Oral: Antagonism of hypotensive effect
    Dexamethasone: Antagonism of hypotensive effect
    Diazepam: Enhanced hypotensive effect
    Digoxin: Increased AV block and bradycardia
* Epinephrine: Severe hypertension
    Ergotamine: Increased peripheral vasoconstriction
    Ether, Anaesthetic: Enhanced hypotensive effect
    Fludrocortisone: Antagonism of hypotensive effect
    Fluphenazine: Enhanced hypotensive effect
    Furosemide: Enhanced hypotensive effect
    Glibenclamide: Masking of warning signs of hypoglycaemia such as tremor
    Glyceryl trinitrate: Enhanced hypotensive effect
    Halothane: Enhanced hypotensive effect
    Hydralazine: Enhanced hypotensive effect
    Hydrochlorothiazide: Enhanced hypotensive effect
    Hydrocortisone: Antagonism of hypotensive effect
    Ibuprofen: Antagonism of hypotensive effect
    Insulins: Enhanced hypoglycaemic effect; masking of warning signs of hypoglycaemia such as tremor
    Isosorbide dinitrate: Enhanced hypotensive effect
    Ketamine: Enhanced hypotensive effect
    Levodopa: Enhanced hypotensive effect
    Levothyroxine: Metabolism of propranolol accelerated (reduced effect)
* Lidocaine: Increased risk of myocardial depression; increased risk of lidocaine toxicity
    Mefloquine: Increased risk of bradycardia
    Metformin: Masking of warning signs of hypoglycaemia such as tremor
    Methyldopa: Enhanced hypotensive effect
    Neostigmine: Antagonism of effect of neostigmine
* Nifedipine: Severe hypotension and heart failure occasionally
    Nitrous oxide: Enhanced hypotensive effect
* Prazosin: Enhanced hypotensive effect; increased risk of first-dose hypotensive effect of prazosin
    Prednisolone: Antagonism of hypotensive effect
* Procainamide: Increased risk of myocardial depression
    Pyridostigmine: Antagonism of effect of pyridostigmine
* Quinidine: Increased risk of myocardial depression
    Reserpine: Enhanced hypotensive effect
    Rifampicin: Metabolism of propranolol accelerated (significantly reduced plasma concentration)
    Sodium nitroprusside: Enhanced hypotensive effect
    Spironolactone: Enhanced hypotensive effect
    Suxamethonium: Enhanced muscle relaxant effect
    Theophylline: Avoid concomitant use on pharmacological grounds (bronchospasm)
    Thiopental: Enhanced hypotensive effect
    Vecuronium: Enhanced muscle relaxant effect
* Verapamil: Asystole, severe hypotension and heart failure

Pyridostigmine

    Alcuronium: Antagonism of muscle relaxant effect

    Atropine: Antagonism of effect

    Biperiden: Antagonism of effect

    Chloroquine: Chloroquine has potential to increase symptoms of myasthenia gravis and thus diminish effect of pyridostigmine

    Clindamycin: Antagonism of effects of pyridostigmine

    * Gentamicin: Antagonism of effect of pyridostigmine

    Lithium: Antagonism of effect of pyridostigmine

    Procainamide: Antagonism of effect of pyridostigmine

    Propranolol: Antagonism of effect of pyridostigmine

    Quinidine: Antagonism of effect of pyridostigmine

    * Streptomycin: Antagonism of effect of pyridostigmine

    Suxamethonium: Effect of suxamethonium enhanced

    Vecuronium: Antagonism of muscle relaxant effect

Pyridoxine

    Levodopa: Antagonism of levodopa unless carbidopa also given

Pyrimethamine

    * Methotrexate: Antifolate effect of methotrexate increased

    * Phenytoin: Antagonism of anticonvulsant effect; increased antifolate effect

    * Sulfadiazine: Increased risk of antifolate effect

    * Sulfamethoxazole+Trimethoprim: Increased antifolate effect

    * Trimethoprim: Increased antifolate effect

Pyrimethamine+Sulfadoxine *see* Sulfadoxine+Pyrimethamine

Quinidine

    * Acetazolamide: Cardiac toxicity of quinidine increased if hypokalaemia occurs; acetazolamide reduces excretion of quinidine (occasionally increased plasma concentration)

    * Alcuronium: Enhanced muscle relaxant effect

    * Amitriptyline: Increased risk of ventricular arrhythmias

    Antacids (Aluminium hydroxide; Magnesium hydroxide): Reduced quinidine excretion in alkaline urine (plasma-quinidine concentration occasionally increased)

    * Artemether+Lumefantrine: Increased risk of ventricular arrhythmias

    * Atenolol: Increased risk of myocardial depression

    Bupivacaine: Increased myocardial depression

    Chloroquine: Increased risk of ventricular arrhythmias

    * Chlorpromazine: Increased risk of ventricular arrhythmias

    * Cimetidine: Increased plasma concentration of quinidine

    * Clomipramine: Increased risk of ventricular arrhythmias

    * Digoxin: Plasma concentration of digoxin increased (halve maintenance dose of digoxin)

    * Fluphenazine: Increased risk of ventricular arrhythmias

    * Furosemide: Cardiac toxicity of quinidine increased if hypokalaemia occurs

    * Haloperidol: Increased risk of ventricular arrhythmias

    * Hydrochlorothiazide: Cardiac toxicity of quinidine increased if hypokalaemia occurs

    * Lidocaine: Increased myocardial depression

    * Mefloquine: Increased risk of ventricular arrhythmias

    * Nelfinavir: Increased risk of ventricular arrhythmias (avoid concomitant use)

    Neostigmine: Antagonism of effect of neostigmine

    Nifedipine: Reduced plasma-quinidine concentration

    Phenobarbital: Metabolism of quinidine accelerated (reduced plasma concentration)

    * Phenytoin: Accelerated metabolism (reduced plasma-quinidine concentration)

    * Procainamide: Increased myocardial depression

    * Propranolol: Increased risk of myocardial depression

    Pyridostigmine: Antagonism of effect of pyridostigmine

    * Rifampicin: Accelerated metabolism (reduced plasma-quinidine concentration)

Quinidine (Continued)

* Ritonavir: Increased plasma-quinidine concentration (increased risk of ventricular arrhythmias—avoid concomitant use)
* Suxamethonium: Enhanced muscle relaxant effect
* Timolol: Increased risk of myocardial depression
* Vecuronium: Enhanced muscle relaxant effect
* Verapamil: Increased plasma-quinidine concentration (extreme hypotension may occur)
* Warfarin: Anticoagulant effect may be enhanced

Quinine

* Artemether+Lumefantrine: Increased risk of ventricular arrhythmias
  Chloroquine: Increased risk of ventricular arrhythmias
  Cimetidine: Metabolism of quinine inhibited (increased plasma concentration)
* Digoxin: Plasma concentration of digoxin increased
* Mefloquine: Increased risk of convulsions, but should not prevent the use of intravenous quinine in severe cases

Reserpine

Acetazolamide: Enhanced hypotensive effect
Alcohol: Enhanced hypotensive effect
Amiloride: Enhanced hypotensive effect
Amitriptyline: Enhanced hypotensive effect
Atenolol: Enhanced hypotensive effect
Captopril: Enhanced hypotensive effect
Chloral hydrate: Enhanced hypotensive effect
Chlorpromazine: Enhanced hypotensive effect; increased risk of extrapyramidal effects
Clomipramine: Enhanced hypotensive effect
Clonazepam: Enhanced hypotensive effect
Contraceptives, Oral: Antagonism of hypotensive effect
Dexamethasone: Antagonism of hypotensive effect
Diazepam: Enhanced hypotensive effect
Fludrocortisone: Antagonism of hypotensive effect
Fluphenazine: Enhanced hypotensive effect; increased risk of extrapyramidal effects
Furosemide: Enhanced hypotensive effect
Glyceryl trinitrate: Enhanced hypotensive effect
Haloperidol: Enhanced hypotensive effect; increased risk of extrapyramidal effects
Halothane: Enhanced hypotensive effect
Hydralazine: Enhanced hypotensive effect
Hydrochlorothiazide: Enhanced hypotensive effect
Hydrocortisone: Antagonism of hypotensive effect
Isosorbide dinitrate: Enhanced hypotensive effect
Ketamine: Enhanced hypotensive effect
Levodopa: Enhanced hypotensive effect; antagonism of antiparkinsonian effect
Methyldopa: Enhanced hypotensive effect; increased extrapyramidal effects
Nifedipine: Enhanced hypotensive effect
Nitrous oxide: Enhanced hypotensive effect
Prazosin: Enhanced hypotensive effect
Prednisolone: Antagonism of hypotensive effect
Propranolol: Enhanced hypotensive effect
Sodium nitroprusside: Enhanced hypotensive effect
Spironolactone: Enhanced hypotensive effect
Thiopental: Enhanced hypotensive effect
Timolol: Enhanced hypotensive effect
Verapamil: Enhanced hypotensive effect

Rifampicin

Amitriptyline: Plasma concentration of amitriptyline possibly reduced (reduced antidepressant effect)
Antacids (Aluminium hydroxide; Magnesium hydroxide): Reduced absorption of rifampicin

Rifampicin (Continued)

* Azathioprine: Manufacturer reports interaction (transplants possibly rejected)

  Chloramphenicol: Accelerated metabolism of chloramphenicol (reduced plasma-chloramphenicol concentration)

* Ciclosporin: Accelerated metabolism (reduced plasma-ciclosporin concentration)

  Cimetidine: Accelerated metabolism of cimetidine (reduced plasma-cimetidine concentration)

  Clomipramine: Plasma concentration of clomipramine possibly reduced (reduced antidepressant effect)

  Clonazepam: Metabolism of clonazepam possibly accelerated (possibly reduced plasma concentration)

* Contraceptives, Oral: Accelerated metabolism of oral contraceptives (reduced contraceptive effect)

  Dapsone: Reduced plasma-dapsone concentration

* Dexamethasone: Accelerated metabolism of dexamethasone (reduced effect)

  Diazepam: Metabolism of diazepam accelerated (reduced plasma concentration)

  Doxycycline: Plasma-doxycycline concentration possibly reduced

  Efavirenz: Reduced plasma concentration of efavirenz (increase efavirenz dose)

* Fluconazole: Accelerated metabolism of fluconazole (reduced plasma concentration)

* Fludrocortisone: Accelerated metabolism of fludrocortisone (reduced effect)

* Glibenclamide: Possibly accelerated metabolism (reduced effect) of glibenclamide

* Haloperidol: Accelerated metabolism of haloperidol (reduced plasma-haloperidol concentration)

* Hydrocortisone: Accelerated metabolism of hydrocortisone (reduced effect)

* Indinavir: Metabolism enhanced by rifampicin (plasma-indinavir concentration significantly reduced—avoid concomitant use)

* Levonorgestrel: Accelerated metabolism of levonorgestrel (reduced contraceptive effect)

  Levothyroxine: Accelerated metabolism of levothyroxine (may increase levothyroxine requirements in hypothyroidism)

* Lopinavir: Reduced plasma concentration of lopinavir (avoid concomitant use)

* Medroxyprogesterone: Accelerated metabolism of medroxyprogesterone (reduced contraceptive effect)

* Nelfinavir: Plasma concentration of nelfinavir significantly reduced (avoid concomitant use)

  Nevirapine: Reduced plasma concentration of nevirapine

* Nifedipine: Accelerated metabolism of nifedipine (plasma concentration significantly reduced)

* Norethisterone: Accelerated metabolism of norethisterone (reduced contraceptive effect)

* Phenytoin: Accelerated metabolism of phenytoin (reduced plasma concentration)

* Prednisolone: Accelerated metabolism of prednisolone (reduced effect)

  Propranolol: Metabolism of propranolol accelerated (significantly reduced plasma concentration)

* Quinidine: Accelerated metabolism (reduced plasma-quinidine concentration)

* Saquinavir: Accelerated metabolism of saquinavir (reduced plasma concentration—avoid concomitant use)

  Theophylline: Accelerated metabolism of theophylline (reduced plasma-theophylline concentration)

* Verapamil: Accelerated metabolism of verapamil (plasma concentration significantly reduced)

* Warfarin: Accelerated metabolism of warfarin (reduced anticoagulant effect)

Ritonavir

* Amitriptyline: Plasma concentration possibly increased by ritonavir
* Carbamazepine: Plasma concentration possibly increased by ritonavir
* Chloral hydrate: Plasma concentration possibly increased by ritonavir
* Chlorpromazine: Plasma concentration possibly increased by ritonavir
* Ciclosporin: Plasma concentration possibly increased by ritonavir
* Clomipramine: Plasma concentration possibly increased by ritonavir
* Clonazepam: Plasma concentration possibly increased by ritonavir
* Codeine: Ritonavir possibly increases plasma concentration of codeine
* Contraceptives, Oral: Accelerated metabolism (reduced contraceptive effect)

  Dexamethasone: Plasma concentration possibly increased by ritonavir
* Diazepam: Plasma concentration possibly increased by ritonavir (risk of extreme sedation and respiratory depression—avoid concomitant use)

  Efavirenz: Increased risk of toxicity (monitor liver function)
* Ergotamine: Increased risk of ergotism (avoid concomitant use)

  Erythromycin: Plasma concentration possibly increased by ritonavir
* Fluconazole: Plasma concentration possibly increased by ritonavir

  Fludrocortisone: Plasma concentration possibly increased by ritonavir
* Fluphenazine: Plasma concentration possibly increased by ritonavir
* Haloperidol: Plasma concentration possibly increased by ritonavir

  Hydrocortisone: Plasma concentration possibly increased by ritonavir

  Ibuprofen: Plasma concentration possibly increased by ritonavir

  Indinavir: Ritonavir increases plasma concentration of indinavir
* Morphine: Ritonavir possibly increases plasma concentration of morphine

  Nelfinavir: Combination may lead to increased plasma concentration of either drug (or both)
* Nifedipine: Plasma concentration possibly increased by ritonavir
* Pethidine: Increased plasma-pethidine concentration (risk of toxicity—avoid concomitant use)

  Prednisolone: Plasma concentration possibly increased by ritonavir
* Quinidine: Increased plasma-quinidine concentration (increased risk of ventricular arrhythmias—avoid concomitant use)
* Saquinavir: Ritonavir increases plasma concentration of saquinavir
* Theophylline: Accelerated theophylline metabolism (reduced plasma concentration)
* Verapamil: Plasma concentration possibly increased by ritonavir
* Warfarin: Plasma concentration possibly increased by ritonavir

Rubella vaccine *see* Vaccine, live

Salbutamol

  Acetazolamide: Increased risk of hypokalaemia with high doses of salbutamol

  Dexamethasone: Increased risk of hypokalaemia if high doses of dexamethasone given with high doses of salbutamol

  Fludrocortisone: Increased risk of hypokalaemia if high doses of fludrocortisone given with high doses of salbutamol

  Furosemide: Increased risk of hypokalaemia with high doses of salbutamol

  Hydrochlorothiazide: Increased risk of hypokalaemia with high doses of salbutamol

  Hydrocortisone: Increased risk of hypokalaemia if high doses of hydrocortisone given with high doses of salbutamol
* Methyldopa: Acute hypotension reported with salbutamol infusion

  Prednisolone: Increased risk of hypokalaemia if high doses of prednisolone given with high doses of salbutamol

  Theophylline: Increased risk of hypokalaemia with concomitant use of high doses of salbutamol

Saquinavir

  Carbamazepine: Possibly reduced plasma-saquinavir concentration

  Dexamethasone: Possibly reduced plasma-saquinavir concentration

  Efavirenz: Efavirenz significantly reduces plasma concentration of saquinavir
* Ergotamine: Possible increased risk of ergotism (avoid concomitant use)

  Fluconazole: Plasma concentration of saquinavir possibly increased

Saquinavir (Continued)
    Indinavir: Indinavir increases plasma concentration of saquinavir
    Nelfinavir: Combination may lead to increased plasma concentration of
        either drug (or both)
    * Nevirapine: Plasma concentration of saquinavir reduced (avoid conco-
        mitant use)
    * Phenobarbital: Plasma concentration of saquinavir possibly reduced
    Phenytoin: Plasma-saquinavir concentration possibly reduced
    * Rifampicin: Accelerated metabolism of saquinavir (reduced plasma
        concentration - avoid concomitant use)
    * Ritonavir: Ritonavir increases plasma concentration of saquinavir
Sodium hydrogen carbonate
    Lithium: Increased excretion; reduced plasma-lithium concentration
Sodium lactate compound solution see Potassium salts; Sodium
hydrogen carbonate
Sodium nitroprusside
    Acetazolamide: Enhanced hypotensive effect
    Alcohol: Enhanced hypotensive effect
    Amiloride: Enhanced hypotensive effect
    Amitriptyline: Enhanced hypotensive effect
    Atenolol: Enhanced hypotensive effect
    Captopril: Enhanced hypotensive effect
    Chloral hydrate: Enhanced hypotensive effect
    Chlorpromazine: Enhanced hypotensive effect
    Clomipramine: Enhanced hypotensive effect
    Clonazepam: Enhanced hypotensive effect
    Contraceptives, Oral: Antagonism of hypotensive effect
    Dexamethasone: Antagonism of hypotensive effect
    Diazepam: Enhanced hypotensive effect
    Ether, Anaesthetic: Enhanced hypotensive effect
    Fludrocortisone: Antagonism of hypotensive effect
    Fluphenazine: Enhanced hypotensive effect
    Furosemide: Enhanced hypotensive effect
    Glyceryl trinitrate: Enhanced hypotensive effect
    Halothane: Enhanced hypotensive effect
    Hydralazine: Enhanced hypotensive effect
    Hydrochlorothiazide: Enhanced hypotensive effect
    Hydrocortisone: Antagonism of hypotensive effect
    Ibuprofen: Antagonism of hypotensive effect
    Isosorbide dinitrate: Enhanced hypotensive effect
    Ketamine: Enhanced hypotensive effect
    Levodopa: Enhanced hypotensive effect
    Methyldopa: Enhanced hypotensive effect
    Nifedipine: Enhanced hypotensive effect
    Nitrous oxide: Enhanced hypotensive effect
    Prazosin: Enhanced hypotensive effect
    Prednisolone: Antagonism of hypotensive effect
    Propranolol: Enhanced hypotensive effect
    Reserpine: Enhanced hypotensive effect
    Spironolactone: Enhanced hypotensive effect
    Thiopental: Enhanced hypotensive effect
    Timolol: Enhanced hypotensive effect
    Verapamil: Enhanced hypotensive effect
Sodium valproate see Valproic acid
Soluble insulin see Insulins
Spironolactone
    Acetylsalicylic acid: Antagonism of diuretic effect
    Alcohol: Enhanced hypotensive effect
    Amitriptyline: Increased risk of postural hypotension
    * Artemether+Lumefantrine: Increased risk of ventricular arrhythmias if
        electrolyte disturbance occurs
    Atenolol: Enhanced hypotensive effect
    * Captopril: Enhanced hypotensive effect (can be extreme); risk of severe
        hyperkalaemia
    Carbamazepine: Increased risk of hyponatraemia

Spironolactone (Continued)
    Chloral hydrate: Enhanced hypotensive effect
    Chlorpromazine: Enhanced hypotensive effect
  * Ciclosporin: Increased risk of hyperkalaemia
    Cisplatin: Increased risk of nephrotoxicity and ototoxicity
    Clomipramine: Increased risk of postural hypotension
    Clonazepam: Enhanced hypotensive effect
    Contraceptives, Oral: Antagonism of diuretic effect
    Dexamethasone: Antagonism of diuretic effect
    Diazepam: Enhanced hypotensive effect
  * Digoxin: Enhanced effect of digoxin
    Ether, Anaesthetic: Enhanced hypotensive effect
    Fludrocortisone: Antagonism of diuretic effect
    Fluphenazine: Enhanced hypotensive effect
    Glyceryl trinitrate: Enhanced hypotensive effect
    Halothane: Enhanced hypotensive effect
    Hydralazine: Enhanced hypotensive effect
    Hydrocortisone: Antagonism of diuretic effect
    Ibuprofen: Risk of nephrotoxicity of ibuprofen increased; antagonism of
        diuretic effect; possibly increased risk of hyperkalaemia
    Isosorbide dinitrate: Enhanced hypotensive effect
    Ketamine: Enhanced hypotensive effect
    Levodopa: Enhanced hypotensive effect
  * Lithium: Reduced lithium excretion (increased plasma-lithium concentra-
        tion and risk of toxicity)
    Methyldopa: Enhanced hypotensive effect
    Nifedipine: Enhanced hypotensive effect
    Nitrous oxide: Enhanced hypotensive effect
    Potassium salts: Risk of hyperkalaemia
  * Prazosin: Enhanced hypotensive effect; increased risk of first-dose
        hypotensive effect of prazosin
    Prednisolone: Antagonism of diuretic effect
    Propranolol: Enhanced hypotensive effect
    Reserpine: Enhanced hypotensive effect
    Sodium nitroprusside: Enhanced hypotensive effect
    Thiopental: Enhanced hypotensive effect
    Timolol: Enhanced hypotensive effect
    Verapamil: Enhanced hypotensive effect
Stavudine
    Doxorubicin: Doxorubicin may inhibit effect of stavudine
  * Zidovudine: Intracellular activation of stavudine may be inhibited (avoid
        concomitant use)
Streptomycin
  * Alcuronium: Enhanced muscle relaxant effect
    Amphotericin: Increased risk of nephrotoxicity
  * Ciclosporin: Increased risk of nephrotoxicity
  * Cisplatin: Increased risk of nephrotoxicity and possibly of ototoxicity
  * Furosemide: Increased risk of ototoxicity
  * Neostigmine: Antagonism of effect of neostigmine
  * Pyridostigmine: Antagonism of effect of pyridostigmine
  * Suxamethonium: Enhanced muscle relaxant effect
    Vancomycin: Increased risk of nephrotoxicity and ototoxicity
  * Vecuronium: Enhanced muscle relaxant effect
Sulfadiazine
  * Ciclosporin: Plasma-ciclosporin concentration possibly reduced;
        increased risk of nephrotoxicity
  * Glibenclamide: Enhanced effect of glibenclamide
    Methotrexate: Risk of methotrexate toxicity increased
    Phenytoin: Plasma-phenytoin concentration possibly increased
  * Pyrimethamine: Increased risk of antifolate effect
  * Sulfadoxine+Pyrimethamine: Increased risk of antifolate effect
    Thiopental: Enhanced effects of thiopental
  * Warfarin: Enhanced anticoagulant effect

Sulfadoxine+Pyrimethamine
* Ciclosporin: Increased risk of nephrotoxicity
* Glibenclamide: Enhanced effect of glibenclamide
* Methotrexate: Antifolate effect of methotrexate increased; risk of methotrexate toxicity increased
* Phenytoin: Plasma-phenytoin concentration possibly increased; increased antifolate effect
* Sulfadiazine: Increased risk of antifolate effect
* Sulfamethoxazole+Trimethoprim: Increased antifolate effect
  Thiopental: Enhanced effects of thiopental
* Trimethoprim: Increased antifolate effect
* Warfarin: Enhanced anticoagulant effect

Sulfamethoxazole+Trimethoprim
* Azathioprine: Increased risk of haematological toxicity
* Ciclosporin: Increased risk of nephrotoxicity; plasma-ciclosporin concentration possibly reduced by intravenous trimethoprim
  Digoxin: Plasma concentration of digoxin possibly increased
* Glibenclamide: Enhanced effect of glibenclamide
  Lamivudine: Plasma concentration of lamivudine increased (avoid concomitant use of high-dose sulfamethoxazole+trimethoprim)
* Mercaptopurine: Increased risk of haematological toxicity
* Methotrexate: Antifolate effect of methotrexate increased; risk of methotrexate toxicity increased
* Phenytoin: Antifolate effect and plasma-phenytoin concentration increased
  Procainamide: Increased plasma-procainamide concentration
* Pyrimethamine: Increased antifolate effect
* Sulfadoxine+Pyrimethamine: Increased antifolate effect
  Thiopental: Enhanced effects of thiopental
* Warfarin: Enhanced anticoagulant effect

Sulfasalazine
  Digoxin: Absorption of digoxin possibly reduced

Suxamethonium
  Cyclophosphamide: Enhanced effect of suxamethonium
  Digoxin: Risk of arrhythmias
* Gentamicin: Enhanced muscle relaxant effect
  Lidocaine: Action of suxamethonium prolonged
  Lithium: Enhanced muscle relaxant effect
  Magnesium (parenteral): Enhanced muscle relaxant effect
  Neostigmine: Effect of suxamethonium enhanced
* Procainamide: Enhanced muscle relaxant effect
  Propranolol: Enhanced muscle relaxant effect
  Pyridostigmine: Effect of suxamethonium enhanced
* Quinidine: Enhanced muscle relaxant effect
* Streptomycin: Enhanced muscle relaxant effect

Tamoxifen
* Warfarin: Enhanced anticoagulant effect

Testosterone
  Glibenclamide: Hypoglycaemic effect possibly enhanced
  Insulins: Hypoglycaemic effect possibly enhanced
  Metformin: Hypoglycaemic effect possibly enhanced
* Warfarin: Enhanced anticoagulant effect

Theophylline
  Acetazolamide: Increased risk of hypokalaemia
  Allopurinol: Plasma-theophylline concentration possibly increased
  Atenolol: Avoid concomitant use on pharmacological grounds (bronchospasm)
  Carbamazepine: Accelerated metabolism of theophylline (reduced effect)
* Cimetidine: Metabolism of theophylline inhibited (plasma-theophylline concentration increased)
* Ciprofloxacin: Increased plasma-theophylline concentration; possible increased risk of convulsions
  Contraceptives, Oral: Delayed excretion of theophylline (increased plasma concentration)
  Dexamethasone: Increased risk of hypokalaemia

Theophylline (Continued)

* Erythromycin: Inhibition of theophylline metabolism (increased plasma-theophylline concentration); if erythromycin given by mouth, also decreased plasma-erythromycin concentration
* Fluconazole: Plasma-theophylline concentration possibly increased

Fludrocortisone: Increased risk of hypokalaemia

Furosemide: Increased risk of hypokalaemia

Halothane: Increased risk of arrhythmias

Hydrochlorothiazide: Increased risk of hypokalaemia

Hydrocortisone: Increased risk of hypokalaemia

Isoniazid: Plasma-theophylline concentration possibly increased

Ketamine: Increased risk of convulsions

Lithium: Increased lithium excretion (reduced plasma-lithium concentration)

* Nalidixic acid: Possible increased risk of convulsions
* Nifedipine: Possibly enhanced theophylline effect (possibly increased plasma-theophylline concentration)
* Ofloxacin: Possible increased risk of convulsions

Phenobarbital: Metabolism of theophylline accelerated (reduced effect)

Phenytoin: Accelerated metabolism of theophylline (reduced plasma concentration)

Prednisolone: Increased risk of hypokalaemia

Propranolol: Avoid concomitant use on pharmacological grounds (bronchospasm)

Rifampicin: Accelerated metabolism of theophylline (reduced plasma-theophylline concentration)

* Ritonavir: Accelerated theophylline metabolism (reduced plasma concentration)

Salbutamol: Increased risk of hypokalaemia with concomitant use of high doses of salbutamol

Timolol: Avoid concomitant use on pharmacological grounds (bronchospasm)

Tobacco: Tobacco smoking increases theophylline metabolism (reduced plasma-theophylline concentration)

Vaccine, Influenza: Plasma-theophylline concentration occasionally increased

* Verapamil: Enhanced theophylline effect (increased plasma-theophylline concentration)

Thioacetazone+Isoniazid *see* Isoniazid

Thiopental

Acetazolamide: Enhanced hypotensive effect

Amiloride: Enhanced hypotensive effect

Amitriptyline: Increased risk of arrhythmias and hypotension

Atenolol: Enhanced hypotensive effect

Captopril: Enhanced hypotensive effect

Chloral hydrate: Enhanced sedative effect

* Chlorpromazine: Enhanced hypotensive effect

Clomipramine: Increased risk of arrhythmias and hypotension

Clonazepam: Enhanced sedative effect

Diazepam: Enhanced sedative effect

* Fluphenazine: Enhanced hypotensive effect

Furosemide: Enhanced hypotensive effect

Glyceryl trinitrate: Enhanced hypotensive effect

* Haloperidol: Enhanced hypotensive effect

Hydralazine: Enhanced hypotensive effect

Hydrochlorothiazide: Enhanced hypotensive effect

Isoniazid: Possible potentiation of isoniazid hepatotoxicity

Isosorbide dinitrate: Enhanced hypotensive effect

Methyldopa: Enhanced hypotensive effect

Nifedipine: Enhanced hypotensive effect

* Prazosin: Enhanced hypotensive effect

Propranolol: Enhanced hypotensive effect

Reserpine: Enhanced hypotensive effect

Sodium nitroprusside: Enhanced hypotensive effect

Spironolactone: Enhanced hypotensive effect

Thiopental (Continued)

Sulfadiazine: Enhanced effects of thiopental

Sulfadoxine+Pyrimethamine: Enhanced effects of thiopental

Sulfamethoxazole+Trimethoprim: Enhanced effects of thiopental

Timolol: Enhanced hypotensive effect

Vancomycin: Hypersensitivity-like reactions can occur with concomitant intravenous vancomycin

* Verapamil: Enhanced hypotensive effect and AV delay

Timolol *NOTE*. Systemic absorption may follow topical application of timolol to the eye

Acetazolamide: Enhanced hypotensive effect

Alcohol: Enhanced hypotensive effect

Amiloride: Enhanced hypotensive effect

Captopril: Enhanced hypotensive effect

Chloral hydrate: Enhanced hypotensive effect

Chlorpromazine: Enhanced hypotensive effect

Clonazepam: Enhanced hypotensive effect

Diazepam: Enhanced hypotensive effect

Digoxin: Increased AV block and bradycardia

* Epinephrine: Severe hypertension

Ergotamine: Increased peripheral vasoconstriction

Ether, Anaesthetic: Enhanced hypotensive effect

Fluphenazine: Enhanced hypotensive effect

Furosemide: Enhanced hypotensive effect

Glibenclamide: Masking of warning signs of hypoglycaemia such as tremor

Glyceryl trinitrate: Enhanced hypotensive effect

Halothane: Enhanced hypotensive effect

Hydralazine: Enhanced hypotensive effect

Hydrochlorothiazide: Enhanced hypotensive effect

Insulins: Enhanced hypoglycaemic effect; masking of warning signs of hypoglycaemia such as tremor

Isosorbide dinitrate: Enhanced hypotensive effect

Ketamine: Enhanced hypotensive effect

Levodopa: Enhanced hypotensive effect

* Lidocaine: Increased risk of myocardial depression

Mefloquine: Increased risk of bradycardia

Metformin: Masking of warning signs of hypoglycaemia such as tremor

Methyldopa: Enhanced hypotensive effect

* Nifedipine: Severe hypotension and heart failure occasionally

Nitrous oxide: Enhanced hypotensive effect

* Prazosin: Enhanced hypotensive effect; increased risk of first-dose hypotensive effect of prazosin

* Procainamide: Increased risk of myocardial depression

* Quinidine: Increased risk of myocardial depression

Reserpine: Enhanced hypotensive effect

Sodium nitroprusside: Enhanced hypotensive effect

Spironolactone: Enhanced hypotensive effect

Theophylline: Avoid concomitant use on pharmacological grounds (bronchospasm)

Thiopental: Enhanced hypotensive effect

* Verapamil: Asystole, severe hypotension and heart failure

Tobacco

Theophylline: Tobacco smoking increases theophylline metabolism (reduced plasma-theophylline concentration)

Trimethoprim

* Azathioprine: Increased risk of haematological toxicity

* Ciclosporin: Increased risk of nephrotoxicity; plasma-ciclosporin concentration possibly reduced by intravenous trimethoprim

Digoxin: Plasma concentration of digoxin possibly increased

Lamivudine: Plasma concentration of lamivudine increased (avoid concomitant use of high-dose trimethoprim)

* Mercaptopurine: Increased risk of haematological toxicity

* Methotrexate: Antifolate effect of methotrexate increased

Trimethoprim (Continued)
* Phenytoin: Antifolate effect and plasma-phenytoin concentration increased

  Procainamide: Increased plasma-procainamide concentration
* Pyrimethamine: Increased antifolate effect
* Sulfadoxine+Pyrimethamine: Increased antifolate effect

  Warfarin: Possibly enhanced anticoagulant effect

Vaccine, Influenza

  Phenytoin: Enhanced effect of phenytoin

  Theophylline: Plasma-theophylline concentration occasionally increased

  Warfarin: Effect of warfarin occasionally enhanced

Vaccine, Live

  Asparaginase: Avoid use of live vaccines with asparaginase (impairment of immune response)
* Azathioprine: Avoid use of live vaccines with azathioprine (impairment of immune response)

  Bleomycin: Avoid use of live vaccines with bleomycin (impairment of immune response)

  Chlorambucil: Avoid use of live vaccines with chlorambucil (impairment of immune response)

  Chlormethine: Avoid use of live vaccines with chlormethine (impairment of immune response)
* Ciclosporin: Avoid use of live vaccines with ciclosporin (impairment of immune response)

  Cisplatin: Avoid use of live vaccines with cisplatin (impairment of immune response)

  Cyclophosphamide: Avoid use of live vaccines with cyclophosphamide (impairment of immune response)

  Cytarabine: Avoid use of live vaccines with cytarabine (impairment of immune response)

  Dacarbazine: Avoid use of live vaccines with dacarbazine (impairment of immune response)

  Dactinomycin: Avoid use of live vaccines with dactinomycin (impairment of immune response)

  Daunorubicin: Avoid use of live vaccines with daunorubicin (impairment of immune response)

  Dexamethasone: High doses of dexamethasone impair immune response; avoid use of live vaccines

  Doxorubicin: Avoid use of live vaccines with doxorubicin (impairment of immune response)

  Etoposide: Avoid use of live vaccines with etoposide (impairment of immune response)

  Fludrocortisone: High doses of fludrocortisone impair immune response; avoid use of live vaccines

  Fluorouracil: Avoid use of live vaccines with fluorouracil (impairment of immune response)

  Hydrocortisone: High doses of hydrocortisone impair immune response; avoid use of live vaccines
* Immunoglobulin, Normal: Avoid use of live vaccine during *3 weeks before* or during *3 months after* injection of normal immunoglobulin (impairment of immune response)

  Mercaptopurine: Avoid use of live vaccine with mercaptopurine (impairment of immune response)

  Methotrexate: Avoid use of live vaccines with methotrexate (impairment of immune response)

  Prednisolone: High doses of prednisolone impair immune response; avoid use of live vaccines

  Procarbazine: Avoid use of live vaccines with procarbazine (impairment of immune response)

  Vinblastine: Avoid use of live vaccines with vinblastine (impairment of immune response)

  Vincristine: Avoid use of live vaccines with vincristine (impairment of immune response)

Vaccine, MMR *see also* Vaccine, live
* Immunoglobulin, Anti-D: Avoid use of MMR vaccine during 3 weeks before or during 3 months after injection of anti-D immunoglobulin (impairment of immune response)

Vaccine, Rabies
  Chloroquine: Concomitant administration of chloroquine may affect antibody response

Valproic acid
  Acetylsalicylic acid: Enhancement of effect of valproic acid
* Amitriptyline: Antagonism (convulsive threshold lowered)
* Carbamazepine: May be enhanced toxicity without corresponding increase in antiepileptic effect; plasma concentration of valproic acid often lowered; plasma concentration of active metabolite of carbamazepine often raised
* Chloroquine: Antagonism of anticonvulsant effect
* Chlorpromazine: Antagonism of anticonvulsant effect (convulsive threshold lowered)
* Cimetidine: Metabolism of valproic acid inhibited (increased plasma concentration)
* Clomipramine: Antagonism (convulsive threshold lowered)
  Erythromycin: Metabolism of valproic acid possibly inhibited (increased plasma concentration)
* Ethosuximide: May be enhanced toxicity without corresponding increase in antiepileptic effect; plasma concentration of ethosuximide sometimes raised
* Fluphenazine: Antagonism of anticonvulsant effect (convulsive threshold lowered)
* Haloperidol: Antagonism of anticonvulsant effect (convulsive threshold lowered)
* Mefloquine: Antagonism of anticonvulsant effect
* Phenobarbital: May be enhanced toxicity without corresponding increase in antiepileptic effect; plasma concentration of valproic acid often lowered; phenobarbital concentration often raised
* Phenytoin: May be enhanced toxicity without corresponding increase in antiepileptic effect; plasma concentration of valproic acid often lowered; plasma concentration of phenytoin often raised (but may also be lowered)
  Warfarin: Anticoagulant effect possibly enhanced
  Zidovudine: Plasma concentration of zidovudine possibly increased (risk of toxicity)

Vancomycin
  Cisplatin: Increased risk of nephrotoxicity and possibly of ototoxicity
  Ether, Anaesthetic: Hypersensitivity-like reactions can occur with concomitant intravenous vancomycin
* Furosemide: Increased risk of ototoxicity
  Gentamicin: Increased risk of nephrotoxicity and ototoxicity
  Halothane: Hypersensitivity-like reactions can occur with concomitant intravenous vancomycin
  Ketamine: Hypersensitivity-like reactions can occur with concomitant intravenous vancomycin
  Nitrous oxide: Hypersensitivity-like reactions can occur with concomitant intravenous vancomycin
  Streptomycin: Increased risk of nephrotoxicity and ototoxicity
  Thiopental: Hypersensitivity-like reactions can occur with concomitant intravenous vancomycin

Vecuronium
  Carbamazepine: Antagonism of muscle relaxant effect (recovery from neuromuscular blockade accelerated)
  Clindamycin: Enhanced muscle relaxant effect
* Gentamicin: Enhanced muscle relaxant effect
  Lithium: Enhanced muscle relaxant effect
  Magnesium (parenteral): Enhanced muscle relaxant effect
  Neostigmine: Antagonism of muscle relaxant effect
  Nifedipine: Enhanced muscle relaxant effect

Vecuronium (Continued)

   Phenytoin: Antagonism of muscle relaxant effect (accelerated recovery
      from neuromuscular blockade)
 * Procainamide: Enhanced muscle relaxant effect
   Propranolol: Enhanced muscle relaxant effect
   Pyridostigmine: Antagonism of muscle relaxant effect
 * Quinidine: Enhanced muscle relaxant effect
 * Streptomycin: Enhanced muscle relaxant effect
   Verapamil: Enhanced muscle relaxant effect

Verapamil

   Acetazolamide: Enhanced hypotensive effect
   Alcohol: Enhanced hypotensive effect; plasma concentration of alcohol
      possibly increased by verapamil
   Alcuronium: Enhanced muscle relaxant effect
   Amiloride: Enhanced hypotensive effect
   Amitriptyline: Possibly increased plasma concentration of amitriptyline
 * Atenolol: Asystole, severe hypotension and heart failure
   Captopril: Enhanced hypotensive effect
 * Carbamazepine: Enhanced effect of carbamazepine
   Chloral hydrate: Enhanced hypotensive effect
   Chlorpromazine: Enhanced hypotensive effect
 * Ciclosporin: Increased plasma-ciclosporin concentration
   Cimetidine: Metabolism of verapamil possibly inhibited (increased
      plasma concentration)
   Clomipramine: Possibly increased plasma concentration of clomipramine
   Clonazepam: Enhanced hypotensive effect
   Contraceptives, Oral: Antagonism of hypotensive effect
   Dexamethasone: Antagonism of hypotensive effect
   Diazepam: Enhanced hypotensive effect
 * Digoxin: Increased plasma concentration of digoxin; increased AV block
      and bradycardia
 * Ether, Anaesthetic: Enhanced hypotensive effect and AV delay
   Fludrocortisone: Antagonism of hypotensive effect
   Fluphenazine: Enhanced hypotensive effect
   Furosemide: Enhanced hypotensive effect
   Glyceryl trinitrate: Enhanced hypotensive effect
   Grapefruit juice: Increased plasma-verapamil concentration
   Haloperidol: Enhanced hypotensive effect
 * Halothane: Enhanced hypotensive effect and AV delay
   Hydralazine: Enhanced hypotensive effect
   Hydrochlorothiazide: Enhanced hypotensive effect
   Hydrocortisone: Antagonism of hypotensive effect
   Ibuprofen: Antagonism of hypotensive effect
   Isosorbide dinitrate: Enhanced hypotensive effect
 * Ketamine: Enhanced hypotensive effect and AV delay
   Levodopa: Enhanced hypotensive effect
   Lithium: Neurotoxicity may occur without increased plasma-lithium
      concentration
   Mefloquine: Possibly increased risk of bradycardia
   Methyldopa: Enhanced hypotensive effect
 * Nitrous oxide: Enhanced hypotensive effect and AV delay
 * Phenobarbital: Effect of verapamil probably reduced
   Phenytoin: Reduced effect of verapamil
 * Prazosin: Enhanced hypotensive effect; increased risk of first-dose
      hypotensive effect of prazosin
   Prednisolone: Antagonism of hypotensive effect
 * Propranolol: Asystole, severe hypotension and heart failure
 * Quinidine: Increased plasma-quinidine concentration (extreme hypoten-
      sion may occur)
   Reserpine: Enhanced hypotensive effect
 * Rifampicin: Accelerated metabolism of verapamil (plasma concentration
      significantly reduced)
 * Ritonavir: Plasma concentration possibly increased by ritonavir
   Sodium nitroprusside: Enhanced hypotensive effect
   Spironolactone: Enhanced hypotensive effect

Verapamil (Continued)

* Theophylline: Enhanced theophylline effect (increased plasma-theophylline concentration)
* Thiopental: Enhanced hypotensive effect and AV delay
* Timolol: Asystole, severe hypotension and heart failure

Vecuronium: Enhanced muscle relaxant effect

Vinblastine

Vaccine, Live: Avoid use of live vaccines with vinblastine (impairment of immune response)

Vincristine

Phenytoin: Reduced absorption of phenytoin

Vaccine, Live: Avoid use of live vaccines with vincristine (impairment of immune response)

Vitamin D *see* Ergocalciferol

Warfarin *NOTE.* Major changes in diet (especially involving salads and vegetables) and in alcohol consumption may affect anticoagulant control

* Acetylsalicylic acid: Increased risk of bleeding due to antiplatelet effect
* Alcohol: Enhanced anticoagulant effect with large amounts of alcohol; major changes in alcohol consumption may affect anticoagulant control

Allopurinol: Anticoagulant effect possibly enhanced

Amoxicillin: Studies have failed to demonstrate an interaction, but common experience in anticoagulant clinics is that INR can be altered by a course of amoxicillin

Ampicillin: Studies have failed to demonstrate an interaction, but common experience in anticoagulant clinics is that INR can be altered by a course of ampicillin

* Azathioprine: Anticoagulant effect possibly reduced
* Carbamazepine: Accelerated metabolism of warfarin (reduced anticoagulant effect)
* Ceftazidime: Possibly enhanced anticoagulant effect
* Ceftriaxone: Possibly enhanced anticoagulant effect

Chloral hydrate: May transiently enhance anticoagulant effect

* Chloramphenicol: Enhanced anticoagulant effect
* Cimetidine: Enhanced anticoagulant effect (inhibition of metabolism)
* Ciprofloxacin: Enhanced anticoagulant effect
* Contraceptives, Oral: Antagonism of anticoagulant effect
* Dexamethasone: Anticoagulant effect possibly altered
* Doxycycline: Anticoagulant effect possibly enhanced
* Erythromycin: Enhanced anticoagulant effect
* Fluconazole: Enhanced anticoagulant effect
* Fludrocortisone: Anticoagulant effect possibly altered
* Glibenclamide: Possibly enhanced hypoglycaemic effects and changes to anticoagulant effect
* Griseofulvin: Metabolism of warfarin accelerated (reduced anticoagulant effect)
* Hydrocortisone: Anticoagulant effect possibly altered
* Ibuprofen: Anticoagulant effect possibly enhanced
* Levonorgestrel: Antagonism of anticoagulant effect
* Levothyroxine: Enhanced anticoagulant effect
* Medroxyprogesterone: Antagonism of anticoagulant effect
* Metronidazole: Enhanced anticoagulant effect
* Minocycline: Anticoagulant effect possibly enhanced
* Nalidixic acid: Enhanced anticoagulant effect
* Norethisterone: Antagonism of anticoagulant effect
* Ofloxacin: Enhanced anticoagulant effect

Paracetamol: Prolonged regular use of paracetamol possibly enhances anticoagulant effect

* Phenobarbital: Metabolism of warfarin accelerated (reduced anticoagulant effect)
* Phenytoin: Accelerated metabolism of warfarin (possibility of reduced anticoagulant effect, but enhancement also reported)
* Phytomenadione: Antagonism of anticoagulant effect by phytomenadione
* Prednisolone: Anticoagulant effect possibly altered
* Proguanil: Possibly enhanced anticoagulant effect

Warfarin (Continued)
* Quinidine: Anticoagulant effect may be enhanced
* Rifampicin: Accelerated metabolism of warfarin (reduced anticoagulant effect)
* Ritonavir: Plasma concentration possibly increased by ritonavir
* Sulfadiazine: Enhanced anticoagulant effect
* Sulfadoxine+Pyrimethamine: Enhanced anticoagulant effect
* Sulfamethoxazole+Trimethoprim: Enhanced anticoagulant effect
* Tamoxifen: Enhanced anticoagulant effect
* Testosterone: Enhanced anticoagulant effect
  Trimethoprim: Possibly enhanced anticoagulant effect
  Vaccine, Influenza: Effect of warfarin occasionally enhanced
  Valproic acid: Anticoagulant effect possibly enhanced

Yellow fever vaccine *see* Vaccine, live

Zidovudine *NOTE.* Increased risk of toxicity with nephrotoxic and myelosuppressive drugs
* Fluconazole: Increased plasma concentration of zidovudine (increased risk of toxicity)
  Ibuprofen: Increased risk of haematological toxicity
  Phenytoin: Plasma-phenytoin concentration increased or decreased by zidovudine
* Stavudine: Intracellular activation of stavudine may be inhibited (avoid concomitant use)
  Valproic acid: Plasma concentration of zidovudine possibly increased (risk of toxicity)

Appendix 2: Pregnancy

During pregnancy the mother and the fetus form a non-separable functional unit. Maternal well-being is an absolute prerequisite for the optimal functioning and development of both parts of this unit. Consequently, it is important to treat the mother whenever needed while protecting the unborn to the greatest possible extent.

Drugs can have harmful effects on the fetus at any time during pregnancy. It is important to remember this when prescribing for a woman of childbearing age. However, irrational fear of using drugs during pregnancy can also result in harm. This includes untreated illness, impaired maternal compliance, suboptimal treatment and treatment failures.

Such approaches may impose risk to maternal well-being, and may also affect the unborn child. It is important to know the 'background risk' in the context of the prevalence of drug-induced adverse pregnancy outcomes. Major congenital malformations occur in 2–4% of all live births. Up to 15% of all diagnosed pregnancies will result in fetal loss. The cause of these adverse pregnancy outcomes is understood in only a minority of the incidents.

During the *first trimester* drugs may produce congenital malformations (teratogenesis), and the greater risk is from third to the eleventh week of pregnancy. During the *second* and *third trimester* drugs may affect the growth and functional development of the fetus or have toxic effects on fetal tissues. Drugs given shortly before term or during labour may have adverse effects on labour or on the neonate after delivery. Few drugs have been shown conclusively to be teratogenic in man but no drug is safe beyond all doubt in early pregnancy. Screening procedures are available where there is a known risk of certain defects.

Prescribing in pregnancy

If possible counselling of women before a planned pregnancy should be carried out including discussion of risks associated with specific therapeutic agents, traditional medicines and abuse of substances such as smoking and alcohol. Folic acid supplements should be given during pregnancy planning because periconceptual use of folic acid reduces neural tube defects.

Drugs should be prescribed in pregnancy only if the expected benefits to the mother are thought to be greater than the risk to the fetus. All drugs should be avoided if possible during the first trimester. Drugs which have been used extensively in pregnancy and appear to be usually safe should be prescribed in preference to new or untried drugs and the smallest effective dose should be used. Well known single component drugs should usually be preferred to multi-component drugs.

The following list includes drugs which may have harmful effects in pregnancy and indicates the trimester of risk. It is based on human data but information on animal studies has been included for some newer drugs when its omission might be misleading.

Absence of a drug from the list does not imply safety.

Table of drugs to be avoided or used with caution in pregnancy

Drug	Comment
Abacavir	Toxicity in *animal* studies; *see* section 6.5.2
Acetazolamide	Not used to treat hypertension in pregnancy First trimester: Avoid (toxicity in *animal* studies)
Acetylsalicylic acid	Third trimester: Impaired platelet function and risk of haemorrhage; delayed onset and increased duration of labour with increased blood loss; avoid analgesic doses if possible in last few weeks (low doses probably not harmful); with high doses, closure of fetal ductus arteriosus *in utero* and possibly persistent pulmonary hypertension of newborn; kernicterus in jaundiced neonates
Aciclovir	Experience limited—use only when potential benefit outweighs risk; limited absorption from topical preparations
Albendazole	Contraindicated in cestode infections; *see* section 6.1.1.1. First trimester: avoid in nematode infections; *see* section 6.1.1.2
Alcohol	First, second trimesters: Regular daily drinking is teratogenic (fetal alcohol syndrome) and may cause growth retardation; occasional single drinks are probably safe Third trimester: Withdrawal may occur in babies of alcoholic mothers
Alcuronium	Does not cross placenta in significant amounts; use only if potential benefit outweighs risk
Allopurinol	Toxicity not reported; use only if potential benefit outweighs risk
Amiloride	Not used to treat hypertension in pregnancy
Aminophylline	Third trimester: Neonatal irritability and apnoea have been reported
Amitriptyline	Manufacturer advises avoid unless essential, particularly during first and third trimesters
Amoxicillin	Not known to be harmful
Amoxicillin + Clavulanic acid	No evidence of teratogenicity
Amphotericin	Not known to be harmful but use only if potential benefit outweighs risk
Ampicillin	Not known to be harmful
Artesunate	First trimester: Avoid
Asparaginase	Avoid; *see also* section 8.2

(Continued)

Drug	Comment
Atenolol	May cause intrauterine growth restriction, neonatal hypoglycaemia, and bradycardia; risk greater in severe hypertension; *see also* section 12.3
Atropine	Not known to be harmful
Azathioprine	Transplant patients immunosuppressed with azathioprine should not discontinue it on becoming pregnant; there is no evidence that azathioprine is teratogenic. Any risk to the offspring of azathioprine-treated men is small
Beclometasone	Benefit of treatment, for example in asthma, outweighs risk
Benzathine benzylpenicillin	Not known to be harmful
Benznidazole	First trimester: avoid
Benzylpenicillin	Not known to be harmful
Betamethasone	Benefit of treatment, for example in asthma, outweighs risk
Bleomycin	Avoid (teratogenic and carcinogenic in *animal* studies); *see also* section 8.2
Bupivacaine	Third trimester: With large doses, neonatal respiratory depression, hypotonia, and bradycardia after paracervical or epidural block
Calcium folinate	Manufacturer advises use only if potential benefit outweighs risk
Captopril	All trimesters: Avoid; may adversely affect fetal and neonatal blood pressure control and renal function; also possible skull defects and oligohydramnios; toxicity in *animal* studies
Carbamazepine	First trimester: Risk of teratogenesis including increased risk of neural tube defects (counselling and screening and adequate folate supplements advised, for example 5 mg daily); risk of teratogenicity greater if more than one antiepileptic used; *see also* section 5.1 Third trimester: May possibly cause vitamin K deficiency and risk of neonatal bleeding; if vitamin K not given at birth, neonate should be monitored closely for signs of bleeding
Ceftazidime	Not known to be harmful
Ceftriaxone	Not known to be harmful
Chloral hydrate	Avoid
Chlorambucil	Avoid; use effective contraception during administration to men or women; *see also* section 8.2
Chloramphenicol	Third trimester: Neonatal 'grey' syndrome
Chlormethine	Avoid; *see also* section 8.2
Chloroquine	First, third trimesters: Benefit of prophylaxis and treatment in malaria outweighs risk; important: *see also* section 6.4.3
Chlorphenamine	No evidence of teratogenicity
Chlorpromazine	Third trimester: Extrapyramidal effects in neonate occasionally reported
Ciclosporin	There is less experience of ciclosporin in pregnancy but it does not appear to be any more harmful than azathioprine
Cimetidine	Use only if potential benefit outweighs risk
Ciprofloxacin	All trimesters: Avoid—arthropathy in *animal* studies; safer alternatives available
Cisplatin	Avoid (teratogenic and toxic in *animal* studies); *see also* section 8.2
Clindamycin	Not known to be harmful
Clomifene	Possible effects on fetal development

(Continued)

Drug	Comment
Clomipramine	Manufacturer advises avoid unless essential, particularly during first and third trimester
Clonazepam	Avoid regular use (risk of neonatal withdrawal symptoms); use only if clear indication such as seizure control (high doses during late pregnancy or labour may cause neonatal hypothermia, hypotonia and respiratory depression)
Cloxacillin	Not known to be harmful
Codeine	Third trimester: Depresses neonatal respiration; withdrawal effects in neonates of dependent mothers; gastric stasis and risk of inhalation pneumonia in mother during labour
Contraceptives, oral	Epidemiological evidence suggests no harmful effects on fetus
Cromoglicic acid	*see* Sodium cromoglicate
Cyclophosphamide	Avoid (use effective contraception during and for at least 3 months after administration to men or women); *see also* section 8.2
Cytarabine	Avoid (teratogenic in *animal* studies); *see also* section 8.2
Dacarbazine	Avoid (carcinogenic and teratogenic in *animal* studies; ensure effective contraception during and for at least 6 months after administration to men or women); *see also* section 8.2
Dactinomycin	Avoid (teratogenic in *animal* studies); *see also* section 8.2
Dapsone	Third trimester: Neonatal haemolysis and methaemoglobinaemia; adequate folate supplements should be given to mother
Daunorubicin	Avoid (teratogenic and carcinogenic in *animal* studies); *see also* section 8.2
Deferoxamine	Teratogenic in *animal* studies; manufacturer advises use only if potential benefit outweighs risk
Desmopressin	Small oxytocic effect in third trimester
Dexamethasone	Benefit of treatment, for example in asthma, outweighs risk; risk of intrauterine growth retardation on prolonged or repeated systemic treatment; corticosteroid cover required by mother during labour; monitor closely if fluid retention
Dextromethorphan	Third trimester: Depresses neonatal respiration; withdrawal effects in neonates of dependent mothers; gastric stasis and risk of inhalation pneumonia in mother during labour
Diazepam	Avoid regular use (risk of neonatal withdrawal symptoms); use only if clear indication such as seizure control (high doses during late pregnancy or labour may cause neonatal hypothermia, hypotonia and respiratory depression)
Didanosine	Avoid if possible in first trimester; increased risk of lactic acidosis and hepatic steatosis; *see* section 6.5.2
Diethylcarbamazine	Avoid: Delay treatment until after delivery
Digoxin	May need dosage adjustment
Diloxanide	Defer treatment until after first trimester
Doxorubicin	Avoid (teratogenic and toxic in *animal* studies); with liposomal product use effective contraception during and for at least 6 months after administration to men or women); *see also* section 8.2

(Continued)

Drug	Comment
Doxycycline	First trimester: Effects on skeletal development in *animal* studies Second, third trimesters: Dental discoloration; maternal hepatotoxicity with large parenteral doses
Efavirenz	Avoid (potential teratogenic affects); *see* section 6.5.2
Eflornithine	All trimesters: avoid
Ephedrine	Increased fetal heart rate reported with parenteral ephedrine
Ergocalciferol	High doses teratogenic in *animals* but therapeutic doses unlikely to be harmful
Ergotamine	All trimesters: Oxytocic effects on the pregnant uterus
Erythromycin	Not known to be harmful
Ether, anaesthetic	Third trimester: Depresses neonatal respiration
Ethinylestradiol	Epidemiological evidence suggests no harmful effects on fetus
Ethosuximide	First trimester: May possibly be teratogenic; risk of teratogenicity greater if more than one antiepileptic used; *see also* section 5.1
Etoposide	Avoid (teratogenic in *animal* studies); *see also* section 8.2
Fluconazole	Avoid in first trimester—multiple congenital abnormalities reported with long-term high doses
Flucytosine	Teratogenic in *animal* studies; manufacturer advises use only if potential benefit outweighs risk
Fluorouracil	Avoid (teratogenic); *see also* section 8.2
Fluphenazine	Third trimester: Extrapyramidal effects in neonate occasionally reported
Furosemide	Not used to treat hypertension in pregnancy
Gentamicin	Second, third trimesters: Auditory or vestibular nerve damage, risk probably very small with gentamicin, but use only if potential benfit out-weighs risk (if given, serum-gentamicin concentration monitoring essential)
Glibenclamide	Third trimester: Neonatal hypoglycaemia; insulin is normally substituted in all diabetics; if oral drugs are used therapy should be stopped at least 2 days before delivery
Griseofulvin	Avoid (fetotoxicity and teratogenicity in *animals*); effective contraception required during and for at least 1 month after administration (**important:** effectiveness of oral contraceptives reduced, *see* Appendix 1); also men should avoid fathering a child during and for at least 6 months after administration
Haloperidol	Third trimester: Extrapyramidal effects in neonate occasionally reported
Halothane	Third trimester: Depresses neonatal respiration
Heparin	All trimesters: Osteoporosis has been reported after prolonged use; multidose vials may contain benzyl alcohol—some manufacturers advise avoid
Hydralazine	Avoid during first and second trimester; no reports of serious harm following use in third trimester
Hydrochlorothiazide	Not used to treat hypertension in pregnancy Third trimester: May cause neonatal thrombocy-topenia

(Continued)

Drug	Comment
Hydrocortisone	Benefit of treatment, for example in asthma, outweighs risk; risk of intrauterine growth retardation on prolonged or repeated systemic treatment; corticosteroid cover required by mother during labour; monitor closely if fluid retention
Ibuprofen	Third trimester: With regular use closure of fetal ductus arteriosus *in utero* and possibly persistent pulmonary hypertension of the newborn. Delayed onset and increased duration of labour
Idoxuridine	Teratogenic in *animal* studies
Imipenem+Cilastatin	Use only if potential benefit outweighs risk (toxicity in *animal* studies)
Indinavir	Avoid if possible in first trimester; theoretical risk of hyperbilirubinaemia in neonate if used at term; *see* section 6.5.2
Insulin	All trimesters: Insulin requirements should be assessed frequently by an experienced diabetic clinician
Iodine	Second, third trimesters: Neonatal goitre and hypothyroidism
Iron Dextran	All trimesters: Avoid (toxicity in *animals*)
Ivermectin	Delay treatment until after delivery; *see also* section 6.1.2.3
Ketamine	Third trimester: Depresses neonatal respiration
Lamivudine	Avoid if possible in first trimester; benefit of treatment considered to outweigh risk in second and third trimesters; *see* section 6.5.2
Levamisole	Third trimester: Avoid
Levodopa+Carbidopa	Toxicity in *animal* studies
Levonorgestrel	In oral contraceptives, epidemiological evidence suggests no harmful effects on fetus In high doses, may possibly be teratogenic in first trimester
Levothyroxine	Monitor maternal serum-thyrotrophin concentration—dosage adjustment may be necessary
Lidocaine	Third trimester: With large doses, neonatal respiratory depression, hypotonia, and bradycardia after paracervical or epidural block
Lithium	First trimester: Avoid if possible (risk of teratogenicity including cardiac abnormalities) Second and third trimesters: Dose requirements increased (but on delivery return to normal abruptly); close monitoring of serum-lithium concentration advised (risk of toxicity in neonate)
Lopinavir with Ritonavir	Avoid if possible in first trimester; avoid oral solution due to high propylene glycol content; *see* section 6.5.2
Magnesium sulfate	Follow hospital regimen in eclampsia; long-term infusion may cause sustained fetal hypocalcaemia
Mebendazole	Toxicity in *animal* studies. Contraindicated in cestode infections; *see* section 6.1.1.1 First trimester: Avoid in nematode infections; *see* section 6.1.1.2
Medroxyprogesterone	First trimester: High doses may possibly be teratogenic
Mefloquine	First trimester: Teratogenicity in *animal* studies; avoid for prophylaxis, *see also* mefloquine and Prophylaxis and Treatment of Malaria, section 6.4.3
Melarsoprol	All trimesters: Avoid

(Continued)

Drug	Comment
Mercaptopurine	Avoid (teratogenic); *see also* section 8.2
Metformin	All trimesters: Avoid; insulin is normally substituted in all diabetics
Methotrexate	Avoid (teratogenic; fertility may be reduced during therapy but this may be reversible); use effective contraception during and for at least 6 months after administration to men or women; *see also* section 8.2
Methyldopa	Not known to be harmful
Metoclopramide	Not known to be harmful
Metronidazole	Avoid high-dose regimens
Minocycline	First trimester: Effects on skeletal development in *animal* studies Second, third trimesters: Dental discoloration; maternal hepatotoxicity with large parenteral doses
Morphine	Third trimester: Depresses neonatal respiration; withdrawal effects in neonates of dependent mothers; gastric stasis and risk of inhalation pneumonia in mother during labour
Nalidixic acid	All trimesters: Avoid—arthropathy in *animal* studies; safer alternatives available
Naloxone	Use only if potential benefit outweighs risk
Nelfinavir	Avoid if possible in first trimester; potential benefit of treatment considered to outweigh risk in second and third trimesters; *see* section 6.5.2
Neostigmine	Third trimester: Neonatal myasthenia with large doses
Nevirapine	Avoid if possible in first trimester; benefit of treatment considered to outweigh risk in second and third trimesters; *see* section 6.5.2
Niclosamide	*T. solium* infections in pregnancy should be treated immediately; *see* section 6.1.1.1
Nifedipine	May inhibit labour; some dihydropyridines are teratogenic in *animals*, but risk to fetus should be balanced against risk of uncontrolled maternal hypertension
Nifurtimox	First trimester: Avoid
Nitrofurantoin	Third trimester: May produce neonatal haemolysis if used at term
Nitrous oxide	Third trimester: Depresses neonatal respiration
Norethisterone	In oral contraceptives, epidemiological evidence suggests no harmful effects on fetus In high doses, may possibly be teratogenic in first trimester
Nystatin	No information available, but absorption from gastrointestinal tract negligible
Ofloxacin	All trimesters: Avoid—arthropathy in *animal* studies; safer alternatives available
Oxamniquine	If immediate treatment not required Schistosomiasis treatment should be delayed until after delivery; *see* section 6.1.3.1
Paracetamol	Not known to be harmful
Penicillamine	All trimesters: Fetal abnormalities reported rarely; avoid if possible
Pentamidine isetionate	Potentially fatal visceral leishmaniasis must be treated without delay. Should not be withheld in trypanosomiasis even if evidence of meningoencephalitic involvement. Potentially fatal *P. carinii* pneumonia must be treated without delay

(Continued)

Drug	Comment
Pentavalent antimony compounds	Potentially fatal visceral leishmaniasis must be treated without delay
Pethidine	Third trimester: Depresses neonatal respiration; withdrawal effects in neonates of dependent mothers; gastric stasis and risk of inhalation pneumonia in mother during labour
Phenobarbital	First, third trimesters: Congenital malformations; risk of teratogenicity greater if more than one antiepileptic used. May possibly cause vitamin K deficiency and risk of neonatal bleeding; if vitamin K not given at birth, neonate should be monitored closely for signs of bleeding; *see* section 5.1
Phenoxymethylpenicillin	Not known to be harmful
Phenytoin	First, third trimesters: Congenital malformations (screening advised); adequate folate supplements should be given to mother (for example folic acid 5 mg daily); risk of teratogenicity greater if more than one antiepileptic used. May possibly cause vitamin K deficiency and risk of neonatal bleeding; if vitamin K not given at birth, neonate should be monitored closely for signs of bleeding. Caution in interpreting plasma concentrations— bound may be reduced but free (or effective) unchanged; *see also* section 5.1
Phytomenadione	Use only if potential benefit outweighs risk—no specific information available
Podophyllum resin	All trimesters: Avoid—neonatal death and terato-genesis have been reported
Polyvidone–iodine	Second, third trimesters: Sufficient iodine may be absorbed to affect the fetal thyroid
Potassium iodide	Second, third trimesters: Neonatal goitre and hypothyroidism
Praziquantel	*T. solium* infections in pregnancy should be treated immediately; *see* section 6.1.1.1. If immediate treatment not considered essential for Fluke infections or Schistosomiasis, treatment should be delayed until after delivery
Prazosin	No evidence of teratogenicity; use only when potential benefit outweighs risk
Prednisolone	Benefit of treatment, for example in asthma, outweighs risk; risk of intrauterine growth retar-dation on prolonged or repeated systemic treat-ment; corticosteroid cover required by mother during labour; monitor closely if fluid retention
Primaquine	Third trimester: Neonatal haemolysis and methae-moglobinaemia. Delay treatment until after deliv-ery
Procarbazine	Avoid (teratogenic in *animal* studies and isolated reports in humans); *see also* section 8.2
Proguanil	Benefit of prophylaxis and of treatment outweighs risk. Adequate folate supplements should be given to mother
Promethazine	No evidence of teratogenicity
Propranolol	May cause intrauterine growth restriction, neonatal hypoglycaemia, and bradycardia; risk greater in severe hypertension
Propylthiouracil	Second, third trimesters: Neonatal goitre and hypothyroidism
Pyridostigmine	Third trimester: Neonatal myasthenia with large doses

(Continued)

Drug	Comment
Pyrimethamine	First trimester: Theoretical teratogenic risk (folate antagonist); adequate folate supplements should be given to the mother. First trimester: avoid in Pneumocystosis and toxoplasmosis; *see also* Sulfadiazine
Quinine	First trimester: High doses are teratogenic; but in malaria benefit of treatment outweighs risk
Retinol	First trimester: Excessive doses may be teratogenic; *see also* section 27.1 [text]
Rifampicin	First trimester: Very high doses teratogenic in *animal* studies Third trimester: Risk of neonatal bleeding may be increased
Ritonavir	*See* Lopinavir with Ritonavir
Salbutamol	For use in asthma *see* section 25.1 [text] Third trimester: For use in premature labour *see* section 22.1
Saquinavir	Avoid if possible in first trimester; potential benefit of treatment considered to outweigh risk in second and third trimesters; *see* section 6.5.2
Silver sulfadiazine	Third trimester: Neonatal haemolysis and methaemoglobinaemia; fear of increased risk of kernicterus in neonates appears to be unfounded
Sodium cromoglicate	Not known to be harmful; *see also* section 25.1 [text]
Sodium valproate	*see* Valproic acid
Spironolactone	Toxicity in *animal* studies
Stavudine	Avoid if possible in first trimester; increased risk of lactic acidosis and hepatic steatosis; *see* section 6.5.2
Streptokinase	All trimesters: Possibility of premature separation of placenta in first 18 weeks; theoretical possibility of fetal haemorrhage throughout pregnancy; avoid postpartum use—maternal haemorrhage
Streptomycin	Second, third trimesters: Auditory or vestibular nerve damage; avoid unless essential (if given, serum-streptomycin concentration monitoring essential)
Sulfadiazine	Third trimester: Neonatal haemolysis and methaemoglobinaemia; fear of increased risk of kernicterus in neonates appears to be unfounded In toxoplasmosis, avoid in first trimester, but may be given in second and third trimester if danger of congenital transmission
Sulfadoxine+Pyrimethamine	In malaria, benefit of prophylaxis and treatment outweigh risk. First trimester: Possible teratogenic risk (pyrimethamine a folate antagonist) Third trimester: Neonatal haemolysis and methaemoglobinaemia; fear of increased risk of kernicterus in neonates appears to be unfounded *See also* section 6.4.3
Sulfamethoxazole + Trimethoprim	First trimester: Theoretical teratogenic risk (trimethoprim a folate antagonist) Third trimester: Neonatal haemolysis and methaemoglobinaemia; fear of increased risk of kernicterus in neonates appears to be unfounded
Sulfasalazine	Third trimester: Theoretical risk of neonatal haemolysis; adequate folate supplements should be given to mother

(Continued)

Drug	Comment
Suramin sodium	In onchocerciasis, delay treatment until after delivery. In *T. b. rhodesiense* treatment should be given even if evidence of meningoencephalopathic involvement
Suxamethonium	Mildly prolonged maternal paralysis may occur
Tamoxifen	Avoid—possible effects on fetal development; effective contraception must be used during treatment and for 2 months after stopping
Testosterone	All trimesters: Masculinization of female fetus
Tetracycline	First trimester: Effects on skeletal development in *animal* studies Second, third trimesters: Dental discoloration; maternal hepatotoxicity with large parenteral doses
Theophylline	Third trimester: Neonatal irritability and apnoea have been reported
Thiopental	Third trimester: Depresses neonatal respiration
Trimethoprim	First trimester: Theoretical teratogenic risk (folate antagonist)
Vaccine, BCG	First trimester: Theoretical risk of congenital malformations, but need for vaccination may outweigh possible risk to fetus (*see also* section 19.3 [contraindications])
Vaccine, Measles	First trimester: Theoretical risk of congenital malformations, but need for vaccination may outweigh possible risk to fetus (*see also* section 19.3 [contraindications and precautions]); avoid MMR
Vaccine, MMR	Avoid; pregnancy should be avoided for 1 month after immunization
Vaccine, Poliomyelitis, live	First trimester: Theoretical risk of congenital malformations, but need for vaccination may outweigh possible risk to fetus (*see also* section 19.3 [contraindications and precautions])
Vaccine, Rubella	Avoid; pregnancy should be avoided for 1 month after immunization
Vaccine, Yellow fever	First trimester: Theoretical risk of congenital malformations, but need for vaccination may outweigh possible risk to fetus (*see also* section 19.3 [contraindications and precautions])
Valproic acid	First, third trimesters: Increased risk of neural tube defects (counselling and screening advised); risk of teratogenicity greater if more than one antiepileptic used; neonatal bleeding (related to hypofibrinaemia) and neonatal hepatotoxicity also reported; *see also* section 5.1 (sodium valproate)
Vancomycin	Use only if potential benefit outweighs risk—plasma-vancomycin concentration monitoring essential to reduce risk of fetal toxicity
Vecuronium	Use only if potential benefit outweighs risk—no information available
Verapamil	*Animal* studies have not shown teratogenic effect; possibility that verapamil can relax uterine muscles should be considered at term; risk to fetus should be balanced against risk of uncontrolled maternal hypertension
Vinblastine	Avoid (limited experience suggests fetal harm; teratogenic in *animal* studies); *see also* section 8.2
Vincristine	Avoid (teratogenicity and fetal loss in *animal* studies); *see also* section 8.2

(Continued)

Drug	Comment
Warfarin	All trimesters: Congenital malformations; fetal and neonatal haemorrhage *See also* section 10.2
Zidovudine	Avoid if possible in first trimester; benefit of treatment considered to outweigh risk in second and third trimesters; *see* section 6.5.2

Appendix 3: Breastfeeding

Administration of some drugs (for example, ergotamine) to nursing mothers may cause toxicity in the infant, whereas administration of others (for example, digoxin) has little effect. Some drugs inhibit lactation (for example, estrogens).

Toxicity to the infant can occur if the drug enters the milk in pharmacologically significant quantities. The concentration in milk of some drugs (for example, iodides) may exceed those in the maternal plasma so that therapeutic doses in the mother may cause toxicity to the infant. Some drugs inhibit the infant's sucking reflex (for example, phenobarbital). Drugs in breast milk may, at least theoretically, cause hypersensitivity in the infant even when concentrations are too low for a pharmacological effect.

The following table lists drugs:
- which should be used with caution or which are contraindicated in breastfeeding for the reasons given above;
- which, on present evidence, may be given to the mother during breastfeeding, because they appear in milk in amounts which are too small to be harmful to the infant;
- which are not known to be harmful to the infant although they are present in milk in significant amounts.

For many drugs insufficient evidence is available to provide guidance and it is advisable to administer only drugs essential to a mother during breastfeeding. Because of the inadequacy of information on drugs in breast milk the following table should be used only as a guide; absence from the table does not imply safety.

WHO POLICY. It is WHO policy to encourage breastfeeding whenever possible, particularly in situations where there is no safe alternative. Advice in the table may differ from other sources, including manufacturer's product literature.

For further information on use of drugs during breastfeeding, see also the WHO document 'Breastfeeding and Maternal Medication', WHO/CDR/95.11.

Table of drugs present in breast milk

Drug	Comment
Abacavir	Breastfeeding recommended during first 6 months if no safe alternative to breast milk
Acetazolamide	Amount too small to be harmful
Acetylsalicylic acid	Short course safe in usual dosage; monitor infant; regular use of high doses could impair platelet function and produce hypoprothrombinaemia in infant if neonatal vitamin K stores low; possible risk of Reye syndrome

(Continued)

Drug	Comment
Aciclovir	Significant amount in milk after systemic administration, but considered safe to use
Alcohol	Large amounts may affect infant and reduce milk consumption
Alcuronium	No information available
Allopurinol	Present in milk
Amiloride	Manufacturer advises avoid—no information available
Aminophylline	Present in milk—irritability in infant reported
Amitriptyline	Detectable in breast milk; continue breastfeeding; adverse effects possible, monitor infant for drowsiness
Amoxicillin	Trace amounts in milk; safe in usual dosage; monitor infant
Amoxicillin + Clavulanic acid	Trace amounts in milk
Amphotericin	No information available
Ampicillin	Trace amounts in milk; safe in usual dosage; monitor infant
Artemether + Lumefantrine	Discontinue breastfeeding during and for 1 week after stopping treatment
Asparaginase	Breastfeeding contraindicated
Atenolol	Significant amounts in milk; safe in usual dosage; monitor infant
Atropine	Small amount present in milk; monitor infant
Azathioprine	Breastfeeding contraindicated
Beclometasone	Systemic effects in infant unlikely with maternal dose of *less than equivalent* of prednisolone 40 mg daily; monitor infant's adrenal function with higher doses
Benzathine benzylpenicillin	Trace amounts in milk; safe in usual dosage; monitor infant
Benzylpenicillin	Trace amounts in milk; safe in usual dosage; monitor infant
Betamethasone	Systemic effects in infant unlikely with maternal dose of *less than equivalent* of prednisolone 40 mg daily; monitor infant's adrenal function with higher doses
Bleomycin	Breastfeeding contraindicated
Bupivacaine	Amount too small to be harmful
Calcium folinate	Manufacturer advises caution—no information available
Captopril	Excreted in milk; safe in usual dosage; monitor infant
Carbamazepine	Continue breastfeeding; adverse effects possible (severe skin reaction reported in 1 infant); monitor infant for drowsiness; *see also* section 5.1
Ceftazidime	Excreted in low concentrations; safe in usual dosage; monitor infant
Ceftriaxone	Excreted in low concentrations; safe in usual dosage; monitor infant
Chloral hydrate	Sedation in infant
Chlorambucil	Breastfeeding contraindicated
Chloramphenicol	Continue breastfeeding; use alternative drug if possible; may cause bone-marrow toxicity in infant; concentration in milk usually insufficient to cause 'grey syndrome'
Chlormethine	Breastfeeding contraindicated
Chloroquine	Amount probably too small to be harmful; inadequate for reliable protection against malaria, *see also* section 6.4.3
Chlorphenamine	Safe in usual dosage; monitor infant for drowsiness

(*Continued*)

Drug	Comment
Chlorpromazine	Continue breastfeeding; adverse effects possible; monitor infant for drowsiness
Ciclosporin	Present in milk—manufacturer advises avoid
Cimetidine	Significant amount—not known to be harmful; monitor infant
Ciprofloxacin	Continue breastfeeding; use alternative drug if possible; high concentrations in breast milk
Cisplatin	Breastfeeding contraindicated
Clindamycin	Amount probably too small to be harmful but bloody diarrhoea reported in 1 infant
Clomifene	May inhibit lactation
Clomipramine	Small amount present in milk; continue breastfeeding; adverse effects possible; monitor infant for drowsiness
Clonazepam	Continue breastfeeding; adverse effects possible; monitor infant for drowsiness; *see also* section 5.1
Cloxacillin	Trace amounts in milk; safe in usual dosage; monitor infant
Codeine	Amount too small to be harmful
Colchicine	Caution because of its cytotoxicity
Contraceptives, oral	Combined oral contraceptives may inhibit lactation—use alternative drug; progestogen-only contraceptives do not affect lactation (start 3 weeks after birth or later)
Cromoglicic acid	*see* Sodium cromoglicate
Cyclophosphamide	Breastfeeding contraindicated during and for 36 hours after stopping treatment
Cytarabine	Breastfeeding contraindicated
Dacarbazine	Breastfeeding contraindicated
Dactinomycin	Breastfeeding contraindicated
Dapsone	Although significant amount in milk risk to infant very small; continue breastfeeding; monitor infant for jaundice
Daunorubicin	Breastfeeding contraindicated
Deferoxamine	Manufacturer advises use only if potential benefit outweighs risk—no information available
Desmopressin	Not known to be harmful
Dexamethasone	Systemic effects in infant unlikely with maternal dose of *less than equivalent* of prednisolone 40 mg daily; monitor infant's adrenal function with higher doses
Diazepam	Continue breastfeeding; adverse effects possible; monitor infant for drowsiness; *see also* section 5.1
Didanosine	Breastfeeding recommended during first 6 months if no safe alternative to breast milk
Digoxin	Amount too small to be harmful
Diloxanide	Manufacturer advises avoid
Doxorubicin	Breastfeeding contraindicated
Doxycycline	Continue breastfeeding; use alternative drug if possible (absorption and therefore discoloration of teeth in infant probably prevented by chelation with calcium in milk)
Efavirenz	Breastfeeding recommended during first 6 months if no safe alternative to breast milk
Eflornithine	Avoid
Ephedrine	Irritability and disturbed sleep reported
Ergocalciferol	Caution with high doses; may cause hypercalcaemia in infant
Ergotamine	Use alternative drug; ergotism may occur in infant; repeated doses may inhibit lactation

(Continued)

Drug	Comment
Erythromycin	Only small amounts in milk; safe in usual dosage; monitor infant
Ethambutol	Amount too small to be harmful
Ethinylestradiol	Use alternative drug; may inhibit lactation; *see also* Contraceptives, Oral
Ethosuximide	Significant amount in milk; continue breastfeeding; adverse effects possible; monitor infant for drowsiness; *see also* section 5.1
Etoposide	Breastfeeding contraindicated
Fluconazole	Present in milk; safe in usual dosage; monitor infant
Flucytosine	Manufacturer advises avoid
Fluorouracil	Discontinue breastfeeding
Fluphenazine	Amount excreted in milk probably too small to be harmful; continue breastfeeding; adverse effects possible; monitor infant for drowsiness
Furosemide	Amount too small to be harmful
Glibenclamide	Theoretical possibility of hypoglycaemia in infant
Haloperidol	Amount excreted in milk probably too small to be harmful; continue breastfeeding; adverse effects possible; monitor infant for drowsiness
Halothane	Excreted in milk
Hydralazine	Present in milk but not known to be harmful; monitor infant
Hydrochlorothiazide	Use alternative drug; may inhibit lactation
Hydrocortisone	Systemic effects in infant unlikely with maternal dose of *less than equivalent* of prednisolone 40 mg daily; monitor infant's adrenal function with higher doses
Ibuprofen	Amount too small to be harmful; short courses safe in usual doses
Imipenem + Cilastatin	Present in milk—manufacturer advises avoid
Indinavir	Breastfeeding recommended during first 6 months if no safe alternative to breast milk
Insulin	Amount too small to be harmful
Iodine	Stop breastfeeding; danger of neonatal hypothyroidism or goitre; appears to be concentrated in milk
Isoniazid	Monitor infant for possible toxicity; theoretical risk of convulsions and neuropathy; prophylactic pyridoxine advisable in mother and infant
Ivermectin	Avoid treating mother until infant is 1 week old
Lamivudine	Present in milk; breastfeeding recommended during first 6 months if no safe alternative to breast milk
Levamisole	Breastfeeding contraindicated
Levodopa + Carbidopa	No information available
Levonorgestrel	Combined oral contraceptives may inhibit lactation—use alternative drug; progestogen-only contraceptives do not affect lactation (start 3 weeks after birth or later)
Levothyroxine	Amount too small to affect tests for neonatal hypothyroidism
Lidocaine	Amount too small to be harmful
Lithium	Present in milk and risk of toxicity in infant; continue breastfeeding; monitor infant carefully, particularly if risk of dehydration
Lopinavir with Ritonavir	Breastfeeding recommended during first 6 months if no safe alternative to breast milk
Lumefantrine	*see* Artemether + Lumefantrine
Mebendazole	No information available
Medroxyprogesterone	Present in milk—no adverse effects reported
Mefloquine	Present in milk but risk to infant minimal

(Continued)

Drug	Comment
Mercaptopurine	Breastfeeding contraindicated
Metformin	Safe in usual doses; monitor infant
Methotrexate	Breastfeeding contraindicated
Methyldopa	Amount too small to be harmful
Metoclopramide	Present in milk; adverse effects possible; monitor infant for adverse effects
Metronidazole	Significant amount in milk; continue breastfeeding; use alternative drug if possible
Minocycline	Continue breastfeeding; use alternative drug if possible (absorption and therefore discoloration of teeth in infant probably usually prevented by chelation with calcium in milk)
Morphine	Short courses safe in usual doses; monitor infant
Nalidixic acid	Continue breastfeeding; use alternative drug if possible; one case of haemolytic anaemia reported
Naloxone	No information available
Nelfinavir	Breastfeeding recommended during first 6 months if no safe alternative to breast milk
Neostigmine	Amount probably too small to be harmful; monitor infant
Nevirapine	Present in milk; breastfeeding recommended during first 6 months if no safe alternative to breast milk
Nifedipine	Small amount in milk; continue breastfeeding; monitor infant
Nitrofurantoin	Only small amounts in milk but could be enough to produce haemolysis in G6PD-deficient infants
Norethisterone	Combined oral contraceptives may inhibit lactation—use alternative drug; progestogen-only contraceptives do not affect lactation (start 3 weeks after birth or later)
Nystatin	No information available, but absorption from gastrointestinal tract negligible
Ofloxacin	Continue breastfeeding; use alternative drug if possible
Oxamniquine	No information available, but considered preferable to avoid
Paracetamol	Small amount present in milk: short courses safe in usual dosage; monitor infant
Pentamidine isetionate	Manufacturer advises avoid unless essential
Pentavalent antimony compounds	Avoid
Pethidine	Short courses safe in usual dosage; monitor infant
Phenobarbital	Continue breastfeeding; adverse effects possible; monitor infant for drowsiness; *see also* section 5.1
Phenoxymethylpenicillin	Trace amounts in milk; safe in usual dosage; monitor infant
Phenytoin	Small amount present in milk; continue breastfeeding; adverse effects possible; monitor infant for drowsiness; *see also* section 5.1
Polyvidone–iodine	Avoid; iodine absorbed from vaginal preparations is concentrated in milk
Potassium iodide	Stop breastfeeding; danger of neonatal hypothyroidism or goitre; appears to be concentrated in milk
Praziquantel	Avoid breastfeeding during and for 72 hours after treatment
Prazosin	Amount probably too small to be harmful
Prednisolone	Systemic effects in infant unlikely with maternal dose of *less than* prednisolone 40 mg daily; monitor infant's adrenal function with higher doses
Primaquine	Avoid; risk of haemolysis in G6PD-deficient infants

(*Continued*)

Drug	Comment
Procainamide	Present in milk; continue breastfeeding; monitor infant
Procarbazine	Breastfeeding contraindicated
Proguanil	Amount probably too small to be harmful; inadequate for reliable protection against malaria, *see* section 6.4.3
Promethazine	Safe in usual dosage; monitor infant for drowsiness
Propranolol	Present in milk; safe in usual dosage; monitor infant
Propylthiouracil	Monitor infant's thyroid status but amounts in milk probably too small to affect infant; high doses might affect neonatal thyroid function
Pyrazinamide	Amount too small to be harmful
Pyridostigmine	Amount probably too small to be harmful
Pyrimethamine	Significant amount—avoid administration of other folate antagonists to infant
Quinidine	Significant amount but not known to be harmful
Retinol	Theoretical risk of toxicity in infants of mothers taking large doses
Rifampicin	Amount too small to be harmful
Ritonavir	*See* Lopinavir with Ritonavir
Salbutamol	Safe in usual dosage; monitor infant
Saquinavir	Breastfeeding recommended during first 6 months if no safe alternative to breast milk
Senna	Avoid; large doses may cause increased gastric motility and diarrhoea
Silver sulfadiazine	Continue breastfeeding; monitor infant for jaundice—small risk of kernicterus in jaundiced infants particularly with long-acting sulphonamides, and of haemolysis in G6PD-deficient infants
Sodium cromoglicate	Unlikely to be present in milk
Sodium valproate	*see* Valproic acid
Stavudine	Breastfeeding recommended during first 6 months if no safe alternative to breast milk
Sulfadiazine	Continue breastfeeding; monitor infant for jaundice—small risk of kernicterus in jaundiced infants particularly with long-acting sulphonamides, and of haemolysis in G6PD-deficient infants
Sulfadoxine + Pyrimethamine	Continue breastfeeding; monitor infant for jaundice—small risk of kernicterus in jaundiced infants and of haemolysis in G6PD-deficient infants (due to sulfadoxine)
Sulfamethoxazole + Trimethoprim	Continue breastfeeding; monitor infant for jaundice—small risk of kernicterus in jaundiced infants and of haemolysis in G6PD-deficient infants (due to sulfamethoxazole)
Sulfasalazine	Continue breastfeeding; monitor infant for jaundice—small amounts in milk (1 report of bloody diarrhoea and rashes); theoretical risk of neonatal haemolysis especially in G6PD-deficient infants
Tamoxifen	Manufacturer advises avoid—no information available
Testosterone	Avoid; may cause masculinization in the female infant or precocious development in the male infant; high doses suppress lactation
Tetracaine	No information available
Tetracycline	Continue breastfeeding; use alternative drug if possible (absorption and therefore discoloration of teeth in infant probably usually prevented by chelation with calcium in milk)
Theophylline	Present in milk—irritability in infant reported; modified-release preparations preferable

(*Continued*)

Drug	Comment
Thiamine	Severely thiamine-deficient mothers should avoid breastfeeding as toxic methyl-glyoxal excreted in milk
Trimethoprim	Present in milk; safe in usual dosage; monitor infant
Valproic acid	Present in milk; continue breastfeeding; adverse effects possible; monitor infant for drowsiness; *see also* section 5.1 (sodium valproate)
Vancomycin	Present in milk—significant absorption following oral administration unlikely
Vecuronium	No information available
Verapamil	Amount too small to be harmful
Vinblastine	Breastfeeding contraindicated
Vincristine	Breastfeeding contraindicated
Warfarin	Risk of haemorrhage; increased by vitamin-K deficiency; warfarin appears safe
Zidovudine	Breastfeeding recommended during first 6 months if no safe alternative to breast milk

Appendix 4: Renal impairment

Reduced renal function may cause problems with drug therapy for the following reasons:

1. The failure to excrete a drug or its metabolites may produce toxicity.
2. The sensitivity to some drugs is increased even if the renal elimination is unimpaired.
3. The tolerance to adverse effects may be impaired.
4. The efficacy of some drugs may diminish.

The dosage of many drugs must be adjusted in patients with renal impairment to avoid adverse reactions and to ensure efficacy. The level of renal function below which the dose of a drug must be reduced depends on how toxic it is and whether it is eliminated entirely by renal excretion or is partly metabolized to inactive metabolites.

In general, all patients with renal impairment are given a *loading dose* which is the same as the usual dose for a patient with normal renal function. *Maintenance doses* are adjusted to the clinical situation. The maintenance dose of a drug can be reduced either by reducing the individual dose leaving the normal interval between doses unchanged or by increasing the interval between doses without changing the dose. The interval extension method may provide the benefits of convenience and decreased cost, while the dose reduction method provides more constant plasma concentration.

In the following table drugs are listed in alphabetical order. The table includes only drugs for which specific information is available. Many drugs should be used with caution in renal impairment but no specific advice on dose adjustment is available; it is therefore important to also refer to the individual drug entries. The recommendations are given for various levels of renal function as estimated by the glomerular filtration rate (GFR), usually measured by the creatinine clearance. The serum-creatinine concentration can be used instead as a measure of renal function but it is only a rough guide unless corrected for age, sex and weight by special nomograms.

Renal impairment is usually divided into three grades:

   mild—GFR 20-50 ml/minute *or* approximate serum creatinine 150–300 micromol/litre

   moderate—GFR 10-20 ml/minute *or* serum creatinine 300–700 micromol/litre

   severe—GFR <10 ml/minute *or* serum creatinine >700 micromol/litre

When using the dosage guidelines the following must be considered:

- Drug prescribing should be kept to a minimum.
- Nephrotoxic drugs should, if possible, be avoided in all patients with renal disease because the nephrotoxicity is more likely to be serious.
- It is advisable to determine renal function not only before but also during the period of treatment and adjust the maintenance dose as necessary.

- Renal function (GFR, creatinine clearance) declines with age so that by the age of 80 it is half that in healthy young subjects. When prescribing for the elderly, assume at least a mild degree of renal impairment.
- Uraemic patients should be observed carefully for unexpected drug toxicity. In these patients the complexity of clinical status as well as other variables for example altered absorption, protein binding or metabolism, or liver function, and other drug therapy precludes use of fixed drug dosage and an individualized approach is required.

Table of drugs to be avoided or used with caution in renal impairment

Drug	Degree of Impairment	Comment
Abacavir	Severe	Avoid
Acetazolamide	Mild	Avoid; metabolic acidosis
Acetylsalicylic acid	Severe	Avoid; sodium and water retention; deterioration in renal function; increased risk of gastrointestinal bleeding
Aciclovir	Mild	Reduce intravenous dose
	Moderate to severe	Reduce dose
Alcuronium	Severe	Prolonged duration of block
Allopurinol	Moderate	100–200 mg daily; increased toxicity; rashes
	Severe	100 mg on alternate days (maximum 100 mg daily)
Aluminium hydroxide	Severe	Aluminium is absorbed and may accumulate NOTE. Absorption of aluminium from aluminium salts is increased by citrates which are contained in many effervescent preparations (such as effervescent analgesics)
Amidotrizoate	*see* Diatrizoates	
Amiloride	Mild	Monitor plasma potassium; high risk of hyperkalaemia in renal impairment; amiloride excreted by kidney unchanged
	Moderate	Avoid
Amoxicillin	Severe	Reduce dose; rashes more common
Amoxicillin + Clavulanic acid	Moderate to severe	Reduce dose
Amphotericin	Mild	Use only if no alternative; nephrotoxicity may be reduced with use of complexes
Ampicillin	Severe	Reduce dose; rashes more common
Atenolol	Moderate	Reduce dose (excreted unchanged)
	Severe	Start with small dose; higher plasma concentrations after oral administration; may reduce renal blood flow and adversely affect renal function
Azathioprine	Severe	Reduce dose
Benzathine benzylpenicillin	Severe	Neurotoxicity—high doses may cause convulsions

(Continued)

Drug	Degree of Impairment	Comment
Benzylpenicillin	Severe	Maximum 6 g daily; neurotoxicity—high doses may cause convulsions
Bleomycin	Moderate	Reduce dose
Captopril	Mild to moderate	Use with caution and monitor response; initial dose 12.5 mg twice daily. Hyperkalaemia and other adverse effects more common
Carbamazepine		Manufacturer advises caution
Ceftazidime	Mild	Reduce dose
Ceftriaxone	Severe	Reduce dose; also monitor plasma concentration if both severe renal and hepatic impairment
Chlorambucil	Moderate	Use with caution and monitor response; increased risk of myelosuppression
Chloramphenicol	Severe	Avoid unless no alternative; dose-related depression of haematopoiesis
Chloroquine	Mild to moderate	Reduce dose (but for malaria prophylaxis see section 6.4.3)
	Severe	Avoid (but for malaria prophylaxis see section 6.4.3)
Chlorphenamine	Severe	Dose reduction may be required
Chlorpromazine	Severe	Start with small doses; increased cerebral sensitivity
Ciclosporin		Monitor kidney function—dose dependent increase in serum creatinine and urea during first few weeks may necessitate dose reduction (exclude rejection if kidney transplant)
Cimetidine	Mild to moderate	600–800 mg daily; occasional risk of confusion
	Severe	400 mg daily
Ciprofloxacin	Moderate	Use half normal dose
Cisplatin	Mild	Avoid if possible; nephrotoxic and neurotoxic
Clindamycin		Plasma half-life prolonged—may need dose reduction
Clonazepam	Severe	Start with small doses; increased cerebral sensitivity
Cloxacillin	Severe	Reduce dose
Codeine	Moderate to severe	Reduce dose or avoid; increased and prolonged effect; increased cerebral sensitivity
Colchicine	Moderate	Reduce dose
	Severe	Avoid or reduce dose if no alternative
Cyclophosphamide		Reduce dose
Dacarbazine	Mild to moderate	Dose reduction may be required
	Severe	Avoid
Daunorubicin	Mild to moderate	Reduce dose
Deferoxamine		Metal complexes excreted by kidneys (in severe renal impairment dialysis increases rate of elimination)

(Continued)

Drug	Degree of Impairment	Comment
Desmopressin		Antidiuretic effect may be reduced
Dextromethorphan	Moderate to severe	Reduce dose or avoid; increased and prolonged effect; increased cerebral sensitivity
Diatrizoates	Mild	Reduce dose and avoid dehydration; nephrotoxic
Diazepam	Severe	Start with small doses; increased cerebral sensitivity
Didanosine	Mild	Reduce dose; consult manufacturer's literature
Diethylcarbamazine	Moderate to severe	Reduce dose; plasma half life prolonged and urinary excretion considerably reduced
Digoxin	Mild	Reduce dose; toxicity increased by electrolyte disturbances
Dimercaprol		Discontinue or use with extreme caution if impairment develops during treatment
Eflornithine		Reduce dose
Ephedrine	Severe	Avoid; increased CNS toxicity
Ergometrine	Severe	Manufacturer advises avoid
Ergotamine	Moderate	Avoid; nausea and vomiting; risk of renal vasoconstriction
Erythromycin	Severe	Maximum 1.5 g daily (ototoxicity)
Ethambutol	Mild	Reduce dose; if creatinine clearance less than 30 ml/minute monitor plasma-ethambutol concentration; optic nerve damage
Fluconazole	Mild to moderate	Usual initial dose then halve subsequent doses
Flucytosine		Reduce dose and monitor plasma-flucytosine concentration—consult manufacturer's literature
Fluphenazine	Severe	Start with small doses; increased cerebral sensitivity
Furosemide	Moderate	May need high doses; deafness may follow rapid i/v injection
Gentamicin	Mild	Reduce dose; monitor plasma concentrations; see also section 6.2.5
Glibenclamide	Severe	Avoid
Haloperidol	Severe	Start with small doses; increased cerebral sensitivity
Heparin	Severe	Risk of bleeding increased
Hydralazine		Reduce dose if creatinine clearance less than 30 ml/minute
Hydrochlorothiazide	Moderate	Avoid; ineffective
Ibuprofen	Mild	Use lowest effective dose and monitor renal function; sodium and water retention; deterioration in renal function possibly leading to renal failure
	Moderate to severe	Avoid
Imipenem + Cilastatin	Mild	Reduce dose

(Continued)

Drug	Degree of Impairment	Comment
Insulin	Severe	May need dose reduction; insulin requirements fall; compensatory response to hypoglycaemia is impaired
Iohexol	Moderate to severe	Increased risk of nephrotoxicity; avoid dehydration
Iopanoic acid	Mild to moderate	Maximum 3 g
	Severe	Avoid
Isoniazid	Severe	Maximum 200 mg daily; peripheral neuropathy
Lamivudine	Mild	Reduce dose; consult manufacturer's literature
Lithium	Mild	Avoid if possible or reduce dose and monitor plasma concentration carefully
	Moderate	Avoid
Lopinavir with Ritonavir		Avoid oral solution due to propylene glycol content; use capsules with caution in severe impairment
Magnesium hydroxide	Moderate	Avoid or reduce dose; increased risk of toxicity
Magnesium sulfate	Moderate	Avoid or reduce dose; increased risk of toxicity
Mannitol		Avoid unless test dose produces diuretic response
Meglumine antimoniate	*see* Pentavalent antimony compounds	
Meglumine iotroxate	Moderate to severe	Increased risk of nephrotoxicity; avoid dehydration
Mercaptopurine	Moderate	Reduce dose
Metformin	Mild	Avoid; increased risk of lactic acidosis
Methotrexate	Mild	Reduce dose; accumulates; nephrotoxic
	Moderate	Avoid
Methyldopa	Moderate	Start with small dose; increased sensitivity to hypotensive and sedative effect
Metoclopramide	Severe	Avoid or use small dose; increased risk of extrapyramidal reactions
Morphine	Moderate to severe	Reduce dose or avoid; increased and prolonged effect; increased cerebral sensitivity
Nalidixic acid	Moderate to severe	Use half normal dose; ineffective in renal failure because concentration in urine is inadequate
Nelfinavir		No information available—manufacturer advises caution
Neostigmine	Moderate	May need dose reduction
Nevirapine		No information available—manufacturer advises avoid
Nitrofurantoin	Mild	Avoid; peripheral neuropathy; ineffective because of inadequate urine concentrations
Ofloxacin	Mild	Usual initial dose, then use half normal dose

(Continued)

Drug	Degree of Impairment	Comment
	Moderate	Usual initial dose, then 100 mg every 24 hours
Penicillamine	Mild	Avoid if possible or reduce dose; nephrotoxic
Pentamidine isetionate	Mild	Reduce dose; consult manufacturer's literature
Pentavalent antimony compounds	Moderate	Increased adverse effects
	Severe	Avoid
Pethidine	Moderate to severe	Reduce dose or avoid; increased and prolonged effect; increased cerebral sensitivity
Phenobarbital	Severe	Avoid large doses
Polyvidone–iodine	Severe	Avoid regular application to inflamed or broken mucosa
Potassium chloride	Moderate	Avoid routine use; high risk of hyperkalaemia
Prazosin	Moderate to severe	Initially 500 micrograms daily; increased with caution
Procainamide	Mild	Avoid or reduce dose
Procaine benzylpenicillin	Severe	Neurotoxicity—high doses may cause convulsions
Procarbazine	Severe	Avoid
Proguanil	Mild	100 mg once daily
	Moderate	50 mg on alternate days
	Severe	50 mg once weekly; increased risk of haematological toxicity
Propranolol	Severe	Start with small dose; higher plasma concentrations after oral administration; may reduce renal blood flow and adversely affect renal function in severe impairment
Propylthiouracil	Mild to moderate	Use three-quarters normal dose
	Severe	Use half normal dose
Pyridostigmine	Moderate	Reduce dose; excreted by kidney
Quinine		Reduce parenteral maintenance dose for malaria treatment
Ritonavir		*See* Lopinavir with Ritonavir
Saquinavir	Severe	Dose adjustment possibly required
Sodium chloride	Severe	Avoid
Sodium hydrogen carbonate	Severe	Avoid; specialized role in some forms of renal disease
Sodium nitroprusside	Moderate	Avoid prolonged use
Sodium valproate	*see* Valproic acid	
Spironolactone	Mild	Monitor plasma K^+; high risk of hyperkalaemia in renal impairment
	Moderate	Avoid
Stavudine	Mild	20 mg twice daily (15 mg if body weight less than 60 kg)
	Moderate to severe	20 mg once daily (15 mg if body weight less than 60 kg)
Streptomycin	Mild	Reduce dose; monitor plasma concentrations
Sulfadiazine	Severe	Avoid; high risk of crystalluria

(*Continued*)

Drug	Degree of Impairment	Comment
Sulfamethoxazole + Trimethoprim	Mild	Use half normal dose if creatinine clearance 15–30 ml/minute; avoid if creatinine clearance less than 15 ml/minute and plasma-sulfamethoxazole concentration cannot be monitored
Sulfasalazine	Moderate	Risk of toxicity including crystalluria—ensure high fluid intake
	Severe	Avoid
Trimethoprim	Moderate	Reduce dose
Valproic acid	Mild to moderate	Reduce dose
	Severe	Alter dosage according to free serum valproic acid concentration
Vancomycin	Mild	Reduce dose—monitor plasma-vancomycin concentration and renal function regularly
Vecuronium	Severe	Reduce dose; duration of block possibly prolonged
Warfarin	Severe	Avoid
Zidovudine	Severe	Reduce dose; manufacturer advises oral dose of 300–400 mg daily

Appendix 5: Hepatic impairment

Liver disease may alter the response to drugs. However, the hepatic reserve appears to be large and liver disease has to be severe before important changes in drug metabolism take place. The ability to eliminate a specific drug may or may not correlate with liver's synthetic capacity for substances such as albumin or clotting factors, which tends to decrease as hepatic function declines. Unlike renal disease, where estimates of renal function based on creatinine clearance correlate with parameters of drug elimination such as clearance and half-life, routine liver function tests do not reflect actual liver function but are rather markers of liver cellular damage.

The altered response to drugs in liver disease can include all or some of the following changes:
- Impaired intrinsic hepatic eliminating (metabolizing) capacity due to lack of or impaired function of hepatocytes.
- Impaired biliary elimination due to biliary obstruction or transport abnormalities (for example rifampicin is excreted in the bile unchanged and may accumulate in patients with intrahepatic or extrahepatic obstructive jaundice).
- Impaired hepatic blood flow due to surgical shunting, collateral circulation or poor perfusion with cirrhosis and portal hypertension.
- Altered volume of distribution of drugs due to increased extracellular fluid (ascites, oedema) and decreased muscle mass.
- Decreased protein binding and increased toxicity of drugs highly bound to proteins (for example phenytoin) due to impaired albumin production.
- Increased bioavailability through decreased first-pass metabolism.
- Decreased bioavailability due to malabsorption of fats in cholestatic liver disease.

In severe liver disease increased sensitivity to the effects of some drugs can further impair cerebral function and may precipitate *hepatic encephalopathy* (for example morphine, pethidine). *Oedema and ascites* in chronic liver disease may be exacerbated by drugs that cause fluid retention (for example acetylsalicylic acid, ibuprofen, prednisolone, dexamethasone).

Usually drugs are metabolized without injury to the liver. A few drugs cause dose-related hepatotoxicity. However, most hepatotoxic reactions to drugs occur only in rare persons and are unpredictable. In patients with impaired liver function the dose-related hepatotoxic reaction may occur at lower doses whereas unpredictable reactions seem to occur more frequently. Both should be avoided.

Information to help prescribing in hepatic impairment is included in the following table. The table contains only those drugs that need dose adjustment. However, absence from the table does not automatically imply safety as for many drugs data about safety are absent; it is therefore important to also refer to the individual drug entries.

Table of drugs to be avoided or used with caution in liver disease

Drug	Comment
Abacavir	No dosage adjustment required in mild hepatic impairment; avoid in moderate or severe hepatic impairment
Acetylsalicylic acid	Avoid—increased risk of gastrointestinal bleeding
Alcuronium	Possibly slower onset, higher dose requirement and prolonged recovery time
Allopurinol	Reduce dose
Aluminium hydroxide	In patients with fluid retention, avoid antacids containing large amounts of sodium; also avoid those causing constipation (can precipitate coma)
Aminophylline	Reduce dose
Amitriptyline	Sedative effects increased (avoid in severe liver disease)
Amoxicillin + Clavulanic acid	Monitor liver function in liver disease. Cholestatic jaundice reported either during or shortly after treatment; more common in patients over the age of 65 years and in males; duration of treatment should not usually exceed 14 days
Azathioprine	May need dose reduction
Bupivacaine	Avoid (or reduce dose) in severe liver disease
Carbamazepine	Metabolism impaired in advanced liver disease
Ceftriaxone	Reduce dose and monitor plasma concentration if both hepatic and severe renal impairment
Chloral hydrate	Can precipitate coma (avoid in severe impairment)
Chloramphenicol	Avoid if possible—increased risk of bone-marrow depression; reduce dose and monitor plasma-chloramphenicol concentration
Chlorphenamine	Sedation inappropriate in severe liver disease—avoid
Chlorpromazine	Can precipitate coma; hepatotoxic
Ciclosporin	May need dose adjustment
Cimetidine	Increased risk of confusion; reduce dose
Ciprofloxacin	Hepatitis with necrosis reported
Clindamycin	Reduce dose
Clomifene	Avoid in severe liver disease
Clomipramine	Sedative effects increased (avoid in severe liver disease)
Clonazepam	Can precipitate coma
Cloxacillin	Cholestatic jaundice may occur up to several weeks after treatment has been stopped; administration for more than 2 weeks and increasing age are risk factors
Codeine	Avoid or reduce dose—may precipitate coma
Contraceptives, oral	Avoid in active liver disease and if history of pruritus or cholestasis during pregnancy
Cyclophosphamide	Reduce dose
Cytarabine	Reduce dose
Dacarbazine	Dose reduction may be required in mild to moderate liver disease; avoid if severe
Daunorubicin	Reduce dose
Dextromethorphan	Avoid or reduce dose—may precipitate coma
Diazepam	Can precipitate coma
Didanosine	Insufficient information but consider dose reduction

(Continued)

Drug	Comment
Doxorubicin	Reduce dose according to bilirubin concentration
Doxycycline	Avoid (or use with caution)
Efavirenz	In mild to moderate liver disease, monitor liver function; avoid in severe hepatic impairment
Ergometrine	Avoid in severe liver disease
Ergotamine	Avoid in severe liver disease—risk of toxicity increased
Erythromycin	May cause idiosyncratic hepatotoxicity
Ether, anaesthetic	Avoid
Etoposide	Avoid in severe hepatic impairment
Fluconazole	Toxicity with related drugs
Fluphenazine	Can precipitate coma; hepatotoxic
Furosemide	Hypokalaemia may precipitate coma (use potassium-sparing diuretic to prevent this); increased risk of hypomagnesaemia in alcoholic cirrhosis
Glibenclamide	Increased risk of hypoglycaemia in severe liver disease; avoid or use small dose; can produce jaundice
Griseofulvin	Avoid in severe liver disease
Haloperidol	Can precipitate coma
Halothane	Avoid if history of unexplained pyrexia or jaundice following previous exposure to halothane
Heparin	Reduce dose in severe liver disease
Hydralazine	Reduce dose
Hydrochlorothiazide	Avoid in severe liver disease; hypokalaemia may precipitate coma (potassium-sparing diuretic can prevent this); increased risk of hypomagnesaemia in alcoholic cirrhosis
Ibuprofen	Increased risk of gastrointestinal bleeding and can cause fluid retention; avoid in severe liver disease
Indinavir	Reduce dose to 600 mg every 8 hours in mild to moderate hepatic impairment; not studied in severe impairment
Iopanoic acid	Avoid in severe hepatic disease
Isoniazid	Avoid if possible—idiosyncratic hepatotoxicity more common
Levonorgestrel	Avoid in active liver disease and if history of pruritus or cholestasis during pregnancy
Lidocaine	Avoid (or reduce dose) in severe liver disease
Lopinavir with Ritonavir	Avoid oral solution because of propylene glycol content; use capsules with caution in mild to moderate hepatic impairment and avoid in severe impairment
Magnesium hydroxide	Avoid in hepatic coma if risk of renal failure
Magnesium sulfate	Avoid in hepatic coma if risk of renal failure
Medroxyprogesterone	Avoid in active liver disease and if history of pruritus or cholestasis during pregnancy
Mefloquine	Avoid for prophylaxis in severe liver disease
Meglumine antimoniate	*see* Pentavalent antimony compounds
Metformin	Avoid—increased risk of lactic acidosis
Methotrexate	Dose-related toxicity—avoid in non-malignant conditions (for example, rheumatic disorders)
Methyldopa	Manufacturer advises caution in history of liver disease; avoid in active liver disease
Metoclopramide	Reduce dose
Metronidazole	In severe liver disease, reduce total daily dose to one-third and give once daily
Minocycline	Avoid (or use with caution)
Morphine	Avoid or reduce dose—may precipitate coma

(*Continued*)

Drug	Comment
Nalidixic acid	Partially conjugated in liver
Nelfinavir	No information available—manufacturer advises caution
Nevirapine	No information available—manufacturer advises avoid
Nifedipine	Reduce dose
Nitrofurantoin	Cholestatic jaundice and chronic active hepatitis reported
Norethisterone	Avoid in active liver disease and if history of pruritus or cholestasis during pregnancy
Ofloxacin	Reduce dose in severe liver disease
Paracetamol	Dose-related toxicity—avoid large doses
Pentavalent antimony compounds	Increased risk of liver damage and hepatic failure in pre-existing liver disease
Pethidine	Avoid or reduce dose—may precipitate coma
Phenobarbital	May precipitate coma
Phenytoin	Reduce dose to avoid toxicity
Prazosin	Initially 500 micrograms daily; increased with caution
Prednisolone	Adverse effects more common
Procainamide	Avoid or reduce dose
Procarbazine	Avoid in severe hepatic impairment
Promethazine	Avoid—may precipitate coma in severe liver disease; hepatotoxic
Propranolol	Reduce oral dose
Propylthiouracil	Reduce dose; *see also* section 18.8
Pyrazinamide	Avoid—idiosyncratic hepatotoxicity more common
Rifampicin	Impaired elimination; may be increased risk of hepatotoxicity; avoid or do not exceed 8 mg/kg daily
Ritonavir	*See* Lopinavir with Ritonavir
Saquinavir	Plasma concentration possibly increased; manufacturer of gel-filled capsules advises caution in moderate hepatic impairment and avoid in severe impairment; manufacturer of capsules containing saquinavir mesilate advises caution in severe impairment
Sodium nitroprusside	Avoid in severe liver disease
Sodium valproate	*see* Valproic acid
Sulfamethoxazole + Trimethoprim	Manufacturer advises avoid in severe liver disease
Suxamethonium	Prolonged apnoea may occur in severe liver disease due to reduced hepatic synthesis of pseudocholinesterase
Testosterone	Preferably avoid—possibility of dose-related toxicity and fluid retention
Theophylline	Reduce dose
Thiopental	Reduce dose for induction in severe liver disease
Valproic acid	Avoid if possible—hepatotoxicity and hepatic failure may occasionally occur (usually in first 6 months)
Verapamil	Reduce oral dose
Vinblastine	Dose reduction may be necessary
Vincristine	Dose reduction may be necessary
Warfarin	Avoid in severe liver disease, especially if prothrombin time already prolonged
Zidovudine	Accumulation may occur